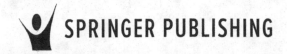
SPRINGER PUBLISHING

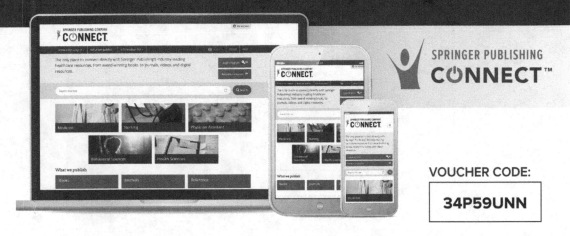
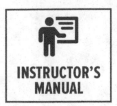

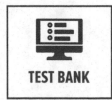

A Population Health Approach to Health Disparities for Nurses

Faye A. Gary, EdD, MS, RN, FAAN, raised in the Jim Crow South and deeply influenced by segregation and discrimination in every facet of her existence, has dedicated her life to eradicating health disparities among vulnerable populations.

Dr. Gary is a Distinguished University Professor and the Medical Mutual of Ohio and Kent W. Clapp Endowed Chair and Professor of Nursing at the Frances Payne Bolton School of Nursing with a secondary appointment in the Department of Psychiatry at the Case Western Reserve University School of Medicine in Cleveland, Ohio. She is also a Distinguished Service Professor Emerita at the University of Florida.

The recipient of numerous awards and honors, Dr. Gary has helped develop and oversee research and training grants totaling more than $24 million. She is the visionary behind the Provost Scholars Program established in 2013. This innovative project pairs secondary students with Case Western Reserve University mentors and tutors.

Dr. Gary was appointed to serve on several federal committees, including the National Advisory Committee on Rural Health and Human Services, the National Institute of Mental Health, and the National Institute on Minority Health and Health Disparities. She was the executive consultant of the Substance Abuse and Mental Health Services Administration (SAMHSA) Minority Fellowship Program at the American Nurses Association. As a W. K. Kellogg Fellow, she has collaborated with fellows from across the nation. She was a member of the board of directors of Mental Health America and served on the Task Force on Ethics and Professional Conduct for the United Nations Commission on Refugees. She has functioned as a consultant to Ministries of Health and other organizations across six continents. Most recently, she has been elected to serve on the board of directors of the International Network of Doctoral Education in Nursing.

A relentless innovator, trailblazer, and impactful scholar with a career spanning a half-century, Dr. Gary's practice, research, scholarship, and prolific publication history have shaped and extended well beyond the field of psychiatric nursing and behavioral health in local and global communities. Informing health policy related to child and adolescent mental health, health disparities, domestic violence, and social justice is the foundation of her legacy.

Marilyn J. Lotas, PhD, RN, FAAN, received her BSN and MEd in clinical psychology from Wayne State University and her MSN in psychiatric nursing and her PhD in nursing with concentrations in family functioning and child development from the University of Michigan. She completed 2 years of postdoctoral education at the University of Pennsylvania as a Robert Wood Johnson Clinical Nurse Scholar focusing on environmental factors influencing the development of preterm infants. At the University of Texas Health Science Center in Houston, she served as professor, assistant dean, and department chair of Target Populations. She established a neonatal nurse practitioner program, which was implemented in Houston and in the Texas Lower Rio Grande Valley, an economically depressed, medically underserved area. At Emory University she served as professor, the Alberta Dozier Williamson Chair in Nursing, and the director of the Office of Research Administration. While there she took leadership in successfully getting approval and funding for a PhD program. From 2000 to 2020 she served on the faculty of the Frances Payne Bolton School of Nursing as an associate professor, associate dean for undergraduate nursing, and director of the BSN program. Within the BSN program, she established a semester abroad program encompassing sites on six continents and including two-way exchanges with universities in Hong Kong, Wuhan, China, and the American Virgin Islands. She redesigned the community health content in the curriculum with courses beginning in the freshman year and culminating in the senior year with coursework on global health and a 300-hour capstone practicum including sites in Cleveland, Ohio, other areas of the United States and internationally through the semester abroad program. She established a 17-year partnership with the Cleveland Metropolitan School District School Nurses directing projects related to childhood obesity and childhood hypertension, and established a lead screening program to address the high rates of lead poisoning in Cleveland's children. From 2011 to 2012 she held a Senior Fulbright Fellowship at the Lebanese American University working with a newly established school of nursing and has consulted widely in the Middle East. She serves on the editorial board of *Neonatal Network* and reviews for multiple journals.

A Population Health Approach to Health Disparities for Nurses

Care of Vulnerable Populations

Faye A. Gary, EdD, MS, RN, FAAN

Marilyn J. Lotas, PhD, RN, FAAN

EDITORS

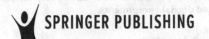

Springer Publishing Company, LLC
11 West 42nd Street, New York, NY 10036
www.springerpub.com
connect.springerpub.com/

Acquisitions Editor: Elizabeth Nieginski
Compositor: Transforma

ISBN: 978-0-8261-8503-7
ebook ISBN: 978-0-8261-8504-4
DOI: 10.1891/9780826185044

SUPPLEMENTS:

 SPRINGER PUBLISHING **CONNECT**™ | A robust set of instructor resources designed to supplement this text is located at http://connect.springerpub.com/content/book/978-0-8261-8504-4. Qualifying instructors may request access by emailing textbook@springerpub.com.

Instructor's Manual ISBN: 978-0-8261-8505-1
Instructor's PowerPoints ISBN: 978-0-8261-8506-8

Printed by BnT

The author and the publisher of this Work have made every effort to use sources believed to be reliable to provide information that is accurate and compatible with the standards generally accepted at the time of publication. Because medical science is continually advancing, our knowledge base continues to expand. Therefore, as new information becomes available, changes in procedures become necessary. We recommend that the reader always consult current research and specific institutional policies before performing any clinical procedure or delivering any medication. The author and publisher shall not be liable for any special, consequential, or exemplary damages resulting, in whole or in part, from the readers' use of, or reliance on, the information contained in this book. The publisher has no responsibility for the persistence or accuracy of URLs for external or third-party Internet websites referred to in this publication and does not guarantee that any content on such websites is, or will remain, accurate or appropriate.

Library of Congress Cataloging-in-Publication Data
Names: Gary, Faye, editor. | Lotas, Marilyn J., editor.
Title: A population health approach to health disparities for nurses : care
   of vulnerable populations / [edited by] Faye A. Gary, Marilyn J. Lotas.
Description: New York, NY : Springer Publishing Company, LLC, [2023]. |
   Includes bibliographical references and index.
Identifiers: LCCN 2022041697 | ISBN 9780826185037 (paperback) | ISBN
   9780826185051 (instructor's manual) | ISBN 9780826185068 (instructor's
   power point) | ISBN 9780826185044 (ebook)
Subjects: MESH: Social Determinants of Health | Vulnerable Populations |
   Health Inequities | Healthcare Disparities | Population Health | Nurses
   Instruction
Classification: LCC RA445 | NLM WA 30 | DDC 362.1089--dc23/eng/20220919
LC record available at https://lccn.loc.gov/2022041697

Contact sales@springerpub.com to receive discount rates on bulk purchases.

Publisher's Note: **New and used products purchased from third-party sellers are not guaranteed for quality, authenticity, or access to any included digital components.**

Printed in the United States of America.

Contents

Contributors

Angela D. Alston, DNP, MPH, APRN-CNP, WHNP-BC, FNP-BC Assistant Professor of Clinical Nursing, Lead Faculty–Women's Health Nurse Practitioner Specialty Track Chief Diversity Officer, Certified Nurse Practitioner, The Ohio State University College of Nursing, Columbus, Ohio

Ena Arce, MSN, RN Health Center Manager, San Jose State University, The Valley Foundation School of Nursing, San Jose, California

Donna Biederman, DPH, RN, FAAN Associate Professor, Duke University School of Nursing, Durham, North Carolina

Latina M. Brooks, PhD, FNP-C, FAANP Assistant Professor and Director of the Doctor of Nursing Practice Program, The Frances Payne Bolton School of Nursing, Case Western Reserve University, Cleveland, Ohio

Robin Brown Director, Concerned Citizens Organized Against Lead (CCOAL), Cleveland, Ohio

Regina Bussing, MD, MSHS Donald R. Dizney Chair in Psychiatry and Professor, University of Florida, College of Medicine, Department of Psychiatry, Gainesville, Florida

Brittney N. Butler, PhD, MPH FXB Health and Human Rights Fellow and David E. Bell Postdoctoral Fellow, Harvard T.H. Chan School of Public Health, Cambridge, Massachusetts

Jacquelyn Campbell, PhD, MSN, FAAN Anna D. Wolf Chair and Professor, Johns Hopkins School of Nursing, Baltimore, Maryland

Rebekah Israel Cross, PhD, MA Student Community Health Sciences, UCLA Fielding School of Public Health, Graduate Student Researcher, Center for the Study of Racism, Social Justice, and Health, Los Angeles, California

Brigette A. Davis, PhD, MPH California Preterm Birth Initiative Postdoctoral Scholar, Reproductive Sciences, School of Medicine, University of California San Francisco, San Francisco, California

Olubukunola Mary Dwyer, JD, MA Clinical Ethicist, Department of Clinical Ethics, University Hospitals, Cleveland Medical Center, Cleveland, Ohio; Clinical Assistant Professor, Department of Bioethics, Case Western Reserve University School of Medicine, Cleveland, Ohio

Irene C. Felsman, DNP, MPH, RN, CGH Assistant Professor, Duke University School of Nursing and Duke Global Health Institute, Durham, North Carolina

Lucine Francis, PhD, RN Assistant Professor, School of Nursing, Johns Hopkins University, Baltimore, Maryland

Rebecca Garcia PhD, MSc, RN, CPsychol FHEA   Interim Associate Head of School for Nursing and Health Professions, School of Health, Wellbeing and Social Care, Faculty of Wellbeing, Education, and Language Studies, The Open University, Milton Keynes, United Kingdom

Faye A. Gary, EdD, MS, RN, FAAN   Distinguished University Professor, Kent W. Clapp Chair and Professor of Nursing and Psychiatry, Case Western Reserve University, Cleveland, Ohio; Distinguished Service Professor, Emerita, University of Florida, Gainesville, Florida

Rosa M. Gonzalez-Guarda, PhD, MPH, RN, CPH, FAAN   Associate Professor, Duke University School of Nursing, Co-Director, Community Engaged Research Initiative, Duke Clinical Translational Science Institute, Durham, North Carolina

Ruby M. Gourdine,* DSW   Professor, Graduate Faculty, Howard University School of Social of Work, Washington, DC

Derek M. Griffith, PhD   Founder and Co-Director of the Racial Justice Institute, Founder and Director of the Center for Men's Health Equity, Professor of Health Systems Administration and Oncology, Georgetown University, Washington, DC

Ningning Guo, DNP, RN, NPD-BC, CCRN-K   Nursing Professional Development Specialist, Stanford Health Care, Center for Education and Professional Development, Palo Alto, California

Michelle DeCoux Hampton, PhD, MS, RN   Director of Academic Nursing and Patient Care Research, Stanford Health Care, Palo Alto, California

Rachel Hardeman, PhD, MPH   Associate Professor, Division of Health Policy and Management, University of Minnesota School of Public Health, Blue Cross Blue Shield Endowed Professor of Health and Racial Equity, Founding Director of the Center for Antiracism Research for Health Equity, Minneapolis, Minnesota

Mona Hassan, PhD, MS, RN   Assistant Professor, College of Nursing, Prairie View A&M University, Houston, Texas

Jesse Honsky, DNP, MPH, RN, PHNA-BC   Assistant Professor, Frances Payne Bolton School of Nursing, Case Western Reserve University, Cleveland, Ohio

June G. Hopps, PhD   Thomas Parham Professor of Family and Children Studies, School of Social Work, University of Georgia, Athens, Georgia

Amie Koch, DNP, FNP-C, RN, ACHPN   Assistant Professor, Duke University School of Nursing, Nurse Practitioner, Lincoln Community Health Center, Durham, North Carolina; Nurse Practitioner, Transitions LifeCare Hospice and Palliative Care, Raleigh, North Carolina

Margaret D. Larkins-Pettigrew, MD, MEd, MPPM, FACOG   Senior Vice President and the Chief Clinical Officer of Diversity, Equity, and Inclusion for Allegheny Health Network/Highmark Health, Pittsburgh, Pennyslvania

Gary L. Lawrence, PhD, RN, MSN, BSN, NRP   Director of Nursing Services, Choctaw Nation Health Services Authority, Talihina, Oklahoma

Linda A. Lewandowski, PhD   Dean and Professor, College of Nursing, Vice-Provost for Health Affairs for Interprofessional and Community Partnerships, University of Toledo, College of Nursing, Toledo, Ohio

---

*Dr. Gourdine died in February, 2022. She remained an active author until her untimely death.

Linda C. Lewin, PhD, PMHCNS-BC   Professor, University of Toledo, College of Nursing, Toledo, Ohio

Kevin Linder, JD   Student, School of Social Work, University of Georgia, Athens, Georgia

Alexis A. Lotas, PhD   Associate Professor, Texas A&M University, Corpus Christi, Texas (Retired)

Marilyn J. Lotas, PhD, RN, FAAN   Adjunct Professor, Frances Payne Bolton School of Nursing, Case Western Reserve University, Cleveland, Ohio (Retired)

Nomsa Magagula, DLitt et Phil, MSc HIS, BEd, CM, RN   Lecturer, Department of General Nursing, General Nursing Science Department, Faculty of Health Sciences, University of Eswatini, Mbabane, Eswatini, Southern Africa

Tengetile R. Mathunjwa-Dlamini, PhD, MS Epi, MNSc, BEd, CM, RN   Associate Professor in Nursing Science, General Nursing Science Department, Faculty of Health Sciences, University of Eswatini, Mbabane, Eswatini, Southern Africa

Eduardo M. Medina, MD, MPH   Clinician, Park Nicollet Clinic Minneapolis, Adjunct Assistant Professor, Department of Family Medicine, University of Minnesota School of Public Health, Minneapolis, Minnesota

Mary Beth Modic, DNP, APRN-CNS, CDCES, FAAN   Clinical Nurse Specialist - Diabetes, Cleveland Clinic, Brecksville, Ohio

Noelene Moonsamy, DNP, APRN, FNP-C   Assistant Professor, Samuel Merritt University, College of Nursing, Oakland, California

Martha Okafor, PhD   Executive Director, COVID-19 Health Equity Task Force, U.S. Department of Health and Human Services, Washington, DC

Terri Ann Parnell, DNP, MA, RN, FAAN   Health Literacy Partners LLC, New York, New York

Gaetan L. Pettigrew, MD   General Obstetrics and Gynecology, University of California San Francisco (UCSF), UCSF Medical Center, San Francisco, California

Liz Piatt, PhD   Assistant Dean, Academic Diversity Success, University College, Center for Undergraduate Excellence, Kent State University, Kent, Ohio

Miamon Queeglay   Research Project Manager, Community Engaged Research and Outreach, Division of Health Policy and Management, University of Minnesota School of Public Health, Minneapolis, Minnesota

Schenita Randolph, PhD, MPH, RN   Associate Professor, Duke University School of Nursing/Co-Director, Duke Center for Research to Advance Healthcare Equity, Durham, North Carolina

Latrice Rollins, PhD, MSW   Assistant Professor, Morehouse School of Medicine, Community Health and Preventive Medicine, Prevention Research Center, Atlanta, Georgia

Rima E. Rudd, ScD, MSPH   Associate of the Department of Social and Behavioral Sciences, Harvard T.H. Chan School of Public Health, Boston, Massachusetts

Nancy Gentry Russell, DNP, MSN, APRN, FNP-BC, CNE   Assistant Professor, School of Nursing, Johns Hopkins University, Baltimore, Maryland

David Satcher, MD, PhD 16th Surgeon General of the United States; Professor, Founding Director, Senior Advisor, The Satcher Health Leadership Institute, Morehouse School of Medicine, Atlanta, Georgia

Rashmi Sharma, MBBS, MIH Fellowship in Disaster Medicine and Emergency Preparedness, PGY-2 Resident at Louisiana State University, Monroe Family Medicine Residency, Shreveport, Louisiana

Phyllis Sharps, PhD, RN, FAAN Associate Dean Emerita, Community Programs and Initiatives, Johns Hopkins School of Nursing, Baltimore, Maryland (Retired)

Ricki Sheldon, EMT, OMS III Arkansas College of Osteopathic Medicine, Fort Smith, Arkansas

J. B. Silvers, PhD Interim Dean and Professor of Banking and Finances, Weatherhead School of Management, Case Western Reserve University, Cleveland, Ohio

Elizabeth Sloand, PhD, RN, PNP-BC, CNE, FAANP, FAAN Professor Emerita, School of Nursing, Johns Hopkins University, Baltimore, Maryland

Carolyn Harmon Still, PhD, MSM, APRN, AGPCNP-BC, FAAN Associate Professor, Frances Payne Bolton School of Nursing, Case Western Reserve University, Cleveland, Ohio

Christopher Strickland, MSW PhD Student, School of Social Work, University of Georgia, Athens, Georgia

Vicken Totten, MD, MS, FACEP, FAAFP Visalia, California (Retired)

Erika S. Trapl, PhD Associate Professor, Department of Population and Quantitative Health Sciences; Director, Prevention Research Center for Healthy Neighborhoods; Associate Director, Community Outreach and Engagement, Case Comprehensive Cancer Center, Case Western Reserve University, Cleveland, Ohio

Veronica E. Villalobos, JD Vice President for Diversity, Equity, and Inclusion, Enterprise Equitable Health Institute, Highmark Health/Allegheny Health Network, Pittsburgh, Pennsylvania

AnnMarie L. Walton, PhD, MPH, RN, OCN, CHES, FAAN Assistant Professor, Duke University School of Nursing, Durham, North Carolina

Christina L. Wilds, DrPH Director, Health Equity and Disparities, Enterprise Equitable Health Institute, Highmark Health/Allegheny Health Network, Pittsburgh, Pennsylvania

Jackson T. Wright Jr, MD, PhD Emeritus Professor of Medicine, Case Western Reserve University, University Hospitals Cleveland Medical Center, Cleveland, Ohio

Kathy D. Wright, PhD, RN, PMHCNS-BC Assistant Professor, Center for Healthy Aging, Self-Management, and Complex Care, College of Nursing, Discovery Themes–Chronic Brain Injury Program, The Ohio State University, Columbus, Ohio

Houssein N. Yarandi, PhD Professor, Center for Health Research, Wayne State University, Detroit, Michigan

Amy Y. Zhang, PhD Associate Professor, Frances Payne Bolton School of Nursing, Case Western Reserve University, Cleveland, Ohio

Foreword

Our country has long struggled with issues of equity as it relates to health and health-care. Driving those issues are a multitude of factors related to social determinants of health, access, and, of course, racism. In light of these challenges, there have been champions that have been leading the charge on this issue for decades now. These champions have made personal and professional sacrifices to advance the field and motivated countless individuals, like myself, to dedicate their lives to tackling issues around health equity and health disparities. They have opened our eyes to potential solutions and pathways that leaders from all walks of life can take to tackle these persistent and deep-rooted problems. The contributors and editors of this book are indeed those champions, experts, and leading authorities on how we should be addressing and improving the health of underserved communities across our country and, in fact, across our world.

The editors of this book embody the deepest understanding of these challenges. Dr. Faye Gary has used her time, skills, and expertise to change how individuals and communities approach many of these intractable challenges. Her strategy has been to cultivate solutions locally while also thinking globally in addressing complex issues such as mental health in African American communities. She also has delved into understanding more about high-risk behaviors impacting vulnerable and underserved communities, particularly younger generations. Her work has served as a foundation for others to build on while also addressing issues related to diversity and the pipeline needed to train the next generation of leaders and academicians to address health disparities. Dr. Marilyn Lotas has served as a professor and department chair of target populations at the University of Texas Health Science Center in Houston, where she implemented neonatal programs for medically underserved areas. Through faculty positions at Emory University, where she was the Albert Dozier Williamson Chair in nursing and head of the office of research administration as well as other faculty positions, she has worked globally to further public health education as well as locally on programs to address childhood obesity, childhood hypertension, and lead screening in the Cleveland community

This deep level of passion and expertise is reflected in the pages of this book, a much-needed and must-read compilation of history, data, evidence, and solutions from a variety of experts spanning the gamut of the top leaders in addressing issues of health disparities and health equity. This book represents a comprehensive viewpoint of the multifaceted nature of the challenges faced in addressing health disparities but more importantly provides a framework and thought pattern about how we continue to move forward and start making progress. This includes understanding not just the significant public health issues related to health disparities but also the social ecological approach, addressing the intersecting dynamics related to environmental ingredients around heart disease as well as the role of local neighborhoods and communities and examining issues around adverse child experiences and the global impact of HIV/AIDS in women. The overall compilation and approach in this book provide a basis for engagement, education, and understanding of a very complex historical challenge that still has its solutions based in the strength and vibrancy of local communities.

A series of recent events has awoken the world to the importance and urgency of tackling health equity. Yet what we must not forget is that these problems are not new and luckily for us there have been talented and devoted researchers and public health leaders who have been working on them for a number of years. This book brings that expertise to light in charting a course forward…and light is what we need most of all.

Garth Graham, MD, PPH, FACC
Director and Global Head of Healthcare and
Public Health Partnerships
Mountain View, California

Preface

Of all the forms of inequality, injustice in health is the most shocking and inhumane.
— Dr. Martin Luther King, Jr.

This book evolved from the editors' decades of experience working with disenfranchised, vulnerable, and underserved populations locally, nationally, and internationally. The book is designed to inform educators, nursing students, clinicians, researchers, and policymakers and to engage the public and those interested in eliminating health disparities. Recognizing that all share the planet, *A Population Health Approach to Health Disparities for Nurses* embraces health-related issues in local, national, and international communities.

In the United States and globally, concern has grown related to inequities in the process and outcomes of healthcare among populations. Despite this concern and associated actions to reduce these inequities, they have persisted. In many cases, they have grown. This book uses the model of population health as a lens for analyzing and understanding the development of health disparities and for beginning to identify areas of needed change. It highlights changes in public policy, attitudes, beliefs, education, and advocacy that will be essential if we are to address these inequities meaningfully.

Over the past several years, issues regarding health disparities have proliferated in the United States and the world community. Too little progress has been made, and entire populations—even within the world's wealthiest countries—scarcely benefit from the scientific advancements in healthcare that are readily available to their more privileged counterparts. Our book examines the social determinants of these well-known disparities; it provides clinical case studies and examples of selected phenomena that should awaken the curiosity of most readers and raise awareness about the possibilities for improved health outcomes across the life course. Sustained action, however, is required for positive change to occur. Albert Einstein succinctly defined our challenge: "No problem can be solved from the same level of consciousness that created it."

The purpose of the book is to provide a scholarly approach to health while highlighting population inequities and health disparities linked through three basic phenomena: healthcare systems, healthcare providers, and patients/consumers, all of whom are connected through the social determinants of health. Leaders worldwide are involved at various levels in supporting health equity, which conjoins with policy and finance. Our textbook illuminates the challenges and opportunities health professionals and policymakers face in multiple settings.

We acknowledge the phenomenal progress made in healthcare, particularly in population and public health, while suggesting that more robust efforts must be made to eliminate the burdens of disease carried by poor and underserved peoples in our local communities and across the world. The book, by design, embraces an interprofessional approach to learning, research, and healthcare delivery. It embraces perspectives from a variety of people, places, and communities, which are embedded throughout this book and provide numerous opportunities for cross-cultural and culturally and linguistically appropriate dialogue and decision-making. It encourages a patient-centered focus, which acknowledges the patient as an active member in the clinical encounter. Our approach includes contributions from various health professionals from around the world. Nurses, physicians, social workers, researchers, epidemiologists, psychologists, and insurance and finance experts are among those who have shared their knowledge supporting interprofessional learning and all aspects of healthcare.

For all who read this book, we hope that you will gain inspiration from the work of the many dedicated professionals who have contributed to it. We hope that the reader will gain an enlightened understanding of health disparities and their stubborn historical and contemporary perspectives and gain inspiration for what is known and what must change. May you be emboldened to question the policies and practices that have driven the research, practice, education, and advocacy that have prevailed in previous years but have not been adequate. Our professional lives have been devoted to improving the human condition. A commitment from each person who is invested in healthcare must occur at a higher level if the entirety of humanity is ever to experience the dignity of basic healthcare. This book provides an opportunity for you to join in this challenging quest.

ORGANIZATION OF THE BOOK

We have organized the book into three sections with a total of 25 distinct chapters, each with their own theoretical and conceptual frameworks, populations of interest, diseases and health conditions, and places and spaces:

- ◆ Section I focuses on the definition, history, and science of population health, which establishes the foundation for the book. This provides the lens through which healthcare systems and health policies are developed and evaluated and through which health inequities and disparities in outcomes can be understood.
- ◆ Section II explores factors that impact the health of individuals, communities, and populations, including the social determinants of health, health literacy, and endemic racism.
- ◆ Drawing from the first two sections, Section III focuses on selected health issues and disparities, exploring the factors that contribute to their development.

Figure 1 further displays the organization of the sections and should help the reader to grasp the comprehensive richness and heftiness of the book and its unique blend of cultural world views, science/research, theory, clinical practice, and decision-making at all levels of healthcare in the United States and globally. The book relies heavily on contributions from

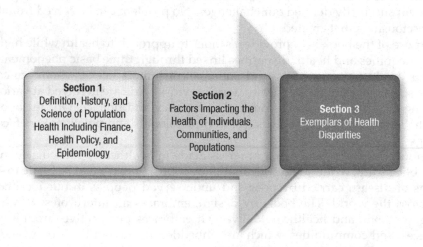

Figure 1 Organization of *A Population Health Approach to Health Disparities for Nurses.*

well-informed professionals representing a variety of disciplines who have amassed robust hands-on work experiences with individuals, families, and communities that are vulnerable and continue to experience a plethora of health disparities.

We have worked with populations across the globe and have integrated their collective experiences throughout the book. Their perspectives provide a professional, impactful, practical, personal, and culturally appropriate approach to eliminating health disparities. This book is designed to become a catalyst for transformative healthcare delivery systems, improved and more diverse workforces, and further engaged and informed patient-centered healthcare.

RESPONSE TO NURSES' ROLES IN ADDRESSING HEALTH DISPARITIES: PAST, PRESENT, AND FUTURE

Since their inception as caregivers, nurses have embraced four distinct roles influencing health outcomes in individuals and communities: education, research, practice, and advocacy. Nurses have long been cognizant of the consequences of educating individuals and communities about risk, methods of protection from and prevention of disease, and the role such education can have in empowering communities. Refinement of interdisciplinary learning among professional groups where nurses have a significant role can be translated into patient advocacy with implications in policy, practice, and research toward reducing health disparities.

Research is designed to promulgate knowledge and evidence-based practice that addresses health promotion, advances certain skill sets, and promotes innovations in patient management within acute and community-based settings. Research in nursing is essential for ensuring the best, most culturally sensitive approach for prevention, diagnosis, treatment, and cure for diseases.

Clinical practice issues include incorporating the social determinants of health into assessment and care planning while endeavoring avoidance of stereotyping, bias, and discrimination. Concerns about patient outcomes abound because racial and ethnic groups and vulnerable persons such as immigrants and the homeless have historically received a poorer quality of care than their more privileged counterparts in the dominant society. Clinical uncertainty, as experienced by the healthcare provider, plays a significant part in creating and maintaining health disparities. Inequities manifest even among those disenfranchised with ample indicators for quality care such as advanced educational achievement, socioeconomic status, and procurement of optimal insurance benefits. The future of equitable healthcare relies upon renewed focus on the social determinants of health: housing, education, employment, environmental justice, climate-related health issues, ethics, and culturally competent care of vulnerable populations.

Advocacy includes advocating for health policies that can improve the quality of care and the equity of care for all populations. It also includes supporting community initiatives that endeavor to educate, increase healthcare resources to underserved and vulnerable communities, and improve health access for all. Nurses witness firsthand the power of efficient access to quality healthcare, as they know all too well that disparities in healthcare are correlated with poor health outcomes. Technology, the rapid transfer of science to practice, social media, and other innovations are profoundly expanding the effectiveness of healthcare. Still, patients will always need individuals who can address their needs in a humane, caring, empathetic, and highly competent manner. Trust and confidence in the nurse and their legacy of care and protection of vulnerable people will continue as the distinguishing feature of nursing around the globe.

Faye A. Gary
Marilyn J. Lotas

Acknowledgments

I wish to acknowledge the contributions of those who have contributed to the development of this book in valuable ways and on multiple levels.

First, over the generations, my family has invested in their children. My parents, Homer and Ollie Gary, and our extended family devoted their time and energy to our well-being. My grandfather, William Primus Gary, taught me and my sister, June, to read. I am grateful for such care and nurturing. My sisters, June Gary Hopps, Gladys Gary Vaughn, Ollie Gary-Christian, and brother, Homer Gary, have been my life mentors. My sons, Michael, Jonathan, William, and Benjamin, are loving supporters and gentle but omnipresent observers who always provide much-appreciated feedback. My granddaughters Nia and Norah share a vibrant perspective about the world and its beauty.

Classmates at Howard Academy, Ocala, Florida, then Florida A&M University, Tallahassee, were reaffirming and supportive during my formative years. At Saint Xavier University, Chicago, my classmates and the graduate faculty in psychiatric nursing embraced who I was and challenged me to what I could become. At the University of Florida, Gainesville, faculty in the department of psychiatry were colleagues, teachers, and friends. I wish to acknowledge the long and trusting friendship and guidance that I received from the late William Jape Taylor, the late Melvin Fregly, the late Hattie Bessent, and Regina Bussing. Associates at the University of Florida, especially Molly Dougherty, Hossein N. Yarandi, and the late Doris W. Campbell, have been trusted colleagues and friends. Their genuine commitment to me as a person, a professional, and a citizen of my community and the world is a remarkable gift to my family and me, which, I hope, will be evidenced for generations to come.

Dean May Wykle at the Frances Payne Bolton School of Nursing recruited me to Case Western Reserve University, and I agreed to a 3-year tenure. Seventeen years later, I am still there. With the assistance of Former Provost William "Bud" Baeslack, Dean May Wykle, and Former East Cleveland City Schools Superintendent Myrna Loy Corley, we developed the Provost Scholars Program, connecting public school students to university mentors and tutors. The program will soon be celebrating its 10th year. It is still thriving and growing because of Katrice Williams, a student coordinator and now practicing attorney and Nancy Kurfess Johnson. They worked tirelessly to assist when additional help was needed. Solid, genuine, and bold commitments from Lee Thompson and Kate Klonowski have helped sustain and advance the program; both are stellar colleagues, mentors, administrators, and advocates for youth.

Finally, we respectfully acknowledge our readers from across the globe. We welcome your comments and recommendations and promise to diligently review and address them in the book's next edition.

With a deep sense of gratitude, thank you!

–FG

I want to thank the many contributors to the book. Their generosity with their time and expertise has made this book possible. I wish to acknowledge my husband Alex Lotas who provided editorial expertise and support. I am grateful to Dr. Joyce Fitzpatrick and Dean May Wykle for their mentorship, support, and guidance. I am grateful to Robin Brown director of Concerned Citizens Organized Against Lead (CCOAL) and Miss Marilyn Burns who have been my partners in the community, friends, and inspirations. I am grateful for the Cleveland Metropolitan School District nurses who have supported my work in the schools. Finally, I am grateful for my sons, Michael and Jeffrey, daughters-in-law, Tammy and Cindy, and my grandchildren Sarah, Cassie, and Zander, who continue to decorate my life.

–ML

Instructor Resources

 A robust set of instructor resources designed to supplement this text is located at http://connect.springerpub.com/content/book/978-0-8261-8504-4. Qualifying instructors may request access by emailing textbook@springerpub.com.

Available resources include:

◆ Instructor's Manual
◆ Chapter-Based PowerPoint Presentations
◆ Mapping to AACN Essentials: Core Competencies for Professional Nursing Education

SECTION I

Definition, History, and Science of Population Health

CHAPTER 1

Social Context for Healthcare

David Satcher, Martha Okafor,* and Faye A. Gary

LEARNING OBJECTIVES

- To examine the social context of healthcare in the United States and globally.
- To provide an overview of healthcare in the global community and in the United States.
- To provide an explication of the role of healthcare in health equity.
- To gaze into the future of healthcare.

INTRODUCTION

The superordinate purpose of this opening chapter of *A Population Health Approach to Health Disparities for Nurses* is to highlight the elements that are critical for improving the nation's health through population health science and the social determinants of health. It features health and healthcare from several perspectives based on theory, research, training, policy, and the viewpoints of the provider, the patient, the family, and the communities. In this chapter, we describe public health and examine what healthcare does and should do to improve the well-being of individuals, families, and communities. This chapter elucidates global and local health issues and the social context where people live, learn, work, play, and pray. This is followed by a discussion of the future of healthcare and the social determinants of health challenges it must confront. Finally, there is an overview of the systems that overlap and help create wicked problems requiring paradigm shifts in priorities and policy.

HEALTHCARE IN THE UNITED STATES

There are many definitions and descriptions of public health. In this chapter, public health is described as a collective effort of a society or community to create and maintain the conditions in which people can be healthy. These conditions include but are not limited to social, cultural, structural, political, institutional, religious, environmental, economic, educational, climate change, and well-being conditions.

The U.S. healthcare system spans the public and private sectors and is primarily regulated by policy decisions that impact individuals, families, and communities. Understanding the complexities and broad implications of the healthcare industry—its management, delivery,

*This author's contributions to this chapter is written in her personal capacity. No official support or endorsement of the content by the US Department of Health and Human Services is intended or should be inferred.

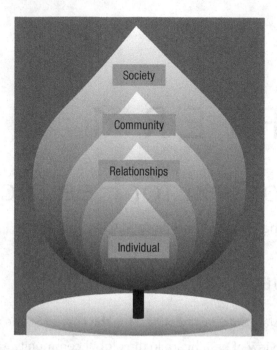

Figure 1.1 Social-ecological model.

Source: Adapted from Centers for Disease Control and Prevention. (2021). The social-ecological model: A framework for violence prevention. www.cdc.gov/violenceprevention/about/social-ecologicalmodel. html.

cost, equity, medical technologies, and other advancements—would not be compelling without factoring in the social determinants of health and consequential outcomes.

The U.S. healthcare system could be described as a patchwork of uneven and incomplete systems and programs from both public and private entities designed to protect and care for the health of all U.S.s populations. Due to the complexities of the healthcare system and the absence of a national public health system, the United States, with one of the world's most advanced economies, has one of the world's most inefficient healthcare systems.

CDC Social-Ecological Model

The Centers for Disease Control and Prevention (CDC, 2021) social-ecological model suggests substantial intersectionality of the individual with interpersonal relationships (e.g., family, relatives, friends); community networks (e.g., neighborhood, school, faith-based place, workplace); and society (e.g., city, state, country, global influences; Figure 1.1). The overlapping features in the model demonstrate how one factor influences another; these influences are present across the life course. The approach supports a prevention perspective that aids in the conceptualization of how best to achieve the desired impact upon specific populations. The utility of this model lies in the clarity with which it portrays the dynamic overlapping of the four domains.

Individual

The level of the individual highlights biological and personal factors that help to produce behavioral and health outcomes. Such factors include age, gender, sexual orientation, education, socioeconomic status, and health behaviors and beliefs. It also includes access to care, including interventions designed to address specific problems such as mental health concerns, substance use, or intimate partner violence (Gary et al., 2021).

Relationship

Interpersonal relationships help to shape beliefs, behaviors, and expectations. The expectations of significant others are highly influential in an individual's decision-making. Healthy relationships can be strengthened through mentoring, coaching, improved parenting and child guidance, and communication enhancement. Conflict resolution and healthy relationships among family and peers promote beneficial outcomes (Okafor et al., 2014).

Community

Community-based places are critical components in the overlapping model. Schools, faith-based institutions, neighborhood organizations, healthcare providers, health systems, and leaders at all levels are essential attributes of developing and maintaining healthy facilitative communities for all people. Safety, at this level, emerges as a dominant concern, especially in underresourced communities and in low- to middle-income countries across the globe. Improved health outcomes are intimately linked to education and access to health services, which are the basis for improved well-being, economic security, and reduced morbidity and mortality. Deterrents to health and well-being include chronic and recalcitrant issues such as poverty; redlining, which impacts access to housing and basic economic resources; food deserts and healthy food insecurities; residential segregation; inadequate schools; limited availability of primary healthcare services; and acceptance/access to harmful substance use/misuse.

Society

The final level of the social-ecological model addresses the comprehensive set of components that help create and maintain health outcomes—ranging from excellent to poor—that are evident over the life course. This includes social norms, cultural practices and beliefs, and historical and ongoing influences such as laws and policies. Collective institutional memories as well as vision regarding the future are other factors for consideration. Economic justice and gainful, reliable employment in healthy environments are also crucial factors that help to determine societal status.

Key elements are crucial in all societies (e.g., healthcare, economics, education, laws, policies, and social norms that help to maintain a civil and orderly society). Flaws in any of the social-ecological levels can create inequities within and across groups in local and global communities. Efforts to improve any of the model components require improvement of the education and health systems and provision of economic opportunities for growth, development, and prosperity.

THE PUBLIC HEALTH SYSTEM OF THE UNITED STATES

The nation's health services are organized and provided by a loosely structured delivery system that is comprised of public and private health insurance programs and subsystems. The public health system nested under the federal government's executive branch is the single largest health insurer in the country. The main component of this public health system is under the Department of Health and Human Services (DHHS). However, other systems in the national government address healthcare issues: the Defense Department, the Veterans Administration, and the Social Security Administration are a few examples. The mission of the DHHS is to protect the health and well-being of the American public through various approaches such as the funding and supporting of health-related research, the promulgation of public policy, and the advancement of best practices in health promotion, disease prevention, and treatment. The Secretary of Health and Human Services is appointed by the President of the United States, along with the Assistant Secretary and the Surgeon General, who is considered America's "top doctor." The DHHS is responsible for a variety of agencies that are critical to health and well-being, including the CDC, the National Institutes of Health (NIH), the Food and Drug Administration (FDA), the Centers for Medicare &

Medicaid Services (CMS), the Substance Abuse and Mental Health Services Administration (SAMHSA), the Health Research and Services Administration (HRSA), and others—the Agency for Toxic Substances and Disease Registry (ATSDR) and the Agency for Healthcare Research and Quality (AHRQ), for example—that might not be as prominent in the public domain, but are nonetheless essential.

The CMS plays a significant role in preserving and advancing the health of people because it administers both Medicare and Medicaid, the two largest public health insurance programs in the nation. Older adults and individuals with disabilities receive support from Medicare, and Medicaid insurance covers essential healthcare services for pregnant people, people with disabilities, and individuals with chronic health conditions (Marmot, 2017; Shultz et al., 2021). Medicaid is jointly financed by both federal and state governments. The federal government matches state Medicaid funds at varied rates based on the state's income and expenditure levels, with the poorer states receiving a higher match from the federal government. SAMHSA provides a spectrum of prevention-to-recovery services for persons living with mental health and substance use disorders. HRSA supports the provision of services for maternal and child health as well as healthcare infrastructure and workforce. The Indian Health Service (IHS) also functions under the auspices of the DHHS. It is designed to provide comprehensive services to Native Americans and Alaska Native people. Cultural competence is associated with the reduction and elimination of health disparities and is highlighted in Healthy People 2020 and Healthy People 2030 (Purnell & Fenkl, 2019). In all of these systems, which are committed to eliminating health disparities and enhancing health equity in local and global communities, leadership remains a crucial element (Satcher, 2020; see Chapter 20 for more information about the IHS).

State, County, and Local Health Systems

While the federal government sets wide-ranging policies, states have the authority, flexibility, and responsibility to develop their state plans and govern the implementation of policies and procedures generated at the legislative and executive levels of government. State plans guide county and city public health departments, and they relate to the state and the federal government, forming a network through which scientific, theoretical, and practical information is shared (Figure 1.2). The three levels of government are also concerned about the specific populations in their jurisdictions, the cultural and political systems that influence policies and practices, and human and material resource allocations. Services are delivered at the individual, family, community, and state levels. Healthcare professionals provide grassroots and essential healthcare designed to reduce mortality and morbidity and enhance well-being.

While this section is focused on the public health system, we feel it is important to mention that the majority of the U.S. population is covered by the private health system. Most members of the population obtain health services through private health insurance that is provided either by their employers or through their direct purchase of nongroup health insurance and self-insured plans. Relatively few members of the population opt out of all insurance programs and remain uninsured or obtain health services through limited charitable healthcare or sporadic services.

Connecting World Health Systems

The World Health Organization (WHO) connects national public health programs and services to global communities. Research and practice models are shared globally with governmental and nongovernmental agencies. The organization is nested in the United Nations (New York); its headquarters are in Geneva, Switzerland; and its mission is addressed through six regional and 150 country offices. Representing the Americas and encompassing the Western Hemisphere is the Pan American Health Organization (PAHO), headquartered in Washington, DC (Shultz et al., 2021).

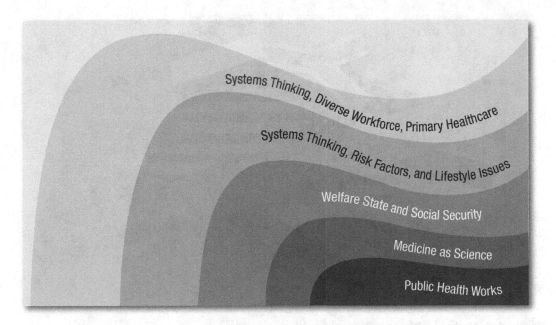

Figure 1.2 The advancement of public health in the United States. Wave One (1800–1819): Public health works such as improved water sanitation and disposal of solid waste; germ theory. Wave Two (1890–1950): Science-based medicine and research. Wave Three (1940–1960): The welfare state and Social Security. Wave Four (1960–2014): Systems thinking, risk factors, and lifestyle issues. Wave Five (2015-future): Systems thinking, diverse workforce, primary healthcare.

Source: Adapted from Lueddeke, G. (2015). *Global population health and well-being in the 21st century: Toward new paradigms, policy, and practice.* Springer Publishing.

WHO produces guidelines designed to facilitate health promotion and disease prevention, such as recommendations for the improvement of physical and emotional well-being (Bull et al., 2020). Another significant contribution facilitated by WHO is the classification of disease across the global community embodied in the *WHO Health Equity Toolkit*, a resource for comparing selected health metrics across world communities that highlight inequities and some of their root causes. It is a resource that provides data about different population groups. It offers valuable evidence for policies, practices, and programs designed to address health inequities and supports work toward the goal of healthcare for all (WHO, 2021). In addition to WHO, there are many nongovernmental agencies across the globe that direct their efforts to public health issues; consider, for example, the American Cancer Society or the Chinese Anti-Cancer Society (Shultz et al., 2021; Xu, 2015).

Classification of Diseases Across the World

Under the auspices of WHO, the classification of disease has evolved into an international method of scientifically categorizing disorders worldwide. The revised system, published in 2018, is titled *The International Statistical Classification of Diseases and Related Health Problems* (ICD-11; Brand et al., 2020; Shultz et al., 2021). The purpose of the ICD-11 is to track the health and illnesses of the world's populations across the life course from birth to death. Diseases are number coded according to broad categories: neoplasms or cancers; infections of the circulatory system; diseases of the respiratory system; and mental, behavioral, and neurodevelopmental disorders. Distinctions are made between infectious or communicable diseases (e.g., those demonstrating vector involvement or transmission from one infected person to another, as with the COVID-19 virus or tuberculosis) and noncommunicable diseases (e.g., those that do not show evidence of being transferred from one person to another, as with asthma or diabetes).

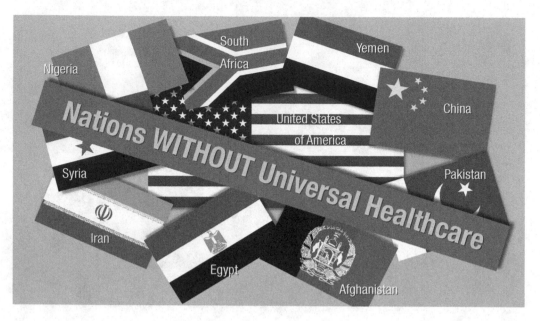

Figure 1.3 Nations without universal healthcare.

Source: Adapted from Shvili, J. (2020, May 30). 10 countries without universal healthcare, *www.worldatlas .com/articles/10-notable-countries-that-are-still-without-universal-healthcare.html*.

Data suggest that communicable diseases are more prevalent among low- and middle-income populations, and noncommunicable diseases are more dominant among upper-middle and high-income populations. About seven of 10 leading causes of mortality are infectious diseases, a trend that is most prevalent in low- and middle-income populations (Shultz et al., 2021). Many chronic diseases, such as heart disease and cancer, which are more common in upper-middle and high-income populations, can possibly be prevented (Marmot, 2017; World Bank, 2022).

Mirror, Mirror on the Wall, Is United States Healthcare the Very Best of All?

In the United States and many other countries, poor health is correlated with a sizeable income gap or gross inequities in resources. Access to healthcare in the United States typically requires insurance—private, public, or out-of-pocket. Healthcare access commonly requires other resources such as transportation, some level of health literacy, and technological competence. The United States boasts the ignominious distinction of being the sole developed nation among the ranks of those countries in the world that deprive their citizens of universal healthcare (Figure 1.3).

When trying to unravel the attributes of the healthcare system n the United States and determine its distinguishing attributes compared with other high-income countries, data from other countries can be informative. A study promulgated by The Commonwealth Fund analyzed data from 71 performance indicators across five domains in 11 countries: access to care, care process, administrative efficiency, equity, and health outcomes (Schneider et al., 2021). Data were generated from each country, along with administrative data from the Organization for Economic Co-operation and Development and WHO. According to their findings, the highest-performing countries were Norway, the Netherlands, and Australia. The second three were the United Kingdom, Germany, and New Zealand. The final three tiers were Sweden, France, Switzerland, and Canada. Despite spending far more of its gross domestic product resources on healthcare, the United States ranked last on four of the five measures, and second on care process (Schneider et al., 2021). A brief description of each of the five domains follows.

Access to Care

This domain focused on affordability and the timeliness of care. Regarding timeliness, residents in countries that ranked high in this domain were more likely to be able to receive same-day medical care, including after-hours assistance. The Netherlands topped the timeliness list, followed by Germany and Norway. The United Kingdom was the leader for affordability. Germany and Norway have insurance that rarely denies claims, and the residents of these two countries were not likely to have difficulty paying for their medical care (Schneider et al., 2021).

Care Process

Regarding care process, the United States earned a commendable rank of two, as did the United Kingdom and Sweden. The key elements in this category are preventive care, safe care, and engagement and patient preferences. Included in the cluster are mammography screening, flu vaccines, and the number of patients who have a consultation with their providers about nutrition, smoking, and alcohol use.

Safe coordination, which includes computerized alerts and medication reviews, were highest in the United States and New Zealand. Coordinated care, however, was highest in New Zealand, Switzerland, and the Netherlands. These same countries, including France, were high performers in measures related to communications between primary care providers and specialists. None of the countries were outstanding when measuring communications between primary care providers, emergency departments, and social services personnel.

The award, however, for addressing patient preferences went to Germany and the United States—even though the United States has the lowest ranking on continuity of care with the same provider. While U.S. residents with chronic health problems were more likely to discuss their goals and treatment options with providers, it is important to recognize that they were less likely to get the needed support from health professionals that they felt they deserved. During the pandemic, providers in Sweden and Australia reported using video consultations with patients more often (Schneider et al., 2021).

Administrative Efficiency

This domain addressed the extent to which healthcare systems reduce the burden of paperwork and government-related tasks that patients and providers must complete related to their care. Norway, Australia, New Zealand, and the United Kingdom ranked at the top of this list. The United States was last as the burden load is heavy; restrictions on insurance and pharmacologic agents are very time-consuming (Schneider et al., 2021).

Equity

Income disparities were extensive in the United States, New Zealand, and Norway. The data were generated from examining access to care, care process, and administrative efficiency across racial and ethnic groups. The countries with the highest equity rankings were Australia, Germany, and Switzerland. Of concern in the United States are the disparities between income groups, including factors such as financial barriers that prevent or delay healthcare, medical payment burdens, and difficulty accessing after-hours care or using web portals for computer-based care. Residents in the United States and Canada more frequently reported larger income differences in patient self-reported experiences (Schneider et al., 2021).

Healthcare Outcomes

This domain refers to health issues that are likely to respond to the healthcare that is received. Australia, Norway, and Switzerland were at the top of the 11-country group. For example, Norway had the lowest infant mortality rate at two deaths per 1,000 live births,

CASE STUDY 1.1: MR. UPJOHN

Upon being laid off from a 20-year career creating advertising materials, Mr. Upjohn lost his company-provided health insurance and could not afford to pay $2,700 per month for COBRA insurance coverage. His state had a limited Medicaid program and did not participate in the Affordable Care Act program, nor did he qualify for Medicare.

Despite picking up various skilled jobs, Mr. Upjohn's finances were tight. Consequently, upon noticing weakness in his legs, Mr. Upjohn tried several home remedies in vain before seeking care through a research and teaching hospital about 60 miles away. This was his most practical option, as private physicians in the area did not typically schedule patients without insurance. A neighbor drove Mr. Upjohn to the hospital emergency department, where he was admitted with a diagnosis of neurodegenerative disease.

Mr. Upjohn's condition continued to deteriorate. Because he had no insurance, the social work/finance department informed him that his resources must be listed as collateral and a potential source for healthcare payment: his car, a small plot of land jointly owned by Mr. Upjohn and two other family members, and his home—where his ancestral family, people who had worked hard and always "paid their way," had lived for more than a century. As his healthcare bills continued to increase, he received invoices from the attending physician, radiology, cardiology, physical therapy, speech therapy, the emergency department, laboratories, pharmacy, and the hospital. Within a short while, his debt approached $75,000.

Mr. Upjohn had always had a stutter. Overwhelmed, his speech became more difficult to understand. He cried. He became depressed. Desperate, Mr. Upjohn requested discharge with detailed written instructions to continue his treatment at home. Family and friends tried to assist in his care, but the instructions were difficult to follow. Home healthcare was unaffordable. Unable to afford the prescribed medications, Mr. Upjohn reverted to home remedies. His condition continued spiraling downward. He eventually had to be admitted to the acute care unit at the research and teaching hospital. Shortly after that, Mr. Upjohn died.

Mr. Upjohn's plight is shared by many people in the United States and worldwide. This book aims to provide insight into the healthcare crisis as it exists and to shine a guiding light toward a brighter future. Our goal is to promote equitable healthcare and well-being for all people wherever they may live.

and Australia had the highest life expectancy after age 65—about 25.6 more years could be expected after a person survived their 60th birthday. By contrast, the United States had the highest infant mortality rate at 5.7 deaths per 1,000 live births. Although, when compared to the other 10 countries, maternal mortality was high in France, it was much lower than the United States (7.6 and 17.4, respectively, per 100,000 live births; see Resources for More In-Depth Information at the end of this chapter; Schneider et al., 2021).

See Box 1.1 for healthcare improvement strategies.

POPULATION HEALTH THINKING

Evolving science and healthcare in recent years have turned the focus toward population health. This requires a paradigm shift from the individual to groups and populations because it "seeks to understand under what circumstances do people experience health and illness, what causes and contributes to their conditions, when and where, in order to improve health

BOX 1.1: Healthcare Improvement Strategies

A brief comparison of the healthcare performance among the world's most resourced countries and the United States reveals deficits suggesting the need for policy and practice changes. The higher-ranking countries reveal characteristics worthy of consideration:

1. Provide universal healthcare for all residents and remove access and cost barriers.
2. Strengthen primary healthcare and deliver high-value and culturally congruent services that are available to individuals and communities, and reduce risks for discrimination, racism, and unequal treatment.
3. Reduce and eliminate administrative burdens that are associated with healthcare delivery and extravagate patients and clinicians from nonclinical and nonhealth-related functions.
4. Reimagine the social services that address the social determinants of health such as housing, transportation, childcare, safer communities, and better schools.
5. Prioritize maternal child health needs for all people across the nation.
6. Offer primary healthcare for all from before conception and through the life course.

Source: Adapted from Schneider, E. C. et al. (2021). Mirror, mirror 2021—reflecting poorly: Health care in the U.S. compared to other high-income countries. *Commonwealth Fund.* https://doi .org/10.26099/01dv-h208.

and achieve health equity" (Okafor, 2019). Population health thinking improves health outcomes for all people by tracking the health of a population and the conditions that optimize equitable health outcomes. While the triggers associated with population health are different from those for specific health and illness among individuals, they include the overall health outcomes of the individual members of the groups that make up the population.

Shifting from an individualistic approach to a population health thinking model suggests that numerous domains are active in producing this outcome and are evident in the four overlapping domains described in the social-ecological model earlier (i.e., individual, relationships, community, and society). When health professionals have insights into the two approaches, substance abuse causes at the individual and the population health levels are different and require reconsideration in program planning, designing interventions, and educating health professionals and the public (Degenhardt et al., 2016; Evans & Bufka, 2020; Marmot, 2017; Shultz et al., 2021). The intersectionality among levels of government and private and philanthropic organizations is evident throughout the other chapters in this book.

Population Health Focus on Youth

Youth tend to model and adopt behaviors that they observe in the activities of daily living of family members, peers, friends, and others in their social networks who are essential to them or who impress them as being cool or popular. During the early to late teen years, peers and individuals outside of the family structure might have as much or more influence on them than their immediate family members. A youth's friends, especially over time, tend to be prominent in their lives and can play significant roles in their decision-making (Henneberger et al., 2021).

In neighborhoods with a surfeit of liquor stores—a common sight in underresourced communities—there is an increased likelihood of frequent alcohol use among adults. The presence of these outlets might also serve as a proxy for the availability of alcohol use among youth. Reducing alcohol consumption among youth will necessitate restricting commercial outlets through amending licensure and zoning requirements for selected

BOX 1.2: A Global Perspective on Mortality

1. Examination of how population health and primary care can be better augmented could help to improve a nation's health.
2. Reflection on the major contributions of developed nations to public health could provide historical and future perspectives for nations seeking direction.
3. Integration of national policies that would promulgate a health-in-all policies approach in agencies/organizations could improve health outcomes worldwide (Lueddeke, 2016).

neighborhood sites. Other approaches include stringently enforcing laws about the consumption of alcohol by minors and educating youth, families, and other leaders in vulnerable neighborhoods about the deleterious consequences of alcohol and other substance use and abuse among teens (Marmot, 2017; Shultz et al., 2021). These measures are population-health focused.

See Box 1.2 for a global perspective on mortality.

GLOBAL AND LOCAL INTERVENTIONS FOR IMPROVED WELL-BEING

WHO has posited that more than 930 million people worldwide are at risk for enduring out-of-pocket health spending that exceeds more than 10% of household budgets (WHO, 2021, April 1). Poverty challenges continue through healthcare costs that place demands on existing families living in poverty, which has the potential for pushing them further into extreme hardships. It is crucial that primary healthcare becomes a key element in guaranteeing the highest quality of healthcare and well-being through a more equitable approach to delivering professional services to all people across the world.

In primary care, health promotion, disease prevention, prompt treatment, and rehabilitation are essential components of theoretical, policy-related, and practical methodologies in health services (Okafor et al., 2018). At the global and local levels, equity is a necessary commitment at the highest levels of government. To be effective, equity must be integrated into the basic fabric of society. To advance health and well-being for all people, the social determinants of health needs must be tackled at every level of government in each community.

For example, people with mental illness are at risk for additional maladies because of the chronic nature of the disorder and because of potential compromises in the education and economic capacity that would typically help them to sustain a better quality of life. Individuals may need transportation to access primary and specialty care. They are entitled to adequate housing in safe and violence-free communities. Interventions should be comprehensive, with one need triggering the call to action for other services that are linked to their comprehensive health demands.

Teams of interprofessional healthcare providers who learn and work together are emerging as the gold standard for delivering health services to diverse populations. Included on such teams are physicians, nurses, navigators, social workers, community health workers, and other volunteers who share a common mission and objective (Castrucci & Auerbach, 2019; Marmot, 2017; Satcher, 2020). Trending patterns include aging at home, use of technology for diagnosing and treating illness conditions, and educating a diverse workforce that mirrors the population needing health services that are delivered in the context of the social determinants of health.

The latter position has emerged in recent years and is linked to the ideology that in local and global communities, all providers must be respectful of and responsive to the cultural needs of individuals and families. The examination and re-engineering of universal policy changes that address the root causes of morbidity and mortality rates and inadequate levels of well-being among vulnerable populations in the world community are critical next steps. These are systemic and policy changes that address the root causes of morbidity and mortality rates among vulnerable populations (Kaholokula, 2020).

Person-centered interventions or personalized healthcare initiatives are notable, and they aid in advancing health and wellness for many, but this approach lacks giving attention to long-term solutions that integrate science and policy, while simultaneously giving the desired consideration to what is needed to address the social determinants of health. Recall that these determinants are entwined in social, economic, and education deficits that aid in the creation and maintenance of these disparities (see Chapter 7 for additional discussion of the social determinants of health).

Person-centered interventions are primarily designed to attend to individuals who reside at the lower points of the health scale; they tend to be queasier and poorer, are less educated, and are often without the necessary health literacy and numeracy knowledge and skills. Unfortunately, they typically present with the most daunting health conditions as well. Their care, if provided, often generates large health expenses—many of which could have been prevented. On the other hand, populations that are not at this lower place, but are someplace in the middle of the health needs continuum, are too often overlooked and do not have access to the essential options needed to adequately provide for their needs (e.g., transportation, time off from work, insurance, computer access and literacy). Over time, delays in seeking and attaining healthcare can catapult them into a downward spiral that creates more morbidity and mortality—at this point, lives are compromised, and health costs for individuals and financial systems are increased. Many health conditions could be prevented if healthcare were universally available to all people (Castrucci & Auerbach, 2019; Gary et al., 2021; Kaholokula, 2020; Marmot, 2017; Okafor et al., 2018; Okafor et al., 2020; Satcher, 2020; Shultz et al., 2021).

One Size Does Not Fit All

Awareness among healthcare professionals and policymakers about ethnic, racial, cultural, and religious diversities; socioeconomic status; and educational opportunities that exist among various populations is fundamental to contextualizing health equity and the improvement of health for all people. These factors often determine individual and community health status. If health equity is to prevail, the health and social needs of specific populations must be taken into consideration in planning and implementing the equitable distribution of goods and services (Emanuel, 2020; Satcher, 2020).

GAZING INTO THE FUTURE OF THE NATION'S HEALTHCARE

The COVID-19 pandemic has exposed gross inequities in the U.S. healthcare system. After years of neglecting the public health infrastructure, opportunities exist for reimagining a system that provides quality and cost-effective care for all people in America. The recent virus and its influence on the daily life of people have highlighted the need for meaningful improvements in the U.S. public health infrastructure and capacity. This reality is illuminated through the challenges that the nation has endured due to COVID-19 and all its negative impacts on health nationwide, including the escalation of mortality and morbidity rates (Emanuel, 2020).

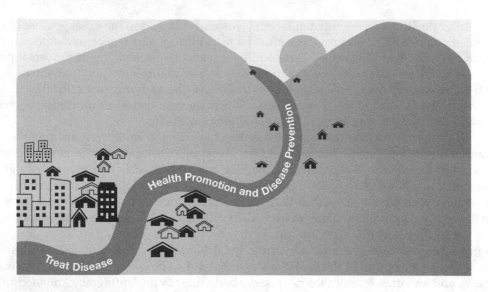

Figure 1.4 Approaches to improve health.

Source: Adapted from Castrucci, B., & Auerbach, J. (2019, January 16). Meeting individual social needs falls short of addressing social determinants of health. *Health Affairs Blog.* https://doi.org/10.1377/forefront.20190115.234942.

States with the healthiest people in the United States include Massachusetts and Hawaii, while those with the unhealthiest people include Arkansas and Mississippi—two states that did not extend the Affordable Care Act (Ellison, 2021). Population health is connected to economic security and the sustained stability of families and communities. Hence, it seems more essential than ever to focus on building a public health infrastructure that involves local, state, and federal planning and program implementation and evaluation that has prevention as the centerpiece. This would benefit from a federal commitment to the creation of a well-coordinated and accountable infrastructure that serves as the foundation for a strong economy, healthy communities, and enhanced well-being for all the nation's people (Maani & Galea, 2020).

Upstream and Downstream Approaches in Population Health

We can use the metaphor of "a river is one way" to conceptualize approaches to improving health outcomes that are cost-effective, timely, and of high quality (Figure 1.4). It is at the intersection of the upstream and downstream places where the social determinants of health are differentiated and manifested. Equity in health for all people is the goal (see Chapter 5 for more discussion about equity).

The upstream approach in healthcare (health promotion and disease prevention) suggests that optimal outcomes can be achieved when antecedents to problems or risk factors are proactively addressed upon the first emergence of a health concern. Through the upstream approach, individuals will have the greatest chance of living a risk-reduced, healthy life. They will be enabled to manage the disease and potential disability promptly, which will be more likely to occur during the later stages of life. The upstream approach helps to avoid the more deleterious consequences of illness, disease, and disability, which are downstream (treatment of disease symptoms) where the more severe levels of poor health are evident (Emanuel, 2020; Shultz et al., 2021; Wakefield et al., 2021).

On the other hand, the downstream approach suggests that the focus will be on treating illnesses and conditions that could have been prevented. The results are increased healthcare needs and higher morbidity and mortality rates among individuals. The downstream prototype also suggests that medical care, as traditionally practiced, has a limited impact on the socially based health disparities as described in the upstream methodology (Castrucci & Auerbach, 2019; Lantz, 2019; Mager & Conelius, 2021; Shultz et al., 2021; Wakefield et al., 2021).

The upstream variables have a direct impact on the health and well-being of individuals and communities across the life course. Laws and policies that improve health in all aspects of daily life at the community level are essential. Midstream, the intersectionality between the social determinants of health and the upstream/downstream prototype is related to variables such as education, income, childhood experiences, housing, nutrition, access to primary care, and safe environments (Okafor et al., 2018). When more attention is given to the social determinants of health, beneficial innovations will emerge midstream at the intersection between the upstream and downstream spaces and places. Specifically, interventions such as assessing for adequate housing, food insecurity, and safety in families and communities could generate data about the individual and the community that would help improve upstream and downstream innovations in healthcare (Gary et al., 2021; Lantz, 2019; Mager & Conelius, 2021; Wakefield et al., 2021).

Vulnerable populations in the United States include young children, older adults, and individuals with chronic illnesses including physical and mental health conditions. Among these populations, neglected oral health can often be an overlooked area that can have deleterious health consequences. These maladies are usually complicated, varied, costly, and evident in urban and rural communities, and they require follow-up over time. To improve healthcare outcomes, a triple approach is necessary: reducing costs, improving the quality of health care, and improving population health (Lantz, 2019).

THE INFLUENCE OF THE SOCIAL DETERMINANTS OF HEALTH ON LONGEVITY

During the 20th century, the United States witnessed phenomenal improvements in health outcomes, with life expectancy increasing by more than 30 years among people in high-income countries like the United States. Of significance was the prevention of infant and early life mortality and morbidity. In the future, gains in life expectancy will probably be less dramatic. The social determinants of health are one of the driving forces that help to account for improved health in the United States. Economic growth, enhanced education, control of infectious diseases (e.g., vaccines, antimicrobials), availability of clean water, and proper disposal of solid waste are primary reasons for these gains (Castrucci & Auerbach, 2019; Kaholokula, 2020; Shultz et al., 2021).

Disease Prevention

In addition to discovering the cures for diseases, health professionals must be encouraged to focus on the prevention of diseases. Discussion of three types of prevention—primary, secondary, and tertiary—should help to illuminate reasonable approaches to improving health across the life course in the United States. These concepts have appeared in the public health science and literature for decades but are seldom adequately implemented (Emanuel, 2020; Maani & Galea, 2020; Okafor et al., 2018; Okafor et al., 2020).

Primary Disease Prevention

At this level, prevention includes plans and actions that forestall, delay, or prevent the development of disease conditions among people/populations. Eliminating a disease is the ideal outcome; smallpox eradication is an example of what can be accomplished through vaccines and health promotion. The intent of primary disease prevention is to engage in planning programs that help to keep people from becoming sick or injured. Such actions are key elements of enhanced population health. Recall that clean water and adequate sanitation are essentials for good health (see Figure 1.2). Across the world community, immunizations and health education/disease prevention have helped to eliminate and reduce diseases and injuries (e.g., administering polio vaccines, promoting safe sex practices, requiring seat belts for youths and adults and special seats for infants and children, promoting oral healthcare; Lueddeke, 2016; Marmot, 2017; Satcher, 2020; Shultz et al., 2021).

Secondary Disease Prevention

This level of intervention centers on early detection and prompt intervention of a disease condition. It also includes diagnosing and treating diseases before a cluster of signs and symptoms are fully evident, which should help to forestall serious illness, decrease the possibility of residual effects, and maximize the possibility of restoring the individual's health status. Timely and effective secondary prevention greatly increases the chances of the person being able to continue functioning productively. Morbidity and mortality rates should be substantially reduced. Screenings for conditions such as hypertension, depression, and cervical cancer combined with rapid administration of interventions as needed are examples of secondary prevention (Basu et al., 2018). Adequate follow-up and lifestyle changes are often required (Basu et al., 2018; Satcher, 2020; Shultz et al., 2021).

Tertiary Disease Prevention

Once the individual has been diagnosed and treated for a disease condition, a focus on tertiary prevention will help to diminish the effect of the injury or illness. Factors that will determine the outcome at this level include the person's genetic makeup, physiological state, lifestyle risk factors, environmental challenges, support systems, and attitudes and behaviors about the illness. The intent at this level is to improve and maintain the person's capacity to function in a family, be employed, and be an active community member. Attainment of the highest possible level of functioning is the goal.

Tertiary care is a major component of all health systems. Organizations that focus on continuity of care for individuals with mental health conditions or substance abuse problems and assisting children and adults with asthma management are examples of tertiary care. Collectively, these three levels of healthcare—primary, secondary, and tertiary—are essential components in any society or health system (Bull et al., 2020; Emanuel, 2020; Marmot, 2017; Satcher, 2020; Shultz et al., 2021; Wakefield et al., 2021).

Wicked Problems

Wicked problems (e.g., healthcare, mental health, substance abuse, climate change, terrorism, education) are complex and have presented challenges to global and local societies for years (Gary et al., 2021). Wicked problems are those that do not have easily identifiable shapes or solutions, are multilayered, and could generate varied solutions, which are difficult or impossible to predict. For example, the component parts of healthcare include elements of law, policy, politics, economics, workforce, culture, geographical location, architectural features, and a plethora of other phenomena. Solving one problem tends to create others. Oftentimes there is one chance to get the solution to a problem right, which seldom happens. These problems are often clouded by limited and contradictory knowledge and science; numerous people or stakeholders may be involved; economics and costs are sure to be a major concern, as are numerous connections that complicate the very nature of the problem. The health status of an individual or a community is linked to access to healthcare, health beliefs and practices, education, economics, transportation, workforce quality, and other factors. The conceptualization of a wicked problem will help to illuminate its complexities (Box 1.3; Baker, 2019; Keijser et al., 2020; Lee, 2018; Rittel & Webber, 1973).

BOX 1.3: Wicked Problems

- Do not have a defined interpretation.
- Have no stopping point.
- Are good or bad (not true or false).
- Are without a test to the problem.
- Are a one-time operation because every attempt has a significant outcome.
- Do not have numerable potential solutions.
- Are unique.
- Each wicked problem is linked to some other indicator of another one.
- Explanations of the inconsistency in explaining the wicked problem are articulated in several ways and the selected narrative is what defines the solution for the problem.
- The person who initiates the action does not have the right to be wrong.

Source: Adapted from Rittel, H. W. J., & Webber, M. M. (1973). Dilemmas in a general theory of planning. *Policy Science, 4*, 155–169. https://doi.org/10.1007/BF01405730

Wicked problems are regarded as unfixable because of the scope and depth of the issues—inequity, disease, mental disorders, substance abuse, high mortality among groups, and famine are examples of global and local wicked problems. A key role of planners and healthcare providers is to work toward mitigating the deleterious impact of wicked problems and to find new solutions that have more advantageous outcomes. Interdisciplinary approaches help to conceptualize and guide planning and actions. Law, medicine, nursing, social work, economics, engineering, pharmacy, statistics, and rigorous scientific methodologies along with tenacity and robustness are essential to grapple with wicked problems (Baker, 2019; Keijser et al., 2020; Lee, 2018; Rittel & Webber, 1973).

SUMMARY

The significant impact of public health on human well-being has been demonstrated in various forms since humans began to commune and live with each other. As an essential societal element, it has undergone an astonishing transformation over the centuries with far-reaching local and global ramifications. The phenomena of health can be conceptualized from several levels as depicted in the social-ecological model that starts with the individual and ends with society—which can be local and global. The five waves of public health began in the early 1800s and continue to this moment: Clean water, the sanitary disposal of solid waste, and the introduction of the germ theory were and continue to be significant components of overall health across the world community (see Figure 1.2). One concrete example of the connectedness of the global community is the role that WHO, a part of the United Nations, has in advancing health, improving practice, and promoting science—as demonstrated through *The International Statistical Classification of Diseases and Related Health Problems*.

Not all nations have adequate health systems. High-income countries such as the United States, England, Australia, South Korea, Taiwan, and others do not necessarily have the best systems. Worldwide, health systems have their attributes and deficits, with outstanding features on some metrics but not others. The United States, the wealthiest country on the planet, does not have a system that provides essential and universal care for its citizens. Nevertheless, it is noted for outstanding innovations and discoveries in health science.

Thinking from a population health model might help to improve the U.S. healthcare system and assist with eliminating health disparities. This approach suggests that even though individual health care is essential, it is also necessary to examine and transform societal systems as depicted in the social-ecological model which highlights the intersectionality of various domains.

As healthcare evolves, more emphasis is being given to health promotion and prevention—an upstream approach. Traditional medical practices that include tertiary care are downstream, and often hospital based. When moving toward the midstream—the intersectionality of the upstream and downstream sections of the streams—the social determinants of health must be carefully addressed. The complexities associated with health and healthcare are further elucidated using the concept of wicked problems, which has been in the scientific literature for decades. It may be used to develop a blueprint that could help all health professionals and citizen scientists re-engineer our overall approach to health and health care delivery in local and global communities.

DISCUSSION QUESTIONS

1. After completing your research, determine which country in the global community has the best healthcare system for health promotion and disease prevention in a primary care setting.
   a. Briefly describe the history of the healthcare system for the country that you have identified.
   b. Based on your research, what lessons can be learned to help the United States improve its care in one or two domains, such as maternal health, childcare, mental health, or substance abuse conditions?
2. How would you describe the healthcare system in the United States?
   a. Identify at least five attributes of the system that support your decision. Document your response.
   b. Describe two shortcomings in the U.S. healthcare system that, if addressed, could improve health outcomes and eliminate health disparities.
3. What similarities and the differences do you notice in the social context of health in the global community compared to that of the United States?
   a. How do public health infrastructure and cost influence healthcare in each context?
4. Numerous theoretical models can depict various components of healthcare in the United States. What two are the most useful for you in your clinical practice, policy development and implementation, intradisciplinary education, and research?
   a. What are the deficits in the models when applied to the population(s) of your interest (e.g., children or individuals with a chronic illness)?
5. How does the concept of health equity relate to population health in a diverse society such as the United States, where there is no universal healthcare for its citizens?
6. Describe advances in public health in the United States and identify the wave that you think has had the most significant impact on health and well-being for the most people.
7. What impact does WHO have on your conceptual thinking about health and healthcare and overall well-being in the world community and the United States?
   a. How are health-related organizations such as the American Medical Association and the American Nurses Association associated with WHO?
8. What are your thoughts about population health thinking, and how could this paradigm influence your work as a health professional? Be specific. Outline your ideas and share them with a colleague.
9. What is your definition of a wicked problem?
   a. Which two wicked problems are you most interested in, and what approaches would you use to address the concerns?
   b. Are there any lessons learned from thinking through the characteristics of a wicked problem?

10. Is your professional work (e.g., as a researcher, clinician, policymaker, or educator) in the upstream, midstream, or downstream domain?
    a. What difference does this make?
    b. Is there a need to rethink your place and space in the metaphor and your professional work?
    c. Design an initiative that focuses on upstream and midstream healthcare interventions, strategies, and practices that prevent a premature cascade of individuals and communities into the downstream, where they are more likely to experience high morbidity and mortality.

ADDITIONAL RESOURCES

This section provides additional resources pertinent for gazing into the future and developing and evaluating new and novel approaches to healthcare for all people.

This site provides a treasure trove of statistics and informative graphics that illustrate the realities of healthcare in the United States as compared to the top-ranking nations in healthcare:

Schneider, E. C., Doty, M. M., Fields, K., & Williams, R. D. -II. (2021, August 4). Mirror, mirror 2021—Reflecting poorly: Health care in the U.S. compared to other high-income countries. Commonwealth Fund. https://doi.org/10.26099/01dv-h208

For more information about the organizational structure of the DHHS, see:

Digital Communications Division. (2021). DHHS Organizational Chart. www.hhs.gov/about/agencies/orgchart/index.html

This site provides an excellent graphic explanation of the interconnectedness of the social determinants and social needs (see Exhibit 1):

Castrucci, B., & Auerbach, J. (2019, January 16). Meeting individual social needs falls short of addressing social determinants of health. Health Affairs Blog. https://shelterforce.org/wp-content/uploads/2019/04/Exhibit_1.png

In this article, Marc Harrison has delineates five priorities that provide a blueprint that could enhance and overhaul the healthcare system:

Harrison, M. (2021, December 15). 5 critical priorities for the U.S. health care system. Harvard Business Review. https://hbr.org/2021/12/5-critical-priorities-for-the-u-s-health-care-system

Boston University School of Public Health collaborated with Sharecare, a digital health company, to rank the status of health risk in the United States through an evaluation of nearly half a million surveys. Massachusetts ranked highest in health quality and Mississippi continued to hold down the lowest rank. You can find the ranking of your state here:

Ellison, A. (2021, September 2). 50 states ranked from healthiest to unhealthiest. Becker's Hospital Review. www.beckershospitalreview.com/rankings-and-ratings/50-states-ranked-from-healthiest-to-unhealthiest-090221.html

The following is a concise and informative explanation of the wicked problem:

Houghton, L. J. (2013, August 11). What is a wicked problem? YouTube. www.youtube.com/watch?v=KmzcmeXTDb8

This interview features Ezekiel Emanuel, bioethicist, and author of the book, *Which Country Has the World's Best Health Care?* He offers suggestions on how the best practices could be gleaned from 10 countries to create a vastly more effective healthcare system in the United States:

Aspen Institute. (2020, June 30). Which country has the world's best health care? A conversation with Zeke Emanuel. YouTube. www.youtube.com/watch?v=5sttFejWXhA

The CBS program *60 Minutes* featured an interview with Catherine Coleman, an activist who is fighting for sanitary sewage disposal in present-day Alabama. This is a short but poignant clip from that interview:

Teklu, A. W. (2021, December 20). 60 Minutes investigates: Americans fighting for access to sewage disposal. YouTube. www.youtube.com/watch?v=jW5u1oGyi5U

REFERENCES

Baker, S. R. (2019). No simple solutions, no single ingredient: Systems-orientated approaches for addressing wicked problems in population oral health. *Community Dental Health*, 36(1), 3–4. https://doi.org/10.1922/CDH_BakerMarch19editorial02

Basu, P., Mittal, S., Bhadra Vale, D., & Chami Kharaji, Y. (2018). Secondary prevention of cervical cancer. *Best Practice & Research Clinical Obstetrics & Gynaecology*, 47, 73–85. https://doi.org/10.1016/j.bpobgyn.2017.08.012

Brand, M., Rumpf, H.-J., Demetrovics, Z., MÜller, A., Stark, R., King, D. L., Goudriaan, A. E., Mann, K., Trotzke, P., Fineberg, N. A., Chamberlain, S. R., Kraus, S. W., Wegmann, E., Billieaux, J., & Potenza, M. N. (2020, June). Which conditions should be considered as disorders in the International Classification of Diseases (ICD-11) designation of "other specified disorders due to addictive behaviors"? *Journal of Behavioral Addictions*. https://doi.org/10.1556/2006.2020.00035

Bull, F. C., Al-Ansari, S. S., Biddle, S., Borodulin, K., Buman, M. P., Cardon, G., Carty, C., Chaput, J.-P., Chastin, S., Chou, R., Dempsey, P. C., Dipietro, L, Ekelund, U., Firth, J., Friedenreich, C. M., Garcia, L., Gichu, M., Jago, R., Katzmarzyk, P. T.,…Willumsen, J. F. (2020). World Health Organization 2020 guidelines on physical activity and sedentary behaviour. *British Journal of Sports Medicine*, 54(24), 1451–1462. https://doi.org/10.1136/bjsports-2020-102955

Castrucci, B., & Auerbach, J. (2019, January 16). Meeting individual social needs falls short of addressing social determinants of health. *Health Affairs Blog*. https://doi.org/10.1377/forefront.20190115.234942

Centers for Disease Control and Prevention. (2021). The social-ecological model: A framework for violence prevention. https://www.cdc.gov/violenceprevention/about/social-ecologicalmodel.html

Degenhardt, L., Stockings, E., Patton, G., Hall, W. D., & Lynskey, M. (2016). The increasing global health priority of substance use in young people. *Lancet Psychiatry*, 3(3), 251–264. https://doi.org/10.1016/s2215-0366(15)00508-8

Ellison, A. (2021, September 2). 50 states ranked from healthiest to unhealthiest. Becker's Hospital Review. https://www.beckershospitalreview.com/rankings-and-ratings/50-states-ranked-from-healthiest-to-unhealthiest-090221.html

Emanuel, E. J. (2020). Which country has the world's best health care? A conversation with Zeke Emanuel. YouTube. https://www.youtube.com/watch?v=5sttFejWXhA

Evans, A. C., & Bufka, L. F. (2020). The critical need for a population health approach: Addressing the nation's behavioral health during the COVID-19 pandemic and beyond. *Preventing Chronic Disease*, 17, E79. http://dx.doi.org/10.5888/pcd17.200261

Gary, F. A., Yarandi, H., Hopps, J. C., Hassan M., Sloand, E. D., & Campbell, J. C. (2021). Tragedy in Haiti: Suicidality, PTSD, and depression associated with intimate partner violence among Haitian women after the 2010 earthquake. *Journal of the National Black Nurses Association*, 32(1), 10–17.

Henneberger, A. K., Mushonga, D. R., & Preston, A. M. (2021). Peer influence and adolescent substance use: A systematic review of dynamic social network research. *Adolescent Research Review*, 6(1), 57–73. https://doi.org/10.1007/s40894-019-00130-0

Kaholokula, J. K. (2020). COVID-19, the disease that has shined a light on health equity. In Goodyear-Ka'ōpua, N., Howes, C., Kamakawiwo'ole Osorio, J. K., & Yamashiro, A. (Eds.), *The value of Hawai'i 3: Hulihia, the turning* (pp. 30–33). University of Hawaii Press. https://scholarspace.manoa.hawaii.edu/bitstream/10125/70171/9780824889159.pdf

Keijser, W., Huq, J.-L., & Reay, T. (2020). Enacting medical leadership to address wicked problems. *BMJ*, 4(1). http://dx.doi.org/10.1136/leader-2019-000137

Lantz, P. M. (2019). The medicalization of population health: Who will stay upstream? *Milbank Quarterly*, 97(1), 36–39. https://doi.org/10.1111/1468-0009.12363

Lee, J. C. (2018). The opioid crisis is a wicked problem. *American Journal on Addictions*, 27(1), 51. https://doi.org/10.1111/ajad.12662

Lueddeke, G. (2016). *Global population health and well-being in the 21st century: Toward new paradigms, policy, and practice*. Springer.

Maani, N., & Galea, S. (2020). COVID-19 and underinvestment in the public health infrastructure of the United States. *Milbank Quarterly*, 98(2), 250–259. https://doi.org/10.1111/1468-0009.12463

Mager, D. R., & Conelius, J. (2021). *Population health for nurses: Improving community outcomes*. Springer.

Marmot, M. (2017). The health gap: The challenge of an unequal world: The argument. *International Journal of Epidemiology*, 46(4), 1312–1318. https://doi.org/10.1093/ije/dyx163

Okafor, M. (2019). Population health. In J. S. Coviello (Ed.), *Health promotion and disease prevention in clinical practice* (3rd ed.). Wolters Kluwer.

Okafor, M., Chiu, S., & Feinn, R. (2020). Quantitative and qualitative results from implementation of a two-item food insecurity screening tool in healthcare settings in Connecticut. *Preventive Medicine Reports, 20*, 101191. https://doi.org/10.1016/j.pmedr.2020.101191

Okafor, M., Ede, V., Kinuthia, R., & Satcher, D. (2018). Explication of a behavioral health-primary care integration learning collaborative and its quality improvement implications. *Community Mental Health Journal, 54*(8), 1109–1115. https://doi.org/10.1007/s10597-017-0230-8

Okafor, M., Sarpong, D., Ferguson, A., & Satcher, D. (2014). Improving health outcomes of children through effective parenting: Model and methods. *International Journal of Environmental Research and Public Health, 11*(1), 296–311. https://doi.org/10.3390/ijerph110100296

Purnell, L. D., & Fenkl, E. A. (2019). *Handbook for culturally competent care: Transcultural diversity and health care.* Springer. https://doi.org/10.1007/978-3-030-21946-8_1

Rittel, H. W. J., & Webber, M. M. (1973). Dilemmas in a general theory of planning. *Policy Sciences, 4,* 155–169. https://doi.org/10.1007/BF01405730

Satcher, D. (2020). *My quest for health equity: Notes on learning while leading (Health equity in America).* Johns Hopkins University Press.

Schneider, E. C., Doty, M. M., Fields, K., & Williams, R. D.-II. (2021, August 4). *Mirror, mirror 2021—reflecting poorly: Health care in the U.S. compared to other high-income countries.* Commonwealth Fund. https://doi.org/10.26099/01dv-h208

Shultz, J. M., Sullivan, L. M., & Galea, S. (2021). *Public health: An introduction to the science and practice of population health.* Springer.

Wakefield, M. K., Williams, D. R., Le Menestrel, S., & Flaubert, J. L. (2021). *The future of nursing 2020–2030: Charting a path to achieve health equity.* National Academies of Sciences. https://doi.org/10.17226/25982

World Bank. (2022). Data: World bank country and lending groups. https://datahelpdesk.worldbank.org/knowledgebase/articles/906519-world-bank-country-and-lending-groups

World Health Organization. (2021). Health Equity Assessment Toolkit (HEAT): Software for exploring and comparing health inequalities in countries. Built-in database edition. Version 4.0. Geneva. https://whoequity.shinyapps.io/heat/

World Health Organization. (2021, April 1). Primary health care. https://www.who.int/news-room/fact-sheets/detail/primary-health-care

Xu, T. (2015). Chinese anti-cancer association as a non-governmental organization undertakes systematic cancer prevention work in China. *Chinese Journal of Cancer Research, 27*(4), 423–427. https://doi.org/10.3978/j.issn.1000-9604.2015.08.01

CHAPTER 2

Definition and History of Population Health

Kathy D. Wright, Angela D. Alston, and Liz Piatt

LEARNING OBJECTIVES

- Examine the theoretical framework and conceptualization of population health.
- Explain the differences among the four definitions of population health.
- Describe public health and its importance in promotion of population health.
- Analyze the elements of the Triple Aim model for population health.
- Identify the significance of the Future of Nursing 2020 to 2030 report to promote health equity.
- Discuss the Healthy People initiative and imminent public health challenges.

INTRODUCTION

Population health begins with an examination of the differences in health outcomes within and between groups of people, and integrates consideration of the social, economic, environmental, and healthcare system factors that contribute to those differences. Government policy that adopts this perspective has the potential to significantly reduce health disparities.

Kindig (2007) asks if population health is a theoretical framework, a concept, or just another way of talking about doing public health. Researchers, public health practitioners, and healthcare professionals concerned with improving the health of populations have debated this question. In this chapter, we discuss all of these possibilities, with an eye toward laying a foundation for the ways in which population health approaches might improve the work of healthcare professionals, especially nurses.

In the first section, we chronicle the development of population heath, outlining the ways that approaching the health of populations have shifted over time, moving from a focus on the health of individuals to community, public, and now population health. While we tend to think of population health as a relatively new phenomenon, it has roots in public health efforts in 18th century Europe to address socioeconomic disparities in health outcomes. Next, we compare and contrast the various definitions of population health and how those definitions have been used in public health, nursing, and healthcare more generally through an examination of Healthy People, the Triple Aim, and the Future of Nursing report.

THEORETICAL FRAMEWORK OF POPULATION HEALTH AND GLOBAL PERSPECTIVE

Population health involves tracking the health of populations and determining what broader policies can disrupt or support the connection between social determinants (economic and social conditions that influence health) and health outcomes for that population. While population health as a discipline is relatively new, population health *thinking* has been an important part of public health from the earliest public health efforts in the late 18th century, as these efforts were born out of observations of the relationship between socioeconomic class, neighborhood environment, economic stability, and health outcomes in a population. In this section, we outline the growth of population health from a way of thinking about how to do public health to a field of inquiry separate from public health.

Many public health historians point to John Snow's epidemiological investigation into cholera outbreaks as one of several events in the mid-19th century that mark the birth of the public health movement in Europe (Ramsay, 2009). Dr. Snow's investigation was a true public health intervention in the sense that he traced the outbreak to a likely source—the handle of a water pump—and removed that source to prevent disease in a population. Other historians, such as Szreter (2003), point to earlier events, such as efforts to address low life expectancy among British citizens living in poverty in the late 18th century and the development of the first accurate life table in 1815. Public health interventions in the 19th century generally lacked a population health focus and were aimed primarily at disease prevention. These include U.S. efforts, such as when nurses worked alongside social workers in New York City's Black and immigrant communities to increase access to care and improve social conditions that were contributing to diseases like tuberculosis, thereby mitigating the spread.

Questions about social determinants of health gained attention again after pioneering British social scientist Richard Morris Titmuss published a series of research papers from 1942 to 1944 that drew attention to the relationships between disease and social conditions such as unemployment. The resulting interest among government officials was funneled into William Beveridge's *Social Insurance and Allied Services* plan. The plan emphasized an access-to-healthcare movement, because quality medical care was viewed to mitigate the effects of inequality on health (Abel-Smith, 1992). This movement led to the establishment of the British National Health Service in 1948, which helped inform the study of population health in the United States (Gorsky, 2015). Government officials' attention generally focused on improving individual risk factors for disease through access to healthcare. The U.S. healthcare system for the delivery of population health focuses on an out-of-pocket model in that there are separate systems for different classes of people (Physicians for a National Health Program, 2021).

Attention again focused on social determinants of health in the United States and Britain in the 1980s. Britain's Department of Health and Social Security produced the Black Report (after chairman Sir Douglas Black, president of the Royal College of Physicians), in 1980, which illustrated that socioeconomic status, housing, and work conditions all had an effect on health outcomes (Gray, 1982). Sir Michael Marmot's first Whitehall Study followed in 1984, showing a strong and persistent association between social class and health despite British citizens having access to universal care (Marmot et al., 1985). The study found that smoking was more common among the working class, especially men, as was coronary heart disease. On the other hand, the 1985 Heckler Report identified race as a social determinant of health in the United States. It documented persistent health disparities experienced by Black Americans and led to the establishment of the U.S. Health and Human

Services Office of Minority Health. Sociologists also contributed to this work through an examination of social inequality as a fundamental cause of health disparities (Link & Phelan, 1995), demonstrating that social class, race, and gender inequities were persistently linked to health outcomes. However, public health and medical professionals and health policy experts were slow to integrate these findings into their work and instead continued to focus on prevention of disease through the improvement of individual risk factors and the treatment of existing disease in acute care in hospitals and clinics. In the United States, for example, public health programs focused on tobacco cessation, getting kids more active in school, and flu vaccination (Institute of Medicine, 1988). Kindig and Magnan (2019) and Valles (2019) date the revival of population health as a field of inquiry in the United States that continues to this day to the publication in 1994 of the edited volume *Why Are Some People Healthy and Others Not? The Determinants of Health Populations* (Evans et al., 1994). Discussing the findings of a 5-year study by the Population Health Program of the Canadian Institute for Advanced Research, Valles (2019) cites themes at recent North American Public Health Association conferences and changes in accreditation standards for public health programs as evidence that population health has become central to public health professionals' work.

THE EVOLVING MEANING OF POPULATION HEALTH

There are many recognized definitions of population health. These definitions have emerged over time and are frequently intertwined within definitions of public health (Figure 2.1). Population health and its initiatives are often closely associated with public health interventions.

Public health can be described as the science of preventing disease that considers physical health and psychological and social well-being (Winslow, 1920). The Centers for Disease Control and Prevention (CDC) describes public health as "the science and art of preventing disease, prolonging life, and promoting health through the organized efforts and informed choices of society, organizations, public and private communities, and individuals" (Winslow, 1920, p. 183). Recent events provide examples of public health and population health: Vaccines are a public health solution; reducing vaccine hesitancy is a population health solution. Both population health and public health are interprofessional disciplines that encompass health of the environment and communities, behavioral and mental health,

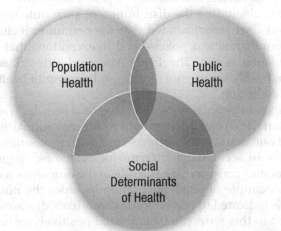

Figure 2.1 This Venn diagram depicts how the definition of population health intersects with the social determinants of health and public health.

TABLE 2.1 Definitions of Population Health

Author, Year	Definition
Kindig and Stoddart, 2003	The health outcomes of a group of individuals, including the distribution of such outcomes within the group.
Stoto, 2013	A holistic focus considerate of a broader array of determinants of health than is typical in healthcare or public health, emphasizing health promotion, disease prevention, and upstream factors other than outcomes alone; there is a shared sense of responsibility for outcomes with diffuse accountability.
Roux, 2016	The consideration of factors (social and biological) that help organizations understand and improve health, with an explicit concern with health equity.
Sharfstein, 2014	Utilization of public health competencies, collaboration with agencies responsible for geographic population, investing in creative and innovative approaches to improve outcomes and participating in activities to address underlying causes of disease.

and public policy. The administration of public health goes well beyond epidemiology in scope. For example, nurses, social service professionals, and health policy makers work alongside epidemiologists and biostatisticians to develop and deliver public health interventions. Population health models are also interprofessional but provide a broad yet narrowed approach to specifically target interventions to improve health outcomes of groups. For example, unsuitable housing conditions that are poorly ventilated or are infested with rodents and other pests are known to impact asthma (Krieger, 2010). A population health strategy would be to broadly address housing as a social determinant of health and to narrowly address health disparities related to asthma prevalence, severity, and, ultimately, long-term outcomes. The COVID-19 pandemic has provided insight into the impact of vaccination and how it can influence work-life conditions. As more of the population becomes vaccinated against COVID-19, safer work environments are created, which is population health. Efforts to educate the public about the purpose and impact of COVID-19 vaccination is a public health initiative.

Table 2.1 provides a range of definitions of population health. Many subsequent definitions have referenced Kindig and Stoddart's (2003) definition: "The health outcomes of a group of individuals, including the distribution of such outcomes within the group" (p. 380). Kindig and Stoddart recommended that the definition include health outcomes, patterns of health determinants, and policies and interventions that link these two areas when examining population health. The Triple Aim model described in the following— focusing on population health, experience of care, and per capita healthcare costs—reflects Kindig and Stoddart's definition.

Stoto's (2013) definition of population health provides a broader framework. Concurring with Kindig and Stoddart (2003) that interventions to address population health must reflect considerations beyond outcomes, Stoto emphasizes health promotion and disease prevention. Stoto also includes an accountability factor for outcomes, suggesting that everyone (government, providers, and consumers) has a role in the outcomes we see with evaluating population health. An example of Stoto's definition includes the human papilloma virus (HPV) vaccine, which is indicated to protect individuals from diseases caused by HPV. The health outcomes related to this virus can be impacted positively or negatively by vaccination status and include cancers of the cervix, vagina, throat, and mouth.

Roux (2016) considers social and biological factors that are necessary for organizations to understand to truly improve health, with a focus on health equity as vital to the definition of population health. As Roux argues, some individuals or groups of people require

2. DEFINITION AND HISTORY OF POPULATION HEALTH

additional resources to have equitable opportunities, and population health depends on understanding the distinction between equality and equity. For example, heat waves are one of the leading weather-related causes of death in the United States (U.S. Environmental Protection Agency [EPA], 2017). Climate change has caused an increase in the occurrence of heat waves that primarily affects lower-income people because they are more likely to live in places where heat waves are increasing or to lack reliable amelioration measures such as central air conditioning and green spaces. New York City's Climate Risk Information Vulnerability Assessment, which is designed to provide comfort and aid to populations who are more vulnerable to extreme weather—chronically ill individuals and those living in poverty—emphasizes the social-biological approach to population health (EPA, 2017). A guide was created that provides best practice recommendations to meteorologists, health officials, and emergency managers on how to implement strategies shown to save lives during excessive heat events. New York City is taking a proactive approach to assessing climate changes by identifying vulnerable populations and how they may be affected by excessive heat to address the health needs of the community. Tactics used to provide comfort and aid in the event of a heat wave include providing weather forecast conditions 1 to 5 days in advance, extending hours at community centers with air conditioning, and suspending utility shutoffs. These strategies are equitable and designed to improve health outcomes for even the most vulnerable populations for conditions that can be forecasted and for which interventions exist.

Like Stoto and Roux, Sharfstein (2014) defines population health as requiring a comprehensive approach that includes collaborating with agencies that have accountability for populations. The emphasis on creative and innovative approaches highlights the need for resource allocation necessary to help drive change, improve outcomes, and address underlying causes of disease and medical conditions. Population health, in Sharfstein's view, is not just the focus on outcomes, or the consideration of factors that may impact health, but the longitudinal approach of using evidence-based interventions and collaborating and investing in strategies, while actively engaging in addressing the causes of disease. While Sharfstein's emphasis on disease prevention may be narrower than other definitions, it provides helpful insight into the importance of health promotion interventions.

The list of social determinants of health published by the World Health Organization (WHO) gives meaning to Sharfstein's definition of population health because a comprehensive approach to understanding factors that impact health is necessary. One factor may have more influence than another, but collectively these social determinants of health give perspective to the complexity of outcomes and how collaborative entities are needed to understand and impact the health of populations, from a longitudinal assessment. These social determinants of health include:

- income and social protection;
- education, unemployment, and job security;
- working life conditions;
- food insecurity;
- housing;
- basic amenities and environment;
- early childhood development;
- social inclusion and nondiscrimination;
- structural conflict; and
- access to affordable health services of decent quality (WHO, 2021).

Silberber et al. (2019) highlighted that social and environmental conditions that influence the health of populations must be considered when defining population health. Examining the Healthy People 2030 framework against Sharfstein's (2014) notion of defining success or failure by not only those served [by a society] but also those left behind suggests the need for a complete view of population health for meaningful intervention and change

(Silberberg et al., 2019; Swarthout & Bishop, 2017). This is the promotion of health equity, which is designed to reduce and eliminate health disparities through a systems approach (Marmot et al., 2008; Matthew, 2018). Meaningful societal change will not occur until we target population health efforts to understand, promote, and ultimately achieve health equity.

APPLICATIONS OF POPULATION HEALTH IN HEALTH AND NURSING PRACTICE

To understand factors that influence population health, all health professionals, including nurses, must consider conditions that influence the daily life and social norms of patients, such as the social determinants of health. Employing a population health approach to clinical practice can be challenging when considering the multidimensional level of complexity that may disproportionally affect certain groups. Consider, for example, the challenges faced by a homeless teenager, a transgender woman, or a male veteran with undiagnosed posttraumatic stress disorder seeking civilian employment. Population health goals and interventions must be compatible with societal or organizational goals and objectives, which may include embedded policies and procedures that need to be initially addressed or considered. Likewise, application must recognize that populations are not unidimensional. Consider the missed opportunities if only race and ethnicity, for example, are considered without also evaluating neighborhood poverty rates or insurance status in embracing a population health approach to communities (Silberberg et al., 2019).

The American Association of Colleges of Nursing (AACN, 2021), in its *Essentials* Domain 3: Population Health, states that "population health spans the healthcare delivery continuum from public health prevention to disease management of populations and describes collaborative activities with both traditional and nontraditional partnerships from affected communities, public health, industry, academia, healthcare, local government entities, and others for the improvement of equitable population health outcomes." The AACN 2013 *Essentials for Core Competencies for Nursing Practice* outlined that undergraduate courses should include aspects of population health through pandemic preparedness, community service experiences, or implementation of evidence-based disease models of care for at-risk groups. Nursing schools have complied and across the nation continue to explore opportunities for nursing students and faculty to engage with communities to best support the unique needs of underrepresented or marginalized groups, including individuals and families in homeless shelters, community refugee agencies, and correctional health settings. Students may even travel abroad to increase cultural awareness for populations that may be represented in the United States but who use or access healthcare very differently in their respective countries or communities. Models of interprofessional care are increasingly cited in the literature, illustrating enhanced learning and better understanding of the role of other health professionals when nursing students are paired with other disciplines, such as medicine, pharmacy, or social work, as part of the clinical experience (Samuriwo et al., 2020). These collaborative learning experiences provide a fundamental foundation for helping different professions understand their role, as part of a team, for affecting population health outcomes in the community served. This concept is not new. In fact, the AACN and the CDC entered the Academic Partnerships to Improve Health cooperative agreement in 2015 to improve healthcare outcomes for individuals and communities. This partnership provides opportunities to strengthen population health education for health science students, including those in nursing, public health, and medicine. It led to the creation of a learning hub hosted by the AACN for nursing students titled "Public/Population Health," which highlights the parallel objectives in public and population health and how these terms are often used interchangeably. Such learning hubs are designed to provide learning opportunities for graduate and undergraduate nursing students related to public/population health.

Students are given opportunities to work with community organizations to address the needs of healthcare communities.

The Triple Aim and the Quadruple Aim

As a response to the increased cost of providing healthcare in the United States, the Institute for Healthcare Improvement (IHI), a global agency, designed the Triple Aim initiative in 2007 to help optimize population health and healthcare systems. This model was also adopted by the Centers for Medicare & Medicaid Services (CMS) and requires an interprofessional team for implementation and evaluation. The Triple Aim model is focused on improving the health of populations, improving the individual experience of care, and reducing the per capita costs of care for populations (Berwick et al., 2008). Objectives include improved patient care and safety, effectiveness in delivery of healthcare, patient-centeredness, timeliness, efficiency, better equity in outcomes, and lower costs. A 2018 article in *U.S. News and World Report* titled "Population Health: The 'North Star' of the Triple Aim" revealed how the foundation laid by the creation of the Triple Aim still has opportunities for growth (Galvin, 2018).

Improving Health of Populations

To apply the Triple Aim model, there is first a need to define the target population and examine data concerning its health (Stiefel & Nolan, 2012). For example, data from the Healthy People 2020 report describe glycemic control by minority populations from 2013 to 2016 (Office of Disease Prevention and Health Promotion, 2021); the rates of poor glycemic control among Hispanic/Latino Americans age 18 years and older with diagnosed diabetes were more than 2.5 times those of non-Hispanic White Americans. By examining such data, the designers of an intervention can better understand disparities that exist among different populations or groups and use these data to specifically target interventions to ameliorate disparities. A "one size fits all" approach to addressing glycemic control in patients, for example, is not appropriate and will not improve the health of populations. Similar data exist when examining race, for example, as a factor for cardiovascular disease risk in patients of Asian descent (Park et al., 2021). Clinicians must understand target populations to appropriately address health outcomes.

For example, applying the Triple Aim model to a community-based diabetes education program would call for adding resources and individual factors to the measurement of the program's success. These resources might include access to healthy foods and a safe environment—factors that typically characterize populations—as well as individual factors, which might include willingness to eat fresh fruits and vegetables, that may be compounded by psychological factors of spirituality and resilience. Improving the health of patients with diabetes requires a comprehensive and integrated approach to understanding the necessity to reduce complications of this devastating disease. It also requires willingness, both to explore the many variables that influence a patient's decision to make healthy life changes and to learn what undertones of bias or judgment a patient may encounter when seeking healthcare services. It is imperative for novice and expert clinicians alike to understand the many variables to be considered in diabetes management and to understand how lack of a comprehensive approach, from the patient's perspective, may continue to lead to rising costs and poorer outcomes for care of this condition.

Improving the Individual Experience

The individual's experience in the healthcare setting is critical to facilitating adherence to treatment, as is support from family and friends. Experience of care received in healthcare settings is often measured with standardized questions from survey tools such as the Consumer Assessment of Healthcare Providers and Health Systems (CAHPS; Agency for Healthcare Research and Quality [AHRQ], 2019). For example, to determine the experience of care for Hispanic/Latino Americans with diabetes, a program would also assess the individual care experience. This would include the aims of the framework from the Institute of Medicine (IOM) to provide safe, effective, timely, efficient, and equitable patient-centered care (AHRQ, 2018). Providing culturally and linguistically appropriate care that does not vary in quality is essential to equitable care of patients. According to AHRQ, few metrics currently examine equity of care, which is a future area of opportunity in examining and improving the patient experience.

Nurses are perfectly poised to lead the measurement of the quality and safety metrics that are the drivers of the experience of care, as measured in the Triple Aim model. Metrics in a hospital might include falls, bedsores, and medication errors. The responsiveness of staff to answering call lights and providing relief from pain are additional patient-centered specific measurements to improve the care experience. In community settings, metrics may include no-show rates, medication compliance, and hospital discharge follow-up visits within a specified period of time.

The Joint Commission (TJC) and the Hospital Standardized Index provide uniform core performance measures that have been used as an accountability metric, and these measures include research (based on evidence-based care), proximity (care performed is related to outcome), accuracy (proper care process), and adverse events (evaluating unintended consequences). Measures are further defined by area of practice, including palliative care, stroke, substance use, and healthcare staffing services. More information on TJC and performance measures can be found www.jointcommission.org/measurement/measures/#592065b7f1d44a5691c528709db19784_bbebaad4025e4900b8f28a00580c26c9. When considering outcomes from a particular hospital, institution, area, or region, these measures can be used to examine the population health strategies needed to improve the health and well-being of individuals and communities.

Reducing the Per Capita Cost of Care for Populations

Reducing cost per capita involves lowering hospitalization and rehospitalization rates and can be done in an interdisciplinary fashion. Healthcare systems providers and management and accounting systems or data informatics can supply information on total expenditures. These may include out-of-pocket costs by the patient, including premiums for private insurance. Indirect costs, such as work absenteeism or patient "no-shows," should also be included in the cost calculation per capita if this information is available. Sometimes, an organization may not have access to that level of data; in these cases, emergency department cost or number of bed days can be a way to examine the cost of care for a population, such as people with diabetes. Lowering the cost of care for patients with diabetes, for example, involves management of the disease but also focusing on possible prevention through lifestyle changes. According to Riddle (2018), the cost of care for U.S. adults with diabetes in 2017 was $237 billion, compared with $116 billion in 2007. In fact, one in four healthcare dollars in the United States are spent on diabetes care. Preventing hospitalizations, increasing access to healthcare providers, and improving housing are population health tactics to reduce per capita cost of care for this population (Riddle, 2018). An interdisciplinary approach is paramount as variables such as transportation, living in food deserts, and financial barriers all play a part in managing this condition and cannot be addressed solely by one discipline.

Quadruple Aim

Improving the health of populations also requires that clinicians are cared for and have the resources to provide quality patient care. For example, nursing burnout is associated with an increased frequency of medication errors and poor patient safety outcomes (Hall et al., 2016). Thus, a fourth aim was added to the Triple Aim to specifically address the care provider (clinician). The Quadruple Aim has all of the same elements as the Triple Aim, but it also includes the clinician's experience—their quality of life (Bodenheimer & Sinsky, 2014). Providers who experience burnout due to being overworked or taxed by administrative demands that inter-fere with the care of patients pose a risk to patient outcomes as well as to providers' own health. A recent study of nurse burnout showed that 31.5% of nurses described burnout as the reason they had left a job within the previous 12 months (Shah et al., 2021). Other reasons given in the study for leaving or considering leaving a job were also related to burnout, such as stressful work environment, inadequate staffing, and lack of good management or leadership.

The COVID-19 pandemic has drawn attention to, and vastly increased rates of, stress and burnout, placing patients at risk of worse mental and physical health outcomes. Organizations can improve clinician experience by implementing team documentation to reduce duplication, standardizing workflows, instituting adequate training to assume new roles, and maintaining adequate staffing ratios (Shah et al., 2021; Bodenheimer & Sinsky, 2014). The stigma associated with mental health disparities creates challenges but can be overcome by societal and organizational acceptance of the normalcy of addressing stress, burnout, or depression, as we would address a broken arm or abdominal pain. As more clinicians become vocal about their experiences and about how organizational support of work-life balance has increased their ability to continue to provide quality health care, we anticipate a positive trend with acceptance of this fourth aim. We must continue to address the needs of providers as we do patients if we are to create a sustainable structure for popu-lation health management. The literature is increasingly evaluating the impact of leadership influence on achieving the Quadruple Aim (Jeffs, 2018; Bowles et al., 2018). It is critical for leaders to acknowledge and support interventions to address the provider experience and encourage providers to speak honestly about their experiences.

Healthy People 2030

The Healthy People initiative began in 1979 as a function of the U.S. Department of Health and Human Services to guide health promotion and disease prevention in the United States (Office of Disease Prevention and Health Promotion [ODPHP], 2021). It provides scientific reports on overall health and well-being measures of the U.S. population every 10 years. The purpose of the report is to (a) increase public awareness and understanding of the deter-minants of health, disease, and disability and the opportunities for progress; (b) provide measurable objectives and goals that are applicable at the national, state, and local levels; (c) engage multiple sectors to take action to strengthen policies and improve practices, driven by the best available evidence and knowledge; and (d) identify critical research, evaluation, and data collection needs (ODPHP, 2021). These data are important for population health for citizens to live healthy, thriving lives, free of preventable disease, disability, injury, and premature death (ODPHP, 2021).

Healthy People 2030 includes 13 new areas not in previous reports: adolescent health; blood disorders and blood safety; dementias; early and middle childhood; genomics; global health; health-related quality of life and well-being; healthcare-associated infections; lesbian, gay, bisexual, and transgender health; older adults; preparedness; sleep health; and social determinants of health. These additions were based on the nation's need to address the latest public health challenges and priorities. The framework for Healthy People 2030 is based on the Secretary's Advisory Committee on National Health Promotion and Disease Prevention Objectives for 2030. Subject matter experts, organizations, and members of the public cre-ated a comprehensive framework that included a focus on health literacy for the first time in the history of the Healthy People initiative (https://health.gov/our-work/healthy-people/healthy-people-2030). See Chapter 8 for an in-depth discussion of health literacy.

The report reveals the need to improve health outcomes in many marginalized groups, including the uninsured, whose low access to health screening and treatment continues to be a problem (ODPHP, 2021). For example, almost two thirds of persons age 50 to 64 years with private health insurance receive colorectal cancer screening, compared with less than a third of their uninsured peers (ODPHP, 2021).

EXHIBIT 2.1: The Vision, Measures, Core Objectives, Developmental Objectives, and Research Objectives for the Healthy People 2030 Initiative

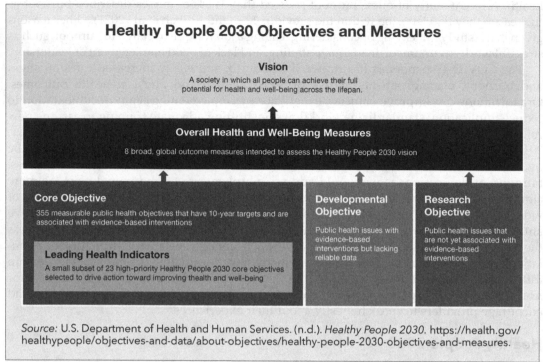

Source: U.S. Department of Health and Human Services. (n.d.). *Healthy People 2030.* https://health.gov/healthypeople/objectives-and-data/about-objectives/healthy-people-2030-objectives-and-measures.

Future Directions

Each decade, the Healthy People initiative continues to improve measures of population health. The 2030 Healthy People initiative includes 355 core—or measurable—objectives, as well as developmental and research objectives to guide healthcare and policy (Exhibit 2.1). The future objectives of these reports are more specific than in times past, and they include the elimination of health disparities, achievement of health equity, and attainment of health literacy to improve the health and well-being of all. The advisory committee has also set national goals and measurable objectives to guide evidence-based policies, programs, and other actions to improve health and well-being. Specifically, the Healthy People 2030 report will include a small subset of 23 high-priority Healthy People 2030 core objectives selected to drive action toward improving health and well-being.

The Next Decade in Nursing and Healthcare: A Conversation About Population Health

What is nursing's role in population health, and what difference can it make in the lives of patients? The National Academies of Sciences, Engineering, and Medicine issued the *Future of Nursing 2020 to 2030: Charting a Path to Advance Health Equity* (2021), which charts the role of nurses to strengthen their awareness of social determinants of health in order to better integrate social care into healthcare. Awareness building relies on the critical assessment of populations that are at risk of adverse health outcomes. The *Future of Nursing 2020 to 2030* report lays out four complementary assessment activities: increasing awareness (of the social risks and assets of the patient/population); adjustment (accommodations to reduce social barriers); alignment (organizing and facilitating activities that help the community); and advocacy (partnering with social care organizations).

Barriers to accessing quality healthcare continue to be a problem. The Camden Core model implemented in Camden, New Jersey, offers an example of nurses and other health professionals partnering with social organizations and the community to improve population health (National Academies of Sciences, Engineering, and Medicine, 2021). It involves a multipronged approach, including community partnerships with churches, outreach programs, and other organizations to provide social and health-related services to the community. Through a technique known as *healthcare hotspotting*, Finkelstein et al. (2020) identified specific areas of Camden that had high hospital readmission rates. In response, the Camden coalition developed a nurse-led care management program to address the after-hospitalization needs of chronically ill people in those areas. They successfully linked patients to needed services such as legal services and community health services. This led to the development of secure, genuine, and continuous partnerships between care teams members and patients and health systems. Thus, it served a critical component of the Triple Aim: the patient experience. Healthcare is moving to the community, where social determinants of health must be considered and outcomes improved. For example, the U.S. Surgeon General's Call to Action to Control Hypertension emphasizes that the goal must be to bring healthcare to where people are—where they live, work and go to school (www.cdc.gov/bloodpressure/CTA.htm).

CONCLUSION

The health outcomes of a group of individuals, including the distribution of such outcomes within the group, is population health. Public health influences population health, and vice versa. Policy recommendations, health education and outreach, and research for disease detection and prevention of injury enable public health to protect and improve a community's health (CDC, 2020).

To fully understand and address population health, practitioners must take a comprehensive, holistic approach. Successful strategies involve various stakeholders, including clinicians, researchers, policymakers, and private and governmental agencies. Population health takes into consideration the most pressing issues within a certain group or community and seeks to create opportunities to effect change that will be beneficial to large groups. However, for those who do not benefit from those interventions, the next task should be to expand views and perspectives to be more inclusive so that society benefits and all people can receive holistic, quality healthcare.

DISCUSSION QUESTIONS

1. Regarding the historical perspective of population health and Snow's attribution an outbreak of cholera to a water pump handle, examine the evolution of the evidence on mask-wearing to prevent the spread of COVID-19. How might the social determinants of health impact the adoption of mask-wearing guidelines?

2. This chapter describes four definitions of population health. Develop your own definition of population health, synthesizing the aspects of those definitions you find most useful. It might include elements that you believe are lacking among the definitions.

3. What objectives would you list that include the social determinants of health? What are the facilitators to creating a functional interdisciplinary team? What steps would you take to engage the community in the dissemination of an evidence-based intervention to reduce a particular chronic disease in marginalized groups? Develop a slide presentation to deliver to an interprofessional group that is undertaking the use of population health to reduce health disparities in chronic illnesses based on your answers to these questions.

4. As a nurse, describe what the fourth aim of the Quadruple Aim means to you. How can you engage your colleagues and your organization to implement the fourth aim?

ADDITIONAL RESOURCES

U.S. Department of Health and Human Services Office of Minority Health (1985). Report of the secretary's task force on Black and minority health (Heckler Report). https://minorityhealth.hhs .gov/heckler30

U.S. Environmental Protection Agency. (2017). Climate change adaptation resource center (ARC-X). Last updated November 13, 2021. https://www.epa.gov/arc-x/new-york-city-assesses-extreme -heat-climate-risk

Wechsler, H., Basch, C. E., Zybert, P., & Shea, S. (1998). Promoting the selection of low-fat milk in elementary school cafeterias in an inner-city Latino community: Evaluation of an intervention. *American Journal of Public Health, 88*(3), 427–433. https://doi.org/10.2105/AJPH.88.3.427

REFERENCES

Abel-Smith, B. (1992). The Beveridge report: Its origins and outcomes. *International Social Security Review, 45*(1–2), 5–16.

Agency for Healthcare Research and Quality. (2018). Six domains for health care quality. https:// www.ahrq.gov/talkingquality/measures/six-domains.html

Agency for Healthcare Research and Quality. (2019). CAHPS Patient experience surveys and guidance. https://www.ahrq.gov/cahps/surveys-guidance/index.html

American Association of College of Nursing. (2013). Public health: recommended competencies and curricular guidelines for public health nursing, a supplement to the essentials of baccalaureate education for professional nursing practice. Author.

American Association of Colleges of Nursing. (2021). The essentials: core competencies for professional nursing education. https://www.aacnnursing.org/Portals/42/AcademicNursing/ pdf/Essentials-2021.pdf

Berwick, D. M., Nolan, T. W., & Whittington, J. (2008). The triple aim: Care, health, and cost. *Health Affairs, 27*(3), 759–769. https://doi.org/10.1377/hlthaff.27.3.759

Bodenheimer, T., & Sinsky, C. (2014). From triple to quadruple aim: Care of the patient requires care of the provider. *Annals of Family Medicine, 12*(6), 573–576. https://doi.org/10.1370/afm.1713

Bowles, J. R., Adams, J. M., Batcheller, J., Zimmerman, D., & Pappas, S. (2018). The role of the nurse Leader in advancing the quadruple aim. *Nurse Leader, 16*(4), 244–248. https://doi.org/10.1016/ j.mnl.2018.05.011

Centers for Disease Control. (2020). What is population health? https://www.cdc.gov/ pophealthtraining/whatis.html

Evans, R. G., Barer, M. L., & Marmor, T. R. (Eds.). (1994). *Why are some people healthy and others not? The determinants of health populations*. Routledge. https://doi.org/10.4324/9781315135755

Finkelstein, A., Zhou, A., Taubman, S., & Doyle, J. (2020). Health care hotspotting—A randomized, controlled trial. *New England Journal of Medicine, 382*(2), 152–162. https://doi.org/10.1056/ NEJMsa1906848

Galvin, G. (2018). Population health: The 'North Star' of the triple aim. *US News and World Report*. https://www.usnews.com/news/healthiest-communities/ articles/2018-05-25/a-decade-later-triple-aim-health-care-framework-offers-lessons-promise

Gorsky, M. (2015). *Health for all: The journey of universal health coverage*. Orient Blackswan.

Gray, A. M. (1982). Inequalities in health. The Black Report: A summary and comment. *International Journal of Health Services, 12*(3), 349–380. https://doi.org/10.2190/XXMM-JMQU-2A7Y-HX1E

Hall, L. H., Johnson, J., Watt, I., Tsipa, A., & O'Connor, D. B. (2016). Healthcare staff wellbeing, burnout, and patient safety: A systematic review. *PLoS One, 11*(7), e0159015. https://doi.org/ 10.1371/journal.pone.0159015

Institute of Medicine. (1988). *The future of public health*. National Academies Press. https://doi. org/10.17226/1091

Jeffs, L. (2018). Achieving the quadruple aim in healthcare: The essential role of authentic. *Complex and Resilient Nurse Leaders (Tor Ont), 31*(2), 8–19. https://doi.org/10.12927/cjnl.2018.25607

Kindig, D. A. (2007). Understanding population health terminology. *Milbank Quarterly, 85*(1), 139–161. https://doi.org/10.1111/j.1468-0009.2007.00479.x

Kindig, D., & Magnan, S. (2019). Can academic population health departments improve population health? *JAMA Network Open, 2*(4), e192205. https://doi.org/10.1001/ jamanetworkopen.2019.2205

Kindig, D., & Stoddart, G. (2003). What is population health? *American Journal of Public Health, 93*(3), 380–383. https://doi.org/10.2105/ajph.93.3.380

Krieger, J. (2010). Home is where the triggers are: Increasing asthma control by improving the home environment. *Journal of Pediatric Allergy, Immunology, and Pulmonology*, 23(2), 139–145. https://doi.org/10.1089/ped.2010.0022

Link, B. G., & Phelan, J. C. (1995). Social conditions as fundamental causes of disease [Extra issue]. *Journal of Health and Social Behavior*, 35, 80–94. https://doi.org/10.2307/2626958

Marmot, M. G., Shipley, M. J., & Rose, G. (1985). The inequalities in death-specific explanation of general pattern? *The Lancet*, 323(8384), 1003–1006. https://doi.org/10.1016/S0140-6736(84)92337-7

Marmot, M., Friel, S., Bell, R., Houweling, T. A., Taylor, S., & Commission on Social Determinants of Health. (2008). Closing the gap in a generation: Health equity through action on the social determinants of health. *The Lancet*, 372(9650), 1661–1669.

Matthew, D. B. (2018). *Just medicine: A cure for racial inequality in American health care*. NYU Press.

National Academies of Sciences, Engineering, and Medicine. (2021). *The future of nursing 2020–2030: Charting a path to achieve health equity*. The National Academies Press. https://doi.org/10.17226/25982

Office of Disease Prevention and Health Promotion. (2021). *HealthyPeople2020—Clinical preventive services*. U.S. Department of Health and Human Services. https://www.healthypeople.gov/2020/leading-health-indicators/2020-lhi-topics/Clinical-Preventive-Services/data

Park, M., Alston, A. D., & Washington-Brown, L. (2021). *Toward rational conversation about race, health risk, and nursing*. American Nurse Journal, 16(1), 5–7, 58.

Physicians for National Health Program. (2021). Health care systems-four basic models. https://www.pnhp.org/single_payer_resources/health_care_systems_four_basic_models.php

Ramsay, A. E. (2009). John Snow, MD: Anaesthetist to the Queen of England and pioneer epidemiologist. *Baylor University Medical Center Proceedings*, 19(1), 24–28. https://doi.org/10.1080/08998280.2006.11928120

Riddle, M. C. (2018). The cost of diabetes care—An elephant in the room. *Diabetes Care*, 41(5), 929–932. https://doi.org/10.2337/dci18-0012

Roux, A. V. (2016). On the distinction—or lack of distinction—between population health and public health. *American Journal of Public Health*, 106(4), 619–620. https://doi.org/10.2105/AJPH.2016.303097

Samuriwo, R., Laws, E., Webb, K., & Bullock, A. (2020). "I didn't realise they had such a key role" Impact of medical education curriculum change on medical student interactions with nurses: A qualitative exploratory study of student perceptions. *Advances in Health Sciences Education*, 25, 75–93. https://doi.org/10.1007/s10459-019-09906-4

Shah, M. K., Gandrakota, N., Cimiotti, J. P., Ghose, N., Moore, M., & Ali, M. K. (2021). Prevalence of and factors associated with nurse burnout in the US. *JAMA Network Open*, 4(2), e2036469. https://doi.org/10.1001/jamanetworkopen.2020.36469

Sharfstein, J. M. (2014). The strange journey of population health. *Milbank Quarterly*, 92(4), 640–643. https://doi.org/10.1111/1468-0009.12082

Silberberg, M., Martinez-Bianchi, V., & Lyn, M. J. (2019). What is population health? *Primary Care Clinics Office Practice*, 46, 475–484. https://doi.org/10.1016/j.pop.2019.07.001

Stiefel, M., & Nolan, K. A. (2012). *A guide to measuring the triple aim: population health, experience of care, and per capita cost* [IHI Innovation series white paper]. Institute for Healthcare Improvement.

Stoto, M. A. (2013, February 21). *Population health in the affordable care act era*. Academy Health. https://community-wealth.org/sites/clone.community-wealth.org/files/downloads/paper-stoto.pdf

Swarthout, M., & Bishop, M. A. (2017). Population health management: Review of concepts and definitions. *American Journal of Health-System Pharmacy*, 74(18), 1405–1411. https://doi.org/10.2146/ajhp170025

Szreter, S. (2003). The population health approach in historical perspective. *American Journal of Public Health*, 93(3), 421–431. https://doi.org/10.2105/ajph.93.3.421

Valles, S. A. (2019). *Philosophy of population health: Philosophy for a new public health era*. Routledge.

Winslow, C.-E. A. (1920). The untilled field of public health. *Modern Medicine*, 2(1306), 183–191. https://doi.org/10.1126/science.51.1306.23

World Health Organization. (2021). *Social determinants of health*. https://www.who.int/health-topics/social-determinants-of-health#tab=tab_1

CHAPTER 3

Health Policy and Finance Across Health Systems

J. B. Silvers

LEARNING OBJECTIVES

- Introduce the basic elements of finance and policy as they relate to disparities.
- Review the origins of disparate access, cost, and quality.
- Consider specific examples of these issues and how they relate to policy and finance.
- Evaluate actions designed to address disparities.
- Understand the ways that payment and policy evolve in response to their effect.

INTRODUCTION

There is no doubt that healthcare policy and finance have a profound effect on the practice of nursing, medicine, and other health professions in the United States and on the development of health disparities. Providers do what is required of them by law, what they are paid to do, and, sometimes, the right thing for ethical or professional reasons. But relying on their good instincts is not enough; policy and payment are also necessary. The details of how policy works and specific ways to pay for care are critical elements in helping vulnerable populations and dealing with disparities.

In this chapter, we start with the basics of both policy and finance within the context of population health. Then we expand into examples of how each may impact the problem and the potential solutions. The chapter also discusses ways to address disparities—some fundamental, and others more subtle. These range from changes in the dominant fee-for-service model to marginal changes in information, subsidies, regulation, and education.

WHAT IS HEALTH POLICY?

Most analyses of policy use the construct of a three-legged stool, with cost, quality, and access as critical supports. We consider each of these. The concern typically has been that we could have two of the supports but would have to sacrifice the third. For instance, high quality and broad access would lead to escalating costs. Or a focus on cost cutting would

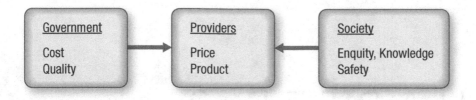

Figure 3.1 Parallel meanings of policy objectives in other spheres.

leave some people out or result in inferior outcomes for all or with a disparate impact on the most vulnerable (Feldstein, 2019). It is only in recent years that policymakers—especially at the federal level—have switched the focus to "value," which is construed as lowering or stabilizing costs while improving measured outcomes. Access is not often part of the discussion of value, although it clearly should be, since value to some but not others is part of the problem (Conrad, 2015). Patients with high deductibles and copayments might put far more emphasis on cost to the detriment of quality or access. On the other hand, those with full coverage, such as low-income individuals on Medicaid, might worry mainly about access because it is sometimes limited for them.

The challenge is in the details. What are costs and to whom, and which of the hundreds of quality measures[1] represent the outcomes of most interest? How much access is enough? The final impact of "value-based purchasing" rests on the incentives that result for each player when these are translated into actual payment. As differential payment based on performance against quality metrics permeates both governmental and private payment systems, the potential grows for bias against those with challenging social determinants of health[2] (SDOH; Garg, 2019). Access to care may be limited since providers find it more difficult to reach these goals for patients with difficult living situations who cannot keep appointments, maintain compliance, and access adequate food, and who may lack transportation and employment or suffer other forms of community trauma.

The Language of Providers

It is interesting to note that the concepts of cost, quality, and access are not unique to government policy objectives but have parallels in all transactions. The cost to the payer is effectively the price to the provider (Reinhardt, 2019). In a similar way, quality is just one attribute of the service delivered. These parallels are shown in Figure 3.1. While the policymaker is trying to manage these at the broad level, providers are making decisions regarding what they charge, what goes into the service, and how many people they can serve. This internal perspective of managers does not necessarily align with community health needs or recognize the health status of people in a particular region or marginalized people. This clearly can lead to a mismatch between what it takes to be successful as a provider and what the community might need. Government action and required disclosure of "community benefit" often come up short in closing the gap.

The conflict between the two perspectives is that trying to reduce the cost to the payer or to the government may mean a reduction in income to the provider. But, on the other hand, in a perfect market, the provider would want to reduce the price to attract more price-sensitive patients. This is the assumption behind the drive for price transparency for

---

1. The National Quality Forum is a nongovernmental organization charged with reviewing and qualifying measures that can be used in value-based payment and evaluation processes (https://www.qualityforum.org/About_NQF/) (Garg, 2019).

2. Social Determinants of Health (SDOH) is a term widely used to describe all of the other conditions where people live, learn, work, and play that affect a wide range of health and quality-of-life-risks (https://www.cdc.gov/socialdeterminants/index.htm).

the consumer. Unfortunately, these "consumers" may not have the ability to pay if not fully covered by insurance, be it from an employer or the government. In a similar way, delivering community benefit probably means higher cost and lower margins to the provider. Furthermore, many managers and clinicians may believe that cutting prices would be contingent on reducing quality. In a private system driven by profits, broad policy objectives to drive actions often leave a gap between what is desirable to society and what can be reasonably expected from providers.

The healthcare market is far from perfect. Prices are rarely truly competitive or visible, and the quality of health services is difficult to judge. On the other hand, greater efficiency could produce good results for all, leaving no policy conflict. It is impossible to generalize which viewpoint is the correct one. Recent government actions to force hospitals to post shoppable service rates on their websites[3] clearly assumes market forces will lead to more price competition with no loss of access or quality. The evidence to support this assumption is mixed (Diamond, 2021), although it is possible that competition in private markets with full transparency will produce results, especially for certain shoppable services. However, the overall impact on healthcare is far from certain.

The point is that there is an intricate dance between policy objectives and how they are interpreted in providers' worlds, where financial constraints and competition for paying patients are very real. Even with the best of intentions by policymakers and providers, the devil is in the details. Simplistic assumptions on the policy side and narrow operational goals of providers will always present a challenge. Professional ethics, personal values, public pressure, and even legal action can help close the gap. But we must realize that institutional survival and bureaucratic inertia can undo even the best-laid plans.

Another complication is that all of this may well be viewed as part of something even greater. For instance, healthcare cost and access may be a proxy for what is equitable in terms of who bears the direct and indirect cost of illness. Should the individual patient, the employer, or society at large pay the bill? Clearly, the ultimate losses are to patients, although employers may lose productivity, and the cost of social support from government may rise in the long run. In a similar way, quality of care as measured in hospitals may be the tip end of the social determinants of health that actually drive worse overall outcomes. The quality metrics that are seen as part of the value equation may result from poor nutrition, housing, education, and other factors—not health services. The increased emphasis on social determinants of health recognizes these interactions, but weaving them into both public policy and organizational incentives is a tricky proposition.

The Policy Cycle

In this chapter, we focus on more traditional policy objectives, realizing that they are part of something much bigger. We try to understand how policymakers attempt to use certain levers to reach their explicit and implicit goals. The primary methods are *payment*, *regulation*, and *taxes*. Sometimes policy simply dictates certain actions or prohibits others through regulation backed up by penalties. Violating accreditation requirements and safety standards or committing fraud may result in corrective actions or even removal of the offending providers. In a similar way, payment is often used as a blunt instrument. We simply do not pay for services that are not preapproved, in some cases, or we pay at a lower rate if certain performance standards are not met. This is an effective way to enforce some policy goals. Tax exemptions for not-for-profit hospitals are loosely contingent on maintaining their charitable objectives, and nontaxable debt is a way to subsidize their financing.

---

3. The Centers for Medicare & Medicaid Services has led in their requirements that hospitals post information regarding their prices in order to make comparisons and shopping easier (https:// www.cms.gov/hospital-price-transparency) (Berwick, 2008).

But the impact may be more subtle if payment is differential depending on other factors such as location (inpatient vs. outpatient vs. telehealth), subsequent events (readmission), episode management (bundled payments), or emergent versus elective care. Here, policymakers hope to influence decisions and processes at the provider level without necessarily demanding specific action. As an example, the fixed-episode payment for a joint replacement under the Bundled Payment for Care Improvement program encourages better outcomes but discourages postacute services, even those necessary for difficult cases, since this is a place where reductions in length of stay are easiest. While this may reduce overall cost, it could result in disparities when there is less family support or a poor living situation. The implicit hope is to influence overall actions toward a particular target (e.g., readmissions, lower infection rates, patient satisfaction) without regard for each specific situation (Lewin Group, 2021).

General Impact of Policy on System Design

Finally, policy might use even broader tax levers to accomplish goals. The largest of these derives from the fact that compensation to workers in the form of health benefits is not taxed as income to them but is deducted from taxable income by employers who offer health insurance to their employees. This creates an enormous subsidy to employer-sponsored health plans, which encourages them to continue their health plans and, perhaps, offer more generous coverage than would otherwise be available (Pauly, 2006). The resulting dependence on employer-sponsored health benefits in the United States as an alternative to a government system has resulted in a patchwork of varying coverage with some left out, especially when the economic cycle results in job loss.

A patient who loses a job or works part time or under contract with no health benefits may be left to fend for themselves. The number of people with employer-sponsored coverage varies widely, largely by the size of the employer. Almost all larger companies cover their workers, but less than a quarter of very small employers (<10) provide health insurance (Employee Benefit Reserch Institute, 2021).

This situation changed substantially with the passage of the Affordable Care Act (ACA) in 2010.[4] This landmark law legislated subsidies and exchanges to reduce premiums to reasonable levels relative to disposable income and to allow comparison of health plans. Previously, employers and insurance companies used mechanisms such as exclusions of services, limited access to expensive drugs, or other methods to reduce their costs. This prompted inclusion of requirements in the ACA on all employer-sponsored plans that prohibited many of the typical access and quality limitations. Thus, pre-existing conditions and other exclusions are gone, leaving a better but imperfect safety net (French, 2016). Yet many are still left uninsured, especially if they live in a state that has not expanded Medicaid coverage to the full range of lower-income people, are undocumented immigrants, or fall into a few other exclusions. The American Rescue Plan (ARP) Act of 2021 expanded coverage and subsidies in a number of important ways as discussed later.[5]

Figure 3.2 illustrates the interaction of these factors in a cycle of interconnected parts, beginning with the policy objective and the lever chosen to accomplish it based on certain assumptions about how affected people will behave. The result of policy depends on the signals given to providers or others to act (e.g., expand capacity, avoid certain patients,

---

4. The Affordable Care Act (ACA) included many reforms that improved access by expanding Medicaid, reducing premiums to a maximum percent of disposable income, eliminating certain insurance practices, creating innovative organizations, and experimenting with alternative forms of payment. The Kaiser Family Foundation has tracked the changes over the years in this Act (https://www.kff.org/health-reform/).

5. A good review of the American Rescue Plan Act of 2021 is available at https://www.kff.org/health-reform/issue-brief/how-the-american-rescue-plan-act-affects-subsidies-for-marketplace-shoppers-and-people-who-are-uninsured/.

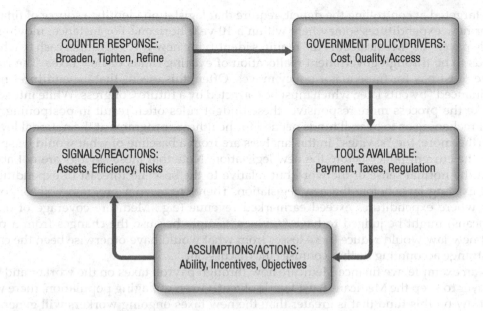

Figure 3.2 Health policy cycle.
Source: Copyright © 2020, J. B. Silvers, Case Western Reserve University, Cleveland, Ohio.

consolidate). For instance, underpayment may produce losses and will signal the need to reduce unprofitable investments (e.g., by closing hospitals or cutting services) even if the underlying needs continue. This has been a continual battle for smaller rural facilities. More than 120 rural hospitals have closed since 2005, with many more in precarious straits, leaving these communities without access.[6]

The result of decisions at the institutional level might be consistent with what the policymakers wanted, or they may result in unexpected consequences. When the results are not consistent with broader societal goals, then the policy may be abandoned or, more often, altered in an attempt to reach the original goal, largely dependent on political and cost considerations. To understand and predict how policy affects the health system and society as a whole, we will need to realistically assess all stages of this process. This chapter provides some examples. The reader is also encouraged to apply the policy cycle to other recommendations in this book to determine what is likely to work in the way that federal and state policymakers intended.

Because policy typically is implemented through a change in the flow of dollars, it is important to turn next to finance in more depth before returning to specifics regarding policy.

WHAT IS FINANCE?

The term *finance* means many things, ranging from how we pay for care globally to where the funds come from for services and new buildings. Because health policy has a potential impact on both, it is useful to distinguish the broadest use of the word from more operational definitions.

In many U.S. policy discussions, the concern is how we can provide funds at the broadest levels through government appropriations. Congressional "pay-go" or "pay-as-you-go"

---

6. See the following for a good account of rural hospitals in trouble https://www.shepscenter.unc.edu/programs-projects/rural-health/projects/north-carolina-rural-health-research-and-policy-analysis-center/.

rules, targeted at controlling the deficit, require that legislation identify a source of financing for new expenditures somewhere within a 10-year horizon.[7] For instance, moving to "single payer" or "Medicare for All" requires identifying new ways to funnel cash to where it needs to be through government reallocation of existing funds or new taxes. The rules say we must pay for these major policy moves. Often, this means that expenditures now are "financed" by cuts later, which must be corrected by a future Congress. While intended to make the process more responsive, these budget rules often result in postponing the day of reckoning as to overall funds needed for healthcare programs at the national level.[8]

Furthermore, the "savings" in this analysis are from a baseline of what would be spent under the current policy before the new legislation. Note that these savings are not absolute in the normal sense of the word but relative to the baseline forecast of expenditures under existing laws before the new legislation. Therefore, even a program with ongoing losses where expenditures exceed earmarked revenue (e.g., Medicare coverage of older Americans) might be judged to have "savings" simply because the changes from a proposed new law would reduce these losses from what would have otherwise been the case. This strange accounting further confuses the discussion.

As an example, we finance Medicare now through payroll taxes on the worker and the employer to keep the Medicare Trust Fund solvent. Given our aging population, there will be a draw on this fund that is greater than the new taxes ongoing workers will generate. Therefore, Medicare will be insolvent by 2024 by current estimates, creating a financing crisis.[9] By the same token, the new $1.9 trillion American Rescue Plan of 2021 requires cuts in Medicare in later years to offset new payments built into this legislation. These unresolved financing issues are left for a future Congress to address.

Tax Policy

This broadest use of the term *financing* misses much of the impact of policy on the system. One of the largest financing factors in healthcare is the dominance of tax-exempt hospitals. Contributions to these core institutions are tax deductible to the donor, interest on their debt is not taxable to the lender, and they are exempt from income tax and, generally, property tax. These strong subsidies are the main reason why this form of organization persists. It all comes from simple provisions in the tax code that were a natural evolution from the origin of hospitals as charities to care for those living in poverty. Originally, they depended totally on contributions rather than insurance payments. Imposing taxes would have made this source of voluntary funding more difficult (Rosenbaum, 2015).

In fact, only after health insurance was established as a reliable source of payment was there substantial growth in taxable investor-owned healthcare providers, other than small facilities started by individual physicians in their own homes in small towns. Medicare payment, in particular, was an accelerator in the 1960s for large for-profit chains, since this source of reliable cash flow was attractive to potential stockholders. This parallel system of investor-owned for-profits and traditional nonprofit tax-exempt hospitals has allowed a contrast as to how much the tax benefits are worth and what society gets in return for them.

Some would like to make these tax subsidies contingent on proof of sufficient community benefit as an incentive to return hospitals to their original charitable focus. Historically, charity care and other tangible social goods were clearly sufficient justification for continuation

---

7. The score keeper for this evaluation of any legislation on the federal deficit is the Congressional Budget Office (https://www.cbo.gov/).

8. The Center on Budget and Policy Priorities provides a good review of the intent and operation of these rules over the years (https://www.cbpp.org/research/federal-budget/the-pay-as-you-go-budget-rule).

9. The annual report of the Medicare Trust Funds Board of Trustees is sent to Congress each year including the forecast of the Office of the Actuary for CMS (https://www.cms.gov/Research-Statistics-Data-and-Systems/Statistics-Trends-and-Reports/ReportsTrustFunds).

of tax-exempt status. However, there is continuing controversy over how far short they fall from matching the economic value of their tax-exempt status (Herring, 2018). Criticism ranges from concerns over *any* profit motive in healthcare (e.g., a governmental system like the National Health Service of the UK) to questions about whether *any* assistance is appropriate (e.g., no tax support at all since for-profit chains do similar work).

However, as all health systems grow larger and rely on financing from the capital markets, the distinctions between for-profit and not-for-profit organizations are blurred. Both issue large debt financing and must earn enough to satisfy these investors. Both use their market power to negotiate high payment rates from insurers (White, 2019). And both have integrated provider networks, including salaried physicians, ancillary services, pharmacy distribution, and even investment arms, to help finance startups and spinoff companies. In other words, it is increasingly difficult to tell the difference, although the potential threat of losing tax advantages is still very potent as a policy lever.

Other goals, such as reducing disparities, improving employment policies, or other less-direct social outcomes (e.g., food distribution, education) also could be incentivized by this pressure to maintain tax-exempt status. Currently, most not-for-profit tax-exempt hospitals struggle to demonstrate that their uncompensated care, education cost, and other categories of social dividends counted by the Internal Revenue Service as community benefits are equal to the value of their tax-exempt status. If the threat of losing this huge subsidy were stronger and more social expenditures counted, there would be much more pressure to broaden the mission of these private organizations. Now, they are not asked to go much beyond the typical health services expected of their investor-owned competitors. There is no penalty for falling short except some bad publicity. Furthermore, most of what counts as "community benefit" is just the difference between what government programs contractually pay for services and the average full cost of providing them (Rosenbaum, 2015). While this undoubtedly is a burden for these providers—especially those who serve many Medicaid patients—it is not the same as classic charity care to those living in poverty or other uncompensated services to society.

As a result of the lower tax-exempt debt cost for not-for-profit tax-exempt hospitals, their investments in buildings, facilities, and equipment have increasingly been financed by borrowing rather than by donations. Although it allows them to expand rapidly, this growing debt also increases their financial risk and imposes the need for higher margins to satisfy lenders who want to ensure repayment. Typically, tax-exempt hospitals must show enough profitability to cover the interest and principal due each year by a minimum of two times up to four times or more.[10] This required cushion of excess earnings is reported as a substantial profit—an ironic result for a not-for-profit organization. Thus, in a roundabout way, health policy implemented through the tax code drives the organizational structure and use of debt by our hospitals. In a further irony, this tax-exempt borrowing typically is used to build capacity largely to serve well-insured patients to generate the profits needed to meet bond requirements regardless of the needs of underresourced populations.

The reliance on private capital markets, in contrast to public financing, as a policy decision has forced providers into this profit-seeking behavior. This was not always the case. In the years after World War II, the U.S. government decided that American hospital capacity was inadequate. Congress passed the Hill-Burton Act in 1946, which provided direct grants to build hospitals in a historic growth spurt. Of most interest is the fact that these grants were to be "paid back" over 20 years via in-kind free services rather than with cash. Specifically, recipients had to certify the provision of charity care of a "reasonable amount" primarily to low-income communities, guaranteeing no discrimination. All of this was a

---

10. The 2019 median annual debt service coverage for U.S. hospitals according to Moody's Investors Service was 4.7 times (i.e., net profit plus interest and principal due divided by interest and principal) as reported in Beckers Hospital Review (https://www.beckershospitalreview.com/finance/45-financial-benchmarks-for-hospital-executives-01242020.html?oly_enc_id=0995H4397367B1U).

precursor to our later health policy initiatives. When it ended in 1975, the Hill-Burton program's objectives were incorporated into Title XVI of the Public Health Service Act.[11]

Direct Payment

In terms of operational impact, the way services are paid at the granular level is a very important factor in how policy actually works—or doesn't. As a major source of operational financing, payment for services and access are the most important direct health policy tool available. Before the creation of Blue Cross and Blue Shield health insurance, payment for patient services was erratic, if it existed at all. Generally, only people who had no means went to hospitals. Therefore, most were sponsored by religious organizations or went to last-resort public hospitals for indigent patients. They had large wards, low standards, marginal expectations, and limited outcomes. They were where indigent patients went to die. People of means typically received private care in their homes until later in the 20th century (Stevens, 1999).

But with the advance of medicine, technology, and clinical knowledge, healthcare services became more valuable and more expensive. Finally, in the 1930s, the United States created a way to spread the cost of episodic and unpredictable care needs across broader populations through the invention of health insurance. Theoretically, everyone could benefit from these increasingly valuable services, but many could not afford them. Thus was born Blue Cross and Blue Shield, largely as creations of hospitals and physicians eager to have a stable source of income. These original insurers were very simple. Fixed premiums were set at the cost per person per month averaged over all enrollees, no matter who they were. This is called *community rating*, and it was the standard for many years. Since the amount of money involved was still relatively small by today's standards, this simple mechanism worked well with minimal operational cost.

Payment was equally simple. Hospitals were paid retrospectively whatever it cost for their services—not a contracted price, discounted rate, or fixed payment per admission, as is now the case. Physicians were "on their honor" as to what they charged but were constrained by a limit relative to what others charged. This cost-based payment for hospitals and "usual and customary rates" for physicians dominated healthcare financing and was even incorporated into Medicare when it was established in 1965. Change was very slow because the forces to maintain the status quo came from physicians acting as fiercely independent businesspeople, hospitals as voluntary community organizations to support them, and lack of political pressure from the middle class, who were reasonably satisfied (Rothman, 1993).

This simple means of financing aggregate payments to providers collapsed under the weight of new competitors and the inherent inflation built into such an unconstrained system. New for-profit insurers realized that they could undercut the average community rate when selling to employers if they enrolled healthier patients, leaving higher-cost patients to be covered by Blue Cross and Blue Shield. Of course, unequal distribution of less-healthy people to some plans and more-healthy ones to others made the use of a single community average premium infeasible. The escalating average premiums for those left behind quickly became uncompetitive with new insurers. As a result, rather than one rate for all patients, premiums had to be adjusted to better reflect the health status of those enrolled in each group. This "experience rating" left those in need of the most care to bear the highest costs—an ironic outcome for a system designed to spread the cost evenly across the whole population.

Under these circumstances, the fundamental assumptions of health insurance are violated. The idea of any type of insurance is that one cannot predict who will need what

---

11. The Hill-Burton Act provided funding for over 4,200 hospitals over its lifetime and pioneered changes in civil rights, public health, and most health policy initiatives, to this day demonstrating that direct financing can be used as a key policy lever. An excellent review of this history can be found in Chapter 1 of a publication by the American College of Healthcare Executives at https://account.ache.org/Cellucci_Ch1-e8991004.

services at the individual level. Alternatively, the average for a larger group can be determined with some confidence. But when the experience of some enrollees is known and is a good predictor of their future expenses, the model falls apart. A patient with cancer or diabetes will have predictably higher future costs than patients without these conditions. Therefore, "pre-existing conditions" were used to screen high-risk patients. This practice was prohibited by the ACA in order to avoid discrimination against these patients and allow them more affordable access. However, for some conditions (e.g., long-term mental health disorders), neither the private insurance system nor governmental targeted direct care have been adequate, leaving a patchwork system of care that often fails.

Changes Under the Affordable Care Act of 2010

As the insurance system evolved, although large employer groups with several hundred employees could effectively average their costs, single enrollees and small groups were subject to the assessments of insurers as to what their individual claims were likely to be. Thus, premiums become erratic and frequently unaffordable for many. This was the genesis of the ACA's insurance exchanges and its subsidy system. The hope was to correct for this failure of the insurance system and allow access for everyone. Insurers receive actuarially fair average premiums overall, and enrollees receive coverage at an affordable cost after subsidies are subtracted, to reduce the net cost to a manageable percentage of their disposable income. Under this system, an individual who, for example, otherwise could have paid a premium of $1000 per month for an unsubsidized health insurance policy might have to pay only $100 if their taxable income was close to the federal poverty level. The federal poverty level is a guideline determined each year by the U.S. Department of Health and Human Services based on what it would take a person or family to have a minimal standard of living.[12] The $900 difference in this example is provided as a subsidy by the federal government. It is paid directly to the insurance company selected by the individual from the offerings on the exchange, but it is construed in the law to be an "advanced tax credit" to the individual.

Through this circuitous method, the individual has what is deemed to be an "affordable" premium (i.e., $100 per month in this example) based on their disposable income, while the insurer receives the amount needed to actuarially cover their expected costs. The hope is that (a) providing choice to the individual will give them satisfactory coverage, while (b) making insurers compete for enrollees will force them to be creative and cost conscious. This is an interesting use of a private market mechanism (the ACA insurance exchanges) to achieve a public purpose (access to insurance coverage). Along with expansion of the existing Medicaid program for those with even less income, many more Americans were insured than before the law's passage, and the premiums stabilized at a reasonable rate in spite of significant challenges by the Trump administration.[13]

This new way to cover neglected parties at a fair rate represents a financing tool of health policy targeted at access and cost from the point of view of individual enrollees. Clearly, lack of insurance for working individuals with low income not working for a larger employer was a disparity that was at least partially corrected by this government action.

The ARP passed by Congress in 2021 goes further by increasing subsidies significantly for middle-income enrollees on the exchanges.[14] The $900 subsidy in the prior example

---

12. The Federal Poverty Guidelines are set annually for each state and used to determine eligibility for various federal assistance programs (https://aspe.hhs.gov/topics/poverty-economic-mobility/poverty-guidelines/prior-hhs-poverty-guidelines-federal-register-references/2021-poverty-guidelines).

13. There were many challenges to the ACA discussed widely in the press such as Silvers, J., "How the G.O.P. Tax Bill Will Ruin Obamacare," https://www.nytimes.com/2017/12/04/opinion/gop-tax-bill-obamacare.html, 12-4-17.

14. The American Recovery Plan had substantial provisions to increase the subsidy levels for middle-income individuals and families that were left with very high premiums for plans they might choose

under the ACA previously would drop in stages to $0 as the purchaser's income rose from 138% to 400% of the federal poverty level. Depending on the specific plan chosen, for someone at 250% of the federal poverty level (i.e., about $26,000 in 2021 for an individual—hardly a high income), the net premium after the ACA subsidy might have risen from $100 a month to perhaps $400 a month, representing a very high portion of their living costs. The ARP provisions increased the subsidy and reduced this net cost radically, to a level that was judged to be much more affordable. In fact, three out of five enrollees now have access to $0 premium plans with the ARP modifications.

Both the ACA and the recent ARP were born out of a concern over access. But the total cost to government has been a continual conservative concern along with the desire of states to control services to those living in poverty. These have longstanding political roots in concerns for states' rights under our federal system and desire for lower taxes. These issues are beyond the scope of this chapter but clearly have made changes very challenging (Mwachofi, 2011). Opposition to further expansion of health service financing to disparate populations is predictable for the same reason. See Chapters 1 and 19 for more in-depth discussion of these issues.

RELATIONSHIP OF POLICY AND FINANCE TO DISPARITITES

We would like to believe that hardly anyone sets out to purposely create disparities. Unfortunately, systemic racism and other biases might suggest otherwise. Our slowness in addressing these issues is also evidence of the relative lack of concern. However, most disparities occur as the unintended consequence of (a) normal market activity or (b) government actions intended to address other societal or political imperatives. It is these, rather than basic flaws in society, that we can address more readily through finance and policy initiatives. Actions to address disparities must be different depending on the causes of the disparities.

Government sometimes acts to address a failure or imperfection in private markets where individual buyers and seller interact (Pinotti, 2012). Generally, competitive markets are efficient ways to provide goods and services to the most people in the most efficient manner. When something goes wrong, the role of the government may be to change the rules slightly to help correct the problem. This might require more full disclosure of prices, features, or risks to allow purchasers to be fully informed before they buy. But in some cases of market failure, government may have to use a heavy hand in prohibiting actions or even banning some of the players. Changing the law to provide price subsidies or impose taxes might be an example of the first, while antitrust action is in the latter category.

This range exists in health policy also (Mwachofi, 2011). The movement to post prices of healthcare services and the subsidies of premiums under the ACA exchanges are ways to overcome access issues. But increasing concerns over consolidation among provider systems to gain market power over insurers may curtail free negotiations to drive down prices (Scheffler, 2021). Some health policy actions may have an indirect or secondary impact on disparities (e.g., avoiding overpricing care to those with pre-existing conditions). Other examples might include expanding capacity in general or primary care, broadening coverage, changing payment, or other actions for all, including underserved populations.

The special case of pharmaceuticals deserves additional comment because this market is so controversial. The argument of drug companies is that they need unfettered pricing and resulting high profits to justify and finance their research into effective therapies. Thus, we

on the ACA insurance exchanges (https://aspe.hhs.gov/topics/poverty-economic-mobility/poverty-guidelines/prior-hhs-poverty-guidelines-federal-register-references/2021-poverty-guidelines).

give monopolies to them during the life of their patents with no restraint on prices. This, plus the questionable role of "middlemen" (pharmacy benefit managers) between insurers and manufacturers and direct-to-consumer advertising, almost guarantees high prices, excess demand, and political influence to continue these arrangements. While the rest of the world engages in various regulations of the industry, the United States continues to avoid conflict and pays an exceptionally high price (Engleberg, 2015). The result is limited access for disadvantaged groups that cannot afford drugs due to their insurance status or inability to meet cost-sharing requirements. In this case, the market failure is due to a lack of meaningful public policy and the political power of an industry that has a lot to gain.

Other actions are direct and have an immediate impact. These include legislative mandates carrying penalties for violation (e.g., Health Insurance Portability and Accountability Act of 1996 [HIPAA] violations of patient privacy), patient safety criteria to be a provider (e.g., Medicare Conditions of Participation), and direct targeted funding to help disadvantaged groups (e.g., Indian Health Service healthcare facilities, Federally Qualified Health Centers, others delivering direct services to identifiable groups).

Health Policy With Indirect Impact on Disparities

The most frequent way the country has addressed disparities is by changing the system for everyone. Thus, Medicare was created to ensure services to older Americans independent of their means. Medicaid took over fragmented state financing of payment for care to people living in poverty, whether they needed a lot or a little. This trickle-down way to help is probably more politically palatable than other methods, although it is not necessarily targeted at specific subgroups in need. Medicare clearly helped older citizens, many of whom were in great need. But part of its political strength is that it benefited all older adults equally. The concept of solidarity, where all are treated the same, is important and helps explain the popularity of broad all-inclusive actions. Targeting help to only one particular vulnerable subgroup requires more political persuasion than offering benefits to all voters.

Medicaid

An example of this political difficulty is the expansion of Medicaid—America's health program for people living in poverty. Initially, this program was seen as an intermediate step in relieving U.S. states of the cost of programs for their most needy, but also as a transition to an insurance system that would cover everyone. But as a voluntary state-run approach, it has been administered in very different ways across the states. For instance, Arizona took 17 years to establish a Medicaid program after federal legislation enabled it. The latest example is the reluctance of 12 states to expand Medicaid to a broader range of income levels even though virtually all of the cost of the newly enrolled population is paid by the federal government under the ACA. The 12 states have some of the sickest people in the nation, where access is a major concern and care is rationed. Clearly citizens of these states were disadvantaged by this reluctance.[15] The attitudes of legislatures toward people living in poverty and the perceived long-term fiscal limits clearly differ among the states. This is further illustrated by the actual or threatened imposition of work requirements for those applying for Medicaid in several states.[16]

15. Arizona's original reluctance being the last state to establish a Medicaid program after passage of the law (https://en.wikipedia.org/wiki/Arizona_Health_Care_Cost_Containment_System) and the slow expansion of Medicaid under the ACA in conservative states (https://www.kff.org/medicaid/issue-brief/status-of-state-medicaid-expansion-decisions-interactive-map/) illustrate this.

16. MultiplestateshaveappliedforwaiverstoimposeworkrequirementsforMedicaideligibilityalthough these have been challenged in the courts (https://www.kff.org/report-section/work-among-medicaid-adults-implications-of-economic-downturn-and-work-requirements-issue-brief/).

Health policy also may be limited by differing social expectations about those who benefit. The result may be an increase in disparities. Thus, while states generally do not limit coverage to children, they vary widely as to Medicaid coverage of adults. Most support the Children's Health Insurance Program, favoring this disadvantaged group. We want to help kids when they are sick no matter what their economic plight—but we do not necessarily want to help working-age unemployed people. Meanwhile, this same concern may be lacking when children face living conditions that may compromise their health (e.g., lead water pipes).

Direct Specialized Providers

Our health policy sometimes attempts to help those in need by financing specialized delivery organizations—although the level of support has varied across the political cycle. Perhaps the oldest such targeted program investment is the Indian Health Service, providing care to those living on reservations. Critics always have argued that the Indian Health Service is underfunded, leading to serious problems and suggesting a cultural bias as well as a failure to meet treaty terms. Tribal members might also enroll in Medicare or Medicaid if they live off the reservation. The result is a patchwork approach to this underserved group. See Chapter 19 for a more in-depth discussion of American Indian and Alaska Native healthcare.

In a similar way, federally qualified health centers (FQHCs) were created as a response to complaints that mainline hospitals and doctors were not serving inner-city residents and migrant workers adequately. Rather than fixing problems with existing systems, policymakers chose to go around them and provide more targeted access through new ambulatory centers. Under the war on poverty initiated in the 1960s, FQHCs were not financed through healthcare mechanisms like Medicaid but by special direct funding through the Office of Economic Opportunity—an agency charged with addressing poverty, not health. Now FQHCs receive direct grants from the Health Resources and Services Administration.

Some services have been targeted directly to veterans (e.g., Veterans Administration facilities), to active-duty military personnel (e.g., military hospitals and clinics), to patients with uncommon conditions (e.g., public health service hospitals for tuberculosis), and even to members of Congress. These are generally well supported, with concerns mainly over access and waiting times. The point is that they are representative of direct care rather than reliance on general delivery systems to the rest of the population.

This strange, disjointed financing is evidence of the barriers the general delivery system faces in trying to reach various groups. The hope, once again, was that providing capacity would result in better health. Even now, FQHCs are seen as unique vehicles to reach difficult populations with free or sliding scale rates to ensure access and reduce cost for health services, health promotion, and prevention.[17] Over time, they have begun to rely more on Medicaid and now look much more like other ambulatory care centers. On the other hand, there is evidence that FQHCs are an important part of community development beyond just health services. It is likely that their unique role in their urban, rural, and homeless communities will continue and be coordinated with other providers increasingly under pressure to provide community benefit (Hilt, 2019).

The Unintended Impact on Disparities From Payment

A change in the method of payment also might impact one group differently than another. A disproportionate number of minorities are covered by Medicaid since their economic and health status is, on average, worse than that of the rest of the population.[18] This means that

17. For more description of FQHCs, see (https://bphc.hrsa.gov/about/index.html).
18. The Kaiser Family Foundation tracks the characteristics of this disadvantaged population and provides comparative data on the Medicaid programs (https://www.kff.org/medicaid/issue-brief/10-things-to-know-about-medicaid-setting-the-facts-straight/).

payment changes in the United States will hit these groups more directly. The most dramatic way this happens is systematic underpayment by Medicaid programs in the states who set the rates and methods used. The degree of underpayment relative to the national average can be quite wide, with a low of 49% in New Hampshire and a high of 169% in Washington, DC.[19] Inevitably these differential rates in poorly paid states will result in inferior staffing, facilities, operations, and care that impact the minority communities served more than the general population. While Medicaid has tended to be a poor payer since its beginning, there definitely is a correlation with more conservative state governments reflecting their political and value judgments (Baker, 2016).

But even within one program, the method of payment can create disparities. The advanced payment methods (APM) recently established by Medicare can produce these inadvertently. Most APM programs attempt to adjust payment for the severity of need. But these risk adjustments are usually based on prior utilization and current diagnosis rather than other factors that make life more difficult for disadvantaged groups. *Social determinants of health* are one way to describe living conditions that may impact need, results, and ongoing health status of individuals or subgroups. The problem is that incorporating these factors into payment is difficult to do, but not including them leads to differential access and outcomes for some. On one hand, it is reasonable that all providers should be held to the same standards of quality and outcomes as measured by the metrics used in these programs. On the other hand, shortfalls in these same measures may be driven by social determinants not the quality of care provided.

An example might help. It has been widely accepted for years that the stress of poor living conditions, low income, food insecurity, and other social determinants of health are associated with poor health outcomes (Guerwich, 2020). As a result, if payment does not recognize the underlying nature of the population adequately, then a provider can be penalized by poor quality measures for such groups. This is a big problem since most payment now includes some penalties for poor outcomes, which might come from social determinants of health rather than the care provided. (For instance, high all-cause 90-day hospital readmission rates might result from poor support and inadequate living conditions rather than poor care.) The "natural" reaction, then, is to avoid serving this element of the population. Yet we don't want to discourage care to patients with these social determinants (Crook, 2021).

As a result, urban and public hospitals often are penalized for high readmissions, infections, and even mortality rates that come from living conditions, lack of support, or lifestyle. The dilemma is that policymakers do not want to condone poor outcomes for these affected populations. So the issue becomes: What is a valid and fair recognition of the underlying social conditions that affect results of care, and how big an incentive is appropriate to encourage striving for results that are equal despite any such handicaps? The issue will not be resolved easily.

But even more insidious is the tendency to avoid discretionary care to some individuals, such as those suffering from diabetes or other chronic conditions. For these patients, it might be difficult to have positive results even if clinical care is of high quality. For instance, the most popular Medicare episodic payment program, Bundled Payment for Care Improvement for joint replacement, has had positive financial results for many hospitals entering this voluntary program. But the sources of cost improvement have come mainly from reducing the days in postacute recovery in skilled nursing facilities, as well as from ruling out candidates for new joints who may have less likelihood of good recovery. This difference in care paths and selection bias are understandable given the financial incentives

---

19. The Medicaid and CHIP Payment and Assess Commission (MACPAC) reviews these programs and provides advice to Congress. This study came from them at (https://www.macpac.gov/publication/medicaid-hospital-payment-a-comparison-across-states-and-to-medicare/) (Guerwich, 2020).

presented to providers who are under financial stress. But the result may be to exclude subgroups with chronic conditions, lack of home support, or comorbidities, even if the patient would be helped with such surgery. The result is a clear potential for increased disparities as an unintended consequence.

The stated goal of the federal government is to have as many people as possible covered by programs that use value-based payment with such quality measures. As a result, we may be growing new disparities and reinforcing existing ones. The danger is that access may be increasingly based on payment methods rather than clinical factors as these payment methods are expanded. The only solution is to make doubly sure that the implicit financial incentives do not exacerbate the problem.

For instance, rather than using raw outcome metrics, most analysts rely on actual versus expected outcomes where social determinants of health, prior clinical conditions, or other factors beyond the control of the provider are used to statistically adjust the target to recognize the unique needs of different populations (Juhnke, 2016; Nerenz, 2021). For instance, for a particular condition, the average 90-day readmission rate for all patients in all facilities might be 3%. But when put into a regression equation with covariates for age, diagnosis, and other factors, the predicted rate for a specific group of patients might be 4%. The latter, then, would be used to compare with actual outcomes for a population with these characteristics. Thus, a hospital with a 3.5% actual readmission rate would be seen as favorable to the target of 4% even if its raw numbers exceed the general population (Lane-Fall, 2013).

Direct Government Action on Disparities

Occasionally, there are direct assaults on disparities, either targeted directly at healthcare needs or as the side effect of other objectives. Perhaps the one that had the biggest impact on the health system was the Civil Rights Act of 1964, which banned racial discrimination in all sorts of institutions, including hospitals, colleges and universities, and public schools—but not churches and private clubs. Until then it was typical to have segregated care in separate multibed wards or even separate facilities.

This now had to change, although the timetable was not rapid. Coincidental with this attack on discrimination, Congress expanded the Hill-Burton subsidies and loan guarantees that helped build new facilities in the postwar period of the 1950s and 1960s. As a result, a hospital building boom occurred. While this clearly was focused on expanding capacity and improving care to all, the focus also for the first time was on building semiprivate rooms to replace large, segregated wards, which were now prohibited. Unfortunately, this new configuration allowed segregation to continue on a by-room basis. While access was arguably better than before, this form of disparity continued, thus undoing some of the intent of the Civil Rights Act. Our move toward equity was very hesitant in most institutions, including health systems and public and private schools.

The Office of Civil Rights in the Department of Health and Human Services continues to monitor compliance with regulations of all sorts, but most important is their review of communication and privacy regarding all minority groups, including those who speak languages other than English. For example, hospitals must provide language services to allow full access and care to those with limited English proficiency. Perhaps even more important is the government's attention to patient confidentiality under HIPAA. Strict rules and penalties are applied to ensure that patient information is not shared beyond what is needed for clinical care. While not targeted at one specific group, this effort has prevented potential discrimination toward patients with HIV/AIDS or other conditions or treatments that might be viewed negatively by some in society.

The section of the federal government directly tasked with addressing areas of differential need is the Health Resources and Services Administration (HRSA) of the Department of Health and Human Services. Besides the FQHCs, HRSA runs more than 90 programs and funds more than 3,000 grantees to meet healthcare needs not addressed elsewhere. These include direct care to targeted groups, training of health professionals, funding of staff in shortage areas, overseeing of organ donations, compensating for vaccination harm, and so forth. Most of these are intended to step in where the delivery system fails. Such failure might be either inadequate resources, as in the Indian Health Services, or gross market failure, such as poor distribution of organs for transplantation.

Other areas of government action may be important for disparities even though they are not intended to focus on these specifically. Legal actions against specific violations of the law probably are at the top. Perhaps most obvious are malpractice suits that address harm to individuals or, in the case of a class action, to identifiable groups. Most litigants have suffered due to an error of omission or commission. While such lawsuits are generally not focused on classically underserved groups alone, they may have that result if the aggrieved overlap. Other legal actions, such as those over lead in the water in Flint, Michigan, a predominantly African American community, may indirectly be an effort to address disparities. Even antitrust actions to prevent the loss or downgrading of a facility in a minority or rural community could potentially fit this description. Alternatively, allowing a proposed merger to proceed might allow a needed upgrading or reconfiguration of a failing hospital. The results may cut both ways regarding service to needy populations by financially stressed providers and opportunistic investors (Gaynor, 2014).

Antitrust enforcement will continue to be an issue as hospital systems consolidate, physician practices are purchased, and new entrants from insurance and pharmacy chains change the landscape of care (Scheffler, 2021). Many of these acquisitions are followed by streamlining and downsizing or refocusing delivery to more profitable sectors. Approval of these changes of ownership typically does not consider the impact on communities of color or other underserved communities. To the extent that the "losers" in these transactions are in areas of higher need but lower purchasing power, with no political power and no social capital, existing disparities may be exacerbated. However, it is not unreasonable to include consideration of the impact on underserved communities as part of the evaluation by the Justice Department, although this is not currently on any agenda because antitrust is dominated by legal and economic factors.

FUTURE CHALLENGES TO FINANCE AND POLICY REGARDING HEALTH DISPARITIES

The tools of finance as levers to implement policy will continue to be a key part of how we address disparities. All of the individual approaches discussed previously will continue to be important. But there are overarching issues that will continue to challenge our approach to minimizing disparities. The big ones are (a) how we deal with differing underlying risks among individuals and across population groups, (b) institutional racism and unconscious bias in the healthcare system, and (c) social determinants of health.

Inherent Differences in Risk Across Populations

The understandable desire to pay for value versus just volume in healthcare will not abate. But the definition of value is problematic. Now we have a fairly simplistic view of healthcare value, using relevant but imprecise metrics of quality and process as a proxy for value. But this does not recognize the fact that in most markets, the participants judge the product or service from their own perspective and vary as to what is more important in determining value. This determines how they choose and what they are willing to pay (Kahneman, 2000).

In a similar way, a disadvantaged group may be concerned with certain aspects of care (e.g., access, clinical quality) more than others (e.g., safety, resource use). Within major categories of value metrics used in value-based payment schemes, the group may consider some much more important (e.g., physician communication vs. whether their hospital room was quiet at night). Uniformly applying one set of measures may lead to care that is seen as less valuable to a specific population of concern. Value in most markets is relative, not absolute, since individuals vary in taste, need, and willingness to pay. However, in healthcare where there are absolutes (mortality and infection rates, for instance), it is harder to accept this. Therefore, we will continue to wrestle with whether there is an ultimate goal of health services and find it very difficult to differentiate its meaning for various groups. As a result, policy and payment can only reflect imperfectly what each person may value most. The obvious solution is to ask members of each group directly.

But even more problematic is the potential exclusion of some patients altogether based on the prior probability of having poor statistical results. A patient with diabetes and a higher body mass index (BMI) may never receive a knee replacement and thus be may restricted to a sedentary life. Unless we figure out how to do a better job of measuring risk and correcting for it in payment processes, this will continue to be a danger.

Institutional Racism and Unconscious Bias

There is probably no other factor more important than racism as a cause of disparities in healthcare. The insidious part of this is that most people in healthcare probably do not see how this might play out. We are largely past the obvious racism that showed up vividly in segregated facilities and other institutions across America. Now there is generally good access to care, except where a group is excluded by other factors such as insurance (e.g., work requirements) or location (e.g., closure of rural or urban facilities). But people of color still have poorer outcomes even if they have insurance, a high level of education, and access to healthcare. Targeting governmental regulations, payment, and review processes in an attempt to change these outcomes may be exceptionally difficult since they are driven by other factors. Among these are the diversity and training of health professionals who still are predominantly White (see www.ncbi.nlm.nih.gov/pmc/articles/PMC3863700).

It may be only through broad societal approaches to understanding and education that these deep-seated issues can be fully addressed. On the other hand, systematic bias in hiring and promotion all through the delivery system can be addressed through required disclosures and even differential payment. Simply training staff to recognize bias is a good start. In other words, where it is possible to measure the direct impact of racism, there is a chance to partially address it. On the other hand, if we don't provide the education and incentives for each healthcare provider and institution to change the way they staff, promote, provide care, and design systems one by one, then widespread change will not be possible. It's not through some general change in the environment, but in the hearts and minds of each provider and policymaker and through sources of financing, that systemic racism is eliminated.

Social Determinants of Health

One glimmer of hope in addressing social determinants of health lies in developing better ways to measure it at a population level and pay for it accordingly. Health systems that receive a higher percentage of payment that is at risk for population-level cost and outcomes have more freedom to invest in whatever it takes to achieve these goals. Recently, even Medicare Advantage plans that receive a flat amount per member per month are now allowed to spend some of it on housing, food, and other ways to address social determinants of health. With the proper incentives, providers will do this voluntarily since the link between these interventions and overall cost and outcome metrics make it a good investment. Accountable Care Organizations and other care covered by alternative payment schemes will follow. This will make a difference if these initiatives are proven to be serious and effective ways to address underlying social determinants of health. However, such efforts must persist for years, not months, until they are effective.

Beyond what healthcare institutions can do, there is the issue of changing the self-defeating behavior of some individuals suffering from disparities. Poor choices of food (often in food deserts), alcoholism and drug use (diseases of despair), gun violence (resulting from inadequate laws), and others add to the health problems of many Americans. But these may often be worse for lower sociodemographic groups. The solutions will rarely be healthcare delivery interventions alone. In the near term, the tools of behavioral economics that are designed to make it easy to do the right things can help. For instance, how food is presented and sold can have a major impact on choices (Thaler, 2008). Making it easier to learn about insurance options on the public health insurance exchanges, and making it automatic or easy to enroll in Medicaid, might help. In addition, addressing education deficits and income inequality that prevent progress are critical rather than just looking to healthcare as the focus of change.

CONCLUSIONS

Some might be tempted to think that all of our disparity issues can be corrected through policy ("Just make them do it") or finance ("Just pay them to do it"). Unfortunately, these are only tools with limited effectiveness that can be used with varying degrees of skill and success in targeted situations. They also are probably most useful in changing marginal decisions and actions of those who are already prepared to change. Thus, the attitude and understanding of both those suffering from disparities and those who seek to eliminate them is the underlying prerequisite for change. It even may be that we are in an eternal battle with no final success, since correcting one disparity may reveal or even lead to another. Much like our recent experience with COVID-19 and its variants, we can learn from one crisis how better to intervene in the next one or even prevent it. But we have to look at the evidence and remain vigilant and inventive.

The bottom line is that it is a journey to solve our problems with disparities rather than a fixed destination. Yet having a clear view of the path ahead will help, along with a perspective on which tools may be more effective. Improving our healthcare and making it available to all requires knowledge and determination. If we apply as much effort to the practice of improvement as we do to the science of biomedical discovery, all things are possible.

DISCUSSION QUESTIONS

1. Using the policy cycle (Figure 3.2), trace the evolution of hospital payment from simple cost-based systems to complicated Medicare value-based payment. Why did the major changes happen?
2. Consider specific disparities in each of the three policy areas (cost, quality, and access) and the most effective methods that have been used to address them. Why were some more successful than others?
3. Argue for or against the following statement: We would like to believe that no one sets out to purposely create disparities.
4. Identify one disparity created indirectly as a result of an attempt to address some other policy objective, and another arising from more fundamental societal factors. How can each type be addressed?

ADDITIONAL RESOURCE

www.ncbi.nlm.nih.gov/pmc/articles/PMC3863700

REFERENCES

Baker, A. E. (2016, July). Counterproductive consequences of a conservative ideology: Medicaid expansion and personal responsibility requirements. *American Journal of Public Health, 106*(7), 1181–1187.

Berwick, D. E. (2008, May/June). The triple aim: Care, health, and cost. *Health Affairs, 27*(3), 759–769.

Conrad, D. (2015, November 9). The theory of value-based payment incentives and their application to health care. *Health Services Research, 50*(52), 2057–2089.

Crook, H. E. (2021, February). How are payment reforms addressing social determinants of health? Policy implications and next steps. *Milbank Memorial Issue Brief*, 1–19.

Diamond, D. (2021, July 16). Nearly all hospitals flout federal requirements to post prices, report finds. *Washington Post*.

Employee Benefit Research Institute. (2021). Workplace health coverage benefits: Facts and figures. EBRI.

Engleberg, A. (2015, October 29). How government policy promotes high drug prices. *Health Affairs Blog*.

Feldstein, P. (2019). Health policy issues: An economic perspective (7th ed.).American College of Healthcare Executives.

French, M. E. (2016, June 5). Key provisions of the patient protection and Affordable Care Act (ACA): A systematic review and presentation of early research findings. *Health Services Research, 51*(5), 1735–1771.

Garg, A. E. (2019, April). Addressing social determinants of health: Challenges and opportunities in a value-based model. *Pediatrics, 143*(4), 2018–2355.

Gaynor, M. (2014, June). Competition policy in health care markets: Navigating the enforcement and policy maze. *Health Affairs, 33*(6), 1088–1093.

Guerwich, D. E. (2020, February 19). Addressing social determinants of health within healthcare delivery systems: A framework to ground and inform health outcomes. *Journal of General Internal Medicine, 35*(5), 1571–1575.

Herring, B. (2018, February 13). Comparing the value of nonprofit hospitals' tax exemption to their community benefits. *Inquiry: The Journal of Health Care Organization, Provision, and Financing, 55*, 1–11.

Hilt, A. (2019, March). Evolving roles of health care organizations in community development. *AMA Journal of Ethics, 21*(3), 201–206.

Juhnke, C. E. (2016). A review on methods of risk adjustment and their use in integrated healthcare systems. *International Journal of Integrated Care, 16*(4).

Kahneman, D. E. (2000). Choices, values, and frames. Cambridge University Press.

Lane-Fall, M. E. (2013). Outcomes measures and risk adjustment. *International Anesthesiology Clinics, 51*(4), 10–21.

Lewin Group. (2021). CMS bundled payments for care improvement advanced model: Year 2 evaluation report. Center for Medicare and Medicaid Services.

Mwachofi, A. E. (2011, August 11). Health care market deviations from the ideal market. *Sultan Qaboos University Medical Journal, 11*(3), 328–337.

Nerenz, D. E. (2021, April 5). Adjusting quality measures for social risk factors can promote equity in health care. *Health Affairs, 40*(4), 637–644.

Pauly, M. (2006). The tax subsidy to employment-based health insurance and the distribution of well-being. *Law and Contemporary Problems, 69*(4), 83–101.

Pinotti, P. (2012, August). Trust, regulation and market failures. *Review of Economics and Statistics, 94*(3), 650–658.

Reinhardt, U. (2019). Priced out: The economic and ethical costs of American health care. Princeton Univ Press.

Rosenbaum, S. E. (2015, July). The value of the nonprofit hospital tax exemption was $24.6 billion in 2011. *Health Affairs, 34*(7), 1225–1233.

Rothman, D. (1993). A century of failure: Health care reform in America. *Journal of Health Politics Policy and Law, 18*(2), 271–286.

Scheffler, R. A. (2021, July 20). Consolidation of hospitals during the COVID-19 pandemic: Government bailouts and private equity. *Milbank Quarterly Opinion*, 1–4.

Stevens, R. (1999). *In sickness and in wealth: American hospitals in the twentieth century*. Johns Hopkins Press.

Thaler, R. A. (2008). *Nudge: Improving decisions about health, wealth, and happiness*. Yale University Press.

White, C. E. (2019). *Prices paid to hospitals by private health plans are high relative to medicare and vary widely*. RAND Corporation.

CHAPTER 4

Major Public Health Issues

Jacquelyn Campbell, Phyllis Sharps, Elizabeth Sloand, Nancy Gentry Russell, and Lucine Francis

LEARNING OBJECTIVES

- Describe the Centers for Disease Control and Prevention's Social Determinants of Health framework as an organizing framework for major public health problems.

- Examine the impact of three specific social determinants (economic stability, social and community context, and neighborhood and built environment) on persistent health disparities that are related to selected major public health issues.

- Describe the relationship of racism with economic stability, social and community context, and the built environment.

- Discuss how poverty, unemployment, and underemployment relate to child and family health.

- Explain how housing instability affects health outcomes including mental illness, chronic health conditions, substance use, and high-risk health behaviors.

- Identify the specific interventions, advocacy strategies, and research that public health professionals can develop and implement to address economic stability, social and community context, and the neighborhood and built environment as related to public health issues.

This chapter uses concepts from the Centers for Disease Control and Prevention's (CDC) Social Determinants of Health (SDOH) framework to describe their influence and impact on selected current major public health issues. The chapter includes recommended strategies for public health practice, scholarship, and policy advocacy.

INTRODUCTION

This chapter highlights major public health issues impacting public health practice, population health, research, and policy. Important concepts and updates from Healthy People 2030 (HP 2030) and the SDOH framework are used to organize some of the most significant public health issues discussed in this chapter.

HP 2030 is the national plan for addressing the most critical public health priorities and challenges. The foundational principles for HP 2030 that have guided the development include the following:

◆ Health and well-being of the population and communities are essential to a fully functioning, equitable society.
◆ Achieving full potential for health and well-being for all provides valuable benefits to society, including lower healthcare costs and more prosperous and engaged individuals and communities.
◆ Healthy physical, social, and economic environments strengthen the potential to achieve health and well-being.
◆ Promoting and achieving the nation's health and well-being is distributed among all stakeholders at the national, state, and local levels, including the public, for-profit, and not-for-profit sectors.
◆ Working to attain the full potential for health and well-being of the population is a component of decision-making and policy formulation across all sectors (CDC, 2021a).

HP 2030 focuses on the health of the nation, with continued emphasis on promotion of health and well-being, reducing health disparities, promotion of equity, and emphasis on shared responsibility for the nation's health across all sectors. HP 2030 groups the leading indicators for the nation's health across 12 topics: access to health services; clinical preventive services; environmental quality; injury and violence; maternal, infant and child health; mental health; nutrition; physical activity and obesity; oral health; reproductive and sexual health; social determinants; and substance abuse and tobacco (CDC, 2021a). The HP 2030 framework groups the objectives into three categories: core, developmental, and research objectives. There are 355 measurable core objectives, which have 10-year targets and evidence-based interventions developed using nationally representative data, and are valid and reliable (CDC, 2021a). The 114 developmental objectives also have evidence-based interventions but no reliable baseline data. The 40 research objectives have no associated evidence-based interventions (CDC, 2021a). These objectives will be used to monitor the nation's progress toward meeting the outcomes associated with the objectives and indicators of improved national health and well-being.

The SDOH framework was first incorporated into Healthy People in 2020, highlighting its importance and emphasizing that environmental conditions related to where people are born, live, learn, work, play, worship, and age significantly influence health. HP 2030 continues to emphasize and incorporate the SDOH framework as an ideal method to organize the intersectionality of public health issues and environmental health conditions, health behaviors, and individual influences. Focusing on public health issues in this manner integrates major concepts fundamental to public health practice and theoretical frameworks, such as persons, populations, environment, health, and systems of healthcare. It also lends itself well to the recommendations and implications for public health practice, scholarship, and advocacy (Figure 4.1).

OVERVIEW OF THE SOCIAL DETERMINANTS OF HEALTH FRAMEWORK

The SDOH framework was developed to acknowledge that health is influenced by homes, schools, workplaces, neighborhoods, and communities (CDC, 2021a). The SDOH framework recognizes that there are economic and physical conditions in the places where people live, attend school, work, and play that have great impact on health. The CDC first used the SDOH framework to establish the Healthy People 2020 objectives and has continued to incorporate the framework for HP 2030 goals for the nation's health. The HP 2030 objectives

Social Determinants of Health

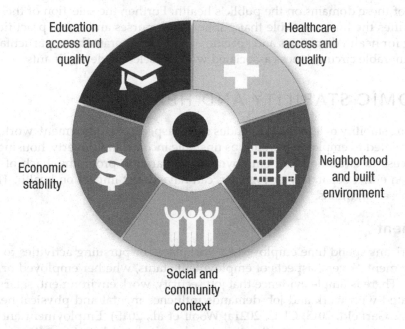

Figure 4.1 Social Determinants of Health framework.

Source: U.S. Department of Health and Human Services, Office of Disease Prevention and Health Promotion. (n.d.). *Healthy People 2030.* https://health.gov/healthypeople/objectives-and-data/social-determinants-health.

include many objectives that address the SDOH framework, with 10-year targets to monitor the achievement of the objectives (CDC, 2021a). The HP 2030 objectives along with the SDOH are designed to help the nation as well as local communities in setting specific targets and using evidence-based interventions to monitor data related to outcomes.

The SDOH framework has five key determinants: (a) economic stability, (b) education access and quality, (c) social and community context, (d) healthcare access and quality, and (e) neighborhood and built environment. Each determinant involves specific, important public health issues that can become the target of disease prevention and health promotion initiatives. *Economic stability* includes employment, food insecurity, housing instability, and poverty. *Education* includes early childhood education, high school graduation, higher education, and language and literacy. *Social and community context* includes civic participation, discrimination, incarceration, and social cohesion. *Healthcare* includes key issues such as access to healthcare, access to primary care, and health literacy. The fifth determinant, *neighborhood and built environment*, includes crime and violence, environmental conditions, quality of housing, and access to nutritious foods.

In this chapter, three of the determinants and related major public health issues are highlighted: economic stability, social and community context, and neighborhood and built environment. Many of the underlying SDOH that significantly influence population health and major public health issues are intertwined and intrinsically related to economic and social interactions and the communities where people reside. The economic stability section discusses the major public health issues of employment, food insecurity, housing instability, and poverty. Some public health issues related to racism and discrimination, family violence, incarceration, and social cohesion are discussed as they are influenced by the social and community context determinant. Important public health issues as they pertain to the neighborhood and built environment determinant include a discussion of important public health issues related to access to food, crime and violence, environmental conditions, and quality of housing. These three determinants have been selected to highlight the impact and interaction of these domains on the public's health. Further, the selection of these determinants magnifies the important role that public health nurses and nurse practitioners have in assessing for health disparities and specific ways to ameliorate them, particularly among those in vulnerable circumstances associated with the selected determinants.

ECONOMIC STABILITY AND HEALTH

The economic stability determinant includes many aspects of employment, work, and other conditions related to employment, such as unstable income and poverty, housing, food status, and access to education and employment preparation programs. Each of these conditions, taken either separately or together, can have direct impact on health. This section examines these conditions.

Employment

Many Americans spend time employed at workplaces or pursuing activities to help them gain employment. Several aspects of employment status, whether employed or not, influence health. There is ample evidence that job security, work environment, salary, and benefits associated with work and job demands influence mental and physical health status (Antonisse & Garfield, 2018; CDC, 2021a; Woolf et al., 2015). Employment and adequate financial compensation, along with other employee-related benefits, often provide better health-related options to the employee than the options available to the unemployed. Recent data from the Kaiser Family Foundation [KFF] (2021) reveal that about 49% of the U.S. total population has employer-sponsored health insurance. Their data also show that states in the Midwest and Northeast have higher percentages of people benefiting from employer-sponsored health insurance than states in other geographical regions of the country (KFF, 2021). Medical care coverage and other paid benefits also vary depending on type of job and full-time and part-time worker status. The 2020 data from the U.S. Bureau of Labor Statistics (BLS, 2020a) indicate that of civilian workers (individuals working more than 1 hour per week for a wage or salary, at least 15 hours per week unpaid in a family business or farm, or self-employed), 51% had access to medical plans and 78% had paid sick leave. Among workers in private industry, 48% had access to medical care plans and 75% had access to paid sick leave, which is low compared with state and local government workers, 89% of whom had access to medical care plans and 91% to paid sick leave. Access to other benefits, such as paid family leave, holidays, wellness programs, and contributions to retirement plans (BLS, 2020a) vary across categories and may minimize pay disruptions and also increase options for maintaining stable housing in desirable locations that offer access to wholesome food, quality public and private education for children, higher education, places to exercise safely, and other resources that promote good health and lessen risks for disabling and chronic diseases. Most Americans are employed, with the highest rate of 61% reported prior to the full impact of the 2020 pandemic (BLS, 2020a). The average U.S. jobless rate, which has been impacted by the 2020 COVID-19 pandemic, stands at 5.4% (BLS, 2022).

Rates of employment have some variability across racial/ethnic groups and gender. Labor force participation is similar across racial groups, with Asian Americans at 63.5%, White Americans at 62.8%, and Black Americans at 62.3%. Ethnic group data describing labor force participation indicate slight variability with Native Hawaiians/Other Pacific Islanders at 68.5%, people of two or more races at 66.6%, Hispanic Americans at 66.3%, and American Indian/Alaska Natives with the lowest rates at 59.6% (BLS, 2019). Gender labor force participation data show that Hispanic American adult males are the largest employed race and ethnicity group (80.2%). and Black American adult men have a lower rate of labor force participation (68%). Among women, labor force participation reveals that Black American adult women have the highest employment rate (62.4%), followed by Hispanic American women (59.4%), and Asian American women (58.6%), with White American women having the lowest labor force participation rate at 57.6% (BLS, 2019). Unemployment also varies by race and ethnic group, and the data reveal that American Indians/Alaska Natives and Black Americans have the highest unemployment rates at 6.5% and Asian Americans have the lowest unemployment rates at 3% (BLS, 2019). Racial unemployment rates from lowest to highest rates are Asian Americans 3%, White Americans 3.5%, Hispanic Americans 4.7%, Native Hawaiian/Other Pacific Islander 5.3%, two or more races 5.5%, Black Americans 6.5%, and America Indian/Alaska Natives 6.6%.

Examining the educational status of the workforce reveals that two thirds of those in the U.S. labor force have at least some college education. Specifically, 60% of Asian Americans and 43% of White Americans in the workforce had obtained at least a bachelor's degree, compared with 28% of Black Americans and 20% of Hispanic Americans, who had attained at least a bachelors' degree. In contrast, 26% of Hispanic Americans had less than a high school education compared with 7% of Black Americans, 6% of Asian Americans, and 4% of White Americans with less than a high school education (BLS, 2017). In general, women in the workforce have obtained less education than men. The exception is at the doctoral degree level, which more women (78.2%) have achieved compared with men (76.6%) Higher education status is associated with increased participation in the labor force, increased likelihood of managerial or professional jobs with higher salaries, more work-associated benefits (BLS, 2017, 2019), and improved health outcomes. Earnings increase with educational level; those with master's degrees and professional degrees earn about three times more (>$1,600/wk) than those with less than high school diplomas ($504/wk; BLS, 2017).

Many research studies provide ample evidence of the important benefits to health and well-being for those who are employed (Antonisse & Garfield, 2018; Khullar & Chokshi, 2018; DeRigne et al., 2016). Benefits often associated with employment include health insurance, paid sick leave, parental leave, maternity leave, and family medical leave that allows time off to care for other family members without losing a job (U.S. Department of Labor, 2017). Data from 2017 indicated that 70% of civilian workers, 67% of private industry workers, and 89% of local and state government employees had health insurance. Two main benefits of health insurance that promote health include (a) greater access to affordable medical care and (b) greater financial security, which can prevent the downward spiral of unpaid medical bills that may lead to bankruptcy and can threaten ability to pay for food, childcare, housing, and other life essentials (Sommers et al., 2017). Some employers offer maternity leave, either paid or unpaid; for women who have access to maternity leave, positive outcomes have been documented for women and children, such as less time off from work and school and less time working while sick (Burtle & Bezruchka, 2016). In a recent review of the relationship between work and health using more than 50 publications and other resources, there was strong evidence that overall, work is good for health and well-being—it reduces the risk for depression and it improves mental health (Antonisse & Garfield, 2018).

Unemployment has also been shown to affect physical and mental health (CDC, 2021a). Limited research has shown that unemployment, unstable work, or poor working conditions may have a negative effect on health. While there are fewer studies of the adverse impact of poor working conditions on health, there is growing evidence of these associations (Conway et al., 2017; Khullar & Chokshi, 2018). Work-related accidents from poorly maintained equipment, repetitive lifting, or pushing heavy equipment can result in accident-related injuries. Exposures to certain industrial chemicals, pesticides, asbestos, and aerosols can lead to adverse health outcomes (Egerter et al., 2008). More recent studies provide additional evidence of workplace exposures and adverse health outcomes related to respiratory and pulmonary diseases (Clarke et al., 2021; Silver et al., 2021). Work-related injuries and environmental exposures result in absences from work and potential income loss, long-term disability, and, in extreme cases, fatalities (Marrone & Swarbrick, 2020). Access to long- and short-term disability insurance varies with employment status (full time or part time) and employer (civilian, private, or government) and affects employees' ability to maintain work status as well as stability in their living situation (BLS, 2019).

Some work-related factors have been associated with psychological stress and other adverse physical and mental health outcomes, including demanding and high-pressure environments, high levels of interpersonal conflict, evening/night shift work or working longer than 8 hours per day, working multiple jobs, and having to withstand difficult work cultures, conditions, and environment (Conway et al., 2017; McHugh et al., 2019). Employees struggling with stress are at increased risk for depression, and their stress may spill over into family interactions, thereby increasing risk for domestic conflicts as well as impaired job performance (Sabbath et al., 2015; Smith et al., 2017). Some employees adopt unhealthy coping behaviors such as smoking and alcohol and drug misuse, both of which may influence job performance, other accidents, and the ability to maintain and support healthy family functioning and well-being (Sabbath et al., 2015). Gender and racial/ethnic backgrounds also relate to adverse work experiences. Some studies suggest that work has different impacts on women's health compared with men's health and that women may experience more stress and fear for personal safety due to male harassment (Logan & Walker, 2017; Quinn & Smith, 2018). More people of color, 20%, are employed in jobs that require heavy lifting and operating machinery, which increases their risk for injury and illness, compared with 13% of White people (Doede, 2016). Other differences in job activities or roles, such as lack of autonomy (nonsupervisory positions), minimal flexibility in work hours, and occupational exposures, may also be associated with anxiety, depression, physical pain, missed days from work, and decreased life expectancy (Doede, 2016; Goh et al., 2015; Ingram et al., 2021). The jobs and roles with lower levels of autonomy and minimal flexibility are often disproportionately held by racial and ethnic minorities.

Researchers have seldom studied unemployment and its impact on health. Low or no income is associated with fewer resources to meet housing, food, and health-related needs, further increasing risk for adverse health outcomes (Berkowitz & Basu, 2021). People who are unemployed report feelings of depression, anxiety, low self-esteem, demoralization, worry, and physical pain (Antonisse & Garfield, 2018). Other studies show that people who are unemployed report more stress-related illnesses such as high blood pressure, stroke, heart attack, heart disease, and arthritis (Antonisse & Garfield, 2018).

A recent study of the increased federal payments of unemployment insurance during the 2020 pandemic provided evidence that provision of this benefit was associated with lower risk for unmet health-related social needs, for delayed healthcare, and for depressive and anxiety symptoms, and may have helped to mitigate economic disruption related to joblessness (Berkowitz & Basu, 2021).

Recommended Strategies and Interventions

The HP 2030 goal for economic stability, "Help people earn steady incomes that allow them to meet their needs," underscores the importance of work. Work can have positive impacts on health and well-being, as well as provide access to money, benefits, and other resources that promote and maintain health for individuals and families. Conversely, poor and unsafe workplaces and unemployment can have negative consequences for physical and mental health. Nurses and all health professionals can advocate for livable wages that promote accessing secure stable housing in safe neighborhoods, adequate food, and adequate educational resources, all of which are necessary for health, well-being, and improved quality of life. All health professionals can advocate for work-related health insurance and workplace health and wellness programs (Robert Wood Johnson, 2018), particularly focusing on people holding lower-wage jobs, or advocate for national universal health insurance. They can also advocate for safe workplaces, including aspects related to equipment, exposures, interpersonal interaction management, workplace safety, and adequate recreational and exercise opportunities (Sorenson et al., 2018). Additional research is needed to better understand the beneficial aspects of work for health and the adverse effects of unsafe work environments, underemployment, and unemployment.

Unstable Income and Poverty

Poverty is a closely related aspect of economic stability in the SDOH framework. Poverty is the condition in which an individual or a community lacks sufficient funds or resources to secure adequate housing, food, clothing, medical care, and other essentials (Giannarelli et al., 2021). In the United States, poverty is defined and measured by the Census Bureau using primarily economic metrics. The U.S. national poverty indicator is based on family income and family size. For example, in 2021, for a family of four, the poverty level is $26,500. In the U.S., 34 million people, or 10.9% of the population, live in poverty (U.S. Census Bureau, 2019). Prior to the 2020 pandemic, poverty rates had dropped consistently for the 5 years between 2014 and 2019 (Giannarelli et al., 2021). The 2020 pandemic increased the U.S. 2021 poverty rate to 13.7% (Giannarelli et al., 2021).

Poverty in the United States varies across racial and ethnic groups, gender, age, family size, and state of residence. States with the highest rates of poverty are primarily in the South and include Mississippi, 19.4%; Louisiana, 18.4%; New Mexico, 16.0%; Arkansas, 15.0%; West Virginia, 14.9%; Kentucky, 14.6%; Alabama, 14.4%; and South Carolina, 13.9%. The states with the lowest poverty rates are concentrated primarily in the Mid-Atlantic and Northeast regions and include New Hampshire, 4.9%; Minnesota, 6.8%; Delaware, 6.9%; Utah, 7.1%; New Jersey, 7.3%; Maryland, 7.5%; Washington, 7.8%; Massachusetts, 8.1%; and Kansas and Wisconsin, 8.5% (Amadeo & Estevez, 2021). Women have higher poverty rates (12.9%) compared with men (10.6%); children have higher rates (16.2%) compared with seniors (9.7%), and people living with disabilities have the highest rates at 25.7% (U.S. Census Bureau, 2019). Poverty rates vary across racial/ethnic groups. Native Americans have the highest rate (25.4%), Hispanic Americans have a 21.9% rate, African Americans have a 18.1% rate, and White Americans and Asian Americans have the lowest rates at 10% or less (U.S. Census Bureau, 2019; Giannarelli et al., 2021). Poverty rates for children in the United States decreased from 16.2% in 2018 to 14.4% in 2019 (Kearney, 2019). UNICEF reported that among 41 member countries, child poverty rates varied widely, with Iceland reporting the lowest rates at 10.4% and Turkey reporting the highest rates at 33%. The United States was fourth from the bottom of the UNICEF's list of countries with a child poverty rate of 30% (UNICEF, 2020). Poverty rates for children vary across racial and ethnic groups, similar to adult rates. Black American and Hispanic American children had the highest poverty rates (26% and 21%, respectively) and White American and Asian American children are at 8.3% and 7.3%, respectively. Children living in a mother-only family had a poverty rate of 41%, compared with 8% among children in two-parent families (Kearney, 2019). In general, families headed by women of color have the highest poverty rates. Children residing in Black woman-headed families experienced the highest poverty rate (35%), compared with Hispanic Americans (34%), White Americans (26%), and Asian Americans (22%) for woman-headed families (Single Mothers, 2021). Like poverty among adults, child poverty rates are highest in states in the South (45.1%), followed by the West (23%), with the lowest rates in the Midwest (18.3%; Children's Defense Fund, 2019). A recent report, *The Basic Facts About Child Poverty* (Haider, 2021), identifies many reasons for the persistent U.S. childhood poverty. Reasons include: (a) the U.S. economic system is not designed to support families (i.e., cost of raising children); (b) jobs do not guarantee a standard of living that supports basic family needs; (c) economic inequality; (d) stagnant wages, labor market discrimination, and inequality in wages especially for Black Americans and women; (e) occupation segregation and wage gaps, with Black Americans and women disproportionately represented in low-wage jobs (Shaw et al., 2016); (f) lack of family-work policies that support caregivers, such as paid family and sick leave (Heymann et al., 2021); (g) unemployment; (h7) barriers to employment, including former incarceration (Western & Sirois, 2019); (i) immigration status regardless of citizenship status (Maurer, 2020); and (j) inequalities related to LGBTQ status (Mirza et al., 2018) and disabilities (BLS, 2020b). Other factors that impact children living in poverty are the conditions associated with poverty. These factors include segregated neighborhoods of concentrated poverty and low-resource schools not able to meet children's learning needs. The schools often enforce disciplinary polices that disproportionately target low-income, disabled, and Black students, and are ultimately linked to high school dropout rates. Children dropping out of school lead to increased incarceration and has created what has become known as the "school-to-prison pipeline" (Aronowitz et al., 2021; Goldstein et al., 2021). While there has been some narrowing of the educational gaps for Black and Hispanic Americans, America Indian children have not fared as well. The long-term historical impact of the American Indian Boarding Schools initiative lingers (Native Americas, 2015). Native American/Alaska Native (NA/AN) children make up 1% of the children in K-12 public schools. Ninety-five percent NA/AN youth attend public schools, and a smaller number attend schools administered by the Bureau of Indian Education (BIE; Cai, 2020). Decades after the American Indian Boarding Schools initiative, the gap in education achievement for NA children remains. NA students are the only group in which there has been no improvement in math and reading scores (Cai, 2020). On average, NA/AN youth have the lowest high school graduation rates (74% compared with the national average of 85%; Cai, 2020), and even fewer enroll in colleges (Cai, 2020). The plight of these youth may also be related to high rates of poverty, attendance at low-resource schools, the impact of digital divide, and lack of NA/AN teachers (Cai, 2020; Haider, 2021; Table 4.1).

Poverty has been shown to have important effects on individual and family health due to a lack of consistent financial and other resources associated with health maintenance and health promotion. People living in poverty often reside in neighborhoods with structural barriers that have also been associated with poorer health outcomes. They often reside in communities with poor-quality, high-density, and overcrowded housing; higher crime rates; less access to fresh, nutritious foods; higher density of fast-food restaurants and alcoholic beverage stores; poorer-quality public schools; and a built environment that does not allow for safe health promotion activities (Khullar & Chokshi, 2018). Oftentimes, people experiencing poverty reside in communities that have high levels of pollutants, high noise levels, and lack of green space (Khullar & Chokshi, 2018; Twohig-Bennett & Jones, 2018). These living conditions increase risks for chronic diseases, which contribute to the persistent health

TABLE 4.1 Department of Health and Human Services Poverty Guidelines for 2021*

Number of Persons in Family/Household	Poverty Guideline
1	$12,800
2	$17,420
3	$21,960
4	$26,500
5	$31,040
6	$35,580
7	$40,120
8	$44,660

*2021 Poverty guidelines for the 48 contiguous states and the District of Columbia. For families/households with more than 8 persons, add $4,540 for each additional person.
Source: U.S. Department of Health and Human Services, Federal Register Notice, February 1, 2021. https://aspe.hhs.gov/poverty-guidelines.

disparities related to hypertension, cardiovascular disease, cancers, obesity, and behavioral health conditions, further contributing to major public health problems. Poverty has a significant impact on children, often with long-term consequences. Children growing up in poverty have poorer physical and mental health, are more likely to reside in segregated neighborhoods with high adult unemployment, and are more likely to attend lower-quality schools with limited resources (Kearney, 2019). Children living in poverty often reside in neighborhoods that do not have resources that support outside enrichment activities and sports and are not safe for outdoor activities, which are conditions that may lend themselves to early-onset obesity (Kearney, 2019).

The onset of negative health consequences during childhood can influence adult onset of health conditions associated with cardiometabolic problems (Khullar & Chokshi, 2018). The landmark CDC-Kaiser Adverse Childhood Experiences (ACEs) study provided compelling research data showing the impact on adult health (Anda et al., 2008). ACEs include *abuse* (emotional, physical, sexual), *household dysfunction* (witnessing mother abused, household substance abuser, mental illness in the household, parental separation or divorce) and *neglect* (emotional, physical). Data have shown that children with 4+ ACEs have almost three times poorer health compared to those with no ACEs (Boullier & Blair, 2018). Adult chronic conditions such as hypertension, diabetes, cardiometabolic conditions, mental health, and use of psychotropic drugs are increased compared to those with no ACES (Boullier & Blair, 2018). These childhood adverse situations and conditions can cascade downward and hinder opportunities for high-school graduation and post high-school education and thereby result in fewer opportunities for adult roles with adequate employment and income and access to housing, food, and other resources that promote quality of life and lifelong health and wellness (Kearney, 2019; Cai, 2020).

Recommendations for Policies and Interventions to Address Poverty

Public health professionals and social service agents are keenly aware of the impact of poverty on the health of individuals, children, families, and communities (Brown et al., 2019). They can play key roles in helping others understand the health impacts of policy and can be strong advocates for policy changes that strengthen the health of those living in poverty. There are several existing policies in the form of federal and state government aid that are designed to help protect families against the negative health consequences of poverty. Many federal government entitlement programs use the Federal Poverty Level to determine eligibility to receive these benefits: Supplemental Nutrition Assistance Program (SNAP) for families earning 130% or lower of the poverty level; Medicaid and the Affordable Care Act (ACA), which provides low-cost health insurance to families earning between 138% and 400% of the poverty level; and the Children's Health Insurance Program (CHIP) for families at or below 200% of the poverty level (Benefits, 2019; Giannarelli et al., 2021; U.S. Government, 2020). Other policy initiatives are designed to support individuals and families struggling with poverty and support positive behavioral changes or otherwise promote health; these include "sin taxes" on cigarettes or sweet beverages; higher minimum wages to help individuals and families survive; the Earned Income Tax Credit designed to support working families with children; and the expansion of state Medicaid programs (Czapp & Kovach, 2015; Khullar & Chokshi, 2018). To date, 12 states have declined participation in the Medicaid Expansion (KKF, 2021; Ali et al., 2015). The 12 states are primarily in the South and Midwest, where poverty rates are higher. Many people living in these areas remain uninsured with limited access to treatment for behavioral health disorders, including mental health and substance use disorder and mental illnesses (Ali et al., 2015).

Medicaid includes prenatal and postpartum care in its core adult services. Medicaid funding has financed 43% of all births. Additionally, among the states choosing not to offer the ACA Medicaid Expansion, postpartum care beyond 60 days is not covered. If all states offered the Medicaid expansion specifically to expand postpartum care for women and infants beyond 60 days, there would likely be a significant decrease in maternal and child health disparities (Katch, 2020). In clinical practice arenas, public health nurses, social workers, and public health clinicians can specifically screen for socioeconomic conditions of families and communities to determine resources that are present and accessible, as well as barriers to accessing resources. Working with individuals, families, or communities, public health nurses and public health nurse practitioners can develop realistic plans of action. For example, they can help families find relief programs in their communities, such as food banks or infant diaper distribution sites, or assist in locating free or low-cost legal assistance to address housing or utility debt relief and to develop plans for self-help and autonomy. Those who have recently obtained health insurance may also need help with navigating the health system to obtain health services (Czapp & Kovach, 2015).

Nurses and all professionals, regardless of settings, can advocate for culturally sensitive clinical practice that includes understanding cultural practices related to health, using language-congruent providers or certified medical interpreters, and offering written, digital, and virtual resources at appropriate literacy levels and in languages consistent with the population being served (Czapp & Kovach, 2015). Public health nurses, public health professionals, and community organization staff persons can advocate for culturally competent, community-based research that further explores the impact of poverty on health and evidence-based programs that help ameliorate the negative health consequences of poverty. A broad agenda that includes findings from culturally responsive community-based research, as well as impact of existing programs on family and childhood poverty, barriers for families, better definitions, and data collection methods for indicators of poverty will be essential for developing plans to reduce and eliminate the causes of the poverty and to improve overall quality of life (Le Menestrel & Duncan, 2019).

Housing Instability

The relationship between housing instability and poor health outcomes has been extensively documented (Cutts et al., 2015; Levinson Publications Group, 2004). People having housing instability experience increased morbidity related to chronic health conditions, mental illness, substance use, and risky health behaviors compared with peers who are housed. They also experience increased all-cause mortality (Cutts et al., 2015). Data also show that minority racial and ethnic groups (Black, Hispanic, and Asian Americans) have higher housing hardships (Fernald, 2021; Sandel et al., 2018). The lack of affordable housing and current housing policies in the United States is linked to the increase in housing instability, particularly among Black, Latino, and Native Americans. Black Americans are more likely than White Americans (or Americans of any other race/ethnicity) to be extremely low-income renters, falling at or below the poverty line for household income (Aurand et al., 2020). Twenty percent of Black American households where homes are rented have household incomes at or below the poverty line (Aurand et al., 2020). Low-income renters who are Black or Hispanic Americans used governmental supplements during the pandemic toward food (60%), utilities (63%), and rent (53%). Even with this support, however, these Americans were the most burdened with rental payments (Fernald, 2021). The 2020 U.S. Census (Center on Budget and Policy, 2021) shows that these patterns related to Black and Hispanic American renters were present before the pandemic and were also exacerbated by the pandemic. The 2020 U.S. Census showed that at least 60 million people, or 25% of all adults, were having difficulty paying rents/mortgages, with Black and Latino Americans reporting this difficulty at much higher rates (44%) than Asian (22%) and White Americans (20%). Among adults with children living in the household, 33% had difficulty meeting rent or mortgage expenses, compared with 22% of households without children (Center on Budget and Policy Priorities, 2021).

Adverse effects of the 2020 COVID-19 pandemic, particularly loss of employment, have only worsened this problem, further increasing housing instability. Other issues disproportionately experienced by people of color that increase vulnerability to housing instability include exposure to community and family violence, substance use disorders, hypertension, cardiovascular conditions, and mental and physical disabilities, all of which have increased during the global pandemic crisis (Center on Budget and Policy Priorities, 2021; Sandel et al., 2018; Taylor, 2018). Decreased access to needed resources and services further compounds housing instability for those in poverty, particularly in Black American, Hispanic American, and American Indian/Native American populations.

Recommended Advocacy for Addressing Housing Instability

Re-envisioning of the U.S. national housing policy is critically needed. Public health professionals, through their local and national professional associations, can join the efforts of other community advocates for new approaches and strategies to alleviate housing challenges, including preparing background information and data regarding health issues and giving testimony. Important actions and policy remedies include addressing the legal and structural barriers that support racial segregation in housing. Nurses and all other health professionals can advocate for subsidies, housing choice vouchers, and tax incentives that promote affordable housing inventories and provide low-income individuals and families with more and better viable housing choices. Public health nurses join with other public health professionals to provide housing education and counseling to individuals and families, so they have the information needed to make informed choices and take advantage of available resources (Fernald, 2020).

Food Insecurity in the United States

Food insecurity (FI), defined as reduction of food intake or disrupted eating patterns due to limited access to funds or resources, currently affects nearly 14 million households in the United States (Coleman-Jensen et al., 2020). FI disproportionately affects people of color, people living in poverty, single people with children, middle-aged and older adults, and adults with disabilities and multiple chronic diseases (Coleman-Jensen et al., 2020; Lopez-Landin, 2013; Maynard et al., 2019). Despite efforts to provide food safety nets through federal nutrition programs such as SNAP, FI persists due to the increasing costs of nutritious foods and the presence of food deserts that are pervasive in low-resourced and low-income communities (Brownell & Frieden, 2009; Putnam et al., 2002).

The health effects of FI are far-reaching. At times, people experiencing FI are compelled to purchase cheaper foods that are less nutritious, consequently consuming foods higher in sugar, fat, and salt (Leung et al., 2014). Poor diet is a risk factor for multiple chronic diseases, including heart disease, dysglycemia, cancer, brain diseases, and obesity (National Center for Chronic Disease Prevention and Health Promotion, 2021). Pandemic-related school closings created major food insecurity for children who were dependent on school breakfasts and lunches (Kinsey et al., 2020).

Recommendations and Strategies for Addressing Food Insecurity

The provisions outlined in the American Nurses Association (ANA) Code of Ethics show that nurses have an ethical mandate and obligation to respect human dignity, care for the environment, and promote health and wellness within the lens of social justice (ANA, 2015). Thus, nurses can and should address FI within multiple spheres of influence, including practice, education, research, and advocacy. Across these spheres, screening for SDOH, including FI, and coordinating care to connect persons to resources is a practical and effective approach.

Screening is relatively simple and quick, so that nurses and other healthcare providers who are pressed for time in their practices can do the screening. There is a two-item FI screener, shown to be just as valid and reliable as multi-item FI screeners, that can easily be used in practice and research (Hager et al., 2010). The two items in the screener are as follows:

1. Within the past 12 months, we worried whether our food would run out before we got money to buy more.
2. Within the past 12 months, the food we bought just didn't last and we didn't have money to get more.

The responses to these two statements identify households as being at risk for FI if they indicate that either or both two statements are "often true" or "sometimes true" (vs. "never true").

Nurses in all roles can work to locate accessible community-based organizations that offer food or assist with addressing other SDOH, such as employment and education. One example of a nurse-led, hospital-based intervention that addresses FI is the *Rush Surplus Project*, implemented in Chicago (Grenier & Wynn, 2018). The Rush Surplus Project is a nurse-led collaboration project between Rush Oak Park Hospital and community-based organizations, including schools, childcare centers, and a food pantry. The project aims to "improve the nutritional health of the community through the distribution of surplus food from hospital cafeterias to food insecure families" through repackaging unserved prepared foods from the hospital cafeteria and capitalizing on volunteer support to distribute to families in need. The project is supported by multiple foundations that helped it expand into schools and other locations that serve low-income families. The project has provided hunger relief to about 8,400 families per day and has reduced food and environmental waste. Efforts such as the *Rush Surplus Project* are a testament to what nurses can do in both hospital and community settings. Nurses and public health professionals can also leverage professional organizations with policy influence, such as the ANA, the American Academy of Nursing, the American Public Health Association, and others, to advocate for supportive policies and to vote for those who champion continued and increased budgets for federal nutrition assistance programs.

SOCIAL AND COMMUNITY CONTEXT AND HEALTH

The *social and community context* determinant of health focuses on where people live and work. This aspect of the SDOH includes the interactions and relations between people and the connections that people have with others in their living, work, and social situations. It includes discrimination, civic participation, incarceration, and social cohesion.

Racism and Health

In examining discrimination, we must closely consider racism and its impact on health. There are many definitions of race; however, a definition offered by Harrell (2000) is useful because it integrates concepts from psychology, sociology, and anthropology. Racism is defined as:

> a system of dominance, power, and privilege based on racial group designations; rooted in historical oppression of a group defined or perceived by dominant group members as inferior, deviant or undesirable; and occurring in circumstances where members of the dominant group create or accept their societal privilege by maintaining structures, ideology, values, and behaviors that have the intent or effect of leaving the nondominant group members relatively excluded from power, esteem status and/or equal access to societal resources. (Harrell, 2000; Hicken et al., 2018)

Racial designations are primarily a social categorization based on nationality, ethnicity, phenotype, or other markers of social differences, factors that also reflect different access to power and resources in society (Williams et al., 2019). Racism is based on ideological ideas of the inherent superiority of Whites and the inherent inferiority of people of color, including American Indians, Alaska Natives, Native Hawaiians/Pacific Islanders, Latinx/Hispanic people, and Black people (Jones, 2018).

Racism is a major cause of adverse health outcomes among ethnic and racial minority populations and of inequities in the healthcare system (Williams et al., 2019). Racism in the United States is pervasive in institutional and governmental policies and laws and interacts with individual behaviors and attitudes of racism, all of which contribute to persistent health disparities and inequities for people of color (Williams et al., 2019). As discussed previously, employment status, poverty, housing instability, and food insecurity and their impact on health are all conditions that have been associated with institutional and structural racism. Lack of access to health insurance, and discrimination and prejudice toward people of color, are associated with adverse physical and mental health. Data show that the racism experienced by people of color is a fundamental cause of persistent health inequalities, such as high rates of infant mortality (Alhusen et al., 2017; Braveman et al., 2018; Lorch & Enlow, 2015), decreased life expectancy (Cunningham et al., 2017), continued poorer performance on many of Healthy People 2020 indicators (CDC, 2017). Racism contributes to psychological and physiological stress processes that account for the adverse effects of racism on physical and mental health throughout the lifespan (Bailey et al., 2017). Most research about the effects of racism on health have focused on perceived discrimination and provides evidence of adverse impact on mental health (Williams, 2018), inflammation, cellular aging, and blood pressure (Cunningham et al., 2017).

The structural racism in the healthcare system throughout the United States has also contributed to health disparities. The mistrust that many Black Americans and other groups such as Native Americans, who have experienced systemic racism, have toward the healthcare system, including providers, is often a barrier to access and use of treatment, resources, and advice offered (Boulware et al., 2003). Through the history of medicine and biomedical research, use of enslaved people to test treatment and surgical procedures, and experiments such as the Tuskegee Syphilis study and the Henrietta Lacks cell research, have eroded the trust of Black Americans and other people of color in the healthcare system (Boulware et al., 2003; Wells & Gowda, 2020). Studies have shown that prejudice, bias, and discrimination are part of medical care and result in discrepancies in procedures, treatments, and recommendations for care for people of color (Wells & Gowda, 2020). Many people of color may prefer healthcare providers of color, but institutional and structural racism have been barriers for enrollment and training of health providers of color (Shen et al., 2018). See Chapter 16 for a discussion about workforce issues in the health professions.

Recommended Strategies and Advocacy

There is a continued need for research that examines the multiple forms of racism and how they interact and affect health (Ford et al., 2018). All public health professionals can advocate for and ensure that curricula include antiracism training and that accrediting bodies of health professionals mandate cross-cultural education standards based on implicit bias theory and evidence-based educational tools (Ford et al., 2018). Advocacy is needed for full approval and funding for existing antiracism legislation, public health antiracism research investments, and improving the evidence base on racial inequities in healthcare. Barriers to admission into health professional programs need to be identified and eliminated to help diversify the workforce. Importantly, strong nursing and public health advocacy is needed to rescind federal, state, and local policies and practices that prohibit diversity, equity, and antiracism training as well as education on the history of racism in all health professions (American Public Health Association [APHA], 2020).

Social Cohesion

Public health nurses and healthcare practitioners well understand that distal factors play an important role in individual and community health, and two such distal factors are social cohesion and social capital. Social cohesion, according to Chan et al. (2006, p. 290), may be defined as the "vertical and horizontal interaction among members of society that include trust, a sense of belonging and the willingness to participate and help." Similarly, Kawachi & Berkman (2000) define social cohesion as the "extent of connectedness and solidarity among groups in society" and includes two dimensions: "a sense of belonging to a community and the relationships among members within the community itself." There is some controversy regarding the difference between social cohesion and social capital; the terms are often used synonymously and can also be considered domains of one another (Carpiano, 2006; Carrasco & Bilal, 2016).

Social cohesion is an important factor in the health of individuals, communities, and societies. Community trust, reciprocity, and solidarity have been shown to be related to health outcomes and morbidity and mortality due to infant death, cancers, and cardiac diseases (Kawachi & Berkman, 2000). While social cohesion is considered a group characteristic, it is protective against physical and mental disease in individuals. A recent study of Congolese (Africa) refugees that explored the poor social cohesion that often is part of the refugee experience is an example (Chiumento et al., 2020). The refugees were settled into two different refugee camps, one in Uganda and one in Rwanda, and poor social cohesion was found to be closely associated with poor mental health and suicidal ideation among participants at both sites (Chiumento et al., 2020). The findings confirmed that among these traumatized people who had fled the political conflict in their home country, community and family social connectedness were critical for psychosocial well-being and good mental health.

Another example of the importance of social cohesion in promoting public health is described by Qin et al. (2021), who researched the impact of neighborhood-level factors, such as social cohesion, on older adults' ability to live independently based on their ability to perform activities of daily living (ADLs) and independent activities of daily living (IADLs). Using national data of more than 7,000 older adults living on their own in the community, they found that social cohesion protected the ability of these older adults to perform their ADLs and IADLs independently. Neighborhood social cohesion was characterized by helpful, caring, trustful neighbors, and their presence was associated with better mental and physical health outcomes. The researchers also found that older adults from minority populations (African American and Hispanic American) and women had more limitations in their ADLs and IADLs, which suggests the importance of considering social cohesion when working with these populations and addressing public health disparities in these communities.

Recommended Strategies and Interventions

Given the importance of social cohesion in achieving optimal public health, public health nurses and practitioners can promote social cohesion at the individual, family, community, and systems levels in accordance with the Public Health Intervention Wheel (Minnesota Department of Health, 2019). Collaboration, one of the 17 interventions that compose the wheel, is a key public health nursing intervention that can effectively be used to promote social cohesion. Collaboration of health departments with community organizations was used to decrease the burden of the 2020 COVID-19 pandemic in vulnerable populations in Baltimore, Maryland (Baltimore Sun; Deville, 2021). Health departments and healthcare institutions partnered with faith-based community programs, which can be strong centers of social engagement, to provide COVID-19 testing and vaccination clinics to vulnerable populations with higher rates of COVID-19 infection in the city, thus leveraging social cohesion to decrease public health disparities. A similar effort engaged faith leaders in the San Bernardino area of

California who served the urban Black population and specifically addressed COVID-19 testing barriers related to transportation and computer literacy (Abdul-Mutakabbir et al., 2021). These examples also illustrate how important it is for nurses to understand the critical role that faith-based communities may play in many communities and the potential for working on health issues with faith-based communities and leaders.

In the clinical practice arena, public health nurses and public health practitioners can build on and enhance social cohesion in school nursing and school-based health centers. In these settings, they can intervene through health teaching, health screening, case management, and community organizing while also engaging parents in all these activities. Through advocacy, public health professionals can actively promote and maintain community advisory boards in healthcare settings such as school-based health centers, community health centers, occupational health sites, boards of health, and hospitals. These community advisory boards can help build on and enhance social cohesion for the benefit of the population served.

NEIGHBORHOOD AND BUILT ENVIRONMENT AND HEALTH

Research has shown that neighborhoods are an important determinant of health and impact health as much as the characteristics of individuals residing in the neighborhood (Gomez et al., 2015). The built environment is also critical to health and includes manufactured structures such as buildings, homes, transportation systems, streets, walkways, open spaces, urban spaces, and any physical structures or infrastructures created by human beings (Gascon et al., 2016; Gilbert & Stephens, 2018). Three specific aspects of the neighborhood and built environment are discussed here and include environment and greenspace, quality of housing, and community violence.

Environment and Green Space

In the already-classic 2017 *Lancet* article on structural racism and health inequities, Bailey et al. cite environmental and occupational health inequities as major contributors to health inequities for populations of color. Examples include strategic placement of bus garages and toxic waste sites in or close to neighborhoods where people of color are concentrated, often because of historic redlining (Bravo et al., 2016; Krieger 2014; Mohai et al., 2009); selective government failure to prevent lead leaching into drinking water (as in Flint, Michigan, in 2015 and 2016); and disproportionate exposure of workers of color to occupational hazards (Siqueira et al., 2014). Municipal governments have disinvested in these communities while investing in neighborhoods where there is more affluence (Richards, 2020).

Green space (e.g., parks, trees) is scarcer in urban communities, most often where people of color reside (Twohig-Bennett & Jones, 2018). Greenness has been associated with both lower levels of community violence and better health indices (Mancus & Campbell, 2018). Green space is linked to lower levels of aggression (Kuo & Sullivan, 2001) and improved stress response to experiencing violence among residents (Mancus et al., 2020). Additionally, green space mitigates urban heat island effect, air pollution, and noise pollution (Livesley et al., 2016) and is associated with improved health outcomes such as decreased mortality from cancer, respiratory illness such as childhood asthma, and kidney disease (James et al., 2016).

Recommended Strategies and Advocacy

In addition to the strategies noted to increase the quality of housing, stricter guidelines related to air quality, drinking water, highway construction, and placement of factories must be developed and enforced to protect vulnerable communities. Nurses and other health care leaders can also advocate for increased investment in green space as a critical policy initiative that includes the building and maintenance of large-scale urban gardens as a way to increase green space and decrease food deserts. Other advocacy can be done to promote boarding up empty homes and cleaning up buildings. The proper disposal of trash and garbage is also a concern—clean streets and sidewalks without litter could be maintained by community dwellers, which could galvanize community members and promote a sense of cohesion and belonging.

Quality of Housing

As discussed previously, quality of housing is a key health issue. This is particularly true for those who may spend most of their time at home and/or who are at increased susceptibility to certain toxins and exposures found in the home, such as children, older adults, and those with a disability or who are immunocompromised (World Health Organization [WHO], 2018). There are many aspects of housing quality that can affect a person's health, including "air quality, home safety, space per individual, and the presence of mold, asbestos, or lead," as well as the design and age of the home (Office of Disease Prevention and Health Promotion [ODPHP], n.d., para. 1]. This section highlights two housing factors, air quality and lead, and their relationship to health.

The health effects of poor air quality and lead in housing can be significant (WHO, 2018). Poor housing and indoor air quality is associated with high asthma morbidity in pediatrics (Hughes et al., 2017). In addition to respiratory health, poor indoor air quality can affect numerous other health systems and contribute to early death (WHO, 2018). There are many causes of poor indoor air quality, including inadequate ventilation, which is a key contributor to negative health outcomes (Wimalasena et al., 2021). Dampness and mold growth inside homes are associated with adverse respiratory effects (ODPHP, n.d.; WHO, 2018). Poor housing conditions and lack of maintenance may result in lead exposure, which can cause severe health consequences, including neurological and developmental damages, particularly among children (ODPHP, n.d.; WHO, 2018). The age of the home is also relevant with respect to childhood lead poisoning since many homes built before 1978 contain lead paint (CDC, 2019; 2021b).

Recommended Strategies and Advocacy

As noted previously, public health nurses and public health practitioners play an important role in addressing SDOH, and this includes the quality of housing. Public health personnel should understand and incorporate knowledge of housing quality as a SDOH into practice (National Advisory Council on Nurse Education and Practice [NACNEP], 2019). Addressing and screening for SDOH, including quality of housing, can improve individual and population health outcomes (American Academy of Pediatrics [AAP], 2021; NACNEP, 2019). Policy is another important avenue by which quality of housing and overall population health can be improved. The Health Impact Assessment (HIA) is one approach that can be used to "judge the potential health effects of a policy, program or project on a population, particularly on vulnerable or disadvantaged groups" (WHO, 2021, para. 1). HIAs have been shown to facilitate inclusion of health in housing policies and improve decision-maker and stakeholder relations (Bever et al., 2021). Public health nurses and colleagues can advocate for the use of HIAs and housing policies that intentionally consider and promote health. Working together with school nurses and other community activists to advocate for health programs like lead screening in schools is another strategy that moves healthcare closer to where people live, work, and go to school.

Community Violence

Violence is pervasive in our society and has increasingly demanded more attention from our citizens. National professional organizations have acknowledged violence as a major and persistent public health problem (APHA, 2018; NAS, 2016; American Psychiatric Nurses Association, 2020). The CDC asserts that violence affects individuals, families, and communities, regardless of age, race, and socioeconomic status (CDC, n.d., a). Healthy People 2030 lists prevention of violence and reducing its consequences as a major public health goal for the nation. Much of the violence in the United States is driven by the prevalence of guns and therefore has been received and responded to as a criminal problem, with police, criminal justice, and legal remedies posed as solutions.

Violence is defined as the intentional use of physical force or power to threaten or to act against oneself, another person, or a group or community (WHO, 2020). Violence is described as a health issue resulting from contextual, biological, environmental, systematic, and social stressors (Ferrari et al., 2014). The typology of interpersonal violence includes family and community. Family violence includes physical, sexual, and psychological abuse; deprivation; or neglect against a child, partner, or elder. Community interpersonal violence includes these types of violent acts against an acquaintance or a stranger (WHO, 2020).

Statistics regarding the impact of violence include cost to society and to individuals. It is estimated that family and domestic (child, elder, partner) violence affects the health of 10 million people each year (Huecker et al., 2022). Recent statistics indicate that annually there were more than 39,700 firearm-related deaths, including 23,941 suicides that were committed with firearms, 14,861 people who died from firearm homicides, and approximately 115,000 people who suffered from nonfatal firearm injuries (CDC, n.d., b). Annually, about 3% of firearm deaths are unintentional, undetermined, from legal intervention, or from public mass shootings (UC Davis, 2022). Violence is costly to the nation, to the healthcare system, and to the health of individuals and families. Health impact and healthcare costs are related to premature deaths, years of potential life lost, disability and disability-adjusted life years lost, poor mental health, high medical costs, and lost productivity (CDC, 2022). An annual average estimate of the cost of crime to the nation is more than $2.6 trillion annually. It is also estimated that the cost of crime for each individual taxpayer is about $3,200 per year (Spivak et al., 2019). The cost estimates include individual direct out-of-pocket expenses and direct costs related to police response, medical and behavioral healthcare, victim services, court and child welfare proceedings, incarcerations and other sanctions, and the value of stolen goods and damaged property (Miller et al., 2021).

As with many of the other SDOH and public health issues discussed previously, violence is related to persistent disparities for certain populations and communities. Individuals, families, and communities of color have higher rates of certain types of violence and related health consequences. Spies (2021) report uses Bureau of Justice Statistics throughout to describe the difference in crime data by race. Violence victimization rates reported to police were lower for White Americans (37%) compared with Black and Latinx Americans (49%). Rates of victimization, arrest, and incarceration vary by race. Recent FBI data indicate that Black Americans are overrepresented among people arrested for nonfatal crimes (33%) and serious nonfatal crimes (36%) relative to their proportion in the population (13%; Spies, 2021). Latinx Americans, similarly, are overrepresented among those arrested for nonfatal crimes at 18% compared with their representation in the population (14%; Spies, 2021). White Americans were underrepresented among those arrested for nonfatal crimes at 46% relative to their proportion in the population (52%). In terms of arrests for violent crimes, similar racial disparities exist. Differences in rates are associated with complex contextual conditions that have an adverse impact on communities of color. These individuals and their families often reside in segregated communities, with high unemployment, poor school systems including high dropout rates, inadequate housing, and limited access to healthcare (APHA, 2018). These conditions are also associated with economic instability, largely related to low-wage jobs, which directly affects individuals and families when they attempt to secure adequate and stable housing, access healthful foods, and access high-quality healthcare and other resources that support health and well-being (APHA, 2018). Another devasting impact on these communities is related to the high arrest and incarceration rates of men of color, who are often fathers, thus depriving families of potential income and parental support (Martin, 2017; Sheats et al., 2018). Often individuals and families residing in such conditions cope using tobacco use, alcohol use, overuse/misuse of prescription and other illicit drugs, and overeating, further contributing to health disparities (Meyer et al., 2014). One other concerning issue is the number of single parents with little support from anyone (although some agencies assist). These parents may struggle and sometimes experience feelings of despair and hopelessness.

Recommended Strategies and Advocacy

Violence is a major public health problem, and applying public health approaches and strategies has been recommended and endorsed by many public health, medical, and nursing professional agencies and professional organizations. Applying the traditional four-step public health approach to violence prevention includes (a) defining the specific violence problem to be prevented; (b) identifying risk and protective factors related to the specific violence problem; (c3) identifying existing evidence-based prevention programs that can be used or modified, or if developing new programs, using data and information from steps a and b to develop strategies and plan related evaluation methods; and (d) if the strategy works, ensuring widespread adoption by determining who else would benefit and how to scale up and by identifying funding resources (CDC, 2021b).

The public health approach recognizes that violence is not an adverse outcome of "bad people" but that violence results from exposure to several risk factors, including those described in this chapter, and that it is a learned behavior (Morrissey, 2016; Rich, 2020). Public health approaches stress prevention, and an important part of the prevention strategy is fostering people, families, and communities with resilience and empowerment strategies to counteract the risks and stressors that challenge them. As such, public health strategies include addressing inequalities and injustices aimed at reducing racial bias and addressing environmental and community factors that increase susceptibility to violence (APHA, 2018). Policymakers, governments, and communities must work together to address environmental and neighborhood factors such as schools, employment, housing, safe places, green spaces, and social cohesion, all of which build resistance and the ability to address risks and challenges related to violence (APHA, 2018). Several evidence-based violence prevention programs have reported promising outcomes. Some programs—for example, universal violence prevention programs—are offered regardless of risk for violence; other programs are aimed at at-risk groups, such as children and teenagers vulnerable to gang involvement (*Chicago Program; Safe Streets*; Webster et al., 2013), parents at risk for child abuse and/or neglect (*Nurse Family Partnership*; Olds & Ammaniti, 2006), partners at risk for partner abuse, or families at risk for elder abuse (McDaniel et al., 2014).

Nurses have a long history of involvement in developing and advocating for prevention of various aspects of violence. The Chicago Parent Program, developed by three nurses in collaboration with parents of young children from low-income Black and Latinx families, aimed to prevent violence by enhancing parenting skills and reducing the use of corporal punishment (Gross et al., 2009). Another nurse-developed and nurse-led violence prevention program is the Domestic Violence Enhanced (DOVE) Program, a public health nurse home visit intervention program that provides education, strategies, and resources to pregnant people who have experienced past intimate partner violence. These program strategies aim to prevent further violence victimization of the individuals and to keep them, their unborn babies, and their children safe, and it has proven to be an impactful program (Sharps et al., 2016). Other approaches to violence prevention recommend patient-centered, trauma-informed, and recovery-oriented care, all of which are practices that nurses can provide and advocate for (Glass et al., 2017; Reif et al., 2020; Williams et al., 2020).

Nurses can advocate in many other ways for public health strategies, programs, and funding that address violence. One example of nurse advocacy to decrease violence in action is the American Academy of Nursing's public call for a National Commission on Mass Shootings (2018). Nurses can also advocate for funding that supports the expansion

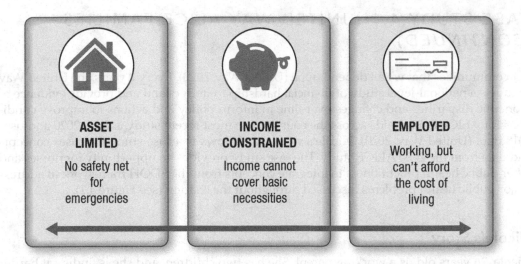

Figure 4.2 What is ALICE?
Source: Adapted from United Way of Central Maryland. www.uwcm.org/alice.

and implementation of evidence-based programs such as Cure Violence (Butts et al., 2015), Healing Hurt People (Rich, 2020), and Safe Streets (Wen & Goodwin, 2016). Advocating for funding that supports school-based suicide prevention and hospital-based violence prevention programs are other nurse-worthy causes. For best effectiveness, developing and supporting cross-sector collaborations will lead to more holistic approaches to address risk for violence. Such collaborations should include leaders from healthcare institutions, health departments, universities, nonprofits, family and child support agencies, faith-based organizations, and law enforcement (APHA, 2018; Rich, 2020). Other important action steps identified by APHA (2018) include educating and training nurses and other healthcare professionals about violence, including how to listen and assess potential violent circumstances, and make appropriate referrals and linkages before violence erupts in hospitals, schools, family homes, and other community spaces. Specific training for partner violence, child abuse, and elder abuse screening is important, and nurses can take leadership roles in this training. Nurses can advocate for funding to support the CDC's establishing a surveillance database that allows monitoring and tracking of violence as it occurs in communities, thus increasing the understanding of patterns of occurrence, risks of violence, and what was effective in mitigating or preventing violence. Violence is deeply entrenched in U.S. society, and the best ways to address it will require a holistic and integrated approach that includes public health, law enforcement, health systems, improved public education in underresourced communities, and widespread violence prevention education.

CASE STUDY 4.1: UNITED WAY ALICE FAMILIES

ALICE is an acronym for individuals who are Asset Limited, Income Constrained, and Employed (Figure 4.2). ALICE individuals may work one 40-hour per week job or several part-time jobs, with an income above their state's federal poverty level, but do not earn enough income to afford a "bare-bones budget" or to pay for necessities such as housing, food, healthcare, childcare, and transportation as described by the United Way of Maryland (2020). They are often described as the "working poor," because their income does not cover the cost of basic needs such as housing, food, transportation, childcare, healthcare, clothing, technology, and leisure activities. ALICE is the childcare worker, the retail cashier at the grocery store, the salesperson at the big box discount store, or the home-health aide, for example—the people in

(continued)

CASE STUDY 4.1: UNITED WAY ALICE FAMILIES (*CONTINUED*)

our communities that we all depend upon (United Way, 2020). Every 2 years, the United Way conducts a national-level study of financial hardship to understand and provide evidence of economic disparities and changes over time to inform policy and actions to improve conditions for ALICE households across the country. The most recent study is from 2020 and uses 2018 data (United Way, 2020). Nicole's story that follows is a case study that uses concepts and data from the 2020 ALICE study. The case study provides an opportunity for nurses and other public health practitioners to integrate concepts from the SDOH framework to address major public health problems discussed throughout the chapter (see Figure 4.1).

Nicole's Story

Nicole, 26 years old, is a working parent. She has two children, and she is finding it harder and harder to make ends meet for her family. Nicole makes $31,680 annually as a hotel front desk manager in a suburban county in Maryland. Her children are Samantha, 2 years old, and Jeffrey, 6 weeks old. The new baby has stretched the already-tight family budget even more. Daycare for Samantha and Jeffrey costs $1,600 month, and the rent on Samantha's 750 square foot, two-bedroom, one-bathroom apartment was recently raised from $1,550 per month to $1,625 per month. Nicole would like to stay in this apartment because she can drop her children off at daycare on her walk to the bus stop, and there is a playground on the premises of the apartment complex. But Nicole worries that if the rent increases again she may need to think about moving. Although she was entitled to remain at home for a 6-month unpaid maternity leave, she has recently returned to work. Nicole started saving money as soon as she learned she was pregnant, because she knew she wanted to take time off after the baby was born. But the money ran out after 5 weeks, so she had to return to work earlier than she wanted to. Nicole is increasingly concerned because things like groceries, diapers, and other necessities are becoming so much more expensive.

Nicole has carefully considered her work situation. She left her previous job because she received no indication of a salary increase in the future. She had worked at her previous job for 5 years, was never late, and never took a sick day, and her annual evaluations were always positive. The only benefits her previous job and the current job offer are free dental cleanings and minor dental work for her and her family. Her current position offers 50 cents more per hour than her previous job, which helps with the household income. Nicole has been told that her family's income is too high to qualify for help from the government, but she knows it is definitely not enough to survive without some assistance. Nicole's husband, Wallace, works at an Amazon warehouse, where he earns $32,387 annually. Nicole and Wallace both drive for Lyft when not working their full-time jobs to help bring some much-needed extra money into their household. Nicole describes herself as the kind of person who always pays her bills, but it is becoming increasingly more difficult to stay on top of everything (United Way, 2020).

Analysis of Case Study

1. Use the information in Table 4.2 to allocate Nicole's household income to meet projected expenses.
2. How does Nicole's budget compare with the estimated expenses needed for a household survival budget? Where are the gaps?
3. What are the public health concerns for this family related to:
   a. Economic stability

(*continued*)

CASE STUDY 4.1: UNITED WAY ALICE FAMILIES (*CONTINUED*)

       b. Social and community context
       c. Neighborhood and built environment
    4. What qualities exist within this family that might contribute to their resilience?
    5. What community resources could be identified and made available to help this family?
    6. What local or federal policies would be important for nurses to advocate for regarding ALICE families like Nicole's family?
    7. What other information, such as social history and past and current health history, is missing that would help the public health nurse further assess this family's needs and plan their care?

Discussion of Case Study

Nicole's family is an example of many ALICE households across the nation. Nicole and Wallace work jobs that many people depend on. During the 2020 COVID-19 pandemic, people in these types of jobs became known as essential workers, and these are the same workers that were previously labeled the "working poor." Nicole and Wallace each work 40 hours or more each week. Their combined income of $64,067 exceeds the 2021 Federal Poverty level income of $26,500, but it is not enough money to meet the estimated survival income for Maryland families, based on the United Way estimate. This family is economically very vulnerable because if they experience one major unexpected event that negatively impacts their income, such as a major illness or hospitalization, a cascade of adverse events is likely. They would potentially experience even more economic instability that could launch more events that would push them into poverty, or perhaps make them unable to maintain their basic needs such as housing, food, healthcare, and appropriate care of their children.

Using Table 4.2, nurses can take a closer look at how this family might allocate their income, which mirrors the dilemmas ALICE families face. The combined income for this family is $64,067. Estimated federal taxes for this family is about $13,213 bringing their federal adjusted gross income (AGI) to $50,854. Estimated Maryland income tax for this family is about $3,123, which further reduces their net income to $47,731. This will give them an average monthly budget of $3,977 to meet all expenses identified in Table 4.2 for this family. Budget expenses already include $1,625 for housing and $1,600 for childcare expenses, totaling $3,225. The family now has about $752 to meet all other monthly expenses.

Survival budgets calculated by United Way vary by state. In this example, the 2018 survival budget for a family residing in Maryland was estimated at $87,156, which shows that Nicole's family has a short fall of $23,089. This family is a clear example of an ALICE family, with income that is above the poverty limit but insufficient to meet all needs and inadequate to save for family emergency situations.

Several federal programs are aimed at helping families like Nicole's, such as the Earned Income Tax Credit (EITC). The EITC aims to provide low- and moderate-income families a tax break by reducing the taxes owed and, in some cases, may increase tax refunds to eligible taxpayers with qualifying children. The 2018 Adjusted Gross Income (AGI) for a family with two eligible children to qualify was $51,492. Eligible taxpayers are considered those with minor children or disabled dependents. Nicole's family income of $64,067 exceeds the income threshold. SNAP might also be helpful; however, again, Nicole's family income exceeds the income threshold level of $34,500. This illustrates how some ALICE families "fall through the cracks" because they have unmet living needs due to limited economic resources, but sometimes do not qualify for programs in the U.S. "safety net" such as AGI and SNAP.

This case study of an ALICE family helps illustrate how economic instability increases a family's vulnerability to major public health problems. Their limited income impacts their

(*continued*)

CASE STUDY 4.1: UNITED WAY ALICE FAMILIES (*CONTINUED*)

ability to secure sufficient and nutritious food and limits their living options in terms of housing types and neighborhoods. They are on a very tight budget so if Nicole or Wallace loses their employment or is unable to work due to health issues, or if they face a major family crisis that requires additional funds, their vulnerability for housing instability and food insecurity also increases. Family crises that disrupt individuals and families are not unusual and could be in the form of an unexpected medical bill or a car breakdown. These crises can tip the family balance and cause less healthful situations, such as poorer nutrition, living in a crowded setting with relatives, or dropping out of a literacy program.

A public health nurse working with this family can consider a multitude of areas to assess as they identify resources to help them survive, thrive, and be safe. Nurses must assess the neighborhood and the quality of the current home and related safety concerns—for example, exposure to lead or other toxins. If the family is considering moving to secure lower rent, would there be other neighborhoods where they will feel safe and have high-quality housing? In considering childcare, does the family qualify for programs such as Head Start or Early Head Start, or are there other programs that offer subsidies that this family may be eligible for? Nicole may want to consider other employment settings where she could use and grow her current skills and receive good options for health insurance. Are there job programs or adult education options available to Nicole and Wallace that appeal to them and would help them secure a better future and more options for their family, such as job and career centers?

TABLE 4.2 Average Household Survival Budget in Maryland, 2018

Monthly Costs	Survival Budget for 2 Adults, 1 Infant, 1 Preschooler	Nicole's Family of 2 Adults, 1 Infant, 1 Preschooler
Housing	$1,542	$1,625
Child care	$1,317	$1,600
Food	$884	–
Transportation	$779	–
Healthcare	$832	–
Technology	$75	–
Miscellaneous	$660	–
Taxes	$1,174	$13,213 annually or $1,101 monthly
Monthly total	$7,263	$4,326
Annual total	$87,156	$51,912
Hourly wage (needed to support the survival budget)	$43.58	$31.50

CONCLUSIONS

This chapter examines three aspects of the SDOH and their associations with major public health problems and persistent health disparities and inequities. Underlying many major public health problems is the pervasive racism in the United States that affects every aspect of society, its history, structures, and institutions, including healthcare systems. Specific strategies for nursing actions, advocacy, and interventions are offered throughout the chapter. While some of the strategies and examples may seem to target low-income and diverse communities, strategies and policies that alleviate inequities for these groups will also help to alleviate inequalities for other groups (APHA, 2020).

ADDITIONAL RESOURCES

Bureau of Labor Statistics. (2017). Employee-reported workplace injury and illness 2016. https://www.bls.gov/news.release/archives/osh_11092017.pdf

Creamer, J. (2020). Poverty rates for blacks and hispanics reached historic lows in 2019: Inequalities persist despite decline in poverty for all major race and hispanic origin groups. https://www.census.gov/library/stories/2020/09/poverty-rates-for-blacks-and-hispanics-reached-historic-lows-in-2019.html

Kang, S. (2015). Inequality and crime revisited: Effects of local inequality and economic segregation on crime. *Journal of Population Economics*, 29(2), 593–626. https://doi.org/10.1007/s00148-015-0579-3

Manca A. R. (2014) Social cohesion. In A.C. Michalos (Ed.). Encyclopedia of quality of life and well-being research. Springer. https://doi.org/10.1007/978-94-007-0753-5_2739

Office of the Assistant Secretary for Planning and Evaluation. (2018). 2018 Poverty guidelines. https://aspe.hhs.gov/2018-poverty-guidelines

Office of the Assistant Secretary for Planning and Evaluation. (2021). 2021 Poverty guidelines. https://aspe.hhs.gov/2021-poverty-guidelines

U.S. Department of Health and Human Services. (2010). Secretary's advisory committee on health promotion and disease prevention objectives for 2020. Healthy people 2020: An opportunity to address the societal determinants of health in the United States. http://www.healthypeople.gov/2010/hp2020/advisory/SocietalDeterminantsHealth.htm

REFERENCES

Abdul-Mutakabbir, J. C. et al. (2021). A three-tiered approach to address barriers to COVID-19 vaccine delivery in the black community. *The Lancet*. https://doi.org/10.1016/S2214-109X(21)00099-1

Alhusen, J. L., Bower, K., Epstein, E., & Sharps, P. (2017). Racial discrimination and adverse birth outcomes: An integrative review. *Journal of Midwifery and Women's Health*, 61(6), 707–720. https://doi.org/10.1111/jmwh.12490

Ali, M. M., Mutter, R., & Teich, J. L. (2015). State participation in the Medicaid Expansion provision of the Affordable Care Act: Implications for uninsured individuals with behavioral health condition. Substance Abuse and Mental Health Services Administration, Center for Behavioral Health Statistics and Quality.

Amadeo, K., & Estevez. (2021). *U.S. poverty rate by demographics*. https://www.thebalance.com/us-poverty-rate-by-state-4585001

American Academy of Pediatrics. (2021). Social determinants of health. https://www.aap.org/en-us/advocacy-and-policy/aap-health-initiatives/Screening/Pages/Social-Determinants-of-Health.aspx

American Nurses Association. (2015). The ANA code of ethics for nurses with interpretative statements (2nd ed.). Washington, DC: America Nurses Association.

American Psychiatric Nurses Association. (2020). Violence prevention. https://www.apna.org/news/violence-prevention/

American Public Health Association. (2018). Violence is a public health issue: Public health is essential to understanding and treating violence in the U.S. https://apha.org/policies-and-advocacy/public-health-policy-statements/policy-database/2019/01/28/violence-is-a-public-health-issue

American Public Health Association. (2020). Structural racism is a public health crisis: Impact on the black community. https://www.apha.org/policies-and-advocacy/public-health-policy-statements/policy-database/2021/01/13/structural-racism-is-a-public-health-crisis

Anda, R. F., Brown, D. W., Dube, S. R., Bremner, J. D., Felitti, V. J., & Giles, W. H. (2008). Adverse childhood experiences and chronic obstructive pulmonary disease in adults. *American Journal of Preventive Medicine*, 34(5), 396–403. https://doi.org/10.1016/j.amepre.2008.02.002

Antonisse, L. & Garfield, R. (2018). The relationship between work and health: Findings from a literature review. https://www.kff.org/medicaid/issue-brief/the-relationship-between-work-and-health-findings-from-a-literature-review/

Aronowitz, S. V., Kim, B., & Aronowitz, T. (2021). A mixed-studies review of the school-to-prison pipeline and a call to action for school nurses. *The Journal of School Nursing: The Official Publication of the National Association of School Nurses*, 37(1), 51–60. https://doi.org/10.1177/1059840520972003

Aurand, A., Emmanuel, D., Threet, D., Ikra, R., & Yentel, D. (2020). *THE GAP: The affordable housing gap analysis 2016*. Washington, DC: The National Low Income Housing Coalition. https://reports.nlihc.org/sites/default/files/gap/Gap-Report_2020.pdf

Bailey, Z. D., Krieger, N., Agenor, M., Graves, J., Linos, N., & Bassett, M. T. (2017). Structural racism and health inequalities in the USA: Evidence and interventions. *Lancet*, 389(1000777), 1453–1463. https://www.thelancet.com/action/showPdf?pii=S0140-6736%2817%2930569-X

Benefits. (2019). Assistance for low-income families. https://www.usa.gov/benefits

Berkowitz, S. A., & Basu, S. (2021). Unemployment insurance, health-related social needs, health care access and mental health during the COVID-19 pandemic. *JAMA Internal Medicine*, 181(5), 699–702. https://doi.org/10.1001/jamainternmed.2020.7048

Bever, E., Arnold, K. T., Lindberg, R., Dannenberg, A. L., Morley, R., Breysse, J., & Pollack Porter, K. M. (2021). Use of health impact assessments in the housing sector to promote health in the United States, 2002–2016. *Journal of Housing and the Built Environment*. https://doi.org/10.1007/s10901-020-09795-9

Boullier, M., & Blair, M. (2018). Adverse childhood experiences. *Paediatrics and Child Health*, 28(3), 132–137.

Boulware, L. E., Cooper, L. A., Ratner, L. E., LaVeist, T. A., & Powe, N. R. (2003). Race and trust in the health care system. *Public Health Reports*, 118(4), 358–65. https://doi.org/10.1016/S0033-3549(04)50262-5

Braveman, P., Heck, K., Egerter, S. et al. (2018). Worry about racial discrimination: A missing piece of the puzzle of black-white disparities in preterm birth? *PloS One*, 12(10), e0186151. https://doi.org/10.1371/journal.pone.0186151

Bravo, M. A., Anthopolos, R., Bell, M. L., & Miranda, M. L. (2016). Racial isolation and exposure to airborne particulate matter and ozone in understudied US populations: Environmental justice applications of downscaled numerical model output. *Environment International*, 92–93, 247–255. https://doi.org/10.1016/j.envint.2016.04.008

Brown, A. F., Ma, G. X., Miranda, J., Eng, E., Castille, D., Brockie, T., Jones, P., Airhihenbuwa, C. O., Farhat, T., Zhu, L., & Trinh-Shervin, C. (2019). Structural interventions to reduce and eliminate health disparities. *American Journal of Public Health*, 109(51). https://doi.org/10.2105/AJPH.2018.304844

Brownell, K. D., & Frieden, T. R. (2009). Ounces of prevention-the public policy case for taxes on sugared beverages. *The New England Journal of Medicine*, 360(18), 1805–1808. https://doi.org/10.1056/NEJMp0902392

Bureau of Labor Statistics. (2017). Employee benefits in the United States. Employee Benefits in the United States-March 2017 (bls.gov).

Bureau of Labor Statistics. (2019). Labor Force Characteristics by Race and Ethnicity, 2018/U.S. Bureau of Labor Statistics, Division of Information and Marketing Services, Washington, DC. https://www.bis.gov/opub/reports/race-and-ethnicity/2018/home.htm

Bureau of Labor Statistics. (2020a). Employee benefits in the United States—2020. https://www.bls.gov/news.release/archives/ebs2_09242020.pdf

Bureau of Labor Statistics. (2020b). Persons with a disability: Barriers to employment and other labor-related issues. https://www.bls.gov/news.release/disabl.nr0.htm

Bureau of Labor Statistics. (2022). *The employment situation—August 2022*. https://www.bls.gov/news.release/pdf/empsit.pdf

Burtle, A., & Bezruchka, S. (2016). Population health and paid parental leave: What the United States can learn from two decades of research. *Healthcare (Basel)*, 4(2), 30. https://doi.org/10.3390/healthcare4020030

Butts, J. A., Roman, C. G., Bostwick, L., & Porter, J. R. (2015). Cure violence: A public health model to reduce gun violence. *Annual Review of Public Health*, 36, 39–53. https://doi.org/10.1146/annurev-publhealth-031914-122509

Cai, J. (2020). *Black students in the condition of education 2020*. National State Boards Association. https://www.nsba.org/Perspectives/2020/black-students-condition-education

Carpiano, R. M. (2006). Toward a neighborhood resource based theory of social capital for health: Can bourdieu and sociology help? *Social Science & Medicine*, 62, 165–175. https://doi.org/10.1016/j.socscimed.2005.05.020

Carrasco, M. A., & Bilal, U. (2016). A sign of the times: To have or to be? Social capital or social cohesion? *Social Science & Medicine*, 159, 127–131. https://doi.org/10.1016/j.socscimed.2016.05.012

Center on Budget and Policy Priorities. (2021). https://www.cbpp.org/research/poverty-and-inequality/tracking-the-covid-19-recessions-effects-

Centers for Disease Control and Prevention. (2017). African American health, CDC vital signs. https://www.cdc.gov/vitalsigns/pdf/2017-05-vitalsigns.pdf

Centers for Disease Control and Prevention. (2019). Lead prevention in children. https://www.cdc.gov/nceh/lead/prevention/children

Centers for Disease Control and Prevention. (2021a). Social determinants of health. https://www.cdc.gov/socialdeterminants/about.html

Centers for Disease Control and Prevention. (2021b). CDC, 2021. Childhood lead poisoning prevention. https://www.cdc.gov/nceh/lead/prevention/sources.htm

Centers for Disease Control and Prevention. (2022). Health and economic costs of chronic diseases. https://www.cdc.gov/chronicdisease/about/costs/index.htm

Centers for Disease Control and Prevention. (n.d., a). Violence prevention. https://www.cdc.gov/violenceprevention/index.html

Centers for Disease Control and Preventions (n.d., b). WISQARS™—Web-based injury statistics query and reporting system. https://www.cdc.gov/injury/wisqars/index.html

Chan, J., To, H.-P., & Chan, E. (2006). Reconsidering social cohesion: Developing a definition and analytical framework for empirical research. *Social Indicators Research*, 75, 273–302. https://doi.org/10.1007/s11205-005-2118-1

Children Defense Fund. (2019). Child poverty in America 2018: State analysis. www.childrendefense.org

Chiumento, A., Rutayisire, T., Sarabwe, E. et al. (2020). Exploring the mental health and psychosocial problems of Congolese refugees living in refugee settings in Rwanda and Uganda: A rapid qualitative study. *Conflict and Health*, 14, 77. https://doi.org/10.1186/s13031-020-00323-8

Clarke, K., Manriquez, A., Sabo-Attwood, T., & Coker, E. S. (2021). A narrative review of occuaptional air pollution and respitartoy health in farmworkers. *International Journal of Environmental Puiblic Health*, 18(4097). https://doi.org/10.3390/ijerph.18084097

Coleman-Jensen, A., Gregory, C. A., & Rabbitt, M. P. (2020). Food security in the US: Key statistics and graphics. https://www.ers.usda.gov/topics/food-nutrition-assistance/food-security-in-the-us/key-statistics-graphics.aspx

Conway, S. H., Pompeil, L. A., Gimeno Porras, D., Follis, J. L., & Roberts, R. (2017). The identification of a threshold of long work hours for predicting elevated risk of adverse outcomes. *American Journal of Epidemiology*, 186(2), 173–183. https://doi.org/1.1093/aje/kwx003

Cunningham, T. J., Croft, J. B., Liu, Y., Lu, H., Eke, P. I., & Giles, W. H. (2017). Racial disparities in age-specific mortality among blacks or African Americans-United States, 1999–2015. *MMWR Morbidity Mortal Weekkly Reports*, 66(17), 444–456. http://doi.org/10.15585/mmwr.mm6617e1External

Cutts, D., Coleman, S., Black, M., Chilton, M., Cook, J., de Cuba, S. E., Heeren, T., Meyers, A., Sandel, M., Casey, P., & Frank, D. (2015). Homelessness during pregnancy: A unique, time-dependent risk factor of birth outcomes. *Maternal and Child Health Journal*, 19(6), 1276–83. https://doi.org/10.1007/s10995-014-1633-6

Czapp, P., & Kovach, K. (2015). Poverty and health-the family medicine perspective (Position Paper). https://www.aafp.org/about/policies/all/poverty-health.html

DeRigne, L., Stoddard-Dare, P., & Quinn, L. (2016). Workers without paid sick leave less likely to take time off for illness or injury compared to those with paid sick leave. *Health Affaris*, 35(3), 520–227. https://doi.org/10.1377/hlthaff.2015.0965

Deville, T. (2021). Partnering with churches, Maryland officials push pop-up clinics as way to address vaccine hesitancy. Baltimore Sun. https://www.baltimoresun.com/coronavirus/bs-md-highlandtown-popup-clinic-20210227-minas4yszbbo3mjw7txvq7b4dm-story.html

Doede, M. S. (2016). Black jobs matter. Racial inequaliti3es in conditions of employment and subsequent health outcomes. *Public Health Nursing*, 33(2), 151–158. https://doi.org/10.111/phm.12241

Egerter, S., Dekker, M., An, J., Grossman-Kahn, R., & Braveman, P. (2008). Work matters for health. Brief Report 4, December. Robert Wood Johnson Foundation. www.commissionhealth.org

Fernald, M. (2020). 2020 State of the nation's housing report. Joint Center for Housing Studies of Havard University. https://www.habitat.org/costofhome/2020-state-nations-housing-report-lack-affordable-housing

Fernald, M. (2021). 2021 State of the nation's housing report. Joint Center for Housing Studies of Havard University. https://www.jchs.harvard.edu/state-nations-housing-2021

Ferrari, G., Agnew-Davies, R., Bailey, J., Howard, L., Howarth, E., Peters, T. J., Sardinha, L., & Feder, G. (2014). Domestic violence and mental health: A cross-sectional survey of women seeking help from domestic violence support services. *Global Health Action*, 7(1). https://doi.org/10.3402/gha.v7.25519

Ford, C. L., Griffith, D. M., Bruce, M. A., & Gilbert, K. (2018). Racism: Science and tools for the public health professional. Washington, DC: American Public Health Association.

Gascon, M., Vrijheid, M., & Nieuwenhuijsen. (2016). The built environment and child health: An overview of current evidence. *Current Environmental Health Report*, 3, 250–257. https://doi.org/10.1007/s40572-016-0094-z

Giannarelli, L, Wheaton, L., & Shantrz, K. (2021). 2021 Poverty projections. https://www.urban.org/sites/default/files/publication/103656/2021-poverty-projections.pdf

Gilbert, J. A., & Stephens, B. (2018). Microbiology of the built environment. *Nature Reviews, 16,* 681. https://doi.org/10.1038/s41578-018-0065-5

Glass, N. E., Perrin, N. A., Hanson, G. C., Bloom, T. L., Messing, J. T., Clough, A. S., Campbell, J. C., Gielen, A. C., Case, J., & Eden, K. B. (2017). The longitudinal impact of an internet safety decision aid for abused women. *American Journal of Preventive Medicine, 52*(5), 606–615. https://doi.org/10.1016/j.amepre.2016.12.014

Goh, J., Pfeffer, J., & Zenios, S. (2015). Exposure to harmful workplace practices could account for inequality in life spans across different demographic groups. *Health Affairs, 34*(10), 1761–1768.

Goldstein, N., Kreimer, R., Guo, S., Le, T., Cole, L. M., NeMoyer, A., Burke, S., Kikuchi, G., Thomas, K., & Zhang, F. (2021). Preventing school-based arrest and recidivism through prearrest diversion: Outcomes of the Philadelphia police school diversion program. *Law and Human Behavior, 45*(2), 165–178. https://doi.org/10.1037/lhb0000440

Gomez, S. L., Shariff-Marco, S., De Rouen, M., Keegan, H. M., Yen, I. H., Mujahid, M., Satariano, W. A., & Glaser, S. L. (2015). The impact of neighborhood social and built environment factors across the cancer continuum: Current research, methodological considerations, and future directions. *Cancer, 121*(14), 2314–2330. https://doi.org/10.1002/cncr.29345

Grenier, J., & Wynn, N. (2018). A nurse-led intervention to address food insecurity in Chicago. *Online Journal of Issues in Nursing, 23*(3), 1–8. https://doi.org/10.3912/OJIN

Gross, D., Garvey, C., Julion, W., Fogg, L., Tucker, S., & Mokros, H. (2009). Efficacy of the Chicago Parent Program with low-income African American and Latino parents of young children. *Prevention Science, 10*(1), 54–65. https://doi.org/10.1007/s11121-008-0116-7

Hager, E. R., Quigg, A. M., Black, M. M., Coleman, S. M., Heeren, T., Rose-Jacobs, R., Cook, J. T., Ettinger de Cuba, S. A., Casey, P. H., Chilton, M., Cutts, D. B., Meyers, A. F., & Frank, D. A. (2010). Development and validity of a 2-item screen to identify families at risk for food insecurity. *Pediatrics, 126*(1). https://doi.org/10.1542/peds.2009-3146

Haider, A. (2021). The basic facts about children in poverty. The Center for American Progress. https://www.americanprogress.org/issues/poverty/reports/2021/01/12/494506/basic-facts-children-poverty/

Harrell, S. P. (2000). A multidimensial conceptulilzation of race-related stress: Implications for well-being of people of color. *American Journal of Orthopsychiatry, 70,* 42–57. https://doi.org/10.1037/h0087722

Heymann, J., Sprague, A., Earle, A., McCormack, M., Waisath, W., & Raub, A. (2021). U.S. sick leave in global context: U.S. eligibility rules widen inequalities despite readily available solutions. *Health Affairs, 40*(9), 1501–1509. https://doi.org/10.1377/hlthaff.2021.00731

Hicken, M. T., Kravitz-Wirtz, N., Durkee, M., & Jackson, J. S. (2018). Racial inequalities in health: Framing future research. *Social Science & Medicine, 199,* 11–18. https://doi.org/10.1016/j.socscimed.2017.12.027

Huecker, M. R., King, K. C., Jordan, G. A., & Smock, W. (2022). Domestic violence. In *StatPearls.* StatPearls Publishing.

Hughes, H. K., Matsui, E. C., Tschudy, M., Pollack, C. E., & Keet, C. A. (2017). Pediatric asthma health disparities: Race, hardship, housing, and asthma in a national survey. *Academic Pediatrics, 17*(2), 127–134. https://doi.org/10.1016/j.acap.2016.11.011

Ingram, M., Wolf, A. M. A., Lopez-Galvez, N. I., Griffin, S. C., & Beamer, P. I. (2021). Proposing a social ecological approach to address disparities in occupational exposures and health for low-wage and minority workers employed in small businesses. *Journal of Exposure Science & Environmental Epidemiology, 31,* 404–411. https://doi.org/10.1038/s41370-021-00317-5

James, P., Hart, J. E., Banay, R. F., & Laden, F. (2016). Exposure to greenness and mortality in a nationwide prospective cohort study of women. *Environmental Health Perspectives, 124*(9), 1344–1352. https://doi.org/10.1289/ehp.1510363

Jones, C. P. (2018). Towards the science and practice of anti-racism: Launching a national campaign against racism. *Ethnicity & Disease, 28*(suppl 1), 231–234. https://doi.org/10.18865/ed.28.S1.231

Kaiser Family Foundation. (2021). Health insurance coverage of the total population. https://www.kff.org/other/state-indicator/total-population/

Katch, H. (2020). Medicaid expansion improves postpartum coverage, access to care. *Center on Budget and Policy Priorities.* https://www.cbpp.org/blog/medicaid-expansion-improves-postpartum-coverage-access-to-care

Kawachi, I., & Berkman, L. (2000). Social cohesion, social capital, and health. In I. Kawachi & L. Berkman (Eds.), *Social epidemiology* (pp. 174–190). Oxford University Press.

Kearney, M. (2019). *Child poverty in the U.S.* https://econofact.org/child-poverty-in-the-u-s

Khullar, D., & Chokshi, D. A. (2018). Health, income and poverty: Where we are and what could help. *Health Affairs Health Policy Brief.* https://doi.org/10.1377/hpb20180817.901935

Kinsey, E. W., Hecht, A. A., Dunn, C. G., Levi, R., Read, M. A., Smith, C., Niesen, P., Seligman, H. K., & Hager, E. R. (2020). School closures during COVID-19: Opportunities for innovation in meal service. *AJPH, 110*(11), 1635–1643. https://doi.org/10.2105/AJPH.2020.305875

Krieger, N. (2014). Discrimination and health inequities. *International Journal of Health Services, 44*(4), 643–710. https://doi.org/10.2190/HS.44.4.b

Kuo, F. E., & Sullivan, W. C. (2001). Aggression and violence in the inner city: Effects of environment via mental fatigue. *Environment and Behavior, 33*(4), 543–571. https://doi.org/10.1177/00139160121973124

Le Menestrel, S., & Duncan, G. (2019). A roadmap to reducing child poverty. Washington, DC: National Academies Press.

Leung, C. W., Epel, E. S., Ritchie, L. D., Crawford, P. B., & Laraia, B. A. (2014). Food insecurity is inversely associated with diet quality of lower-income adults. *Journal of the Academy of Nutrition and Dietetics, 114*(12), 1943–1953.e2. https://doi.org/10.1016/j.jand.2014.06.353

Levinson, D., & Publications Group. (2004). Encyclopedia of homelessness. SAGE Publications.

Livesley, S. J., McPherson, G. M., & Calfapietra, C. (2016). The urban forest and ecosystem services: Impacts on urban water, heat, and pollution cycles at the tree, street, and city scale. *Journal of Environmental Quality, 45*(1), 119–124. https://doi.org/10.2134/jeq2015.11.0567

Logan, T. K. & Walker, R. (2017). The gender safety gap: Examining the impact of victimization history, perceived risk, and personal control. *Journal of Interpresonal Violence, 36*(1–2), 603–631. https://doi.org/10.1177/0886260517729405

Lopez-Landin, H. (2013). SNAP access barriers faced by low income 50–59 year olds. American Association of Retired Persons Foundation. https://www.aarp.org/content/dam/aarp/aarp_foundation/2013-dfs/SNAP_White_Paper_Mar_2013.pdf

Lorch, S. A., & Enlow, E. (2015). The role of social determinants in explaining racial/ethnic disparities in perinatal outcomes. *Pediatric Research, 79*(1–2), 141–1347. https://doi.org/10.1038/pr.2015.199

Mancus, G. C., & Campbell, J. C. (2018). Integrative review of the intersection of green space and neighborhood violence. *Journal of Nursing Scholarship, 50*(2), 117–125. https://doi.org/10.1111/jnu.12365

Mancus, G., Cimino, A., Hasan, Z., Sharps, P., Winch, P. J., Tsuyuki, K., Stockman, J., & Campbell, J. C. (2020). Residential greenness positively associated with the cortisol to DHEA ratio among urban-dwelling African American women at risk for HIV. *Journal of Urban Health.* https://doi.org/10.1007/s11524-020-00492-0

Martin, E. (2017). Hidden consequences: The impact of incarceration on dependent children. *National Institute of Justice Journal.* https://nij.ojp.gov/topics/articles/hidden-consequences-impact-incarceration-dependent-children

Marrone, J. & Swarbrick, M. A. (2020). Long-term unemployment: A social determinant underaddressed within community behavioral health programs. *Psychiatric Services, 71*(7), 745–748. https://doi.org/10.1176/appi.ps201900522

Maurer, R. (2020). Removing employment barriers for immigrant workers. Society for Human Resource Management. https://www.shrm.org/resourcesandtools/hr-topics/talent-acquisition/pages/removing-employment-barriers-immigrant-workers.aspx

Maynard, M., Dean, J., Rodriguez, P. I., Sriranganathan, G., Qutub, M., & Kirkpatrick, S. I. (2019). The experience of food insecurity among immigrants: A scoping review. *Journal of International Migration and Integration, 20*(2), 375–417. https://doi.org/10.1007/s12134-018-0613-x

McDaniel, D. D., Logan, J. E. D., & Schneiderman, J. U. (2014). Supporting gang violence prevention efforts: A public health approach for nurses. *The Online Journal of Issues in Nursing, 19*(1). https://www.ncbi.nlm.nih.gov/pmc/articles/PMC4703334/

McHugh, M., French, D. D., Farley, D., Maechling, C. R., Dunlop, D. D., & Holl, J. L. (2019). Community health and employee work performance in the American manufacturing environment. *Journal of Community Health, 44*, 178–184. https://doi.org/10.1007/s10900-018-0570-5

Meyer, O. L., Castro-Schilo, L., &Aguilar-Gaxiola, S. (2014). Determinants of mental health and self-rated health: A model of socioeconomic status, neighborhood safety, and physical activity. *American Journal of Public Health, 104*(9), 1734–1741. https://doi.org/10.2105/AJPH.2014.302003.

Miller, T. R., Cohen, M. A., Swedler, D. I., Ali, B., Hendrie, D. V. (2021). Incidence and costs of personal and property crimes in the USA, 2017. *Journal of Benefit-Cost Analysis, 12*(1). https://dx.doi.org/10.2139/ssrn.3514296

Mirza, S. A. et al. (2018). The State of the LGBTQ Community in the Labor Market: Pre-June 2018 Jobs Day Release. Center for American Progress. https://www.americanprogress.org/issues/economy/news/2018/07/05/453094/state-lgbtq-community-labor-market-pre-june-2018-jobs-day-release/

Morrissey, J. (2016). Violence: A community health approach. *Journal of the Catholic Health Association of the United States, Health Progress.* www.chausa.org

Mohai, P., Pellow, D., & Roberts J. T. (2009). Environmental justice. *Annual Review of Environmental Resources, 34,* 405–430. https://doi.org/10.1146/annurev-environ-082508-094348

National Academies of Sciences, Engineering, and Medicine. (2016). Community violence as a population health issue: Proceedings of a workshop—in brief. Washington, DC: The National Academies Press. https://doi.org/10.17226/23668

Native Americans. (2015). Education of first people: Native American students left behind. https://theredroad.org/issues/native-american-education/

Minnesota Department of Health. (2019). Public health interventions: Applications for nursing practice (2nd ed.). https://www.health.state.mn.us/communities/practice/research/phncouncil/docs/PHInterventions.pdf

National Advisory Council on Nurse Education and Practice. (2019). Integration of social determinants of health in nursing education, practice, and research. *16th Report to the Secretary of Health and Human Services and the U.S. Congress.* https://www.hrsa.gov/sites/default/files/hrsa/advisory-committees/nursing/reports/nacnep-2019-sixteenthreport.pdf

National Center for Chronic Disease Prevention and Health Promotion. (2021). Poor nutrition. Centers for Disease Control and Prevention. https://www.cdc.gov/chronicdisease/resources/publications/factsheets/nutrition.htm

Office of Disease Prevention and Health Promotion. (n.d.). Quality of housing: Healthy people 2030. U.S. Department of Health and Human Service. https://health.gov/healthypeople/objectives-and-data/social-determinants-health/literature-summaries/quality-housing

Olds, D., & Ammaniti, M. (2006). The nurse-family partnership: An evidenced-based preventive intervention. *Infant Mental Health Journal, 27,* 5–25.

Putnam, J., Allshouse, J., & Kantor, L. S. (2002). U.S. per capita food supply trends: More calories, refined carbohydrates, and fats. *Food Review, 25*(3), 2–15. https://doi.org/10.22004/ag.econ.234624

Qin, W., Wang, Y., & Cho, S. (2021). Neighborhood social cohesion, physical disorder, and daily activity limitations among community-dwelling older adults. *Archives of Gerontology and Geriatrics, 93.* https://doi.org/10.1016/j.archger.2020.104295

Quinn, M. M., & Smith, P. M. (2018). Gender, work, and health. *Annuals of Work Exposures and Health, 62*(4), 389–392. https://doi.org/10.1093/annweh/wxy019

Reif, K., Jaffe, P., Dawson, M., & Straatman, A. L. (2020). Provision of specialized services for children exposed to domestic violence: Barriers encountered in Violence Against Women (VAW) services. *Children and Youth Services Review, 109,* 104684. https://doi.org/10.1016/j.childyouth.2019.104684

Rich, J. (2020). Healing hurt people. Center for Nonviolence and Social Justice. https://drexel.edu/cnvsj/healing-hurt-people/overview/

Richards, M. (2020). Who benefits from public green space? Scientific American. https://www.scientificamerican.com/article/who-benefits-from-public-green-space/

Sharps, P. W., Bullock, L. C., Campbell, J., Alhusen, J., Ghazarian, S., Bhandari, S., & Schminkey, D. (2016). Domestic violence enhanced prenatal home visits: The DOVE randomized clinical trial. *Journal of Women's Health, 25*(11), 1129–1138.

Sabbath, E. L., Mejia-Guevara, I., Noelke, C., & Berkman, L. F., (2015). The long-term mortality of combined job strain and family circumstances: A life course analysis of working American mothers. *Social Science & Medicine, 146,* 111–119. https://doi.org/10.1016/j.socscimed.2015.10.024

Sandel, M., Sheward, R., Ettinger de Cuba, S., Coleman, S. M., Frank, D. A., Chilton, M., Black, M., Heeren, T., Pasquariello, J., Casey, P., Ochoa, E., & Cutts, D. (2018). Unstable housing and caregiver and child health in renter families. *Pediatirics, 14*(2), e2020172199. https://doi.org/10.1542/peds.2017-2199

Shaw, E. et al. (2016). Undervalued and underpaid in America: Women in low-wage, female-dominated jobs. Washington, DC: Institute for Women's Policy Research. https://iwpr.org/job-quality-income-security/undervalued-and-underpaid-in-america/

Sheats, K. J., Irving, S. M., Mercy, J. A., Simon, T. R., Crosby, A. E., Ford, D. C., Merrick, M. M., Annor, F. B., & Morgan, R. E. (2018). Violence-related disparities experienced by black youth and young adults: Opportunities for prevention. *American Journal of Preventive Medicine, 55*(4), 462–469. https://doi.org/10.1016/j.amepre.2018.05.017

Shen, M. J., Peterson, E. B., Costas-Muniz, R., Hernandez, M. H., Jewell, S. T., Matsoukas, K., & Bylund, C. L. (2018). The effects of race and racial concordance on patient-physician communication: A systematic review. *Journal of Racial and Ethnic Health Disparities, 5*(1), 117–140. https://doi.org/10.1007/s40615-017-0350-4

Silver, S. R., Alacron, W. A., & Li, J. (2021). Incident chronic obstructive pulmonary disease associated with occupation, industry, and workplace exposure in the health and retirement study. *American Journal of Industrial Medicine, 64,* 26–38. https://doi.org/10.1002/ajim.23196

Single Mother Statistics. (2021). https://singlemotherguide.com/single-mother-statistics/

Siqueira, C. E., Gaydos, M., Monforton, C., Slatin, C., Borkowski, L, Dooley, P., Liebman, A., Rosenberg, E., Shor, G., & Keifer, M. (2014). Effects of social, economic, and labor policies on occupational health disparities. *American Journal of Industrial Medicine*, 57, 557–72. https://doi.org/10.1002/ajim.22186

Sommers, B. B., Gawande, A. A., Baicker, K. (2017). Health insurance coverage and health-what the recent evidence tells us. *New England Journal of Medicine*, 377(8), 586–593. https://doi.org/10.1056/NEJMsb1706645

Sorenson, G., Sparer, E., Williams, J., Gundersen, D., Boden, L. I., Denneriein, J. T., Hashimoto, D., Katz, J. N., McLellan, D. L., Okechuwu, C. A., Pronk, N. P., Revette, A., & Wagner, G. R. (2018). Measuring best practices for workplaces safety, health and wellbeing: The workplace integrated safety and health assessment. *Journal of Occupational Environmental Medicine*, 60(5), 430–439. https://doi.org/10.1097/JOM.0000000000001286

Smith, T. D., Hughes, K., DeJoy, D. M., & Dyal, A. A. (2017). Assessment of relationships between work stress, work-family conflict, burnout and firefighter safety behavior outcomes. *Safety Science*, 103(2018), 287–292. https://doi.org/10.1016/jssci.2017.12.005

Spies, L. A. (2021). Department of justice data on violent crime and race. https://www.crimeinamerica.net/department-of-justice-data-on-violent-crime-and-race/

Spivak, H., Jenkins, E., VanAudenhove, K., Lee, D., Kelly, M., & Iskander, J. (2019). A public health approach to the prevention of intimate partner violence. *Centers for Disease Control and Prevention Morbidity and Mortality Weekly Report*, 63(2), 38–41. https://www.cdc.gov/mmwr/preview/mmwrhtml/mm6302a4.htm

Taylor, L. (2018). Housing and health: An overview of the literature. *Health Affairs Health Policy Brief*. https://doi.org/10.1377/hpb20180313.396577

Twohig-Bennett, C., & Jones, A. (2018). The health benefits of the great outdoors: A systematic review and meta-analysis of greenspace exposure ad health outcomes. *Environmental Research*, 166, 628–637. https://doi.org/10.1016/j.envres.2018.06.030

United Nations Children's Emergency Fund: UNICEF. (2020). https://www.unicef.org/reports/unicef-annual-report-2020

United Way. (2020). ALICE report: A study of financial hardship in Maryland. https://www.uwcm.org/alice/

U.C. Davis. (2022). *Gun violence: UC Davis researches causes, trends, solutions.* https://www.ucdavis.edu/news/gun-violence-uc-davis-researches-causes-trends-solutions

U.S. Census Bureau. (2019). How the US measures poverty, US Census Bureau; Income, Poverty and Health Insurance Coverage in the United States. Washington, DC.

U.S. Government. (2020). Government benefits. https://www.usa.gov/benefits

Webster, D. W., Whitehill, J. M., Vernick, J. S., & Curriero, F. C. (2013). Effect of Baltimore's safe streets program on gun violence: A replication of Chicago's cease fire program. *Journal of Urban Health*, 90(21)7–40. https://doi.org/10.1007/s11524-012-9731-5

Wen, L. S., & Goodwin, K. E. (2016). Violence is a public health issue. *Journal of Public Health Management and Practice*, 22(6), 503–505. https://doi.org/https://10.1097/phh.0000000000000501

Wells, L., & Gowda, A. (2020). A legacy of mistrust: African Americans and the US healthcare system. *Proceedings of UCLA Health*, 24. https://proceedings.med.ucla.edu/index.php/2020/06/12/a-legacy-of-mistrust-african-americans-and-the-us-healthcare-system/

Western, B., & Sirois, C. (2019). Racialized re-entry: Labor market inequality after incarceration. *Social Forces*, 97(4), 1517–1542. https://doi.org/10.1093/sf/soy096

Williams, D. R. (2018). Stress and the mental health of populations of color: Advancing our understanding of race-related stressors. *Journal of Health & Social Behavior*, 59(4), 466–485. https://doi.org/10.1177/0022146518814251

Williams, D. R., Lawrence, J. A., & Davis, B. (2019). Racism and health: Evidence and needed research. *Annual Review Public Health*, 40, 105–25. https://doi.org/10.1146/annurev-publichealth-040218-043750

Williams, J. R., Gonzalez-Guarda, R. M., Halstead, V., Martinez, J., & Joseph, L. (2020). Disclosing gender-based violence during health care visits: A patient-centered approach. *Journal of Interpersonal Violence*, 35(23-24), 5552–5573. https://doi.org/10.1177/0886260517720733

Wimalasena, N. N., Chang-Richards, A., Wang, K. I., & Dirks, K. N. (2021). Housing risk factors associated with respiratory disease: A systematic review. *International Journal of Environmental Research and Public Health*, 18(6), 2815. https://doi.org/10.3390/ijerph18062815

Woolf, S. H., Aron, L., Dubay, L., Simon, S. M., Zimmerman, E., & Luk, K. (2015). How are income and wealth linked to health and longevity? Urban Institute and Virginia Commonwealth University. https://www.urban.org/research/publication/how-are-income-and-wealth-linked-health-and-longevity

World Health Organization. (2018). WHO Housing and health guidelines. https://apps.who.int/iris/bitstream/handle/10665/276001/9789241550376-eng.pdf

World Health Organization. (2020). Definition and typology of violence. https://www.who.int/violenceprevention/approach/definition/en/

World Health Organization. (2021). Health impact assessment. https://www.who.int/health-topics/health-impact-assessment#tab=tab_1

CHAPTER 5

Epidemiology and Health Disparities

Faye A. Gary and Hossein N. Yarandi

LEARNING OBJECTIVES

◉ Explain historical trends in the American health system and relate these trends to contemporary issues in health outcomes.

◉ Discuss factors that influence human health and outcomes from the epidemiological methodology perspective.

◉ Compare and contrast the differences between health equality and health equity and give two examples of each.

◉ Apply the three approaches to health generated by the World Health Organization (WHO) to common health issues in local and global communities.

◉ Explain the epidemiological triad in the context of COVID-19 and Healthy People 2023 and the social determinants of the health model.

INTRODUCTION

As a primary core in public health and other disciplines involved in the measurement of health outcomes (Curley, 2020), epidemiology is "the study of the distribution and determinants of health-related states or events (including disease), and the application of this study to the control of diseases and other health problems" (Last, 1988). Other disciplines are interwoven into this approach to science, such as biostatistics, biology, anthropology, geography, economics, nursing, sociology, and others, which serve as backdrops for creating epidemiological data and community profiles (Tapia, 2003). Epidemiology is often considered the basic science of public health aimed at the prevention of disease and the promotion of health. Epidemiology focuses on social interactions of human activities that affect health and examines the social and behavioral factors associated with health and illness.

EPIDEMIOLOGY: BASIC PUBLIC HEALTH SCIENCE

Factors that impact human health may include social hardships (e.g., poverty, lack of health insurance, discrimination) and lifestyle practices (e.g., smoking, unhealthy eating habits, alcohol and substance use). Epidemiology considers how well-established exposures (e.g., environmental exposures such as noise, water, and air pollutants) occur within the social system. This leads to the identification of social characteristics that affect the pattern of disease and health status in a society and an understanding of its mechanisms. Some important concepts of epidemiology are social inequalities, social relationships, social capital, and work stress (Braveman, 2006; Curley, 2020; Donkin, 2014; Marmot et al., 2008).

Epidemiologists explore the access of populations to public health services and examine the effects of inequalities on health (Box 5.1). They can contribute to the process of health management and the reduction of inequities in health. Epidemiologists can make a useful contribution to health services research by identifying social inequality factors that influence health and healthcare. Social inequality factors like education or income can influence access, utilization, and quality in healthcare (Donkin, 2014; Ghebreyesus, 2020; Satcher, 2020; Shultz et al., 2021). Social relationships networks influence help-seeking behavior, utilization of health services, compliance or adherence to medical treatment, and outcomes. They also provide social, emotional, and financial support to individuals and families (Hamilton, 2021; World Health Organization [WHO], 2008; Shultz et al., 2021).

Social inequality is the existence of unequal opportunities and rewards for different social positions or status within a group or society. It involves structured and recurrent patterns of unequal distributions of goods, wealth, opportunities, rewards, and punishments. Income, wealth, power, occupational prestige, schooling, ancestry, and race distinguish important dimensions of social inequality.

Social inequality goes hand in hand with social stratification. Discrimination at individual, community, and institutional levels is a major cause of social inequality with respect to race, ethnicity, class, gender, and sexuality. Social inequality can manifest in two ways:

◆ Inequality of conditions (unequal distribution of income, wealth, and material goods)
◆ Inequality of opportunities (unequal access to education, healthcare, and cultural resources, including differential treatment by the judicial system)

Social inequality can be studied under three dimensions: structural conditions, ideological supports, and social reforms. *Structural conditions* include measurable factors that contribute

BOX 5.1: Two Among Many Views of Social Inequality: Functionalist Theory and Conflict Theory

Functionalist Theory

- Those who receive more training should obtain more rewards.
- Advancement should be the result of individual ability or achievement.

Conflict Theory

- Social inequality prevents and hampers individual and community progress.
- Individuals and groups within a society maximize their own wealth and power.
- Those in power maintain the status quo by limiting those who are powerless.

Source: Adapted from Lenski, G. E. (2013). *Power and privilege: A theory of social stratification.* University of North Carolina Press.

to social inequality. Educational attainment, wealth, poverty, occupation, and power are all measurable factors that lead to social inequality between individuals and groups of people. *Ideological supports* comprise ideas and assumptions that support the social inequality present in a society. Examination of these aspects of society illuminates how things such as formal laws, public policies, and dominant values reinforce social inequality and help sustain it. Organized resistance, protest groups, and social movements are examples of *social reforms* designed to help shape or change social inequality that exists in a society. Social reforms gain impetus through the exposition of the origins, impact, and long-term effects of inequality (Donkin, 2014; Garrigues, 2021; Ghebreyesus, 2020; Lueddeke, 2015; Marmot, 2017; Matthew, 2018).

Social relationships affect mental health, physical health, health behaviors, and mortality risk. People seek social relationships at work and in communities, educational settings, religious organizations, online communities, and other social contexts. These relationships have immediate and long-term cumulative effects on physical and mental health. Depriving people of social relationships can be physically and psychologically devastating (Donkin, 2014; Garrigues, 2021; Kunitz, 2004; Lenski, 2013; Lueddeke, 2015; WHO, 2008; Zheng, 2018).

Social capital includes the network of relationships, norms, and social trust that facilitate coordination and cooperation for mutual benefit. Social capital is frequently cited in health research, affirming the positive relationship between socioeconomic status and individual health status. This relationship remains an important factor in maintaining good health. Social capital has been used as a means of understanding how income inequality might be associated with health disparities.

Community organizations play important roles in facilitating health outcome. For example, African American and Hispanic American churches initially demonstrated hesitancy about becoming involved with those swept up in the HIV/AIDS epidemic, but with exposure to more scientific data, were able to assist affected individuals and their families (Kunitz, 2004). Health practices of relatives and friends can also have a profound influence on help-seeking behaviors and support for treatment. These relationships can work to the benefit and detriment of certain groups at a particular time. From another perspective, social capital may be valuable in facilitating various actions and behavioral changes such as voting, getting mammography screening, or getting the vaccine for COVID-19 (Kunitz, 2004; Marmot, 2017; Snowden & Graaf, 2021).

Work stress, a common feature of most occupations, may result from work overload, time pressures, interpersonal conflicts, inadequate compensation, threat of job layoff, and unemployment. *Stress* has been defined as physical and emotional factors that can accumulate to cause physical or mental disorders. Frequently, stress has been studied in relation to cardiovascular disease, substance use, posttraumatic stress disorder, work-related anxiety disorders, chronic diseases, and impaired immune function. More than ever before, rapid changes in work expectations and settings pose a threat to the health of workers. Nurses and physicians have some of the highest levels of stress in healthcare systems (Donkin, 2014; Pihkala, 2020; Rodriquez et al., 2017; Wells, 2011).

Climate trauma is related to crises that permeate events occurring worldwide. A distinguishing feature of climate trauma is the threat to the global environment impacting all living plants and animals on earth. The reality suggests that there is a shared human connection created by climate trauma that links all of humanity—and represents a period of the environmental record when the daily activities of humans begin to have a substantial negative impact on flora and fauna ecosystems, the atmosphere, and the entire planet. It has the potential to activate past traumas, including personal, cultural, historical, political, and intergenerational phenomena. Climate trauma has not yet been acknowledged as being manifest across the world community—yet its effects permeate all life forms.

Examples of manifestations of climate trauma are numerous. Catastrophes have the capacity to create instant acute psychological trauma—physical injury, death, destruction of personal property, loss of jobs and meaningful employment, terror, shock, anxiety, depression, isolation, and a plethora of emotions. Migration and displacement of families and large populations are common outcomes. Intense concerns about the future of a community, or a nation, or the world are topics of consideration (Clayton et al., 2014; Pihkala, 2020; Woodbury, 2019). Local, state, national, and international governments will need to develop community-relevant plans to respond quickly and efficiently to the perils of climate change, which include the physical environment and the psychological and emotional short- and long-term needs of individuals and families (Sheehan et al., 2017).

EQUALITY, EQUITY, AND POPULATION-FOCUSED HEALTHCARE

Health disparities, health inequality, and health inequities (Box 5.2) are terms that are often used interchangeably in the literature and in clinical practice. Researchers have sought to provide clarity about these concepts (Braveman, 2006).

Health disparities and *health inequalities* are terms linked to the categories of differences in health status that have the most critical impact on an individual's health and that could hypothetically be manipulated by law or policy. Groups that experience health disparity or health inequality have systematically and persistently experienced prejudice and discrimination. They have been exposed to biases in general society and when interacting with healthcare providers. The health outcomes among these populations are worse than those of their more affluent counterparts in society, who might enjoy advantages of wealth, status, or race, for example (Braveman, 2006; Matthew, 2018).

Health equity, on the other hand, refers to the intent to reduce and eliminate health disparities through a systems approach among health institutions, as shown in Figure 5.1 (Marmot et al., 2008; Matthew, 2018). Evidence is available to support findings that people living in poverty in U.S. communities—and globally—experience more illness, infectious

BOX 5.2: Causes of Health Disparities, Health Inequality, and Health Inequities

- Economic disadvantage
- Racial/ethnic/minority status
- Disorders and disabilities
  - Physical
  - Intellectual
  - Psychiatric
- Gender identities other than cisgender heterosexual male
- Female gender
- GLBTQIA+ identity
- Age
  - Older adults
  - Children
    - Immigrants, migrants, and their families
    - Zip code
  - Rural
  - Disadvantaged urban areas
  - Native reservations

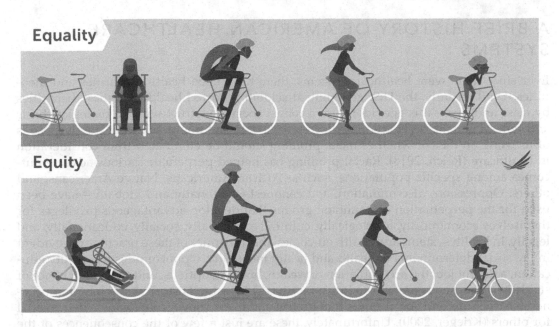

Figure 5.1 Health equality versus health equity.

Source: Robert Wood Johnson Foundation. (2017). *Visualizing health equity: One size does not fit all.*
www.rwjf.org/en/library/infographics/visualizing-health-equity.html.

disease, and disability than their more resourced counterparts. Basic health needs such as ample food and clean water are critical, along with decent shelter and the proper disposal of solid waste. Access to quality healthcare is essential (Marmot, 2015). Health equity suggests that the focus must be on the "causes of the causes" and an in-depth review of the two basic structures: (a) the fundamental constructs of a society's social order or hierarchy, and (b) the conditions in an environment that create and maintain unhealthy circumstances for those who live there (Braveman, 2006; Hess, 2020; Marmot, 2007; Matthew, 2018).

Examples of how the absence of health equity can quickly express itself have been demonstrated in COVID-19 morbidity and mortality rates among the nation's vulnerable populations (Khazanchi et al., 2020; Satcher, 2020). Other disease conditions, such as malnutrition, smoking, alcohol use, hypertension, physical inactivity, obesity, and risky sexual behaviors, are local and global causes of noncommunicable diseases, most of which are preventable (Murray et al., 2013). In the context of equity, one must ask, "What are the causes of these conditions? How did they happen?"

Examples of future trends of global burdens are associated with caring for an aging population and the persistent proliferation of HIV/AIDS in some global geographical areas (U.S. Department of Health and Human Services [DHHS], 2020). Health outcomes will depend on how mortality is addressed through social and economic structures and investments in people living in poverty and in communities at all levels. Equity will occur when the available resources are adjusted in accordance with human needs (Ghebreyesus, 2020; Marmot et al., 2008; Mathers & Loncar, 2006; Matthew, 2018; Shultz et al., 2021).

Population-focused healthcare involves the turning of attention to various risk factors (demographic factors such as age, race/ethnicity, and geographical locale), data analyses, and interpretation of findings; these produce profiles that highlight the existence of health disparities. These elements are essential because they are used to help determine how variables will be measured and monitored and how funding agencies (including the federal government and private or community-based organizations) might allocate resources (Braveman, 2006; Marmot et al., 2008; Tapia, 2003).

A BRIEF HISTORY OF AMERICAN HEALTHCARE SYSTEMS

Ever since there were healthcare systems, there have been health disparities and inequities. Until recently, the U.S. government seldom reported health statistics/disparities by class and race—this is evidence of a robust social construct with no biological basis and reflects genetic diversity (Smedley et al., 2009). One might ask what the purpose is of focusing on race or whether racial profiling should be eliminated from consideration in healthcare (Reich, 2018). Racial profiling has helped perpetuate various adverse outcomes among specific populations, such as African Americans, Native Americans, and others. Oppression, discrimination, and conquest—nationally and globally—have been used for the perpetuation of dominant groups that develop advantageous privileges for themselves economically, ideologically, culturally, politically, socially, educationally, and legally. In health systems and health outcomes, the dynamics of these practices are evident in the social determinants of health and health inequality. Opportunities for quality education, a decent job, the accumulation of wealth, housing options, and the maintenance of stable neighborhoods are woven into a race-based tapestry. Historical and long-term economic structures and social status that protect and favor some groups can be detrimental for others (Krieger, 2000). Unfortunately, these are just a few of the consequences of the social construct of race.

More specific data about the health status of the American people could better inform researchers, policy makers, educators, and the general public, thereby assisting all individuals in their pursuit of healthier, longer, and more satisfying lives (Meyer et al., 2013). Recently, researchers have suggested that a more efficacious approach to eliminating health disparities might be through using model-based health promotion interventions that are grounded in culturally and historically oriented factors. Pender's model of health promotion, for example, is a broad approach that focuses on identifying and supporting habits and lifestyles that lead to optimal health (Pender, 2011; Murdaugh et al., 2018).

The Heckler Report represents one of the first national attempts to delineate the health status of minority people in America despite disparities that have existed for more than four centuries (Bediako & Griffith, 2008; Heckler, 1985; Thomas & Casper, 2019). Smedley et al. (2009), in their book *Unequal Treatment: Confronting Racial and Ethnic Disparities in Healthcare*, warned that the overall poor health status of minority people in the United States had not appreciably changed over the previous 20 years. Federal initiatives such as *Healthy People 2000* and *Healthy People 2020* continue to shed light on the severity and long-standing devastating impact of poor health outcomes among minority populations and other disadvantaged groups (Centers for Disease Control and Prevention [CDC], 1990; Koh et al., 2014). *Healthy People 2030* continues the assessment of the nation's health with hope for progress (Box 5.3; National Academies of Sciences, Engineering and Medicine [NASEM], 2019, 2020; DHHS, 2020).

BOX 5.3: Healthy People 2030's Five Domains to Guide Implementation of Social Determinants of Health

1. Economic stability
2. Education
3. Healthcare access and quality
4. Neighborhood and built community environment
5. Social and community context

GLOBAL PREVENTION OF HEALTH INEQUITIES

Despite an abundance of affordable and effective life-saving technologies, medicines, and knowledge, inequities in health outcomes continue to expand globally. This is largely due to insufficient attention to illness prevention and the broader social determinants of health. Healthcare aims should focus on developing systems within health services to collaboratively monitor and improve health policy and provide a framework for improved measurement of social capital processes and impacts.

Primary Prevention

The 1978 Alma-Ata Declaration represented the culminating recommendations of the International Conference on Primary Healthcare held in Alma-Ata, Kazakh Soviet Socialist Republic (currently Kazakhstan). It became a worldwide landmark in the reformation of healthcare delivery systems. Prior to this, primary healthcare had been conceptualized as a hospital-based phenomenon with a focus on biomedical practice. WHO (Box 5.4) incorporated the principles of the Alma-Ata Declaration into the goal *Health for All*, heralding a transformative paradigm shift toward providing community- and family-oriented care highlighting the elimination of health disparities. Using this expanded and reconfigured primary care design, the prevailing emphasis would be on the unique needs of individuals and families in communities with the goal of the improvement of overall well-being (Ghebreyesus, 2020).

The 2018 Astana Declaration on Primary Healthcare (Kazakhstan), unanimously endorsed by members of WHO, reaffirmed the global need for enhanced primary care, sustainable health systems, and availability of universal health coverage. The declaration advised that primary care should offer a variety of services supporting the individual and the family. Promotion, prevention, early detection, prompt treatment, rehabilitation, and palliative care are core components of this approach. Linking personalized care to population healthcare is an important pathway to the elimination of health disparities, reaffirming the aspiration of *Health for All* (Ghebreyesus, 2020; Marmot et al., 2008; Satcher, 2020).

Secondary Prevention

Specifically, secondary prevention involves actions that bring about prompt and efficient assessment and treatment as soon as there is some suspicion of an illness condition. The intent is to cure or effectively manage a disease as promptly and efficiently as possible when persons have preclinical signs and symptoms or suspect that "something" might need attention. Screenings for depression, anxiety, bone density, or cholesterol levels in community clinics and hospitals are some common examples of secondary prevention (Ghebreyesus, 2020; Marmot et al., 2008; Matthew, 2018).

BOX 5.4: The World Health Organization's Approaches to Global Health and Well-Being

WHO has been instrumental in advancing three approaches to address health and well-being across the global community:

1. *Primary prevention*: Preventing occurrence of injury or disease.
2. *Secondary prevention*: Reducing consequences of injury or disease.
3. *Tertiary prevention*: Helping with long-term management of injury or disease.

Tertiary Prevention

Tertiary prevention is embedded in the theory and practice of public health models. In general, it is the promotion of ongoing treatment and management of illnesses, especially chronic conditions. The approach involves the following features, all of which should ideally take into consideration families and other support services:

◆ Working to improve prognosis
◆ Monitoring and preventing the exacerbation of signs and symptoms
◆ Decreasing the potential for disability
◆ Restoring the individual to the highest possible level of functioning

Professionals in the field should strive to ensure best practices; evidence-based science should be used to facilitate healthcare and decision-making (Dodd et al., 2014; Starfield et al., 2008). Inculcated in the three levels of prevention are methods for prediction and prevention of disease, which is the core of epidemiology (Curley, 2020; Shultz et al., 2021).

See Box 5.5 for a list of public health milestones.

PROJECTING DISEASE RISKS AND PREVENTION

A critical function of epidemiology is the study of etiology, the natural history of disease and methods for providing care across the life course. Several models for thinking have been developed to explain how diseases occur and behave. One model, the epidemiological triad, can be used to explain the transmission of diseases such as influenza and COVID-19 (Figure 5.2). This model provides a straightforward way to understand how diseases cause health problems by highlighting interactions among an agent (disease), a host (a vulnerable person/animal), and the environment that facilitates the interaction among them. Controlling of the disease will occur when there is a disruption in the triangle, which thwarts the spread of the disease (Mpolya et al., 2009; Tsui et al., 2020). The host includes noninfected people/animals. Their age, gender, comorbidities, susceptibility, and sometimes race may be included in documentation. The agent is the disease, which is described according to strain, pathogenicity, and virulence. The environment provides exposure to droplets, surfaces, ingested substances, and air movement. The interruption between one of the three elements in the triad is needed to reduce and eliminate the continued spread of disease.

BOX 5.5: Public Health Milestones

- COVID-19 pandemic response
- Vaccines: polio, diphtheria, tetanus, pertussis, and other preventable diseases
- Marked reduction of tobacco use
- Reduction in heart disease
- Early detection and treatment of cancer
- HIV/AIDS prevention and treatment
- Early childhood health and nutrition
- Fluoridated water; better oral health

Source: Adapted from Research America. (2020). *Public health milestones.* www.researchamerica.org

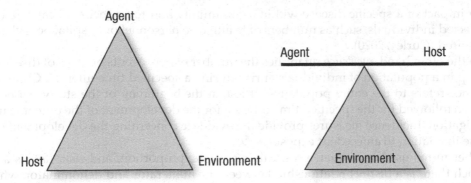

Figure 5.2 Epidemiological triad.

Source: Adapted from U.S. Department of Health and Human Services. (2012). *Principles of epidemiology in public health practice (3rd ed.).* ww.cdc.gov/csels/dsepd/ss1978/SS1978.pdf.

BOX 5.6: The ABCs of Epidemiology

A principal objective in epidemiology is to identify the causes of disease. Classically, the definition of causality is one of pure determinism in which a constant, unique, and perfectly predictable connection is postulated between two factors X and Y. X is a cause of Y means any manipulation or change in X alone induces a subsequent change in Y.

More specifically, this definition of causation requires two criteria: specificity of cause and specificity of effect. The former indicates that X is the only cause of Y, and the latter indicates that Y is the only effect of X.

The specificity of cause criterion implies that two other conditions must also be met: X is both a necessary and sufficient cause of Y. X is a necessary cause if all changes in Y must be preceded by changes in X; conversely, X is a sufficient cause if all changes in X inevitably induce changes in Y.

It should be noted that the two sufficient and necessary conditions are theoretically independent. That is, a factor may be a necessary but not sufficient cause, a sufficient but not necessary cause, both necessary and sufficient, or neither necessary.

Source: Adapted from Pearl, J. (2009). *Causality: Models, reasoning, and inference (2nd ed.).* Cambridge University Press.

EPIDEMIOLOGICAL METHODOLOGY

Measurement is essential in epidemiology (Box 5.6). It is a prerequisite for any epidemiological investigation to quantify the occurrence of disease. The fundamental concerns of epidemiologists are the measurement, the analysis, and the interpretation of an observed set of new events, incident cases of disease, deaths from one or more causes, or new occurrences of any health-related event. The information interpretation and the decisions made in the care of patients depend on measurement (Keyes & Galea, 2016).

The three main groups of measures in epidemiology are *frequency, association,* and *potential impact.* Incidence and prevalence are the most significant frequency measures and can be obtained when both morbidity and mortality of diseases are studied. In descriptive epidemiology, these measures are fundamental and involve studying how the disease is distributed in the population.

Prevalence is defined as the proportion of the population that are cases at a point in time. Thus, prevalence can be thought of as the status of the disease in a population at a point in time. Prevalence measures are most useful for healthcare providers to assess the public health impact of a specific disease within a community and to project medical care needs for affected individuals, such as numbers of health care personnel or hospital beds that will be required (Curley, 2020).

On the other hand, *incidence* quantifies the number of new events or cases of disease that develop in a population of individuals at risk during a specified time interval. Cumulative incidence refers to the entire population at risk at the beginning of the study period that has been followed for the specified time interval for the development of the outcome under investigation. Incidence measures provide the evidence concerning the development of the disease in relation to antecedent exposures.

Other terms used in frequency measures are rate, proportion, and risk. *Rate* is a ratio in which there is a distinct relationship between the numerator and denominator, where a measure of time is an intrinsic part of the denominator, such as number of miles per hour. *Risk* is the probability of an individual's developing a given disease or experiencing a health status change over a specified period. And *proportion* is a type of ratio in which those who are included in the numerator must also be included in the denominator, such as the proportion of women older than 50 years who have had a hysterectomy.

The strength of the statistical relationship between a given study factor and a disease are assessed using measures of association. Measures of association involve a direct comparison of frequency measures for different values or categories of the study factor. The study population is divided into two or more groups, each of which can be compared to a single category designated as the reference group. Preferably, the reference group should be large enough to provide precise frequency estimates, and it should be relatively homogeneous so that comparisons are meaningful. Odds ratio and relative risk are the most significant measures of association that are used in analytical epidemiology.

The *relative risk* estimates the magnitude of an association between exposure and disease and indicates the likelihood of developing the disease in the exposed group relative to those who are not exposed. It is defined as the ratio of the incidence of disease in the exposed group divided by the corresponding incidence of disease in the nonexposed group. Its value can be one, more than one, or less than one. A relative risk equal to one indicates that the incidence rates of disease in the exposed and nonexposed groups are identical and thus that there is no association observed between the exposure and the disease in the data. A relative risk of more than one indicates a positive association (i.e., an increased risk among those exposed to a factor). And a relative risk of less than one indicates an inverse association (i.e., a decreased risk among those exposed).

Odds ratio is defined as the ratio of odds of being exposed if having disease to those of being exposed if disease-free. It is based on odds rather than risks. In a case-control study (or retrospective), where participants are selected based on disease status, it is usually not possible to calculate the risk of development of disease given the presence or absence of exposure. Instead, the odds ratio should be calculated for data in a case-control study. On the other hand, the relative risk will be a proper measure of association in a cohort (or prospective) study.

Other terms used for the measure of association are attributable risk and attributable risk percent. *Attributable risk* is a measure of association that provides information about the absolute effect of the exposure or the excess risk of disease in those exposed compared with those nonexposed. This measure is defined as the difference between the incidence rates in the exposed and nonexposed groups and is used to quantify the risk of disease in the exposed group that can be considered attributable to the exposure by removing the risk of disease that would have occurred anyway due to other causes. The interpretation of the attributable risk is dependent on the assumption that a cause/effect relationship exists between exposure and disease. There would be no association between exposure and disease if the attributable risk equals zero. On the other hand, there would a causal association between the exposure and disease if the attributable risk is more than one, which indicates the number of cases of the disease among the exposed that can be attributed to the exposure itself, or the number of cases of the disease among the exposed that could be eliminated if the exposure were eliminated. The attributable risk can be useful as a measure of the public health impact of a particular exposure.

The attributable risk exposure as a proportion (or percentage) of total risk in the exposed group is known as the *attributable risk percent*. The attributable risk, which is often expressed as a percentage, estimates the proportion of the disease among the exposed that is attributable to the exposure, or the proportion of the disease in that group that could be prevented by eliminating the exposure.

Measures of potential impact reflect the expected contribution of a study factor to the frequency of a disease in a particular population. It is a combination of frequency and association measures that are derived from case-control and cohort studies in order to understand and to help compare the population impact of different interventions. Examples of measures of potential impact could be predicting the impact of removing a hazardous exposure from the population; the number of persons with a disease that must be treated to achieve one beneficial outcome or to prevent one adverse outcome; and the number of people that are exposed to the particular exposure or risk factor. In general, it is important to consider that the relevance of calculating the frequency, association, and potential impact measures depends on the study design (Kestenbaum, 2019).

Relative risk is a measure of the strength of the association between an exposure and disease and provides information that can be used to judge whether a valid observed association is likely to be causal. In contrast, the attributable risk provides a measure of the public health impact of an exposure, assuming that the association is one of cause and effect. The magnitude of the relative risk alone does not predict the magnitude of the attributable risk. For example, cigarette smoking is a much stronger risk factor for mortality from lung cancer than for coronary heart disease. However, if smoking is causally related to both diseases, the elimination of cigarettes would prevent far more deaths among smokers from coronary heart disease than from lung cancer. Although the death from lung cancer is a relatively rare occurrence, the annual death rate for coronary heart disease is much higher. Therefore, the potential public health impact of smoking cessation on mortality will be far greater for coronary heart disease than for lung cancer (Aschengrau & Seage, 2018).

Unravelling Our Understanding of COVID-19

COVID-19 is a pandemic with unique characteristics that should be understood as one develops policy and information for education and prevention. Community-based efforts to eradicate the COVID-19 virus include vaccines, antiviral therapy, testing, education, masking, social distancing, handwashing, isolation, and travel/visit restrictions (Tsui et al., 2020). Narrative 5.1 provides a succinct overview of the situation facing epidemiologists.

NARRATIVE 5.1: EPIDEMIOLOGY OF COVID-19, BY NICHOLAS K. SCHILTZ, PhD

Coronavirus disease 2019 (COVID-19) is an ongoing global pandemic caused by the severe acute respiratory syndrome coronavirus 2 (SARS-CoV-2). The pandemic began in late 2019 and has continued into 2021, with more than 607 million cases and more than 6.4 million deaths worldwide as of September 2022 (WHO, n.d.).

COVID-19 spreads quickly as it has a relatively high basic reproduction number (R0), estimated at 5.7 (Sanche et al., 2020). This means that each person with the disease will on average infect 5 to 6 new people. For comparison, seasonal flu has an R0 of about 1.3 (Biggerstaff et al., 2014). The virus spreads person-to-person via respiratory droplets and can be transmitted by asymptomatic carriers.

(continued)

NARRATIVE 5.1: EPIDEMIOLOGY OF COVID-19, BY NICHOLAS K. SCHILTZ, PhD (*CONTINUED*)

Most of the efforts to control the disease have been nonpharmaceutical interventions aimed at reducing the effective R0 and hence slowing the spread of disease. These interventions have included recommendations or mandates calling for social distancing; wearing a face mask in public; business and school closures; working at home; increased vigilance of hand washing; and frequent cleaning and disinfecting of surfaces (Ayouni et al., 2021). Several COVID-19 vaccines were approved in late 2020, which provide acquired immunity to the SARS-CoV-2 virus.

The burden of COVID-19 has not been equal across populations. While infection rates are similar across age groups, the risk of hospitalization and death increases drastically with older age (Centers for Disease Control and Prevention [CDC], 2021a). There are significant disparities in COVID-19 infection rates and outcomes by race and ethnicity in the United States. Mortality rates due to COVID-19 are 1.8 times higher among American Indians/Alaska Natives (Arrazola et al., 2020), 1.9 times higher among Black Americans/African Americans (CDC, 2021b), and 2.3 times higher among Hispanic Americans compared with White Americans (CDC, 2021b). The incidence of COVID-19 varies globally, as Europe, the United States, and Latin America have experienced higher fatality rates compared with Asian and African nations. The cause of these differences is not known but could be due to differences in population age, underreporting, or past immune system exposures (Sorci et al., 2020).

SOCIAL DETERMINANTS OF HEALTH

In recent years, the social determinants of health have been used to help illuminate a series of events that occur when people who are disadvantaged concerning socioeconomic status have less favorable health outcomes and shorter life expectancies than their more advantaged counterparts (Donkin, 2014; Marmot et al., 2008). Specifically, the social determinants of health refer to economic stability, access to and quality of education, access to and quality of healthcare, neighborhood and environment, and social and community context of individuals and populations (see Figure 4.1 in Chapter 4).

People employed in lower-status jobs—essential workers (a frequently used term during the COVID-19 pandemic that includes bus drivers, grocers, maintenance workers, and others)—are more likely to perceive themselves as having poor health. Numerous researchers have observed that definite health risks and undesirable behaviors are evident among disadvantaged populations, such as smoking, poor diet, and limited exercise. Ungratifying working conditions—low autonomy, lack of job satisfaction, and unsafe work environments—thrust individuals into conditions that are unhealthy. These are factors that mitigate against opportunities to improve health status and, in some cases, overall social status (Braveman, 2006; Donkin, 2014; Koh et al., 2014; Marmot et al., 1991; see Chapter 7 for more detailed discussion of health disparities).

The Commission on Social Determinants of Health, created by WHO, concluded with three basic recommendations:

1. Address inequities that occur because of the social conditions related to where individuals work, are educated, and reside.
2. Challenge and fix the inequities that are associated with power, money, privilege, and resources.
3. Measure the problems, collect data, evaluate actions, expand knowledge and skills, develop a workforce that is astute about and attentive to the social determinants of health, and raise public awareness about these essentials that are associated with improving health outcomes and reducing morbidity and mortality (WHO, 2008).

The social determinants of health provide support for the position that health is more than the sum of genetic variations and lifestyles. These are positions that have long been the prevailing sentiments linked to morbidity and mortality. This is especially true in the United States where the health systems—despite being scientifically and technically advanced—are not always equally accessible to all persons (Marmot, 2015).

Implicit bias is still evident during clinical encounters and needs to be acknowledged and addressed (Matthew, 2018). Implicit bias can dominate all aspects of the provider's interactions with the patient. Race and ethnicity are the communication starting points, including the provider's knowledge and skillsets about the illness phenomena and different perceptions regarding the patient's racial or ethnic group. Factors such as biased perceptions, biased use of statistical data, and biased clinical encounters between the provider and the patient collectively influence the patient's diagnosis and plan of care. These factors sway the patient's sense of bias after the medical assessment has occurred. A sense of satisfaction, trust, adherence to the proposed therapeutic plan, and self-management of the disease are desirable outcomes: These are some of the critical elements needed to reduce health disparities and enhance the embodiment of health equity (Matthews, 2015).

The National Institute of Minority Health and Health Disparities (NIMHD) research framework is an important tool for highlighting variabilities among specific populations (e.g., race/ethnicity, socioeconomic status, age, sexual orientation, mental health status, immigrant status, geography, disability; Alvidrez et al., 2019). This framework could be used to refine perspectives in research, practice, and policy (Exhibit 5.1).

The NIMHD research framework has five domains of influence that are manifested over the life course: biological, behavioral, physical/built environment, sociocultural environment, and health systems (see Exhibit 5.1). Corresponding to these domains are four levels of influence: individual, interpersonal, community, and societal. All of the

EXHIBIT 5.1: National Institute on Minority Health Disparities Research

Framework					
		Levels of Influence*			
		Individual	**Interpersonal**	**Community**	**Societal**
Domains of Influence (Over the Lifecourse)	**Biological**	Biological Vulnerability and Mechanisms	Caregiver–Child Interaction Family Microbiome	Community Illness Exposure Herd Immunity	Sanitation Immunization Pathogen Exposure
	Behavioral	Health Behaviors Coping Strategies	Family Functioning School/Work Functioning	Community Functioning	Policies and Laws
	Physical/Built Environment	Personal Environment	Household Environment School/Work Environment	Community Environment Community Resources	Societal Structure
	Sociocultural Environment	Sociodemographics Limited English Cultural Identity Response to Discrimination	Social Networks Family/Peer Norms Interpersonal Discrimination	Community Norms Local Structural Discrimination	Social Norms Societal Structural Discrimination
	Health Care System	Insurance Coverage Health Literacy Treatment Preferences	Patient–Clinician Relationship Medical Decision-Making	Availability of Services Safety Net Services	Quality of Care Health Care Policies
Health Outcomes		Individual Health	Family/ Organizational Health	Community Health	Population Health

Source: National Institutes of Health on Minority Health and Health Disparities. (n.d.). *NIMHD research framework.* www.nimhd.nih.gov/about/overview/research-framework/nimhd -framework.html.

domains and levels of influence are interconnected. This model can be applied to any population or community, and it provides the researcher with the option to adapt the model to fit the characteristic of the population they are studying and the purposes of their research.

Healthy People 2030 and the Social Determinants of Health

The amelioration of social disparities can become overwhelming when one realizes the enormity of the issues that require attention. It is imperative that epidemiologists recognize the interconnectedness of factors on multiple levels so that they might arrive at conclusions that are valid. As seen in the illustration of the fishbowl dilemma (Figure 5.3), recommendations to replace the dirty water in the fishbowl would not have solved the problem that sickened the fish unless the crack in the glass had also been repaired. And neither of those remedies would have helped because there was no food either (Keyes & Galea, 2016). So it is with efforts to bring about equity. "Band-aid" approaches simply do not work. Effective solutions require the wisdom of careful consideration from a broad perspective. A broad perspective involves grappling with needs and solutions as they play out at the level of individuals, their families, and the communities that give them support, all the way through to local, state, national, and global organizations, programs, and policies that are designed to improve the human condition (Artiga & Hinton, 2018). The goal must be to provide equity so that people and societies can thrive to their full potential.

Over the past two decades, the social determinants of health have come to the forefront in healthcare. The social determinants of health help to delineate the differences likely to be experienced by members of specific populations, such as access to quality healthcare, a valuable education, and thriving and safe neighborhoods. The traditional impetus to improve health is shifting from healthcare systems to a broader approach and the recognition that other critical factors influence health. This approach includes the influence of social, economic, environmental, and behavioral factors on health outcomes. It emphasizes the composite circumstances in the environments where people are born, live, learn, work, play, worship, and age that affect a wide range of health, functioning, and quality-of-life outcomes and risks (DHHS, 2020).

In creating the major components of Healthy People 2030, the social determinants of health were highlighted, with emphasis on the following:

Economic stability increases the likelihood of individuals to be healthy. It can typically provide them with the purchasing power to obtain the necessities for maintenance of a reasonably good level of health.

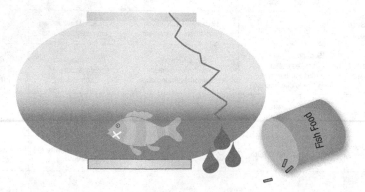

Figure 5.3 Epidemiological interconnectedness.
Source: Adapted from Keyes, K.M., Galea, S. (2016). *Population health science.* Oxford University Press.

Education plays a beneficial life-long role in the social determinants of health. As a rule, people who have achieved higher levels of education live longer. Children from underresourced communities commonly have deficits in reading and math, compromising their efforts for graduating from high school, restricting their potential for completing college, and negatively impacting their economic stabilily (Haycock, 2010).

Healthcare access and quality are essential for improving health and eliminating health disparities. This particular goal is focused on helping individuals to obtain quality healthcare services that are timely and culturally appropriate. Unlike other developed nations, not having proper health insurance is a major barrier in the United States, where one in 10 people do not have health insurance (Berchick et al., 2018; DHHS, 2020). Other barriers include lack of transportation, lack of a primary care provider, and limited access to healthcare professionals and communications, whether in person or virtually (DHHS, 2020). Facilitation of communication between the provider and the patient is essential for the elimination of health disparities.

Neighborhood and built community environments encompass those spaces where individuals make their homes, find jobs, receive their education, form social networks, and engage in recreation. Improving the quality of these spaces significantly impacts the health, safety, and well-being of people across the life course (Berchick et al., 2018; DHHS, 2020). Too many people live in communities where violence is at an unacceptable rate, safe recreational and walking space are lacking, air quality is poor, and water—though essential for sustaining life—is not readily available or is contaminated. These risk factors are more likely to exist in urban and rural neighborhoods where minority people and other Americans living in poverty reside (Hess, 2020). Adequate laws and policies, along with interventions with measurable metrics at the local, regional, state, and national levels, are required for the improvement of living conditions among disadvantaged populations.

Social and community context highlights the value of healthy interpersonal relations among family, friends, colleagues, and neighbors. Within these structures are nested support systems and reference groups. When neighborhoods are safe and people have basic amenities necessary for healthy living, health outcomes are more likely to be favorable. Conversely, where racial and religious discrimination exist, it is more likely that crime, poor schools, and inadequate housing will be evident, basic determinants of health will be compromised, and life expectancy and general well-being will suffer. Some people are "caught" in circumstances, and even when there is a desire to improve individual health habits, the goals that lead to healthier lives might not always be attainable (Rodriquez et al., 2017).

Flint, Michigan, Water Crisis

Fundamental issues confronting epidemiologists include identification of the causes of new cases of diseases through systematic scientific approaches, documentation of deaths, and being alert to any emerging health-related threats. Clean water, the primary source of life, should be available to all people and all communities in the United States, the wealthiest country in the world. Instead, the Flint community's contaminated water placed residents at risk and compromised health outcomes, including blood lead levels among children. Clean water is essential to health; reliable access reduces medical expenses and missed days of employment and school, which have implications for the community's economic stability. The Flint water crisis has had a profoundly harmful impact on the people of that community. Anxiety and depression continue to be evident. Basic epidemiological principles have been violated. Trust among residents and health systems and local and state governments has been eroded, much like the rusty pipes that carried the contaminated water to Flint residents (Boufides et al., 2019; James, 2017; Satcher, 2020; Shultz et al., 2021; Weiss-Laxer et al., 2020). A poignant detailing of the efforts of activists in Flint, Michigan, are found in Narrative 5.2.

NARRATIVE 5.2: CLEAN WATER IN FLINT? STILL WAITING!

A Flint, Michigan, activist, E. Hill De Loney, MA, relates an account of resolution of a recent crisis that was sought through the combined epidemiological efforts of valiant private citizens, community leaders, and scientists from the local university:

Flint had faced public health crises in the past but this one in 2014 … . The water coming out of our faucets was cloudy … . It was brown … . And it stank!

When the Flint city emergency manager changed the source of Flint's water to the Flint River, municipal water quality became disturbing and unfit for consumption. Immediately, people inundated the city administrators with their observations. People were becoming ill, missing work, seeking medical care, and getting depressed. Parents worried about skin rashes on children who were being bathed in city water. Some people reported upset stomachs and headaches. Others reported losing their hair in clumps.

In response to the situation, Flint's faith-based ministers hastily aligned with local non-profits, collected data about the contaminated water, and presented their findings to local officials. The response: The water is fine; it is drinkable. No further comment was provided. Eventually, the city did issue a "boil water advisory"; again, without additional explanation.

Community members and organizations consulted university scientific experts who documented and communicated the public health threat of contaminated water to the citizens of the community. We went to see our governor and other state officials in Lansing. We presented our findings: that when the city emergency manager changed our water source to the Flint River, the result was unfit to drink—contaminated by corroded pipes and lead—all done to save the city a few dollars. Our questions, our pleas, our scientific evidence, including samples taken directly from faucets, were ignored. Their verdict: Flint water is safe to drink.

After about 18 months, and based on the clinical evidence among children that she treated, a local pediatrician conducted tests and found lead in Flint's water. It was her "discovery" that seemed to get the attention of officials in Lansing and Flint. Slowly, we began to see some action. Now, the nation and the world is aware of Flint's water debacle.

We citizens of Flint still have unanswered questions. Why were our community-based data and observations ignored for more than 48 months? Is this a political, ethical, legal, public health issue, tinged with arrogance and indifference about the (primarily African American) people of Flint? How will the permanent scars that have unnecessarily tarnished the lives of people in our community, and interrupted the future of our children for generations, be repaired? How could this have happened in America?

Discussion Questions

1. Name at least three strategies that nurses and other healthcare professionals can use to establish meaningful dialogue among community members and policymakers to address their concerns.
2. After research of state and local policies that address issues regarding water in your area:
   a. Determine if lead is an issue in your community.
   b. Verify whether fluoride is added to your water as a means of enhancing oral health.
   c. In the community where you practice, ascertain the risk of pollutants getting into the water system. Be specific.

DISCUSSION QUESTIONS

1. What do you think are the benefits of developing knowledge and skills that bolster an in-depth understanding of population health and health disparities–related curiosity and critical thinking from local and global perspectives?

2. Considering the projected Healthy People 2030 goals and objectives, what are your predictions about outcomes in three areas that are most significant in your projected practice, research, and policy activities as you develop and enhance your professional career in nursing and other health professions?

3. After reviewing the Alma Ata Declaration (Health for All), the Report of the Secretary's task force on Black and Minority Health, and the Social Determinants of Health documents, discuss your thoughts about (1) barriers and facilitators associated with national and state (yours) efforts to provide health care to all people and improved health outcomes, (2) how you can address the critical components of these documents in your area of clinical practice (e.g., pediatrics, women's health, mental health promotion) and (3) how would you determine the impact of your efforts?

4. Do you think that developing a blueprint for population health that is culturally congruent with a particular group is more complex than focusing on the individual health models standard in the United States? Your country? For starters, discuss the population health model in your state, and determine its assets and deficits. Are there some population groups that benefit? How is equity addressed? What proposed changes would you make? Provide a rationale based on data and science.

5. Identify a community/state (population) and apply the NIMHD research framework in your efforts to delineate the variables that you think would fit in each of the four levels of influence and the domains for an impact that occurs over the life course. For example, if the model were applied to migrant workers in California or Florida, what would be significant variables in the framework? Alternatively, if you were planning to improve the overall health of individuals with severe mental illness and histories of substance use and abuse, what would your framework highlight? Using the Flint Water content, apply the NIMHD research framework and make a practical plan of action that involves scientists, clinicians, and community people.

6. Identify a health problem in your community/state/nation and (1) write down the problem and (2) compose an accompanying research question that someone could develop to examine the problem. Determine what groups/individuals should be engaged with you in developing a culturally relevant intervention that is collaborative and impactful. How would your research reflect the goals and objectives of Healthy People 2030?

7. Apply the epidemiologic triad to a disease that is of interest to you. What plans could be made by nurses to break the interactions among the agent (disease), the host (vulnerable person or animal), and the environment (the facilitating force) that are necessary to control the disease? What societal beliefs and practices ought to be considered when making your plans? Be specific.

ADDITIONAL RESOURCES

This slide presentation from the CDC includes extensive notes providing a thorough explanation of epidemiology. It is a valuable resource, comprehensive, concise, and well worth the reader's time:

Centers for Disease Control and Prevention. (2018). *Introduction to epidemiology*. www.cdc.gov/training/publichealth101

The framework described in this article can be adapted to the community or the population to be served; it enables development of a profile based on the people to be served. This is a detailed description of the design and use of the minority health and health disparities research framework:

Alvidrez, J., Castille, D., Laude-Sharp, M., Rosario, A., & Tabor, D. (2019). The national institute on minority health and health disparities research framework. *American Journal of Public Health*, *109*(S1), S16–S20. https://doi.org/10.2105/AJPH.2018.304883

For COVID-19 statistics that are animated and continuously updating in real time:

Dong, E., Du, H., & Gardner, L. (2020). An interactive web-based dashboard to track COVID-19 in real time. *Lancet, 20*(5), 533–534. https://doi.org/10.1016/S1473-3099(20)30120-1

An excellent fact sheet for application of Healthy People 2030 principles:

Healthy People 2030. (2020). *Use healthy people 2030 in your work.* https://health.gov/healthypeople/tools-action/use-healthy-people-2030-your-work

A discussion of how to interpret the genetic validation of racial classification:

Reich, D. (2018, March 23). *How genetics is changing our understanding of "race".* New York Times. www.nytimes.com/2018/03/23/opinion/sunday/genetics-race.html

More information on events in Flint, MI:

Kennedy, M. (2016, April 20). *Lead-laced water in Flint: A step-by-step look at the makings of a crisis.* National Public Radio. www.npr.org/lead-laced-water-in-flint

Centers for Disease Control and Prevention. (2016). *Community assessment for public health emergency response: Flint water crisis.* www.cdc.gov/nceh/casper/pdf-html/flint_water_crisis_pdf.html

REFERENCES

Alvidrez, J., Castille, D., Laude-Sharp, M., Rosario, A., & Tabor, D. (2019). The national institute on minority health and health disparities research framework. *American Journal of Public Health, 109*(S1), S16–S20. https://doi.org/10.2105/AJPH.2018.304883

Arrazola, J., Masiello, M. M., Joshi, S., Dominguez, A. E., Poel, A., Wilkie, C. M., Bressler, J. M., McLaughlin, J., Kraszewski, J., Komatsu, K. K., Pompa, X. P., Jespersen, M., Richardson, G., Lehnertz, N., LeMaster, P., Rust, B., Metobo, A. K., Doman, B., Casey, D., … Landen, M. (2020, December 11). COVID-19 mortality among American Indian and Alaska native persons—14 states, January–June 2020. *Morbidity and Mortality Weekly Report, 69*(49), 1853–1856. https://doi.org/10.15585/mmwr.mm6949a3

Artiga, S., & Hinton, E. (2018). *Beyond healthcare: The role of social determinants in promoting health and health equity* (Issue Brief). Kaiser Family Foundation. Beyond Healthcare: The Role of Social Determinants in Promoting Health and Health Equity | KFF.

Aschengrau, A., & Seage, G. (2018). *Essentials of epidemiology in public health* (4th ed.). Jones & Bartlett Learning.

Ayouni, I., Maatoug, J., Dhouib, W., Zammit, N., Fredj, S. B., Ghammam, R., & Ghannem, H. (2021). Effective public health measures to mitigate the spread of COVID-19: A systematic review. *BMC Public Health, 21*, 1015. https://doi.org/10.1186/s12889-021-11111-1

Berchick, E. R., Hood, E., & Barnett, J. C. (2018). *Health insurance coverage in the United States: 2017.* United States Census Bureau. https://www.census.gov/content/dam/Census/library/publications/2018/demo/p60-264.pdf

Biggerstaff, M., Cauchemez, S., Reed, C., Gambhir, M., & Finelli, L. (2014). Estimates of the reproduction number for seasonal, pandemic, and zoonotic influenza: A systematic review of the literature. *BMC Infectious Diseases, 14*, 480. https://doi.org/10.1186/1471-2334-14-480

Boufides, C. H., Gable, L., & Jacobson, P. D. (2019). Learning from the flint water crisis: Restoring and improving public health practice, accountability, and trust. *Journal of Law, Medicine & Ethics, 47*(suppl 2), 23–26. https://doi.org/10.1177/1073110519857310

Braveman, P. (2006). Health disparities and health equity: Concepts and measurement. *Annual Review of Public Health, 27*, 167–194. https://doi.org/10.1146/annurev.publhealth.27.021405.102103

Centers for Disease Control. (1990). Healthy people 2000: National health promotion and disease prevention objectives for the year 2000. *Morbidity and Mortality Weekly Report, 39*(39), 689–690, 695–697.

Centers for Disease Control and Prevention. (2021a, February 18). *Risk for COVID-19 infection, hospitalization, and death by age group.* https://www.cdc.gov/coronavirus/2019-ncov/covid-data/investigations-discovery/hospitalization-death-by-age.html

Centers for Disease Control and Prevention. (2021b, February 18). *Risk for COVID-19 infection, hospitalization, and death by race/ethnicity.* https://www.cdc.gov/coronavirus/2019-ncov/covid-data/investigations-discovery/hospitalization-death-by-race-ethnicity.html

Clayton, S., Manning, C. M., & Hodge C. (2014). *Beyond storms & droughts: The psychological impacts of climate change*. Washington, DC: American Psychological Association and ecoAmerica.

Curley, A. L. (2020). *Population-based nursing: Concepts and competencies for advanced practice* (3rd ed.). Springer Publishing.

Dodd, D. R., Sugarman, D. E., & Greenfield, S. F. (2014). Tertiary prevention. In R. L. Cautin, & S. O. Lilienfeld (Eds.), *Encyclopedia of clinical psychology* (pp. 1–5). John Wiley & Sons. https://doi.org/10.1002/9781118625392.wbecp289

Donkin, A. J. (2014). Social gradient. In W. C. Cockerham, R. Dingwal, & S. R. Quah (Eds.), *Wiley Blackwell encyclopedia of health, illness, behavior, and society* (pp. 2172–2178). Wiley Blackwell.

Garrigues, L. J. (2021). Addressing the lens of health inequities and social justice with vulnerable populations. In A. Vermeesh (Ed.), *Integrative health nursing interventions for vulnerable populations* (pp. 11–25). Springer.

Ghebreyesus, T. A. (2020). Strengthening our resolve for primary healthcare. *Bulletin of the World Health Organization, 98*(11), 726–726A. https://doi.org/10.2471/BLT.20.279489

Hamilton, J. B. (2021). Storytelling: A cultural determinant of health among African American cancer patients. *Journal of Cancer Education*. https://doi.org/10.1007/s13187-021-01978-4

Haycock, K. (2010). The education-health link: Why success in school matters to health throughout life. *NASN School Nurse, 25*(3), 116–119. https://doi.org/10.1177/1942602X10363736

Heckler, M. (1985). Report of the Secretary's task force on Black & minority health. U.S. Department of Health and Human Services. http://resource.nlm.nih.gov/8602912

Hess, C. (2020). Residential segregation by race and ethnicity and the changing geography of neighborhood poverty. *Spatial Demography*. https://doi.org/10.1007/s40980-020-00066-3

James, L. (2017). Books: The health gap: The challenge of an unequal world: Unjust sense. *British Journal of General Practice, 67*(662), 415. https://doi.org/10.3399/bjgp17X692429

Kestenbaum, B. (2019). *Epidemiology and biostatistics: An introduction to clinical research* (2nd ed.). Springer.

Keyes, K. M., & Galea, S. (2016). *Population health science*. Oxford University Press.

Khazanchi, R., Beiter, E. R., Gondi, S., Beckman, A. L., Bilinski, A., & Ganguli, I. (2020). County-level association of social vulnerability with COVID-19 cases and deaths in the USA. *Journal of General Internal Medicine, 35*(9), 2784–2787. https://doi.org/10.1007/s11606-020-05882-3

Koh, H. K., Blakey, C. R., & Roper, A. Y. (2014). Healthy people 2020: A report card on the health of the nation. *Journal of the American Medical Association, 311*(24), 2475–2476. https://doi.org/10.1001/jama.2014.6446

Krieger, N. (2000). Refiguring "race": Epidemiology, racialized biology, and biological expressions of race relations. *International Journal of Health Services, 30*(1), 211–216. https://doi.org/10.2190/672J-1PPF-K6QT-9N7U

Kunitz, S. J. (2004). Social capital and health. *British Medical Bulletin, 69*(1), 61–73. https://doi.org/10.1093/bmb/ldh015

Last, J. M. (1988). *A dictionary of epidemiology* (2nd ed.). Oxford University Press.

Lenski, G. E. (2013). *Power and privilege: A theory of social stratification*. University of North Carolina Press.

Lueddeke, G. (2015). *Global population health and well-being in the 21st century: Toward new paradigms, policy, and practice*. Springer.

Marmot, M. (2015). *The health gap: The challenge of an unequal world*. Bloomsbury.

Marmot, M. (2017). The health gap: The challenge of an unequal world: The argument. *International Journal of Epidemiology, 46*(4), 1312–1318. https://doi.org/https://doi.org/10.1093/ije/dyx163

Marmot, M., Friel, S., Bell, R., Houweling, T. A. J., & Taylor, S. (2008). Closing the gap in a generation: Health equity through action on the social determinants of health. *Lancet, 372*(9650), 1661–1669. https://doi.org/10.1016/S0140-6736(08)61690-6

Marmot, M. G., Stansfeld, S., Patel, C., North, F., Head, J., White, I., Brunner, E., Feeney, A., & Smith, G. D. (1991). Health inequalities among British civil servants: The Whitehall II study. *Lancet, 337*(8754), 1387–1393. https://doi.org/10.1016/0140-6736(91)93068-K

Mathers, C., & Loncar, D. (2006). Projections of global mortality and burden of disease from 2002 to 2030. *PLoS Medicine, 3*(11), 442. https://doi.org/10.1371/journal.pmed.0030442

Matthew, D. B. (2018). *Just medicine: A cure for racial inequality in American healthcare*. NYU Press.

Meyer, P. A., Yoon, P. W., Kaufmann, R. B., & Centers for Disease Control and Prevention. (2013). Introduction: CDC health disparities and inequalities report—United States, 2013. *Morbidity and Mortality Weekly Report Supplements, 62*(3), 3–5. http://europepmc.org/abstract/MED/24264483

Mpolya, E. A., Furuse, Y., Nukiwa, N., Suzuki, A., Kamigaki, T., & Oshitani, H. (2009). Pandemic (H1N1) 2009 virus viewed from an epidemiological triangle model. *Journal of Disaster Research, 4*(5), 356–364. https://doi.org/10.20965/jdr.2009.p0356

Murdaugh, C., Parsons, M. A., & Pender, N. (2018). *Health promotion in nursing practice* (8th ed.). Pearson.

Murray, C. J. L., Phil, D., & Lopez, A. D. (2013). Measuring the global burden of disease. *New England Journal of Medicine, 369*(5), 448–457. https://doi.org/10.1056/NEJMra1201534

National Academies of Sciences, Engineering & Medicine. (2019). *Criteria for selecting the leading health indicators for healthy people* 2030 (Ch. 3). National Academies Press. https://doi.org/10.17226/25531

Pender, N. J. (2011). *Health promotion model manual.* University of Michigan. HEALTH_PROMOTION_MANUAL_Rev_5–2011[1].doc (umich.edu).

Pihkala, P. (2020). The cost of bearing witness to the environmental crisis: Vicarious traumatization and dealing with secondary traumatic stress among environmental researchers. *Social Epistemology, 34*(1), 86–100. https://doi.org/10.1080/02691728.2019.1681560

Reich, D. (2018, March 23). How genetics is changing our understanding of 'race'. New York Times. https://www.nytimes.com/2018/03/23/opinion/sunday/genetics-race.html

Rodriquez, E. J., Gregorich, S. E., Livaudais-Toman, J., & Pérez-Stable, E. J. (2017). Coping with chronic stress by unhealthy behaviors. *Journal of Aging and Health, 29*(5), 805–825. https://doi.org/10.1177/0898264316645548

Sanche, S., Lin, Y. T., Xu, C., Romero-Severson, E., Hengartner, N., & Ke, R. (2020). High contagiousness and rapid spread of severe acute respiratory syndrome coronavirus 2. *Emerging Infectious Diseases, 26*(7), 1470–1477. https://doi.org/10.3201/eid2607.200282

Satcher, D. (2020). *My quest for health equity: Notes on learning while leading.* Johns Hopkins University Press.

Sheehan, M. C., Fox, M. A., Kaye, C., & Resnick, B. (2017). Integrating health into local climate response: Lessons from the US CDC climate-ready states and cities initiative. *Environmental Health Perspectives, 125*(9), 094501. https://doi.org/10.1289/EHP1838

Shultz, J. M., Sullivan, L., & Galea, S. (2021). *Public health: An introduction to the science and practice of population health.* Springer.

Smedley, B. D., Stith, A. Y., & Nelson, A. R. (Eds.). (2009). *Unequal treatment: Confronting racial and ethnic disparities in healthcare.* National Academy Press.

Snowden, L. R., & Graaf, G. (2021). COVID-19, social determinants past, present, and future, and African Americans' health. *Journal of Racial and Ethnic Health Disparities, 8*(1), 12–20. https://doi.org/10.1007/s40615-020-00923-3

Sorci, G., Faivre, B., & Morand, S. (2020). Explaining among-country variation in COVID-19 case fatality rate. *Scientific Reports, 10*(1), 18909. https://doi.org/10.1038/s41598-020-75848-2

Starfield, B., Hyde, J., Gérvas, J., & Heath, I. (2008). The concept of prevention: A good idea gone astray? *Journal of Epidemiology and Community Health, 62*(7), 580–583. https://doi.org/10.1136/jech.2007.071027

Tapia, G. (2003). Economics, demography, and epidemiology: An interdisciplinary glossary. *Journal of Epidemiology and Community Health, 57*(12), 929–935. https://doi.org/10.1136/jech.57.12.929

Thomas, S. B., & Casper, E. (2019). The burdens of race and history on Black people's health 400 years after Jamestown. *American Journal of Public Health, 109*(10), 1346–1347. https://doi.org/10.2105/AJPH.2019.305290

Tsui, B. C. H., Deng, A., & Pan, S. (2020). COVID-19: Epidemiological factors during aerosol-generating medical procedures. *Anesthesia & Analgesia, 131*(3), e175–e178. https://doi.org/10.1213/ANE.0000000000005063

U.S. Department of Health and Human Services. (2020). Healthy people 2030: Social determinants of health. Office of Disease Prevention and Health Promotion. https://health.gov/healthypeople/objectives-and-data/social-determinants-health

Weiss-Laxer, N. S., Crandall, A., Hughes, M. E., & Riley, A. W. (2020). Families as a cornerstone in 21st century public health: Recommendations for research, education, policy, and practice. *Frontiers in Public Health.* https://doi.org/10.3389/fpubh.2020.00503

Wells, J. (2011). The impact of stress amongst health professionals. *Journal of Mental Health, 20*(2), 111–114. https://doi.org/10.3109/09638237.2011.556161

Woodbury, Z. (2019). Climate trauma: Toward a new taxonomy of trauma. *Ecopsychology, 11*(1), 1–8. https://doi.org/10.1089/eco.2018.0021

World Health Organization. (2008). *Closing the gap in a generation: health equity through action on the social determinants of health: Final report of the commission on social determinants of health.* https://www.who.int/publications/i/item/WHO-IER-CSDH-08.1

World Health Organization. (n.d.). WHO coronavirus (COVID-19) dashboard. https://covid19.who.int/.

Zheng, R. (2018). What is my role in changing the system? A new model of responsibility for structural injustice. *Ethical Theory and Moral Practice, 21*(4), 869–885. https://doi.org/10.1007/s10677-018-9892-8

SECTION II

Factors Impacting the Health of Individuals, Communities, and Populations

CHAPTER 6

Social Determinants of Health

Rebecca Garcia

LEARNING OBJECTIVES

- Discuss the meaning of social determinants of health.
- Explain the conceptual and operational challenges of defining ethnicity.
- Identify the social determinants for perinatal mortality.
- Examine the limitations of the social determinants of health approach.
- Discuss the concept of intersectionality as an approach to addressing inequalities in health systems.

INTRODUCTION

This chapter presents the social determinants of health (SDOH) framework, sometimes referred to as the wider determinants of health. It helps readers to understand the factors that contribute to individual health outcomes. More than two decades ago, the World Health Organization (WHO) commissioned work on the SDOH, with their publication of "The Solid Facts" (Marmot & Wilkinson, 2003; Wilkinson & Marmot, 1998). Since then, there has been a growing body of health research supporting the SDOH framework, which helps explain health outcomes, and health inequalities in particular (Marmot et al., 2010; Marmot & Wilkinson, 2003; Marmot et al., 2020). This chapter draws on research into inequalities in perinatal mortality as evidenced in England.

The chapter begins by reviewing the concept of health using a broad perspective, then describes the SDOH framework and moves on to apply the SDOH in the context of understanding inequalities in perinatal mortality in Pakistani and Bangladeshi infants who are born in England. Next, the chapter briefly critiques the SDOH before introducing the concept of intersectionality, and suggests how examining the hypothesis helps to advance the SDOH framework in both theoretical and practical ways for providers of health and social care. The term "inequality" is used widely in literature discussing SDOH; however, in some countries, the term "inequity" is used. This chapter uses the term inequality, consistent with United Kingdom and European literature.

UNDERSTANDING HEALTH

Health outcomes are not achieved in a vacuum. Historically, deterministic thinkers such as Watson (1997) and Skinner (1988) believed in a cause-and-effect model of health, singling out biological and chemical processes as the contributors of disease processes and ignoring social and cultural issues contributing to an individual's health outcomes. In more recent times, medical, nursing, and social education have attempted to step away from this perspective and use a biopsychosocial approach (Engel, 1977, 2012). Hence, the thinking has evolved to examine contributions to health, well-being, and illness, which are multifaceted and combine internal factors (e.g., body situated as biological and or psychological processes) and external factors (e.g., socially situated, and psychological interpretation of such external stimuli). Together these factors mediate health outcomes. In this chapter, health is understood as the consequence of biopsychosocial factors contributing to mental and physical well-being.

THE SOCIAL DETERMINANTS OF HEALTH EXPLAINED

The SDOH framework suggests that health outcomes are contextualized within the wider social environment in which a person works, learns, and lives. It also incorporates a life course perspective, acknowledging that influences in early life can predispose an individual to poor health in adulthood and later life (Blane, 2006). The SDOH framework further acknowledges psychosocial processes, recognizing the relationship between external stressors (e.g., financial issues) and internal responses (e.g., biological responses such as raised cortisol; Brunner & Marmot, 2006). Since the original report on the SDOH in 1999, a growing body of research evidence supports the SDOH framework, which has been used to facilitate changes in policy and practice aimed at reducing inequality and improving health outcomes (Marmot et al., 2020). However, progress to address inequalities and improve the health of individuals and societies has been reported to be slow (Marmot et al., 2020).

The SDOH framework acknowledges the wider social, political, economic, and environmental circumstances of individuals that contribute to their overall health outcomes (Brunner & Marmot, 2006; Marmot et al., 2020). It is widely known that access to money and resources, both individually and at a societal level, also contributes to health outcomes, seen by clear deprivation curves that show the least wealthy experiencing worse outcomes than more advantaged individuals in the same society. It is also accepted that exposure to advantages or disadvantages accumulates throughout a person's lifespan, resulting in a psychobiological response and impacting health further and across the life course (Winning et al., 2016). For instance, an individual's perception of a certain stressor will trigger a psychobiological stress response that has been shown to have biological consequences on the body (Hostinar et al., 2017). Therefore, individual health is influenced beyond biological factors and includes a wider set of determinants. These wider determinants interact with social, environmental, and psychosocial processes mediating health outcomes. Furthermore, a clear social gradient for health outcomes is evidenced in the context of where individuals live and the environment in which they interact. For example, those living in deprived or underresourced areas will have worse health outcomes than people of the same age/ethnicity who reside in more affluent regions (Marmot, 2017b). Social gradients are evident across the world and affect life expectancy, disability, and health outcomes. Differences are evident between and within countries. For example, people living in north England have a lower life expectancy (Manchester is 79.6 years) than individuals living in south England (Camden is 86.5 years), who enjoy an extra 7 years of expected life (The Kings Fund, 2020).

Figure 6.1 is adapted from Dahlgren–Whitehead's widely used "rainbow" model, showing the layered SDOH (Dahlgren & Whitehead, 1991). It starts at the *individual level*, which accounts for fixed factors such as hereditary factors: age, sex assigned at birth, and genetic

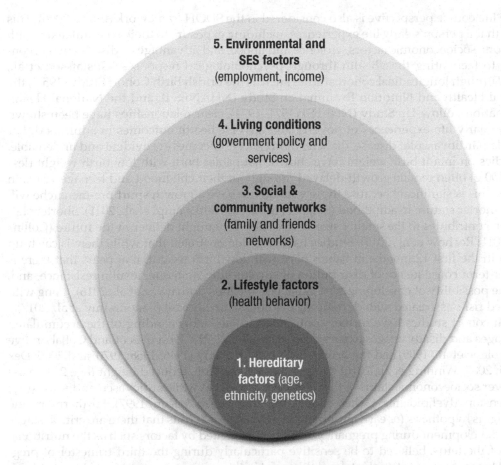

Figure 6.1 The social determinants of health (SDOH) framework.

Source: Adapted from Dahlgren, G., & Whitehead, M. (1991). *Policies and strategies to promote social equity in health background document to WHO–Strategy paper.* In Institutet för Framtidsstudier (Issue September). http://s2.medicina.uady.mx/observatorio/docs/eq/li/Eq_2007_Li_Dahlgren.pdf.

factors. The *second level* in the model represents the contribution of an individual's lifestyle factors, including health behavior, which may be positive and protective of health or negative and contributing to risk factors.

The *third level* represents the individual's social and community networks in which they interact. The *fourth level* considers the working and living conditions and wider community services in the locality where the person lives; for example, housing conditions, education facilities, access to healthcare and basics such as the provision of food and water. The *fifth level* includes the wider environmental, socioeconomic, and cultural factors. The social determinants found in these five levels combine to contribute to the individual's overall health outcome.

While the SDOH framework helps conceptualize contributing factors to health outcomes, the framework does not explain how social determinants are created or maintained. This means that discrete forces that operate both within and across society, such as politics and power dynamics, are not explicit in the SDOH framework (Salway et al., 2010). Power dynamics contribute to the context and empowerment of determinants on different levels in society, such as national or local policies. For example, governments prioritize public health spending, which then increases or reduces access to services and the allocation of resources for certain health promotion and intervention programs. These decisions might also help to perpetuate inequality and poor health outcomes (Patterson, 2014).

The life course perspective is also considered in the SDOH framework (Blane, 2006). This means that a person's early life experiences, including exposure to their accumulated health behaviors, socioeconomic factors, violence and abuse, and advantage or disadvantage, contribute to facilitating their health through psychobiological responses (Gustafsson et al., 2014). Through longitudinal cohort studies such as the British Birth Cohort Study (1958), the National Health and Nutrition Examination Study (NHANES I), and the National Health Examination Follow-Up Study (NHEFS) (1971–1974), clear relationships have been shown between early life experiences of poverty and adverse health outcomes in adulthood. For example, cardiovascular disease, diabetes, and cancer outcomes are evident and undeniable.

Studies on infant birth weight have shown that babies born with low birth weight (less than 2500 g) often remain growth-delayed throughout their childhood and teenage years. In females, this is significant because those who do not have a growth spurt pre-menarche will be of a shorter stature in adulthood (Saigal et al., 2006; Wehkalampi et al., 2011). Shorter stature then contributes to the smaller size of any baby they might deliver in the future (Collins et al., 2011; Rochow et al., 2019). Studies have also demonstrated that while there is catch-up growth in the first 12 months in babies born with low birth weight, it appears that there is a longer-term consequence of distribution of surplus adipose tissue, insulin resistance, and, later, the possibility of developing type 2 diabetes mellitus (Jornayvaz et al., 2016), along with increased risks associated with developing cardiovascular disease (Antonisamy et al., 2017).

Birth cohort studies have further contributed to our understanding of the accumulated advantages and disadvantages experienced in childhood. The West of Scotland Collaborative Study (Blane et al., 1999) and the British Birth Cohort Study (1946, 1958, 1970, and 2000; Dex & Joshi, 2005; Winning et al., 2016) suggest that for children, reduced height (age 2–4 years) and lower socioeconomic status of the family are associated with cardiovascular disease (e.g., hypertension, dyslipidemia; Cohen et al., 2010; Wadsworth & Kuh, 1997). Furthermore, the fetal origins hypothesis (or early programming hypothesis) posits that there are critical stages in fetal development during pregnancy, which are mediated by factors such as the nutritional intake of the fetus, believed to be sensitive particularly during the third trimester of pregnancy. Hence, poor nutritional intake at this point in the pregnancy results in an increased risk of the child developing cardiovascular or endocrine problems in later life (Hsu & Tain, 2019). Taken together, these circumstances demonstrate that the determinants of health are far from straightforward, and a wide range of social factors interact.

INEQUALITIES IN PERINATAL MORTALITY IN PAKISTANI AND BANGLADESHI WOMEN IN ENGLAND

This section starts with a brief explanation of perinatal mortality, and then explains the conceptual challenges with defining ethnicity, before moving on to explore the SDOH framework in the context of inequalities in perinatal mortality in Pakistani and Bangladeshi infants.

Perinatal Mortality

The SDOH framework is the dominant method used in public health to understand inequalities in health. It is also an efficient way to discuss perinatal mortality, which is a significant public health problem across the globe (De Bernis et al., 2016). Perinatal mortality is closely associated with maternal mortality and is accepted to be responsive to temporal changes in healthcare provision and the wider determinants of health, such as general living conditions (e.g., housing, transportation), environmental factors, and overall well-being (WHO, 2015). Consequently, globally perinatal mortality is considered a proxy for the quality of a country's healthcare system and economic resources (Gonzalez & Gilleskie, 2017).

While perinatal mortality figures have declined since 2000, there is a clear social gradient observed across the globe, with less economically developed countries experiencing

TABLE 6.1 Perinatal Mortality Rate by Country and Perinatal Mortality Rate Within Country Regional Variation, by Highest and Lowest Rank, Measured per 1,000 Live Births

	England		**United States**	
National perinatal mortality rate per 1,000 live births	3		4	

Source: World Bank (2019). https://data.worldbank.org/indicator/SH.DYN.NMRT?locations=GB

	Highest	**Lowest**	**Highest**	**Lowest**
Within-country perinatal mortality rate per 1,000 live births	West Yorkshire 6.9[1]	Warwickshire 5.2[1]	Alabama and Mississippi 8.32[2]	New Hampshire 3.07[2]

[1]Office for National Statistics. (2018). www.ons.gov.uk/peoplepopulationandcommunity/birthsdeathsandmarriages/deaths/datasets/infantmortalitybirthcohorttablesinenglandandwales

[2]Centers for Disease Control and Prevention. (2018). www.cdc.gov/nchs/data/databriefs/db316.pdf

higher rates of perinatal mortality (United Nations Inter-agency Group for Child Mortality Estimation, 2020). However, there are also high rates of perinatal mortality observed in high-income countries such as the United States and England. In addition to variances seen *within* the countries, after data are stratified by maternal ethnicity/race or country of birth, inequalities remain (Centers for Disease Control and Prevention [CDC], 2018; Office for National Statistics, 2018). Table 6.1 demonstrates between and within-country differences for England and the United States, indicating inequalities.

"Perinatal" is variously defined, depending on the country, according to an agreed criterion that is linked to the legal definitions of viability. For instance, WHO uses the parameters of 22 completed weeks of gestation and 7 days after birth (WHO, 2021). In the United States, the CDC National Vital Statistics System uses 28 completed weeks of gestation to 7 days post-birth (Gregory et al., 2018), while in England government figures (i.e., from the National Health Service [NHS]) use 24 completed weeks of gestation and 7 days post-birth. Twenty-four weeks of gestation is England's legal threshold of viability, which is also linked to the Abortion Act (1967), referring to the age at which the fetus is thought to be able to survive outside of the uterus (Llamas et al., 2018). In the United States, however, different states have different definitions for viability (Arzuaga & Lee, 2011). Consequently, this means that the legal definition of when a fetus is considered "viable" and able to survive outside the uterus, albeit with medical aid (if this is available), varies depending on country or state law. Viability thresholds are becoming increasingly complex with advances in neonatal intensive care science and technologies supporting the survival of very preterm infants. Mortality and morbidity rates are also far from being straightforward and adequately documented (Raju et al., 2014). Perinatal mortality refers to the death rate of infants in this age range, including stillborn and neonatal deaths (infants born live but who die before 7 days old) and is calculated as a rate out of 1,000 live births. In research terms, the use of various definitions across the globe makes comparisons between and among data sets and populations difficult. (Please note that this chapter uses United Kingdom definitions.)

THE CHALLENGES OF DEFINING ETHNICITY

It is important to understand the impact and challenges of using race or ethnicity as a variable in health research and when considering the SDOH. The terms *race* and *ethnicity* are often used interchangeably. However, these terms are widely debated and poorly understood (Atkin, 2011). Attitudes toward diverse racial or ethnic groups are historically and politically situated, where differences hasvebeen used to justify unequal treatment in minority groups, which may be ethnically defined. The use of these terms has been further compounded by poorly designed research, resulting in misleading findings, laws, and policies that create different opportunities, which provide resources for some and not others. Such practices further contribute to inequalities at all levels of society, including health outcomes (Bhopal, 2007).

The term "race" was previously argued to be biologically determined; however, scholars now agree that to use a particular phenotype characteristic but with cultural attributes (i.e., race) is incorrect because it is socially constructed (Karlsen & Nazroo, 2011; Senior & Bhopal, 1994). On the other hand, "ethnicity" is a term that usually includes religion and language differences, contrasted with the majority population (Bartley, 2008). Therefore, "race" and "ethnicity" are argued as two separate concepts: "Race" is biological and heritable, whereas "ethnicity" implies social and cultural differences (Chaturvedi, 2001). (See Chapter 15, Race, Ethnicity, and Population Health, for a detailed discussion.)

Caution is needed when using ethnicity as a determinant of health. As constructed categories, "race" and "ethnicity" are not risk factors per se, but the associated sociocultural and psychobiological factors (e.g., political, legal, socioeconomic) that are experienced in conjunction with certain ethnicities contribute to enhanced probabilities for risk of poor health outcomes. Race or ethnicity data are collected at national levels (e.g., census data), often through force-choice boxes so that governments can measure, monitor, and deliver service provision on a large scale in predefined categories. However, this practice contributes to inequalities when populations are not properly represented. In addition to the conceptual issues, there are further operational problems due to the heterogeneous categorization systems used in different countries, utilizing forced and fixed options. For example, the category "Asian" in American literature broadly refers to people from southeast Asia, China, the Far East, Japan, Thailand, the Philippines, and Korea (Humes et al., 2011), whereas "Asian" in UK literature specifies people identifying as Indian, Bangladeshi, Pakistani, Chinese, or "Asian other" (Office for National Statistics, 2012). This makes a comparison between groups difficult, and in some instances impossible.

The longitudinal UK Household Survey (2013) found differences among categories by religion, culture, beliefs, behavior, and socioeconomic factors and by the extent to which people assimilate and/or become acculturated to the host country (Nandi & Platt, 2013). It is now widely accepted that ethnicity is self-defined and incorporates physical appearance, shared ancestry and territories, culture, language, and religion (Chattoo & Atkin, 2019). Furthermore, the majority of health services research focuses on ethnic "difference," making comparisons against the majority (typically White) populations (Cohen, 2020). Consequently, by focusing on differences compared with the majority population, this research method unintentionally "others" the minority group. In other words, it "outs" the minority population as "different" from the majority population, which further perpetuates ideas of difference and misses opportunities to understand similarities between and among people.

Culture

It is important to consider the contribution of culture when defining ethnicity. Like ethnicity, culture is a complex and debated concept (Marsella & Yamada, 2010). There are two important distinctions in the debate: culture being constructed from an external human experience; conversely, culture being shared beliefs and practices that unite or separate humans. These approaches have resulted in many definitions being offered to explain "culture," including culture being learned or a learned experience attending to meaning-making, or being an institutional group addressing meaning-making or a collective group of systems and subsequent meanings (Cohen, 2020).

Arguably, culture needs a structural reality—for instance, external objects used to suggest cultural group membership, such as dress code, and a conceptual reality as seen in attitudes toward group membership, which are themselves dynamic and mediate a shared understanding of the cultural identity and subsequent behavior, including a shared language (Markus & Hamedani, 2010). Cultural practices such as accepted marital norms, for instance, being a single mother (associated with poverty and a lack of social support) or consanguineous marriage (associated with genetic risk) are shown to be an increased risk for adverse pregnancy outcomes (Memon & Rahman, 2020). Culture is therefore dynamic and subjective.

Language

Language also contributes to our self-defined culture and ethnicity. Shared meanings of cultural practices such as our attitudes and behaviors are exchanged through common verbal and nonverbal language, body language, dialects, and slang (Markus & Hamedani, 2010). Furthermore, language informs our thinking, and concepts in one language may not be present in another (Triandis, 2010). For instance, the perception of "stress" in English-speaking countries may be different in other languages: In Urdu (Pakistan), *pereshaan* means "tense," and in Bengali (Bangladesh), *oshanti* means "no peace."

Limited language proficiency by ethnic minority women not born in the host country is commonly cited in research to explain barriers to accessing healthcare services (Marie et al., 2019; Phillimore, 2016). Language proficiency may further discriminate against expectant migrant women, with reduced knowledge of local healthcare provisions or perceived or real entitlements, which can act as a barrier to sharing health information. Also, reduced educational attainment and lower levels of health and numeracy literacy often further exacerbate disadvantage (Lu & Halfon, 2003). In the United Kingdom, the NHS offers language translation services to meet the needs of its diverse population. However, Centre for Maternal and Child Enquiries (CMACE; 2015) studies revealed that in 83% of perinatal deaths, there was no professional translation service offered to women who were not proficient in speaking English, resulting in unsatisfactory care (Cross-Sudworth et al., 2015). Consequently, translation services are now routinely offered during antenatal checks for non-English–speaking women accessing maternity care in England. This is offered as part of the NHS maternity care package, and no fee is paid by the pregnant patient.

Reviewing the research evidence on patient experiences of using translation services reveals that interpretation goes beyond the conveyance of information between patients and healthcare staff. There have been questions raised regarding the accuracy of translation services in healthcare practice, in particular with slang or dialects and the subjective experience and subsequent influence of the interpreter. These circumstances have resulted in the standard use of medically trained translation services professionals (Ali, 2003; Regmi et al., 2010). Sometimes, healthcare staff use family members to translate, and this practice has been highlighted as being inappropriate due to the sensitive nature of questions in maternity care (and numerous other health conditions, such as reproductive medicine, contraception, and sexual health). There is also a risk of misinformation due to poor health literacy, or the filtering of information between and among family members (Cross-Sudworth et al., 2015). Research shows that South Asian women may be fearful of stigmatization or breaches of confidentiality if speaking with members of their own community about personal health-related issues (Garcia et al., 2020a). Taken together, it is evident that limited language proficiency is a barrier to accessing quality maternity care; it is also more complex to resolve than by a simple translation. Care is needed when developing potential support services for migrants, and including people from their community during the development of possible service design further offers nuanced understanding. This practice helps to ensure that the proposed support service meets the needs of the patient and is accessible to the migrant family in ways that are appropriate and acceptable to them. For example, a recent breast-screening leaflet was developed in a local area with good intentions, but it used eloquent and elaborative Urdu language that everyday British Pakistani women did not understand and was not therefore helpful. These types of unintended events must be avoided.

Religion

When discussing ethnicity and culture, it is important to consider the implicit and explicit contributions that religion may make to our health beliefs and behaviors (Raman et al., 2016). Religion is also a contested term. Typically, in lay terms, religion may refer to affiliation with a deity, as seen in Christianity or Islam, while Buddhism and Taoism have no deity, making operationalization of religion a challenge (Flannelly et al., 2014). Box 6.1 explores religion and spirituality.

Returning to our example of inequalities in perinatal mortality seen in Pakistani and Bangladeshi infants in the United Kingdom, two dominant religions are present in this population: Christianity (White British) and Islam (Pakistani and Bangladeshi). Religious and cultural beliefs contribute to differences in health beliefs and health behaviors. For example, Muslims may believe that illness is a test from Allah, facilitating cleansing after sinful behavior and offering a future-based reward. The Bible (Christianity), on the other hand, sometimes suggests that illness is a punishment from God. Some Muslims and Christians believe illness is God's will, while others may believe it leads to purification, and adverse pregnancy outcomes may be explained as "the will of God" (Garcia et al., 2020a).

BOX 6.1: Definitions of Religion and Spirituality and the Main Differences Between Them

The difference between religion and spirituality is not well understood (Jones, 2018). The terms are widely contested, and many definitions can be found, depending on the context used. For instance, reflect on texts about the end-of life care or how spirituality or religion might influence health beliefs and health behavior among different populations.

The Cambridge Dictionary (2021) defines religion as having beliefs in God(s) that include worship, but this description fails to acknowledge the subjective experience of religion. Religion is a structured set of shared beliefs and practices which provide guidance for individuals and groups to address the ethical and moral challenges that characterize human life.

On the other hand, "Spirituality is the dynamic dimension of human life that relates to the way persons (individual and community) experience, express and/or seek meaning, purpose and transcendence, and the way they connect to the moment, to self, to others, to nature, to the significant and/or the sacred" (Best et al., 2020, p. 2). Tanyi (2002) claims, "Spirituality is a personal search for meaning and purpose in life, which may or may not be related to religion" (p. 690).

Religion is socially constructed. Therefore, it is not objective or measurable, but instead is a framework of ideas, narratives, practices, and symbols that are used to help people make sense of their world. While religious belief is private, it is often a collective phenomenon (Bidwell et al., 2016). When using religious ideas and symbols the person might follow defined routines as stated in religious texts, in hope, praise, or thanks of a matter that is of concern to them (e.g., health of a close relative). Religion may intersect with cultural beliefs, practices, or behaviors.

Spirituality is also socially constructed. It is subjective and difficult to define and measure. Spirituality, however, is eclectic insofar that ideas are taken from numerous influences that are not necessarily religious. For instance, ideas from Shamans, Buddhism, Taoism, or wise words from a grandparent, a walk in nature, or spending time with close family/friends are all examples of ways that help people make sense of their world and meet their spiritual needs.

Simply stated, religion is a shared experience, whereas spirituality is a private experience (Bidwell et al., 2016; Ross et al., 2018).

Concerning termination of pregnancy (or abortion), some Christians or Muslims may not practice this option because of their faith. For Muslims, it might only be considered if there is a significant risk to the pregnant person (in which case termination needs to be completed within 120 days, consistent with the Islamic fatwa[1]). However, fatwas are commonly misunderstood. Consequently, there is a widely held misunderstanding that Muslim people hold a "no termination of pregnancy" attitude (Shaw, 2012). This then has an impact on the uptake of genetic screening services and is cited as a reason to explain the higher rates of congenital anomalies found in Pakistani infants (Koenig & Al Shohaib, 2014). For example, pregnant Muslims may not intentionally seek anomaly screening because, regardless of the test result, they do not want to undertake a termination of the pregnancy. However, some Muslims may participate in anomaly screening to gain knowledge of a child with congenital anomalies to prepare for the infant, but they will not terminate the pregnancy. Those with unclear immigration status may not access maternity services at all. Together, these circumstances highlight the complex relationships between ethnicity, culture, religion, and immigration status, and their impact on health beliefs and health behaviors that influence birth outcomes.

NARRATIVE 6.1: ASMA'S STORY

A 23-year-old Bangladeshi woman named Asma lives in a large city in northern England. The city has a large population of Pakistani, Bangladeshi, and Indian residents, in addition to other migrants. Asma was born in Bangladesh and speaks Sylheti. Her English language proficiency is quite limited, as the family members speak Sylheti at home and in their community.

Asma was married at age 19 years old to her husband, Hasan, who was age 29 years when they were wedded in a consensual and arranged consanguineous (cousin) marriage. Hasan works as a local restaurant owner. After they were married, Asma moved into Hasan's family home; Hasan being the only son in the family, there was a cultural expectation that he would remain living with his aging parents (Nasreen and Sadiq) to support them through their later years.

In addition to Hasan and his parents, Hasan's younger sister, Fathida, still lives in the parents' home. Fathida is 21 years old and has several medical problems related to genetic malformations. Their home is a moderate-sized, four-bedroom, terraced property in a neglected and underresourced part of town. Asma and Hasan have their own bedroom but share all other living spaces with the rest of the family. As is typical in South Asian families, Asma is expected to contribute to the personal caring, housework, and cooking responsibilities of the family home.

The maternity unit is situated on the other side of the town and requires a 60-minute journey on two buses. Asma prefers to go with her husband using a taxi, so he can help translate English to Sylheti, helping Asma better understand the healthcare staff's communication related to her prenatal visits. However, it is difficult to find an appropriate appointment time as it means Hasan will lose valuable working hours (and income) while he accompanies his wife.

Asma is 29 weeks pregnant with her first baby when she arrives at the hospital. To date, her pregnancy has been fairly uneventful, with only the suffering of morning sickness since she was 10 weeks' pregnant. Although the sickness has continued throughout her pregnancy, Asma's mother-in-law, Nasreen, had assured Asma that this symptom is normal. Nasreen encourages Asma to drink hot buttermilk (melted butter in milk) every day to help with a "smooth delivery" and the delivery of a baby with a "golden skin tone." As a consequence of drinking buttermilk (and other calorie-dense cultural food), Asma has gained excessive weight during the 29 weeks of her pregnancy, despite her feelings of nausea. Asma has attended few of her prenatal checkups and only attended her first appointment when she

(continued)

---

1. A fatwa is a religious rule that becomes enmeshed in Islamic law (sharia) by religious scholars but is not explicitly mentioned in a Hadith or the Qur'an (Koenig et al., 2001).

NARRATIVE 6.1: ASMA'S STORY (*CONTINUED*)

was 16 weeks' pregnant. Consequently, Asma has missed all early screening opportunities and pregnancy care advice. Nevertheless, Asma does not recognize this concern as a potential problem, as pregnancy is considered "normal" for women in her community. Asma has also been busy with housework and looking after Nasreen and Sadiq. In addition, the maternity unit is considered too far away, and she struggles to understand what the staff are trying to communicate. Hence, there are several barriers related to her accessing timely maternity care. In the meantime, at home, other important events are occurring.

It is Sadiq's 70th birthday, and the family has arranged a big gathering to celebrate. Asma has been busy for several days with preparations for the event. She has been cleaning the house and assisting with preparing food. They are expecting more than 20 guests so there is much to be done. All family members are looking forward to the event. However, during the midst of the birthday-related preparations, Asma starts to get stomach cramps and realizes she has not noticed the baby's movements during the past few days. Asma believes that any adverse event is "the will of God," and she places her trust in Allah. Moreover, with the 70th birthday event planned and so many guests expected, she decides it is best not to say anything. As the day wears on, Asma's cramps get worse, and she eventually tells Nasreen and Hasan, but Nasreen advises her that "the baby is asleep," so, with this reassurance, Asma lies down quietly on the sofa. Suddenly, Asma feels dragging pains from her groin that accompany her cramps. She quietly takes herself off to the bathroom so as not to make a fuss and spoil the birthday event. Hasan's cousin, Samira, suddenly calls unexpectedly from the bathroom, "Quickly! Come!" Asma is found barely conscious, with a pool of blood on the floor. An ambulance is immediately called and Asma and Hasan are transported to the nearby hospital. After an examination, it is determined that Asma has started premature labour at 29 weeks and the baby has sadly died.

Discussion Questions

1. How did language impact Asma's healthcare experience?
2. How did cultural beliefs contribute to the sequence of events?
3. What might be done differently in future?

An analysis of the events revealed a series of related factors that contributed to Asma's adverse outcome. For example, her poor understanding of the purpose of attending screening visits resulted in reduced attendance at the prenatal checks, missing opportunities for the identification of potential risk factors for adverse birth consequences. The situation was exacerbated by lack of English language proficiency, meaning she did not feel confident in speaking with staff, which further acted as a barrier to accessing maternity care. Moreover, health staff assumed Asma had an understanding of pregnancy and maternity services and also assumed she had an understanding of pregnancy-related health messages when she did not. Consequently, Asma relied on her mother-in-law's advice regarding her pregnancy, delaying her seeking help and accurate health messages. Furthermore, Asma later recognized that she put the needs of her family ahead of her own needs (as was considered culturally appropriate), which added a further delay to her seeking timely intervention. Asma concluded that in hindsight she did not know very much about pregnancy or any associated risk factors (such as maternal weight, age, hypertension, intrauterine growth restriction, screening tests, late booking, and inadequate prenatal attendance at clinics). She and her family had "normalized" pregnancy and accepted the reality; they put their trust in fate. This example shows a multifaceted and complex series of events contributing to the adverse outcome, involving all levels of the SDOH.

THE SDOH FRAMEWORK AND PERINATAL MORTALITY

The SDOH framework is a good place to start when exploring public health problems such as perinatal mortality. It allows us to understand the wider determinants that mediate inequalities in perinatal mortality (and other public health issues) by taking a broad view of related contributory factors. The SDOH for perinatal mortality is explored in the following, using Dahlgren and Whitehead's model as a framework (see Figure 6.1).

Heritable Factors

Research has shown that there are several individual and heritable factors that adversely contribute to perinatal mortality. These include maternal age, either younger than 20 years or older that 35 years (Kahveci et al., 2018; Walker et al., 2016). In addition, certain ethnic groups appear more at risk in particular locations, such as Pakistani and Bangladeshi people in England (Garcia et al., 2020b), non-Hispanic Black women in the United States (CDC, 2020), and Aboriginal and Torres Strait Islander women in Australia (Australian Institute of Health and Welfare, 2020). Similar patterns are observed across the globe, with disadvantaged communities having higher rates of perinatal mortality than the majority population.

Genetic factors also contribute to perinatal mortality. There are more than 165 identified factors found to contribute to congenital anomalies. These include genetic factors, neural tube defects, chromosomal abnormalities (e.g., Down syndrome), autosomal recessive inheritance disorders (e.g., sickle cell and thalassaemia), metabolic disorders (e.g., diabetes), and exposure to teratogens[2] (Blackwell, 2015; WHO, 2016). While statistics show the most common cause of perinatal mortality is immaturity-related deaths, it is closely followed by congenital anomalies. Interestingly, there is a social gradient component in congenital anomalies in England, with a third more cases identified in women living in under-resourced socioeconomic groups, suggesting that factors related to poverty contribute to genetic anomalies (WHO, 2020). Furthermore, when reviewing termination of pregnancy statistics (postantenatal screening), those from the United Kingdom show that 51% of pregnancy terminations were sought on maternal medical grounds while only 2% were reported to be because of mental or physical disability of the fetus (Department of Health, 2015).

Both globally and in England, Pakistani infants have a higher prevalence of congenital anomalies, perinatal mortality, and burden of disease than infants from other ethnic groups (Kurinczuk et al., 2010; Office for National Statistics, 2014). The exact mechanism that helps to create the condition is unclear, but the commonly cited explanation is a result of consanguinity (WHO, 2020). The identified risk factors that contribute to congenital anomalies include older maternal age, comorbid disease such as diabetes and obesity, and lower socioeconomic position, suggesting complicated mechanisms contributing to genetic factors.

Lifestyle Factors and Health Behavior

The contributions of lifestyle factors and health behaviors to individual health outcomes are widely accepted, with growing bodies of research in specific areas (e.g., smoking and nutritional intake during pregnancy), further supporting the interactions among selected factors. Conner and Norman (2005, p. 2) define health behavior as "activity undertaken for the purpose of preventing or detecting disease or for improved health and well-being." The definition includes accessing health information or remedies from various sources, such as spiritual beliefs, icons, cultural beliefs, herbs, and modern medicine (Tarafder et al., 2013). Cultural practice, customs, past behaviors, peer interactions, and levels of health literacy have been shown to contribute to health beliefs and health

---

2. Pharmacologic teratogens (e.g., thalidomide, sodium valproate, warfarin); chemical teratogens (e.g., alcohol); and infectious teratogens (e.g., rubella, cytomegalovirus, coxsackie, and *Staphylococcus aureus* (Kurinczuk et al., 2010a).

behaviors (Conner & Norman, 2015). These sources of influence on health behaviors are fluid and are dependent on the cultural and situational contexts of the people involved. Health behaviors within the perinatal mortality literature are constrained to behaviors that are mostly considered modifiable. Typically, these are tobacco consumption, alcohol and substance misuse, nutritional intake, monitoring of fetal movements, clinic bookings and keeping of appointments, parity, body mass index, gestational diabetes, hypertension, and consanguinity (Conner & Norman, 2015).

Social and Community Networks

There is an established body of evidence-based research supporting the contribution of social support in health outcomes. For instance, a buffering effect has been shown when migrant individuals and families live in areas with other people from the same ethnic group (Bécares et al., 2012; Halpern & Nazroo, 1999). Furthermore, social support is not static; it changes across the life course. Among families that are separated through migration or natural disasters, social support may be fractured or nonexistent.

Social support can include practical, emotional, and informational resources and is exchanged among family, friends, community networks, and public services. It also includes religious networks (Reid & Herbert, 2014). Family and friends are considered a resource for pregnant patients and may influence birth outcomes by the extent of their social support, information sharing, and social inclusion (which may be perceived as positive or negative; Cross-Sudworth et al., 2015). Researchers have considered the impact of social support after a stillbirth; however, there is a paucity of studies exploring the contribution of social support to the outcome of perinatal mortality (Redshaw et al., 2014). Moreover, research on kinship ties in South Asian families resulted in stereotyped assumptions of social support being available, contributing to less professional support being offered (Katbamna et al., 2004). Consequently, when health professionals and policymakers (erroneously) determine that social support is available, it negates the responsibility of formalized support services and the development of policies that address the problems. The contribution of social support in birth outcomes is complicated but an important consideration to SDOH.

Living Conditions

When considering societal and government policy-level implications on SDOH in perinatal mortality, it is evident that changes at the government level can impact health outcomes. In more recent years, the UK government has paid increased attention to reducing perinatal mortality and addressing inequalities in health. This approach has included changes to legislation as evidenced in the Health and Social Care Act (2012) whereby the government pledged to address inequality in access, service provision, and quality of care (Health and Social Care Act, 2012). Furthermore, legal objectives are evident in the "Mandate for the NHS" to reduce fetal deaths, stillbirths, and neonatal deaths, which makes local NHS services legally accountable for their compliance to the outcomes framework (Department of Health, 2015). The mandate includes reducing inequalities and perinatal mortality. Therefore, tangible attempts to reduce inequality and address perinatal mortality are evidenced in the United Kingdom and filter to local initiatives such as the Infant Mortality National Support Team and the Child Overview Death Panel. These agencies are charged with reviewing local cases of perinatal mortality and responding with improved approaches to evidence-based care.

Environmental, Cultural, and Socioeconomic Factors

We now turn our attention to the influence of determinants linked with socioeconomic, cultural, and environmental factors on perinatal mortality in the United Kingdom. Poverty and deprivation are often used interchangeably in the literature, but it is worth clarifying the distinction between the two concepts. Typically, poverty is associated with financial resources (e.g., used to purchase supplies such as food) and is considered one-dimensional, whereas deprivation refers to the difficulties that occur due to the lack of resources; thus, it is conceptualized as multidimensional (Unwin, 2014). For instance, having access to adequate financial resources enables healthy food choices needed for positive and protective health outcomes. The relationships concerning poverty, deprivation, and adverse birth outcomes are well documented with a clear social gradient observed between/among and within countries (Zeitlin et al., 2016). Statistical data demonstrate that women living in the most deprived areas (in the United Kingdom and United States) have worse birth outcomes (Dibben et al., 2006; Driscoll & Ely, 2019). These patterns of the most deprived areas having worse birth outcomes are observed across the globe and have existed over decades.

Early life experiences of growing up in poverty have been shown to mediate health outcomes, although the mechanism behind this relationship is complicated. Current thinking suggests three explanations: first, the direct consequence of poverty, such as poor living standards or reduced material resources; second, individual health behaviors as a result of living in poverty (includes greater perceived stress); and finally, less engagement with health services (Wickham et al., 2016). These three explanations combined with health behaviors such as smoking, alcohol misuse, poor nutrition, and inadequate exercise exacerbate poor health outcomes (Benzeval et al., 2014). However, a paucity of individual resources alone is not a robust explanation for perinatal mortality. The global social gradient easily explains impoverished families, but it does not explain why Pakistani and Bangladeshi women have worse birth outcomes in England.

Culture mediates how people interpret their social world; a collection of social norms and expectancies envelop the experience of pregnancy. For example, in Pakistani and Bangladeshi families, pregnancy is anticipated following marriage (Koenig & Al Shohaib, 2014) and elevates "social status" within the community (Choudhury & Ahmed, 2011). Commonly, in Pakistani and Bangladeshi families, women hold the role of "homemaker" with the social norm of attending to household matters and family caring responsibilities (Jomeen & Redshaw, 2013; Puthussery et al., 2010). The position impacts the family's financial resources, with small numbers of Pakistani and Bangladeshi women in formal employment positions, as shown in labor market figures (Office for National Statistics, 2020). As mentioned previously, cultural experience is also mediated by language.

This brief review of the SDOH on perinatal mortality in England shows a complex and interrelated picture of birth outcomes, revealing biopsychosocial factors at all levels of the SDOH, contributing to health outcomes. Naba, a Pakistani woman, helps to illuminate the interactions among these issues.

CASE STUDY 6.1: NABA–A WOMAN AT RISK OF PERINATAL MORTALITY

Naba is a 28-year-old British second-generation Pakistani woman who is 32 weeks pregnant with her third child. Her first pregnancy resulted in a stillbirth delivered at 34 weeks; the cause was unknown. She is a nonsmoker, does not take regular exercise, and has a body mass index (using WHO revised Asian metrics) of 28 kg/m² indicating "high risk" (Barba et al., 2004; Garcia et al., 2017).

Naba lives with her husband, who is self-employed as a taxi driver, and her 20-month-old daughter, Rukia. She also lives with her mother-in-law, who has renal problems and her father-in-law who is a type 2 diabetic, in a culturally typical multigenerational family living setting. Naba is not employed and cares for her child and her parents-in-law. Naba's husband earns a small amount over the threshold for the family, which precludes them from receiving any financial aid from the government. Other relatives from her husband's family live close by, while Naba's parents and sisters reside 200 miles away in a different part of the country. Naba and her husband live in a mid-terraced home with three bedrooms. They

(continued)

CASE STUDY 6.1: NABA: A WOMAN AT RISK OF PERINATAL MORTALITY (*CONTINUED*)

live in a disadvantaged part of town, densely populated and run-down, with other migrant settlers from Pakistan or Bangladesh. The area is affordable and offers social support by living close to other people who share their culture and values. However, crime rates are high, and the majority of residents live below the minimum income level. Health outcomes are poor (Marmot, 2017b).

Naba has full access to maternity and medical services in primary and secondary care with the NHS (free at the point of delivery; Box 6.2) in Britain, and her local hospital is 3 miles away, requiring a bus or taxi to get there.

BOX 6.2: Understanding the British Healthcare System

The British government's Department of Health has the responsibility for and oversees the National Health Service (NHS), which is publicly funded through taxation. The service is "free at the point of delivery" for residents entitled to the services. In 2018, the cost of healthcare in the United Kingdom was £214.4 billion (Office for National Statistics, 2018). The government uses an accountability framework, legislated by the National Health Service Act (2006) and documents such as The Long Term Plan, detailing the legal responsibility of service provision. The accountability is mandated by the Secretary of State to local NHS Trusts to pursue defined goals such as improving outcomes for major diseases and long-term conditions (Department of Health, 2015, 2016).

The NHS operates throughout the United Kingdom although it has been separated by nations (Wales, Northern Ireland, Scotland, and England). This example focuses on services delivered through NHS England. Over the years, there have been changes to the structure of the NHS. Health services are offered through the Office for Health Improvement and Disparities (OHID; formerly Public Health England) supporting public health and health protection and NHS England, which commissions primary and secondary care services. NHS services are delivered through primary (district general hospitals), secondary (community-based services including general practitioners), and tertiary care (specialist services including neurosurgery or forensic mental health). At the time of writing, locally organized clinical commission groups have the responsibility of assigning services as deemed necessary in the secondary care sector. These include elective care in a hospital setting, including rehabilitation, urgent or emergency care, community and mental health (including learning disability) health services, and recovery services (for substance misuse).

A CRITIQUE OF THE SDOH FRAMEWORK IN UNDERSTANDING PERINATAL MORTALITY

The SDOH framework is widely accepted and has utility in understanding morbidity and mortality; however, the exact mechanisms behind the inequalities remain unclear. Furthermore, there are limitations to the conceptual and applied functionality of the SDOH framework. Consequently, research has focused on measurable biological or behavioral determinants in perinatal mortality that are considered modifiable, such as smoking cessation or pre-pregnancy weight loss. Therefore, reviewing distal determinants that contribute to the outcome of biological or behavioral factors and the result of direct and indirect advantage or disadvantage is often ignored (Atkin, 2011). Figure 6.2 shows the relationship between proximal and distal determinants in adverse birth outcomes.

The SDOH uses a systems framework that incorporates policy, environment, and community layers. While it acknowledges that interventions for reducing inequalities at one layer will influence another layer (Dahlgren & Whitehead, 1991; Navarro, 2009), the layers

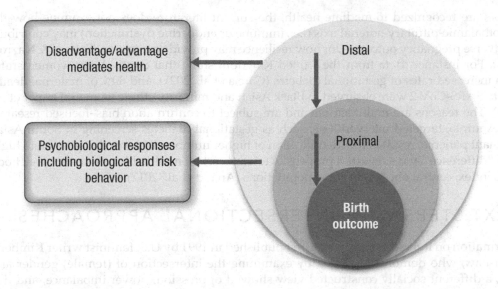

Figure 6.2 The relationships between distal and proximal determinants of birth outcomes.

are conceptualized and operationalized as separate and are not understood to be intersected. A further criticism of the SDOH framework has been the lack of acknowledgment of power dynamics, such as political, discriminatory, or class related, which can be identified at all levels in society but are not represented in the SDOH (Salway et al., 2010). Power dynamics may impact the context and empowerment of numerous factors at different layers (e.g., individual, community, environment). Here is an example: A local government prioritizes public health agendas, mediating access and funding on specific health interventions (Patterson, 2014). Reducing perinatal mortality was not a priority in the United Kingdom until 2015, with the publication of the WHO's sustainable development goals. However, a problem with politically driven priorities is that disadvantaged members of society are often further excluded, and the inequality gap becomes wider (Marmot, 2017a). Moreover, the paucity of acknowledging power dynamics may well be the result of the SDOH framework being conceived in the West, with homogeneous assumptions made on human experience, therefore obscuring the contributions of ethnicity and culture. Inequalities in health are the result of inequitable life circumstances that are then perpetuated by power dynamics, finance, and resources that money can purchase (e.g., education, healthcare) that then continue to intentionally or unintentionally discriminate and perpetuate an inequitable sharing of resources (Marmot, 2015).

The SDOH positions ethnicity in the heritable factors section. However, as mentioned previously, ethnicity is a multifaceted construct and is not grounded in genetics (i.e., biologically) as is the conceptual issue of discussing "race." Ethnicity interacts with all levels of the SDOH; for example, Pakistani and Bangladeshi families tend to reside in areas of high deprivation, with poor quality housing and increased exposure to environmental risks, with resulting increased risks of adverse birth outcomes (Sharp, 2010). Moreover, culture is positioned in the farthest layer from the individual; however, culture being a dynamic concept is also present in every level of the SDOH framework—seen in policy, environment, community, and individual levels—and incorporates shared values influencing beliefs and behavior (Patterson, 2014).

Many of the SDOH factors at each layer are context dependent and are not made explicit. Moreover, discrimination and disadvantage may be experienced across all levels of the framework whereby quality of life will be affected; however, this is not accounted for in the SDOH framework (Brunner & Marmot, 2006). Furthermore, while psychosocial and psychobiological factors are recognized to mediate health, the current literature does not examine how the hypothalamic-pituitary-adrenal axis (i.e., immune or endocrine dysfunction) may contribute to adverse pregnancy outcomes, or how resilience may provide protection (Saffron & Nazroo, 2002). For instance, data from the United Kingdom show that South Asian women suffer from increased rates of gestational diabetes (Garcia et al., 2021), and 80% of maternal deaths due to SARS-CoV-2 were observed in Black Asian and minority ethnic women (Draper et al., 2021). The reasons are multifactorial and are subject to confirmation bias–focused research. For example, targeted interventions, such as gestational diabetes screening in South Asian pregnant patients, result in the identification of higher numbers of cases that goes on to high-light "difference" and suggests a propensity toward certain modifiable risk factors (e.g., body mass index, central obesity) in some populations (Anand et al., 2017).

NEXT STEPS WITH INTERSECTIONAL APPROACHES

Information on intersectionality was first published in 1991 by U.S. feminist writer Kimberlé Crenshaw, who demonstrated that by examining the intersection of (female) gender and race, a different socially constructed view showed oppression, power imbalance, and discrimination. Her work demonstrated that the experience of domestic violence was different for Black women than for White women; White women experienced only sexism, whereas Black women experienced sexism *and* racism (Crenshaw, 1991).

The SDOH framework has been useful to consider some of the determinants of perinatal mortality, but there are both functional and conceptual limitations with this approach. As a result, research has focused on proximal determinants, such as biological factors or lifestyle behaviors. However, the distal determinants and the consequence of disadvantage have been neglected (Garcia, 2017). More needs to be done to recognize and understand the causes of the causes (Marmot & Wilkinson, 2003). Arguably, utilizing an intersectional approach reveals previously obscured factors that may contribute to the experience of perinatal mortality and recognizes this is mediated by intersecting factors such as power dynamics, socioeconomic status, education status, and ethnicity (Viruell-Fuentes et al., 2012).

Much of the current research with Pakistani and Bangladeshi patients in the maternity literature emphasizes differences focused on maternal ethnicity; however, this ignores power dynamics and social relationships, perpetuating "othering," and contributes further to a lack of objective criticism (Garcia, 2017). Furthermore, while epidemiological research highlights risk factors, researchers used predefined categories that are conceptualized as being additive. This then fails to reveal risks that may be more important to the outcome, or conceptualized as multiplicative, and may hide other contributory factors that might not be evident.

By conceptualizing risk using SDOH, the researcher obscures power dynamics that operate at individual, social, or environmental levels, and this hides similarities or differences operating between and within disadvantaged groups, failing to uncover the key determinants for perinatal mortality (Garcia, 2017). Examples may include power imbalance observed in maternity care, *with* power imbalance observed as an ethnic minority, *with* power imbalance being perceived in the uneducated, and so forth. The combined and multiplicative risk effects following the power imbalance experienced by a migrant pregnant patient can then be seen to be substantial. Research now needs to elucidate further to determine how this mechanism works.

Most health research and policies fail to recognize the intersection of various social identities and are unaware of how this conjuncture of multiple determinants at the individual level interacts with structural level health disparities (Bowleg, 2012). For example, how the combination of ethnicity, deprivation, low education attainment, employment options, and poor health literacy interacts with rigid maternity services aimed at middle-class White women, further excluding already marginalized women, is missing from the science (Garcia, 2017). Therefore, intersectionality addresses power dynamics such as privilege and oppression. It considers how these powerful forces interact with structural level services in maintaining inequality. Moreover, using intersectionality to understand health inequalities moves away from victim-blaming—as is often seen in studies that involve ethnicity or culture—and encourages researchers to reconceptualize existing issues and use a broader praxis as is required in health research, therefore being more empowering (López & Gadsden, 2016).

CONCLUSION

The SDOH is a useful way to understand the wider biopsychosocial factors that contribute to health inequalities and health outcomes. It highlights the distal determinants that mediate health in a variety of contexts and considers the wider social environment in which individuals are situated. Perinatal mortality is an example that shows a clear social gradient, as evidenced in Pakistani and Bangladeshi infants in the United Kingdom. However, using ethnicity as a variable in research is not without its conceptual and operational challenges, including considerations of how culture, language, and religion contribute to shaping an individual's subjective experience and engagement in health behaviors. While the SDOH framework has been useful, it is not without its limitations. The intersectional approach offers a more complex conceptual analysis of the wider determinants that mediate health outcomes.

DISCUSSION QUESTIONS

1. Using the social determinants of health framework, what specific risk factors does Naba have for an adverse birth outcome?
2. Identify where inequality may contribute to an adverse birth outcome for Naba.
3. How could a culturally specific plan of care address the major health-related issues that might then improve Naba's overall health and help to ensure that her future childbearing experiences might have a more favorable outcome?
4. Apply the concept of intersectionality to Naba's lived experiences in the United Kingdom. What recommendations could an informed health professional make for policy and practice changes?

REFERENCES

Abortion Act. (1967). https://www.legislation.gov.uk/ukpga/1967/87?view=extent
Ali, N. (2003). Fluency in the consulting room. *British Journal of General Practice*, July, 514–518. http://www.ncbi.nlm.nih.gov/pmc/articles/PMC1314639/pdf/14694661.pdf
Anand, S. S., Gupta, M., Teo, K. K., Schulze, K. M., Desai, D., Abdalla, N., Zulyniak, M., de Souza, R., Wahi, G., Shaikh, M., Beyene, J., de Villa, E., Morrison, K., McDonald, S. D., & Gerstein, H. (2017). Causes and consequences of gestational diabetes in South Asians living in Canada: Results from a prospective cohort study. *CMAJ Open, 5*(3), E604–E611. https://doi.org/10.9778/cmajo.20170027
Antonisamy, B., Vasan, S. K., Geethanjali, F. S., Gowri, M., Hepsy, Y. S., Richard, J., Raghupathy, P., Karpe, F., Osmond, C., & Fall, C. H. D. (2017). Weight gain and height growth during infancy, childhood, and adolescence as predictors of adult cardiovascular risk. *Journal of Pediatrics, 180,* 53–61.e3. https://doi.org/10.1016/j.jpeds.2016.09.059
Arzuaga, B. H., & Lee, B. H. (2011). Limits of human viability in the United States: A medicolegal review. *Paediatrics, 128*(6), 1047–1052. https://doi.org/10.1542/peds.2011-1689
Atkin, K. (2011). Negotiating ethnic identities and health. In H. Graham (Ed.), *Understanding health inequalities* (2nd ed., pp. 125–141). Open University Press.
Australian Institute of Health and Welfare. (2020). Stillbirths and neonatal deaths in Australia, maternal characteristics. https://www.aihw.gov.au/reports/mothers-babies/stillbirths-and-neonatal-deaths-in-australia/contents/overview-of-perinatal-deaths/maternal-characteristics

Barba, C., Cavalli-Sforza, T., Cutter, J., Darnton-Hill, I., Deurenberg, P., Deurenberg-Yap, M., & Gill, T. (2004). Appropriate body-mass index for Asian populations and its implications for policy and intervention strategies. *Lancet*. https://doi.org/10.1016/S0140-6736(03)15268-3

Bartley, M. (2008). *Health inequality: An introduction to theories, concepts and methods*. Blackwell Publishers.

Bécares, L., Shaw, R., Nazroo, J., Stafford, M., Albor, C., Atkin, K., Kiernan, K., Wilkinson, R., & Pickett, K. (2012). Ethnic density effects on physical morbidity, mortality, and health behaviours: A systematic review of the literature. *American Journal of Public Health*, 102(12). https://doi.org/10.2105/AJPH.2012.300832

Benzeval, M., Bond, L., Campbell, M., Egan, M., Lorenc, T., Petticrew, M., & Popham, F. (2014). *How does money influence health?* Joseph Rowntree Foundation. (Issue March 2014). http://www.jrf.org.uk/sites/files/jrf/income-health-poverty-full.pdf

Best, M., Leget, C., Goodhead, A., & Paal, P. (2020). An EAPC white paper on multi-disciplinary education for spiritual care in palliative care. *BMC Palliative Care*, 19(1), 1–10. https://doi.org/10.1186/s12904-019-0508-4

Bhopal, R. (2007). Ethnicity, race and health in multicultural societies: Foundations for better epidemiology, public health and health care. Oxford University Press.

Bidwell, D. R., Bava, S., Gergen, K., & Hosking, D. (2016). *Spirituality, social construction, relational processes*. In D. Bidwell (Ed.). Issue November. Worldshare Books.

Blackwell, C. (2015). The role of infection and inflammation in stillbirths: Parallels with SIDS? *Frontiers in Immunology*, 6(June), 1–8. https://doi.org/10.3389/fimmu.2015.00248

Blane, D. (2006). The life course, the social gradient and health. In M. Marmot & R. Wilkinson (Eds.), Social determinants of health (2nd ed., pp. 54–78). Oxford University Press.

Blane, D., Smith, G. D., & Hart, C. (1999). Some social and physical correlates of intergenerational social mobility: Evidence from the west of Scotland collaborative study. *Sociology*, 33(1), 169–183. https://doi.org/10.1177/S0038038599000097

Bowleg, L. (2012). The problem with the phrase women and minorities: Intersectionality—an important theoretical framework for public health. *American Journal of Public Health*, 102(7), 1267–1273. https://doi.org/10.2105/AJPH.2012.300750

Brunner, E., & Marmot, M. (2006). Social organisation, stress and health. In M. Marmot & R. G. Wilkinson (Eds.), Social determinants of health (2nd ed., pp. 6–31). Oxford University Press.

Cambridge Dictionary. (2021). Spirituality. Cambridge Dictionary. https://dictionary.cambridge.org/dictionary/english/spirituality

Centers for Disease Control and Prevention. (2020). Pregnancy mortality surveillance system. https://www.cdc.gov/reproductivehealth/maternal-mortality/pregnancy-mortality-surveillance-system.htm#trends

Centers for Disease Control and Prevention. (2018). Infant mortality. https://www.cdc.gov/reproductivehealth/maternalinfanthealth/infantmortality.htm

Chattoo, S., & Atkin, K. (2019). 'Race', ethnicity and social policy: Theoretical concepts and the limitations of current approaches to welfare. In G. Craig, K. Atkin, S. Chatoo, & F. R. (Eds.), Understanding "race" and ethnicity: Theory, policy and practice (2nd ed., pp. 19–41). Policy Press.

Chaturvedi, N. (2001). "Ethnicity as an epidemiological determinant—crudely racist or crucially important?' *International Journal of Epidemiology*, 30(5), pp. 925–927. https://doi.org/10.1093/ije/30.5.925

Choudhury, N., & Ahmed, S. M. (2011). Maternal care practices among the ultra poor households in rural Bangladesh: A qualitative exploratory study. *BMC Pregnancy and Childbirth*, 11(1), 15. https://doi.org/10.1186/1471-2393-11-15

Cohen, D. (2020). Methods in cultural psychology. In S. Kitayama & D. Cohen (Eds.), Handbook of cultural psychology (2nd ed., pp. 196–237). The Guildford Press.

Cohen, S., Janicki-Deverts, D., Chen, E., & Matthews, K. (2010). Childhood socioeconomic status and adult health. *Annals of the New York Academy of Sciences*, 1186, 37–55. https://doi.org/10.1111/j.1749-6632.2009.05334.x

Collins, J. W., Rankin, K. M., & David, R. J. (2011). Low birth weight across generations: The effect of the economic environment. *Maternal and Child Health Journal*, 15(4), 438–445. https://doi.org/10.1007/s10995-010-0603-x

Conner, M., & Norman, P. (2005). Predicting health behaviour: A social cognition approach. In M. Conner & P. Norman (Eds.), Predicting health behaviour. (2nd ed., pp. 1–373). Open University Press.

Conner, M., & Norman, P. (2015). Predicting and changing health behaviour: research and practice with social cognition models. In M. Conner & P. Norman (Eds.) (3rd ed.). McGraw Hill. https://www.mheducation.co.uk/predicting-and-changing-health-behaviour-research-and-practice-with-social-cognition-models-9780335263783-emea-group

Crenshaw, K. (1991). Mapping the margins: Intersectionality, identity politics, and violence against women of color. *Stanford Law Review*, *43*(6), 1241–1299. https://doi.org/10.2307/1229039

Cross-Sudworth, F., Williams, M., & Gardosi, J. (2015). Perinatal deaths of migrant mothers: Adverse outcomes from unrecognised risks and substandard care factors. *British Journal of Midwifery*, *23*(10), 734–740. https://doi.org/10.12968/bjom.2015.23.10.734

Dahlgren, G., & Whitehead, M. (1991). Policies and strategies to promote social equity in health Background document to WHO–Strategy paper. In Institutet för Framtidsstudier (Issue September). http://s2.medicina.uady.mx/observatorio/docs/eq/li/Eq_2007_Li_Dahlgren.pdf

De Bernis, L., Kinney, M. V., Stones, W., Ten Hoope-Bender, P., Vivio, D., Leisher, S. H., Bhutta, Z. A., G. lmezoglu, M., Mathai, M., Beliz, J. M., Franco, L., McDougall, L., Zeitlin, J., Malata, A., Dickson, K. E., & Lawn, J. E. (2016). Stillbirths: Ending preventable deaths by 2030. *The Lancet*, *387*(10019). https://doi.org/10.1016/S0140-6736(15)00954-X

Department of Health. (2015). The mandate 2015–2016. April 2015–March 2016. https://www.gov .uk/government/uploads/system/uploads/attachment_data/file/486818/mndate-NHSE-15_16. pdf

Department of Health. (2016). The Government's mandate to NHS England for 2016–17. http:// www.parliament.uk/written-questions-answers-statements/written-statement/Commons/ 2015-12-17/HCWS440

Dex, S., & Joshi, H. (Eds.). (2005). Children of the 21st century. The Policy Press.

Dibben, C., Sigala, M., & Macfarlane, A. (2006). Area deprivation, individual factors and low birth weight in England: Is there evidence of an "area effect"? *Journal of Epidemiology Community Health*, *60*, 1053–1059. https://doi.org/10.1136/jech.2005.042853

Draper, E. S., Gallimore, I. D., Kurinczuk, J. J., & Kenyon, S. (2021). Maternal, newborn and infant clinical outcome review programme MBRRACE-UK perinatal confidential enquiry stillbirths and neonatal deaths in twin pregnancies (Issue January). www.hqip.org.uk/national-programmes

Driscoll, A. K., & Ely, D. M. (2019). National Vital Statistics Reports Volume 68, Number 11 September 25, 2019. https://www.cdc.gov/nchs/products/index.htm

Engel, G. L. (1977, 2012). The need for a new medical model: A challenge for biomedicine. *Psychodynamic Psychiatry*, *40*(3), 377–396. https://www.urmc.rochester.edu/MediaLibraries/ URMCMedia/medical-humanities/documents/Engle-Challenge-to-Biomedicine-Biopsychosicial-Model.pdf

Flannelly, K. J., Jankowski, K. R. B., & Flannelly, L. T. (2014). Operational definitions in research on religion and health. *Journal of Health Care Chaplaincy*, *20*(2), 83–91. https://doi.org/10.1080/088547 26.2014.909278

Garcia, R., Ali, N., Griffiths, M., & Randhawa, G. (2020a). A qualitative study exploring the experiences of bereavement after stillbirth in Pakistani, Bangladeshi and white British mothers living in Luton, UK. *Midwifery*, *91*, 102833. https://doi.org/10.1016/j.midw.2020.102833

Garcia, R., Ali, N., Guppy, A., Griffiths, M., & Randhawa, G. (2017). A comparison of antenatal classifications of "overweight" and "obesity" prevalence between white British, Indian, Pakistani and Bangladeshi pregnant women in England; Analysis of retrospective data. *BMC Public Health*, *17*(1), 308. https://doi.org/10.1186/s12889-017-4211-1

Garcia, R., Ali, N., Guppy, A., Griffiths, M., & Randhawa, G. (2020b). Ethnic differences in risk factors for adverse birth outcomes between Pakistani, Bangladeshi, and White British mothers. *Journal of Advanced Nursing*, *76*(1), 174–182. https://doi.org/10.1111/jan.14209

Garcia, R., Ali, N., Guppy, A., Griffiths, M., & Randhawa, G. (2021). Analysis of routinely collected data: Determining associations of maternal risk factors and infant outcomes with gestational diabetes, in Pakistani, Indian, Bangladeshi and white British pregnant women in Luton, England. *Midwifery*, *94*, 102899. https://doi.org/10.1016/j.midw.2020.102899

Garcia, R. L. (2017). Perinatal mortality in Pakistani, Bangladeshi and White British mothers, in Luton. University of Bedfordshire. http://uobrep.openrepository.com/uobrep/ handle/10547/622733

Gonzalez, R. M., & Gilleskie, D. (2017). Infant mortality rate as a measure of a country's health: A robust method to improve reliability and comparability. *Demography*, *54*(2), 701–720. https://doi .org/10.1007/s13524-017-0553-7

Gregory, E. C. W., Drake, P., & Martin, J. A. (2018). Lack of change in perinatal mortality in the United States, 2014–2016. *NCHS Data Brief*, 316, 1–8.

Gustafsson, P. E., Miguel, S. S., Janlert, U., Theorell, T., Westerlund, H., & Hammarström, A. (2014). Life-course accumulation of neighbourhood disadvantage and allostatic load: Empirical integration of three social determinants of health frameworks. *American Journal of Public Health*, *104*(5), 904–910. https://doi.org/10.2105/AJPH.2013.301707

Halpern, D., & Nazroo, J. (1999). The ethnic density effect: Results from a national community survey of England and Wales. *International Journal of Social Psychiatry*, *46*(1), 34–46. https://doi. org/10.1177/002076400004600105

Health and Social Care Act 2012. (2012). http://www.legislation.gov.uk/ukpga/2012/7/contents/ enacted

Hostinar, C. E., Ross, K. M., Chen, E., & Miller, G. E. (2017). Early-life socioeconomic disadvantage and metabolic health disparities. *Psychosomatic Medicine*, *79*(5), 514–523. https://doi.org/10.1097/ PSY.0000000000000455

Hsu, C.-N., & Tain, Y.-L. (2019). The good, the bad, and the ugly of pregnancy nutrients and developmental programming of adult disease. *Nutrients*, *11*(894), 1–21. https://doi.org/10.3390/ nu11040894

Humes, K. R., Jones, N. A., & Ramirez, R. R. (2011). Overview of race and Hispanic origin: 2010. In United States Census Bureau (Issue March). http://www.census.gov/population/race/

Jomeen, J., & Redshaw, M. (2013). Ethnic minority women's experience of maternity services in England. *Ethnicity & Health*, *18*(3), 280–296. https://doi.org/10.1080/13557858.2012.730608

Jones, K. F. (2018). Spirituality: More than just religion. *Journal of the Australasian Rehabilitation Nurses Association*, *21*(1), 12–14. https://search.informit.org/doi/10.3316/INFORMIT.978149216740268

Jornayvaz, F. R., Vollenweider, P., Bochud, M., Mooser, V., Waeber, G., & Marques-Vidal, P. (2016). Low birth weight leads to obesity, diabetes and increased leptin levels in adults: The CoLaus study. *Cardiovascular Diabetology*, *15*(1), 1–10. https://doi.org/10.1186/s12933-016-0389-2

Kahveci, B., Melekoglu, R., Evruke, I. C., & Cetin, C. (2018). The effect of advanced maternal age on perinatal outcomes in nulliparous singleton pregnancies. *BMC Pregnancy and Childbirth*, *18*(1), 1–7. https://doi.org/10.1186/s12884-018-1984-x

Karlsen, S., & Nazroo, J. (2011). Religion, ethnicity and health inequalities. In H. Graham (Ed.), *Understanding health inequalities* (2nd ed., pp. 103–125). Open University Press.

Katbamna, S., Ahmad, W., Bhakta, P., Baker, R., & Parker, G. (2004). Do they look after their own? *Informal Support for South Asian Carers. Health and Social Care in the Community*, *12*(5), 398–406.

Koenig, H. G., McCullough, M. E., & Larson, D. B. (2001). Handbook of religion and health. *In* H. G. Koenig (Ed.). Oxford University Press.

Koenig, M., & Al Shohaib, S. (2014). Health and wellbeing in Islamic societies: Background, research and applications. Springer New York.

Kurinczuk, J. J., Hollowell, J., Boyd, P. A., Oakley, L., Brocklehurst, P., & Gray, R. (2010). The contribution of congenital anomalies to infant mortality. National Perinatal Epidemiology Unit, Oxford.

Llamas, A., Borkowski, L., & Wood, S. (2018). Public health impacts of state-level abortion restrictions (Issue April). https://publichealth.gwu.edu/sites/default/files/downloads/projects/ JIWH/Impacts_of_State_Abortion_Restrictions.pdf

López, N., & Gadsden, V. L. (2016). Health inequities, social determinants, and intersectionality. *National Academy of Medicine, Perspective*, 1–15. https://nam.edu/wp-content/uploads/2016/12/ Health-Inequities-Social-Determinants-and-Intersectionality.pdf

Lu, M. C., & Halfon, N. (2003). Racial and ethnic disparities in birth outcomes: A life-course perspective. *Maternal and Child Health Journal*, *7*(1), 13–30. https://doi.org/10.102 3/A:1022537516969

Marie, G., Higginbottom, A., Evans, C., Morgan, M., Bharj, K. K., Eldridge, J., & Hussain, B. (2019). Experience of and access to maternity care in the UK by immigrant women: A narrative synthesis systematic review. *BMJ Open*, *9*, 29478. https://doi.org/10.1136/bmjopen-2019-029478

Markus, H. R., & Hamedani, M. Y. (2010). Sociocultural psychology: The dynamic interdependence among self systems and social systems. In S. Kitayama & D. Cohen (Eds.), *Handbook of cultural psychology* (pp. 3–40). The Guildford Press.

Marmot, M., Allen, J., Goldblatt, P., Boyce, T., McNeish, D., Grady, M., & Geddes, I. (2010). Fair society, healthy lives. https://doi.org/10.1016/j.puhe.2012.05.014

Marmot, M., & Wilkinson, R. (2003). Determinants of health. the solid facts. In R. Wilkinson & M. Marmot (Eds.), World Health Organization (2nd ed., Vol. 2, Issue 2). World Health Organization. https://doi.org/10.1016/j.jana.2012.03.001

Marmot, M. (2015). The health gap: The challenge of an unequal world. *The Lancet*, *386*(10011), 2442–2444. https://doi.org/10.1016/S0140-6736(15)00150-6

Marmot, M. (2017a). Social justice, epidemiology and health inequalities. *European Journal of Epidemiology*, *32*(7), 537–546. https://doi.org/10.1007/s10654-017-0286-3

Marmot, M. (2017b). Closing the health gap. *Scandinavian Journal of Public Health*, *45*(7), 723–731. https://doi.org/10.1177/1403494817717433

Marmot, M., Allen, J., Boyce, T., Goldblatt, P., Morrison, J., Michael Marmot, B., Jessica Allen, C., Allen, M., Ntouva, A., Porritt Peter Goldblatt, F., Beswick, L., Bourke, D., Codling, K., Hallam, P., Munro, A., Dixon, J., Bibby, J., Cockin, J., Elwell Sutton, T., … Wiseman, A. (2020). Health equity in England: The Marmot review 10 years on (Vol. 10). http://www.instituteofhealthequity.org/ resources-reports/marmot-review-10-years-on/the-marmot-review-10-years-on-full-report.pdf

Marsella, A. J., & Yamada, A. (2010). Culture and psychopathology: Foundations, issues and directions. In S. Kitayama & D. Cohen (Eds.), Handbook of cultural psychology (pp. 797–821). The Guildford Press.

Memon, K. N., & Rahman, A. A. (2020). Consanguinity: A risk factor for adverse birth outcomes. *International Journal of Current Research*, 8(11), 41132–41137.

Nandi, A., & Platt, L. (2013). Britishness and identity assimilation among the UK's minority and majority ethnic groups. December 2013.

Navarro, V. (2009). What we mean by social determinants of health. *International Journal of Health Services*, 39(3), 423–441. https://doi.org/10.2190/HS.39.3.a

Office for National Statistics. (2012). Ethnicity and national identity in England and Wales (2011) (Issue December). http://www.ons.gov.uk/ons/dcp171776_290558.pdf

Office for National Statistics. (2014). Childhood, infant and perinatal mortality in England and Wales, 2012. http://www.ons.gov.uk/ons/dcp171778_350853.pdf

Office for National Statistics. (2018). Child mortality (death cohort) tables in England and Wales - Office for National Statistics. Child Mortality Data. https://www.ons.gov.uk/peoplepopulationandcommunity/birthsdeathsandmarriages/deaths/datasets/childmortalitystatisticschildhoodinfantandperinatalchildhoodinfantandperinatalmortalityinenglandandwales

Office for National Statistics. (2020). Labour market status by ethnic group A09. https://www.ons.gov.uk/employmentandlabourmarket/peopleinwork/employmentandemployeetypes/datasets/labourmarketstatusbyethnicgroupa09

Patterson, O. (2014). Making sense of culture. *Annual Review of Sociology*, 40(1), 1–30. https://doi.org/10.1146/annurev-soc-071913-043123

Phillimore, J. (2016). Migrant maternity in an era of superdiversity: New migrants' access to, and experience of, antenatal care in the West Midlands, UK. *Social Science and Medicine*, 148, 152–159. https://doi.org/10.1016/j.socscimed.2015.11.030

Puthussery, S., Twamley, K., Macfarlane, A., Harding, S., & Baron, M. (2010). "You need that loving tender care": Maternity care experiences and expectations of ethnic minority women born in the United Kingdom. *Journal of Health Services Research & Policy*, 15(3), 156–162. https://doi.org/10.1258/jhsrp.2009.009067

Raju, T. N. K., Mercer, B. M., Burchfield, D. J., & Joseph, G. F. (2014). Periviable birth: Executive summary of a joint workshop by the Eunice Kennedy Shriver National Institute of Child Health and Human Development, Society for Maternal-Fetal Medicine, American Academy of Pediatrics, and American College of Obstetricians and Gynecologists. In Obstetrics and Gynecology (Vol. 123, Issue 5, pp. 1083–1096). Lippincott Williams and Wilkins. https://doi.org/10.1097/AOG.0000000000000243

Raman, S., Nicholls, R., Ritchie, J., Razee, H., & Shafiee, S. (2016). How natural is the supernatural? Synthesis of the qualitative literature from low and middle-income countries on cultural practices and traditional beliefs influencing the perinatal period. *Midwifery*, 39, 87–97. https://doi.org/10.1016/j.midw.2016.05.005

Redshaw, M., Rowe, R., & Henderson, J. (2014). Listening to parents after stillbirth or the death of their baby after birth (Issue May). https://www.npeu.ox.ac.uk/listeningtoparents

Regmi, K., Naidoo, J., Pilkington, P., Researcher, P., Naidoo, J., & Pilkington, P. (2010). Understanding the processes of translation and transliteration in qualitative research. *International Journal of Qualitative Methods*, 9(1), 16–26.

Reid, C., & Herbert, C. (2014). 'Welfare moms and welfare bums': Revisiting poverty as a social determinant of health. *Health Sociology Review*, 14(2), 161–173. https://doi.org/10.5172/hesr.14.2.161

Rochow, N., Alsamnan, M., So, H. Y., Olbertz, D., Pelc, A., Däbritz, J., Hentschel, R., Wittwer-Backofen, U., & Voigt, M. (2019). Maternal body height is a stronger predictor of birth weight than ethnicity: Analysis of birth weight percentile charts. *Journal of Perinatal Medicine*, 47(1), 22–29. https://doi.org/10.1515/jpm-2017-0349

Ross, L., McSherry, W., Giske, T., van Leeuwen, R., Schep-Akkerman, A., Koslander, T., Hall, J., Steenfeldt, V. Ø., & Jarvis, P. (2018). Nursing and midwifery students' perceptions of spirituality, spiritual care, and spiritual care competency: A prospective, longitudinal, correlational European study. *Nurse Education Today*, 67(May), 64–71. https://doi.org/10.1016/j.nedt.2018.05.002

Saffron, K., & Nazroo, J. Y. (2002). Agency and structure: The impact of ethnic identity and racism on the health of ethnic minority people. 24(1), 1–20.

Saigal, S., Stoskopf, B., Streiner, D., Paneth, N., Pinelli, J., & Boyle, M. (2006). Growth trajectories of extremely low birth weight infants from birth to young adulthood: A longitudinal, population-based study. *Pediatric Research*, 60(6), 751–758. https://doi.org/10.1203/01.pdr.0000246201.93662.8e

Salway, S., Nazroo, J., Mir, G., Craig, G., Johnson, M., Gerrish, K., Sarah, S., James, N., Mir, G., Gary, C., Johnson, M., & Gerrish, K. (2010). Fair society, healthy lives: A missed opportunity to address ethnic inequalities in health. *British Medical Journal*, 340(April). http://www.bmj.com/rapid-response/2011/11/02/fair-society-healthy-lives-missed-opportunity-address-ethnic-inequalities-

Senior, P. A., & Bhopal, R. (1994). Ethnicity as a variable in epidemiological research. *BMJ (Clinical Research Ed.)*, 309(6950), 327–330. https://doi.org/10.1136/bmj.309.6950.327

Sharp, K. (2010). Nursing and the sociology of healthcare. In E. Denny & S. Earle (Eds.), *Sociology for nurses* (2nd ed., pp. 7–28). Policy Press.

Shaw, A. (2012). "They say Islam has a solution for everything, so why are there no guidelines for this?" Ethical dilemmas associated with the births and deaths of infants with fatal abnormalities from a small sample of Pakistani Muslim couples in Britain. *Bioethics*, 26(9), 485–492. https://doi.org/10.1111/j.1467-8519.2011.01883.x

Skinner, B. F. (1988). The selection of behavior: The operant behaviorism of B. F. Skinner ... - Burrhus Frederic Skinner - Google Books. Cambridge University Press. https://books.google.co.uk/books?hl=en&lr=&id=3nY7AAAAIAAJ&oi=fnd&pg=PR13&dq=Burrhus+Skinner+&ots=7fQgZef-J4&sig=KS35BK7×9pSyUPufsQufDpbuzns#v=onepage&q=Burrhus Skinner&f=false

Tarafder, T., Sultan, P., & Rashid, T. (2013). Reproductive health beliefs and perceptions among slum women in Bangladesh. In P. Dalziel (Ed.), 37th Annual Conference of the Australian and New Zealand Regional Science Association International (Issue December, pp. 124–136). Lincoln University, New Zealand.

Tanyi, R. A. (2002). Towards clarification of the meaning of spirituality. *Journal of Advanced Nursing*, 39, 500–509.

The World Health Organization. (2015). Maternal and perinatal health. http://www.who.int/maternal_child_adolescent/epidemiology/profiles/neonatal_child/pak.pdf

The Kings Fund. (2020). What are health inequalities? https://www.kingsfund.org.uk/publications/what-are-health-inequalities

Triandis, H. C. (2010). Culture and psychology: A history of the study of their relationship. In S. Kitayama & J. Cohen (Eds.), Handbook of cultural psychology (pp. 59–77). The Guildford Press.

United Nations Inter-agency Group for Child Mortality Estimation. (2020). Stillbirth rate United Kindom. Kingdom of Great Britain and Northern Ireland. https://childmortality.org/data/United.

Unwin, J. (2014). A UK without poverty. Joseph Rowntree Foundation. https://www.jrf.org.uk/report/uk-without-poverty

Viruell-Fuentes, E. A., Miranda, P. Y., & Abdulrahim, S. (2012). More than culture: Structural racism, intersectionality theory, and immigrant health. *Social Science and Medicine*, 75(12), 2099–2106. https://doi.org/10.1016/j.socscimed.2011.12.037

Wadsworth, M. E., & Kuh, D. J. (1997). Childhood influences on adult health: A review of recent work from the British 1946 national birth cohort study, the MRC National Survey of Health and Development. *Paediatric and Perinatal Epidemiology*, 11(1), 2–20. https://doi.org/10.1046/j.1365-3016.1997.d01-7.x

Walker, K. F., Bradshaw, L., Bugg, G. J., & Thornton, J. G. (2016). Causes of antepartum stillbirth in women of advanced maternal age. *European Journal of Obstetrics & Gynecology and Reproductive Biology*, 197, 86–90. https://doi.org/10.1016/j.ejogrb.2015.11.032

Watson, J. (1997). Behaviourism. Routledge. https://www-routledge-com.libezproxy.open.ac.uk/Behaviorism/Watson/p/book/9781560009948

Wehkalampi, K., Hovi, P., Dunkel, L., Strang-Karlsson, S., Järvenpää, A. L., Eriksson, J. G., Andersson, S., & Kajantie, E. (2011). Advanced pubertal growth spurt in subjects born preterm: The Helsinki study of very low birth weight adults. *Journal of Clinical Endocrinology and Metabolism*, 96(2), 525–533. https://doi.org/10.1210/jc.2010-1523

Wickham, S., Anwar, E., Barr, B., Law, C., & Taylor-Robinson, D. (2016). Poverty and child health in the UK: Using evidence for action. *Archives of Disease in Childhood*, 101(8), 759–766. https://doi.org/10.1136/archdischild-2014-306746

Wilkinson, R., & Marmot, M. (1998). The solid facts. In R. Wilkinson, M. Marmot (Eds.). WHO Regional Office for Europe.

Winning, A., Glymour, M. M., McCormick, M. C., Gilsanz, P., & Kubzansky, L. D. (2016). Childhood psychological distress as a mediator in the relationship between early-life social disadvantage and adult cardiometabolic risk. *Psychosomatic Medicine*, 78(9), 1019–1030. https://doi.org/10.1097/PSY.0000000000000409

World Health Organization. (2016). Congenital anomalies. Fact Sheet 370. http://www.who.int/mediacentre/factsheets/fs370/en/

World Health Organization. (2020). Congenital anomalies. https://www.who.int/news-room/fact-sheets/detail/congenital-anomalies

World Health Organization. (2021). Maternal and perinatal health. WHO; World Health Organization. https://www-who-int.libezproxy.open.ac.uk/maternal_child_adolescent/topics/maternal/maternal_perinatal/en/

Zeitlin, J., Mortensen, L., Prunet, C., Macfarlane, A., Hindori-Mohangoo, A. D., Gissler, M., Szamotulska, K., van der Pal, K., Bolumar, F., Andersen, A-M. N., Olafsdottir, H. S., Zhang, W-H., Blondel, B., & Alexander, S. (2016). Socioeconomic inequalities in stillbirth rates in Europe: Measuring the gap using routine data from the Euro-Peristat Project. *BMC Pregnancy and Childbirth*, *16*, 15–15. https://doi.org/10.1186/s12884-016-0804-4

CHAPTER 7

Health Literacy: Insights for Action

Rima E. Rudd and Terri Ann Parnell

LEARNING OBJECTIVES

- Examine and discuss the history of adult literacy assessments and the emergence of health literacy studies.

- Describe the literacy and health literacy skills of adults in industrialized nations and the social factors associated with limited skills.

- Explain why the early definition of health literacy constrained the health sector response.

- Describe the five components or variables of health literacy.

- Provide at least three examples of how health professionals can improve numeric communication with patients.

- Provide an example of efficacious action that could be undertaken within each of the five components of health literacy.

INTRODUCTION

Communication has always been a vitally important component of efforts to improve individual, public, and population health. Clear exchanges of accessible information among scientists, health practitioners, policymakers, and the public help build knowledge, trust, and a healthy society. Unfortunately, the complex challenges of our time have revealed fractures in important information exchanges. The toll taken by the COVID-19 pandemic, environmental disasters, war and migration, inequities, bias and discrimination, and the politicization of science has also compromised trust and constrained needed dialogues. News abounds with stories of the purposive misinformation on social media and of skepticism related to the veracity of health information. In these fraught times, health messages have been challenged, trust has been diminished, inequities have been exacerbated, and the health and well-being of communities have been profoundly affected. Needless to say, these issues are of deep concern to public health and healthcare practitioners.

Many communication guidelines now draw from health literacy studies to support efforts to improve, repair, and rebuild information exchanges, especially during troubled times. Health literacy is grounded in respectful exchange and can thereby augment our efforts to rebuild trust. In clinical settings, health literacy considerations are improving discussion between and among health professionals and between health professionals and patients with concrete implications for health outcomes (Parnell, 2015). Health literacy in the public health arena is informing program design and evaluation studies in health communication, health promotion, disease prevention, care management, environmental health, and for preparedness and disaster mitigation efforts (Morello-Frosch et al., 2014; Rudd et al., 2003). At the policy level, examination of institutional and system-level characteristics that support or impede access to information, care, and services are informing health policy initiatives and institutional change (Koh et al., 2012). Added attention to health literacy can contribute to ongoing efforts to increase access to information and services and thereby reduce disparities.

The term *health literacy* was formally defined by Nutbeam in the World Health Organization's (WHO) 1998 Health Promotion Glossary. It is defined as the *cognitive and social skills that determine the motivation and ability of individuals to gain access to, understand, and use information in ways that promote and maintain good health* (Nutbeam, 1998). Subsequent research into the links between people's literacy skills and health outcomes has proved fruitful, as described in the following. However, with careful consideration, the 2004 Institute of Medicine (IOM) Committee on Health Literacy called for a new understanding of health literacy. The IOM report noted that we needed to consider health literacy as an interaction between individuals and other key factors rather than as a "characteristic" of individuals (Kindig et al., 2004).

The change in our understanding of health literacy and the broader potential for adjustments and actions at multiple levels is the focus of this chapter. The discussion begins with a brief history of the emergence of health literacy as an area of study and concern. Next, the discussion focuses on how a more nuanced understanding of health literacy enables us to consider multiple focal points for efficacious change. An expansion of our understanding of health literacy calls for the active engagement of health professionals and policymakers. Such engagement, informed by health literacy insights, can bring about needed changes that will increase access to information, care, and services and contribute to a reduction in health disparities.

BACKGROUND

Education has long been acknowledged as a social determinant of health. Literacy, of course, sits at the foundation of education. In addition, early arguments for universal schooling cited literacy as a critical contributor to the creation and maintenance of an informed citizenry. Since the founding of the United Nations, member nations regularly report literacy rates. However, comparisons between and among nations could not be calculated because national measures varied—from a measure of one's ability to sign one's name, for example, to calculations of average years of schooling in the population. Generally, literacy was recognized as problematic in pre-industrialized nations but was taken for granted among industrialized nations because of mandatory schooling.

Literacy Skills of Adults in Industrialized Nations

In the late 1980s, with the widespread introduction of new technologies, educators and economists were eager to assess the readiness of adults in industrialized nations for the challenges of the 21st century. Because there was no uniform measure of literacy as such, a group of education scholars, working with the U.S. Department of Education, Educational

Testing Services, Statistics Canada, and the Organization for Economic Cooperation and Development (OECD) developed a literacy assessment measure that could be used for comparative analyses within and between industrialized nations. This measure focused on people's ability to use the various materials commonly found in their society in order to accomplish everyday tasks. This assessment approach led to the rigorous surveys of adult literacy skills among member countries of the OECD. The stated purpose was to examine the population's readiness to participate in the sophisticated technological and complex social and economic environments ahead. These assessments, first conducted in the 1990s, have been expanded and undertaken every 10 years or so to inform educators, economists, and policymakers.

Each participating country agreed to design a sample representing its national population age 16 to 65 years. For example, the first of these surveys was conducted in the United States with a sample of 26,000 adults. These rigorously designed and carefully sampled surveys, known as the International Adult Literacy Surveys (IALS), were conducted in 22 industrialized nations in the 1990s (Kirsch, 1993; Tuijnman et al., 1995). The surveys were expanded to include additional countries with added measures focused on problem-solving and numeric skills between 2003 and 2006 (Desjardins et al., 2005). A decade later, the newly named PIAAC surveys (Programme for the International Assessment of Adult Competencies) were conducted among 40 nations and were further expanded to include the use of technology (OECD Skills Outlook, 2013, 2017, 2019).

Designed as a 90-minute at-home interview, the adult literacy surveys focus on people's ability to use an array of commonly available materials related to family life, health and safety, leisure activities, work, finance, and civic society. They are carefully described by Kirsch, one of the developers, in a monograph from the Educational Testing Services (Kirsch, 2001). The materials collected for the surveys, in the appropriate legal languages of each country, varied by type. They were classified as continuous texts (prose) or noncontinuous texts (documents). Some materials include numbers and require one or more quantitative operations for a calculation of quantitative skills. Among the materials, for example, might be a sports article, a report of a civic event, directions on how to care for a child's fever, or a magazine health article (all continuous texts). The materials also included commonly available documents (noncontinuous texts, some containing numbers) such as a weather chart, a train schedule, a sales sign, or a medicine label. All materials were rated for level of complexity and difficulty.

The tasks participants were asked to undertake with the materials were directly related to how and why people would use the materials. For example, someone might quickly read a sports article to find the winning team and final score. These tasks would also include identifying a bias in a report or editorial, or determining an appropriate dosage for a child using the information on a medicine box. All tasks were rated for level of difficulty and complexity. For example, the task of interpretation or "reading between the lines" (noting a bias in a report or editorial) is far more difficult than is the task of location, such as finding a final score in a sports article. The calculation of literacy skills included an understanding of the complexities of materials and an analysis of the difficulties of tasks. In addition, the surveys collected extensive background information. Data collection includes parental schooling, books in the home, schooling, work type and frequency, income, age, nativity, ethnicity, geographic location, access to resources, and more.

The published findings from the first wave of surveys conducted in the 1990s within 22 industrialized nations (IALS) were met with shock. Analyses indicated that large percentages of the population of most industrialized nations have limited literacy and math skills. This finding indicated difficulty using commonly available, everyday materials with accuracy and consistency. Thus, literacy and numeracy emerged as problematic issues for these sophisticated nations. Furthermore, analyses indicated that literacy and numeracy skills were not randomly distributed within countries. Social disparities became evident. Analyses of the various surveys, from those in the 1990s to those of 2019, yielded similar problematic findings that literacy is linked to a variety of social factors. Within each participating country, specific population groups were found to have limited literacy and numeracy skills. For example, those with lower skills were more likely to have lower social standing (due to minority or immigrant status, for example), have limited access to resources, or to reside in underresourced areas. Those with stronger skills were more likely to be members of majority population groups, have access to greater resources, and reside in well-resourced geographic locations. The long-held assumptions that universal schooling yields adequate literacy and numeracy skill levels across the populations of industrialized nations were shown to be faulty (Kirsch, 1993; Desjardins et al., 2005; Kirsch, 1993; OECD, 2013, 2019).

Health Literacy Studies

The initial findings for the survey of U.S. adults, published in 1992, and for those of the other 21 industrialized nations throughout the 1990s, inspired health researchers to examine the influence of literacy on health outcomes. The paramount research question was: *Given literacy findings, are there health consequences*? This question was not new to health researchers in the less industrialized or less wealthy nations of Africa, Asia, the Middle East, or South America. For example, in their 1989 public health review article, Grosse and Auffrey examined the links between maternal literacy and health of children and helped established literacy as a major determinant of health (Grosse & Auffrey, 1989). However, this interest in links between literacy and health outcomes represented a new area of inquiry for many health researchers in industrialized nations.

In the United States, health literacy studies began shortly after the results of the first wave of adult literacy survey were published. Within the first decade of health literacy inquiries, links between patients' literacy skills and health outcomes were firmly established (Kindig et al., 2004). Research findings indicated that people with limited literacy skills are less likely to engage in health promotion action or disease prevention activities and are less likely to succeed with chronic disease management. Those with limited or poor literacy skills are more likely to report poor health and are more likely to die at an earlier age than are those with stronger literacy skills (Berkman et al., 2011). Subsequently, health literacy emerged as a new variable for health studies—generating interest among health researchers, practitioners, and policymakers, as can be witnessed in the growth of a substantial body of literature.

Population-based measures of health literacy were assessed soon thereafter and offered the same pattern of results as did the adult literacy surveys. The Health and Adult Literacy Survey (HALS) and the National Assessment of Adult Literacy (NAAL) focused on health-related items and tasks linked to the adult literacy surveys. Analyses indicated that about half of U.S. adults, including those without a high school diploma and those who completed high school, have limited health literacy skills (Kirsch et al., 2004; Kutner et al., 2006; Rudd 2007). Similar results were found for several other countries that applied the HALS analysis to their adult literacy surveys such as Canada (Murray et al., 2007) and the Netherlands (van der Heide et al., 2013). The European Health Literacy Survey (HLS-EU), based on a questionnaire focused on self-perceived health literacy, found that close to half the population in participating countries of the European Union reported problematic or inadequate levels of health literacy (Sorensen et al., 2015). These population measure findings also indicated that health literacy is linked to a variety of social factors. Overall, population groups with lower socioeconomic status and of lower social standing within any given country have lower health literacy skills and/or perceive more difficulty with health-related activities and communications. Consequently, health literacy emerged as a new variable for analyses of health outcomes and health disparities and as a new consideration in efforts to redress inequities (Baur, 2010; Kleinman et al., 2018).

THE EXPANDING CONCEPT OF HEALTH LITERACY

As was noted, health literacy was originally considered to be a characteristic of an individual who has or does not have the ability to access and use information for healthful action. This definition determined what and who would be measured. Based on this understanding, researchers developed quick assessment tools to differentiate between those with limited and those with adequate health literacy skills to study links between literacy and health outcomes. For example, more than 125 assessment tools are currently available online (Health Literacy Toolkit, 2021). These tools support an array of inquiries linking an individual's skills to health outcomes. The implication is that changes in health literacy skills would lead to improved health outcomes. But, as fruitful as these early studies were, they eventually posed a dilemma for health practitioners. How we define a term has implications for where we place our focus, what we measure, how we conceptualize action, and whom or what we expect to change (Rudd et al., 2012).

Practice Dilemma

Health practitioners cannot bear the added responsibility for increasing the literacy skills of their patients. They are not, after all, education or literacy experts. Therefore, the logical policy and practice consequences would be focused on the education sector and would call for improved skill development through primary and secondary schools as well as through adult education programs. However, the growing evidence of increased morbidity and mortality among those with limited literacy skills, as well as evidence of disparities, raises issues of ethics and social justice. Data from research studies linking low literacy skills and poor health outcomes would not allow health experts to bypass the issue and wait for the education sector to improve the public's skills. Ironically, health literacy's initial focus on individuals' skills and abilities proved to be a limiting factor for strategic action.

Unlike the surveys of adult literacy, which had included a careful calculation of the complexity of texts as well as the difficulty of tasks, health literacy studies had not followed suit. Most health literacy studies were based on measures of individual's skills and did not, for the most part, simultaneously consider text or task difficulties. The communication skills of health providers were not simultaneously considered or measured. This was a serious omission that sharply differed from literacy assessments. Often, the health information was treated as a "given" and not as something that was malleable.

An individual's literacy skills are only part of what is called a literacy exchange. For example, one must consider both the skills of the reader and the communication and organization skills of the writer. The quality of the text will change the measure of literacy skills. Technically, one could manipulate literacy results by presenting a reader with simple or complex texts resulting in high literacy outcomes or poor literacy results. Similarly, one cannot measure the skills of the listener without an understanding of the skills of the speaker. The environment or context is an important consideration as well. The task of leisurely reading, for example, in a quiet and safe environment is quite different from the task of rushed reading to sign a form or waiver in a chaotic, noisy, or anxiety-producing setting. Thus, according to literacy experts, any measure of literacy skills has to consider the various elements of the exchange, including the texts and the contexts (Purcell-Gates, 2007). This calls for a new understanding of health literacy as a complex interaction with several key components. Furthermore, this notion of a complex interaction opens the door to an array of actions that can take place in different arenas.

Evolving Concept

The foundation stones for an expanded concept of health literacy were set in the 2003 articulation of U.S. Health Communication Objectives for the nation (Rudd, 2003) and in the 2004 IOM's Committee on Health Literacy (Kindig et al., 2004). The implications were

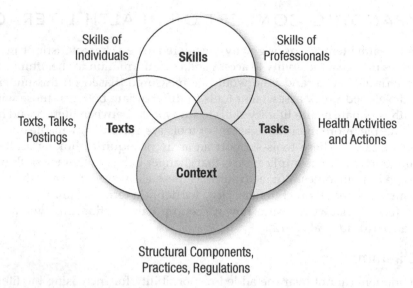

Figure 7.1 Interacting components of health literacy.

explored in the 2007 Surgeon General's Workshop on Health Literacy (Office of the Surgeon General, 2006). Subsequently, the 2010 National Action Plan to Improve Health Literacy outlined government strategy based on an expanded concept (Baur, 2010). The Health Literacy Issues Brief to Inform Development and Implementation of Healthy People 2030 proposed an expanded consideration of health literacy: *Health literacy occurs when a society provides accurate health information and services that people can easily find, understand, and use to inform their decisions and actions* (Kleinman et al., 2018). As Nutbeam noted earlier, health literacy is an evolving concept (Nutbeam, 2008; Rudd et al., 2012).

This expanded understanding of health literacy alters the burden of responsibility. The emphasis is no longer on the adult's ability to obtain and use health information but is instead on the health system's ability to provide accessible and usable information. As a result, the lens of health literacy helps focus on the communication skills of health and healthcare professionals, the clarity and complexity of health information, the difficulties of action steps, and the literacy related characteristics of health institutions and health systems. Figure 7.1 illustrates the interrelated variables that are increasingly being recognized as core components of health literacy.

This interactive model of health literacy proposed by the first author envisions overlapping key components, with the concept of health literacy serving as the central point where all components overlap. Needless to say, many public health or clinical research studies or interventions would be hard-pressed to address all of these components at once. However, health researchers, practitioners, and policymakers are recognizing that health literacy cannot be defined, measured, or ameliorated when attention is paid to only one part of these complex interactions. These insights are forging new paths of inquiry and broadening the scope of proposed remedial practices. New initiatives in health literacy are bringing attention to the proficiencies of the various health professionals as well as to those of the intended audience. Also under consideration are the demands and expectations of health materials and health encounters, as well as the characteristics of health organizations and systems.

Health Literacy Components

Adjustments within each of the five components of the health literacy exchange may increase or hinder health literacy. These components or variables are also interwoven. As noted, one cannot consider the skills of the individual without considering the quality of the text or talk or context. Similarly, efforts to increase the skills of health professionals must simultaneously consider the existing norms and characteristics of the institutions and health system within which they work. Organizational and system-wide characteristics also shape the visitor's or user's experience and, as a result, facilitate or impede access to information, care, and services.

Skills of the Public

The skills of the public are well documented. The findings of the recent survey of adult literacy competencies in the United States were found to be comparable to the findings of earlier surveys. For example, almost one quarter of adults performed at the lowest level for literacy and numeracy and for digital problem solving. Fewer than half performed at adequate to high levels of proficiency. While there were not statistically significant differences based on sex, performance gaps were found based on race/ethnicity, schooling, age, employment participation, and nativity or immigration status (National Center for Education Statistics, 2017). On average, a U.S. adult with a high school education has limited literacy and numeracy skills. At the two extremes, less than 20% of the population evidences strong skills and about 30% very low skills. As health professionals shape their talks and texts, procedures and protocols, they must keep these findings as well as local indicators firmly in mind.

It is vitally important to maintain awareness of the documented skills and abilities of the public to help assess and adjust communications and programs. The American Medical Association has consistently encouraged the use of "universal health literacy precautions," and noted, for example, in 2017: *We know that a large proportion of adults have limited literacy and numeracy skill and therefore need to adopt universal precautions* (Killian & Coletti, 2017). "Universal precautions" here refers to measures taken to safeguard the vulnerable—the majority of U.S. adults who have limited literacy skills. This offers a starting point for practice, and any needed adjustments based on a particular intended audience can follow. We have long known that those with strong literacy skills as well as those with limited skills benefit from discussions, presentations, and materials designed with the application of health literacy principles.

Finally, we note that while numeracy has always been assessed in the literacy surveys, attention to math-related issues in health literacy studies are relatively recent. People grapple with numbers in myriad health-related activities including comparison shopping for safety equipment, checking weather charts, buying food, or reading medicine labels. In healthcare situations, people are expected to understand a test result or vital sign measure in the context of a normal range. They are challenged to undertake risk/benefit analysis for critical decisions. Public health efforts to inform the population focus on risks, refer to statistical findings, and use a variety of data displays. Consequently, we need to recognize that activities that involve hearing, reading, or discussion of numbers may be fraught with difficulties, errors, or misconceptions. Numbers are important for decisions and for health actions but frequently get in the way for many adults and confound other communication difficulties (Apter et al., 2008). Needless to say, miscalculations can lead to tragedy (Box 7.1).

BOX 7.1: Practice Pearls

Needed Support: The K-12 education sector and the adult education sector, both of which need widespread support and advocacy, must improve basic skills. In the interim, adults need health information that is appropriately crafted to what is known of existing skills. Skills levels have been well documented in the various waves of adult literacy surveys since 1992.

Respectful Exchanges: Adults need to be treated with respect and dignity no matter their skills. A "health-literate environment" offers acknowledgment of complexities (*this is not easy; many of my patients have difficulties with this …*) and supports question asking (*many people have questions about this; what questions do you have?*).

Adult Education Insights: Learning best takes place when people feel supported, at ease, and have enough time to take in and process information.

As is noted in the following, a variety of practices can ease the burden on members of the public. These include activities undertaken by health professionals as they write, speak, and listen to patients and members of the public. They relate to the development and design of health materials and to the complexities of health activities. Changes in characteristics of health institutions and systems (which shape professional practice as well as public access) can eliminate unnecessary barriers and ease the burden on members of the public as well.

Skills of Health Professionals

The abilities or competencies of those who provide information in healthcare settings and public health venues have yet to be rigorously and consistently measured with a health literacy lens. Consequently, the contributions of professional skills and practices to health outcomes are currently not as well explored or documented as they might be. Several researchers have been assessing health literacy awareness, practice, and competencies in dentistry, nursing, and medicine. For example, U.S. and international researchers include Maybury, Caiero, Coleman, Karuranga, Coleman, and Groene (Maybury et al., 2012; Cafiero, 2013; Coleman et al., 2013; Karuranga et al., 2017, Groene et al., 2017). Findings indicate the need for continued awareness-raising efforts and skill building. In addition, examinations of curricula in professional schools in the United States and the European Union indicate that health literacy is only partially addressed (Johnson et al., 2014; Wills, 2016). At the same time, attempted interventions have been found to improve clinicians' knowledge and broaden their understanding of and attitudes toward health literacy. They have also improved self-reported confidence in medication counseling, increased effectiveness in using teach back, and improved clinicians' ability to use illustrations and plain language when communicating with patients (Coleman, 2011; Green et al., 2014).

Guidebooks abound. All health writers are urged to follow articulated plain language guidelines, engage in rigorous formative research, pilot test materials, and revise as indicated. In addition, public health and healthcare professionals are being encouraged to be more attentive to mathematical concepts as well as numbers. Studies indicate that math concepts, such as *average* or *normal*, are difficult to grasp; so too is the notion of *risk* or *benefit*. Consequently, all health practitioners are being encouraged to provide visual as well as verbal explanations of risk (Fagerlin et al., 2011). We are asked to do the math for the reader or patient (Apter et al., 2008). We are cautioned to provide words along with numbers (Peters et al., 2007). We must always consider and explain the context—such as comparisons to an average or to an individual's previous tests (Rudd & Baur, 2020). Furthermore, health writers, patient portal designers, and researchers are being asked to consider data displays and the value of different types of graphic representation (Ancker et al., 2006).

Public health and healthcare professionals are consistently asked to be attentive to specialized professional language. Jargon is interfering with the dissemination of information—among specialists, between researchers/scientists and practitioners, and between practitioners and the public. For example, Goto et al. discovered that in the aftermath of the 2011 triple disaster in Fukushima, Japan, public health nurses were losing the trust of the community members they had long served. Part of the problem was that the scientific data being distributed to policymakers, doctors, and nurses were filled with scientific measures and esoteric terms that were not "translated" into everyday language. The nurses who had long served their communities were losing the trust of community members because they could only offer answers to critical questions raised by their patients using the same scientific terms they were offered—untranslated and not applied to everyday life experiences (Goto et al., 2014; Box 7.2).

Quality of Health Information

An informed public needs to have readily available information. Health information, posted online and in print, is intended to help the public understand and take action. To take action, people are expected to access and understand the text, follow directions, consider options,

BOX 7.2: Teaching in Context

Bilingual Skills: Health professionals are being asked to become "bilingual"—to be conversant with colleagues and at the same time, be able to shift to everyday language with patients and community members. After years of specialized training and daily interactions with colleagues, any professional is challenged to automatically switch to "everyday language." We can always ask our audience/patients to help out, noting that we welcome interruption at any time we use a technical term without explanation.

Teach Back: One often cited approach for helpful communication in the clinical encounter is use of the *teach back*. With appropriate teach back, the health professional takes responsibility for the communication. For example, instead of asking do you *understand?*, the clinician is encouraged to ask: *Was I clear? Did I leave anything out?* Then the clinician might say: *To check if I included everything, tell me how you will take your meds tomorrow so that I can see if I skipped over something.*

make decisions, and/or respond to calls to action. While health information is indeed ubiquitous, access has increasingly relied on modern technology, on internet services, and on possession/access to the electronic tools of modern society. This poses a critical equity issue that must be addressed because it limits access to information and services among those who do not have resources.

Attention here is being focused on the notion of "accessibility" once one has obtained the information. Available information is not necessarily accessible information. Health materials that are jargon filled or poorly organized are clearly not accessible. Thousands of studies of health materials, conducted over four decades and across an array of health topics, have consistently documented a substantial mismatch between the literacy skills of the public and the literacy demands of the health materials.

CASE STUDY 7.1: NO TRANSLATION AVAILABLE

On March 11, 2011, Fukushima, Japan, experienced a triple disaster. A 9-magnitude earthquake shook the city. Soon after, at the shore some miles away from the city center, a tsunami hit, with devastating consequences; it took untold numbers of people out to sea. Then the Daiichi nuclear plant lost its entire core cooling capacity for the three reactors. Substantial amounts of radioactive substances were released into the atmosphere. Confusion, distress, and deaths increased. Even as residents along the coast were evacuating, radiation "rained from the skies" and scores more died. Reactor explosions followed in the next few days. Transportation, electricity, water, gas, telecommunications, and radiation monitoring were all disrupted. Information about radiation levels and the evacuation processes were not available.

Stories of action among and between residents and dedicated healthcare personnel are quite amazing and provide profound insights for future planning and disaster mitigation. But this story moves a bit forward in time to the re-establishment of a new "normal" among those who survived and stayed on. In the years following, multiple physical and psychological health issues needed ongoing attention. Public health nurses, situated within the community, played a critical role.

Public health nurses in Japan get to know their population through home visits and regular monitoring activities and address a wide range of complicated health problems. They establish solid relationships and are well trusted. In the early years following the Fukushima disaster, however, they noticed that the level of trust normally accorded them was being eroded. Dr. Aya Goto, a physician overseeing activities of the public health nurses, carefully examined complaints and stories and found that communication issues were the core of the problem. Specifically, scientific observations and reports were not being adapted for

(continued)

CASE STUDY 7.1: NO TRANSLATION AVAILABLE (*CONTINUED*)

nonscientists. Scientists sent reports to inform policymakers; policymakers passed on these reports to inform health practitioners who were expected to inform the public. However, needed "translations" were not provided—neither by the scientists to the policymakers nor by policymakers to practitioners. Many of the terms and measures used in the scientific reports were unfamiliar; the numbers had little meaning; and the concepts and measures were not linked to everyday events. The well-meaning public health nurse could provide numbers but not transform these numbers into advice for the parents who wanted to know if their child could "play outside this week."

Dr. Goto established health literacy workshops for the public health nurses. Participants learned about health literacy studies, findings, and insights. They learned how to evaluate and modify existing health materials as well as how to prepare new texts (for conversations or handouts). They practiced speaking and writing in "plain language." Together with Dr. Goto, several of the nurses participated in the next step: working with a range of experts to translate findings and prepare a glossary of terms for practitioners. This ongoing project aims to make available health information readily accessible.

◆ Imagine a friendly but professional discussion between two people who are sharing important information.
◆ What happens when one of them uses "foreign" words without explanation? Notice that the burden of responsibility falls on the shoulders of the listener, the person who does not understand. Sometimes, admitting this can be embarrassing. In some circumstances, asking for an explanation may not be socially acceptable.
◆ What happens if the speaker does not fully understand the words either? Will this influence tone or affect?
◆ Consider: How do you define and describe *risk?*

Further information about this brief case can be found in the following publications:

1. Goto, A., Rudd, R. E., Alden, L. Y. et al. (2014). Leveraging public health nurses for disaster risk communication in Fukushima City: a qualitative analysis of nurses' written records of parenting counseling and peer discussions. *BMC Health Services Research 14*(1290): 1–9.
2. Goto, A., Rudd, R. E., Yuanghong, L., Yoshida-Komiya, H. (2014). Health literacy training for public health nurses in Fukushima: A case study of program adaptation, implementation and evaluation. *Japan Medical Association Journal, 57*(3):146–153.
3. Lai, A., Goto, A., Rudd, R. E. (2015). Advancing health literacy from a system perspective: Health literacy training for healthcare professionals. *The European Health Psychologist, 17*(6):281–285. 2015.
4. Goto, A., Lai, A.Y., Kumagai, A., Koizumi,S., Yoshida, K., Yamawaki, K., & Rudd, R. E. (2018). Collaborative processes of developing a health literacy toolkit: a case from Fukushima after the nuclear accident. *Journal of Health Communication, 23*(2).

Overall, a large variety of guidelines are readily available to those responsible for "communicating health." All offer similar pieces of advice, the first three of which are: know the intended audience, clearly identify the goal or purpose of the materials or talk, and always provide action steps. Writers as well as speakers are urged to state the main point up front and repeat it at the end. The guidelines encourage the use of a comfortable tone and active voice. Clear writing and speaking are both built from varied but relatively short sentences because complex sentences leave poor readers confused. Clear communication draws on common, everyday language (such as *use* instead of *utilize*) and provides explanations/translations of medical and scientific terms and concepts. Well-organized texts, spoken or written, provide clear cues for the listener or reader. Consequently, chunking of like information, titles and headings, and uncluttered texts ease the reading and searching process. Furthermore, diagrams and pictures can be helpful when well designed to support the key information in the text.

Most of the early assessments of health materials were based on reading grade level tools such as the SMOG (McLaughlin, 1969). Originally designed to help teachers or parents choose appropriate texts for children, these tools offer a superficial measure of suitability because they attend to word length and sometimes, as in the case of the SMOG, sentence length as well. They are helpful in English because long words often have silent letters and are not appropriate for languages such as Italian or Spanish, in which most letters are pronounced. Furthermore, long sentences tend to confuse readers at lower skill levels. In general, reading grade assessments offer initial insight into difficulty of texts but a relatively superficial measure of suitability. The current literature indicates an increased use of more comprehensive efforts to assess health information in print, online, and delivered in clinical encounters. Relatively new tools, such as the Health Literacy Index from the Centers for Disease Control and Prevention (CDC; Baur and Prue, 2014) and the Patient Education Material Assessment Tool (PEMAT) from the Agency for Healthcare Research and Quality (AHRQ; Shoemaker et al., 2014) address key textual issues beyond word or sentence length. Both tools draw from the early work of the Doaks in the development of the more lengthy and detailed SAM (the Suitability Assessment of Materials; Doak et al., 1996). These tools, freely available online, help researchers and practitioners assess health materials at various stages of development and use. The focus is always on a clear statement of purpose, everyday vocabulary, simple sentence structure, clear organization, tested data displays, and an articulation of action steps.

Missing from these assessments are tools that focus on nonprose texts. The PMOSE/IKIRSCH tool (Mosenthal and Kirsch, 1998) was developed for educators to examine the difficulty of displays such as lists, graphs, and charts. It is increasingly being cited in health materials assessment studies. Although a numeracy assessment tool is not yet available, studies are addressing the burden of numbers in texts by identifying frequency of use and consistency with which numbers are presented and indicating whether or not readers are expected to do any calculations (Ancker & Kaufman, 2007; Rudd, 2016). An examination of how numbers are used in health texts would be quite helpful.

The most frequently used tools such as the SAM, the CDC Index, and the AHRQ PEMAT carry insight for materials development as well. All of the tools in use for assessment purposes can readily be converted into guidelines and checklists. They all highlight the importance of pilot testing materials with members of the intended audience and subsequently undertaking revisions. The scientific processes involve rigorous protocols for the development of medicines and medical devices. However, those same mandated processes that include pilot/field testing and needed revisions, for example, are not consistently applied to the development of critical health information. Even though the components of rigorous formative research have long been well articulated in science as well as in health education and communication literature (Fischhoff, 2013), we lack evidence that such processes are regularly followed. Consequently, regulations related to the design of both print and electronic health materials may be called for. A more "scientific" approach to the development and design of health texts will be beneficial to the public.

Critical health information is also delivered in the talks that take place in clinical encounters, community settings, and over the airwaves. For example, Roter offered a conceptual approach for capturing the oral literacy demand in healthcare dialogue, provided reviews of several studies that support the predictive validity of the framework, and proposed ways to both diminish literacy demand and support more effective healthcare exchanges (Roter, 2011). To reestablish trust between public health nurses and their community members in the aftermath of the Fukushima disasters, Goto et al. offered health literacy workshops for public health nurses. They subsequently worked with nurses to develop a glossary of terms to help translate scientific jargon into language that could be used in the community. This helped nurses, for example, to avoid presenting a radiation-related number in isolation. Instead, nurses were able to talk with a parent about the numbers in terms of a child's safe return to an outdoor playground. Needless to say, this is an interim, though much-needed, step until science communicators offer "translations" for the lay public.

Analyses of disaster-related messages and of COVID-19 responses have highlighted communication errors and are leading to proactive efforts to include health literacy expertise in the development of public health messages (Rudd et al., 2003; Rudd & Baur, 2020). The hope is that the recognition of missteps and the accumulated findings of a mismatch between provided health information and the ability of the public to access this information will reinvigorate efforts to promote and perhaps mandate the implementation of long-established guidelines for rigorous formative research (Box 7.3).

Health Tasks

The developers of the adult literacy surveys examined the activities people need to undertake when they use various texts. For example, a patient uses a medicine label to find dosage instructions or locate information such as expiration date. A consumer might compare and contrast critical information such as the safety ratings on two different bicycle helmets. More challenging tasks involve computations or interpretations. For example, a consumer must calculate a price by subtracting the discount. More challenging still, a reader or listener picks up on tone and vocabulary to "read between the lines" and decide if one procedure is more strongly recommended over another. These activities can be considered proximal tasks—those actions involved in the process of using the text, such as locating information.

The more distal tasks are those to be undertaken after people consult the texts. These activities include taking medicine on time, cleaning a wound after reading directions, or using an inhaler based on the results of a peak-flow meter. Health practitioners can deconstruct common health-related activities that patients are expected to undertake. This exercise helps us to list and consider potential difficulties involved. We can make changes in the education process, such as providing opportunities for people to practice under supervision or providing tools to try to ease the burden (Box 7.4).

BOX 7.3: Health Systems and Organizations

Rigorous Processes: Practice guidelines call for treating the "word" with scientific rigor. This involves careful drafting, professional reviews, assessments, pilot testing with members of the intended audience, and revisions, as indicated.

Plain Language: Jargon and undefined specialized terms should be avoided. The Plain Language Act of 2010 can provide guidance to the health sector.

Policies Related to Health Materials: Standards such as evidence of pilot test results and assessment scores for health texts can be set by review boards. In addition, because most health institutions do not produce their own materials, contracts with vendors can include requirements for reports of pilot test processes and assessment scores.

BOX 7.4: Keep Score

A deconstruction process enables us to look closely at actions people are expected to undertake and identify potential problems that can be eased. Reminder calls or texts are now ubiquitous for appointment keeping. Pulmonologists often use tape as a marker on a peak flow meter to indicate when action is needed. A paper chart with a sample pill taped next to the name, purpose, and dosage offers a helpful guide for medicine taking. Pill boxes are used as reminder of medicine to take or indicate those already taken. Numerous decision aids are available for a variety of discussions and determinations of which course of action to take.

The Health Context

Practice norms, articulated policies, and formal regulations shape the activities within institutions and systems. Healthcare institutions, organizations, and systems strongly influence professional practice as well as users' access to information, care, and services. The Health Literacy Committee of the Institute of Medicine, in its 2004 Health Literacy: A Prescription to End Confusion, offered a vision for a "health literate America." The 15 recommendations offered concrete steps for achieving that vision. They included needed initiatives: in government through a variety of federal health-related agencies, through accreditation institutions in education and health, within professional schools and continuing education programs, and by data collection agencies, as well as through healthcare organizations and systems (Kindig et al., 2004).

Introduced in 2007, the Health Literacy Environment of Hospitals and Health Centers offered a mechanism for identifying contextual barriers and facilitating factors (Rudd & Anderson, 2006). The assessment tool provided a schema for rating navigation ease, print communication, the oral exchange, technology, policies, and protocols. Suggestions for corrective actions and examples of efficacious change were also provided. Researchers have used this tool to assess a variety of healthcare environments such as hospitals or dental services within community health centers (Groene & Rudd, 2011; Horowitz et al., 2014; Oelschlegel et al., 2018). Revised, reviewed, and pilot tested, the updated assessment tool HLE^2 was completed with the participation of a health literacy team at the University of Tennessee Medical Center. The revised tool includes an opportunity to assess technological changes and includes a more detailed set of items to examine organizational policies and practices. It continues to include a focus on navigation, culture, and language, and written as well as electronic communication (Rudd et al., 2019). An additional tool, one focused on clinical office settings, built on the original EHL tool. The AHRQ's Universal Tool Kit offers a variety of strategies and assessment tools to aid consideration and change (DeWalt et al., 2010).

In 2012, the Roundtable on Health Literacy focused on the notion of a health-literate organization and set out a list of 10 crucial attributes. These attributes include leadership and links to the mission of the organization, as well as the integration of health literacy into planning, evaluation, patient safety, and quality improvement. This concept of a health-literate organization also includes institutional responsibility for preparing the workforce, for providing information, and for enhancing the engagement of patients, family members, and the community it serves. This call for health-literate organizations garnered international interest and, as a result, a variety of practitioners, managers, and policymakers are engaged in discussions of needed cultural adaptations or modifications for use within their countries and institutions (Brach et al., 2012).

Innovative strategies have been undertaken in a variety of ways. For example, the Public Health Authority of the Regio Emelia region in northern Italy offered two week-long trainings in health literacy for specific staff within 11 hospitals in the region. Each sent two oncology doctors, two nurses, and two hospital communication staff to take part in the training and help launch a region-wide health literacy undertaking. An increased awareness and opportunities to explore a variety of action steps, such as teach back and materials assessments, led to institutional as well as regionwide changes (IOM, 2013). After examining barriers to information, care, and services in the Māori health sector, the New Zealand Ministry of Health focused on health literacy as a vehicle for reducing inequalities and inequities for New Zealand's Māori population (IOM, 2013).

In addition, new initiatives are being forged in the broader public health arena. A health literacy perspective has been offering insights for a diverse set of public health issues and for the design of both research inquiries and implementation programs. In environmental health literacy, for example, researchers and practitioners are examining health literacy–related barriers in water quality, emergency response, food safety, air quality, and disaster

BOX 7.5: Place Matters

Take a Tour: A walking tour of a local hospital or of your own institution or agency offers insights into barriers that visitors might face. Meet with a colleague at a nearby transportation stop and take a walk to the entry. Consider what eased or hindered the journey. Determine a location within the institution that neither of you has visited before and as you walk about, make note of words on signs and wayfinding tools. A structured walking interview is available on line at: www.hsph.harvard.edu/healthliteracy.

preparedness (Hoover, 2019). They are similarly examining systemic issues that may facilitate or stymie access to information, engagement, and decision-making in this broader arena. For example, the legislative context that shapes state and local water regulations is available to all but filled with legal jargon that is often difficult for citizens to decipher (Simonds et al., 2019). This leads to limited access to needed information that, in turn, could stymie action (Ramirez-Andreotta et al., 2016; Box 7.5).

CONCLUSIONS: EFFICATIOUS ACTION

Practitioners and policymakers can work to remove literacy-related barriers and further strengthen the needed work to improve health for all. Efforts to improve health literacy include improving the communication skills of health professionals, clarifying health materials, easing tasks, and identifying and removing systemic barriers. The focus of attention in research and in practice is shifting from an analysis of the skills and deficits of individuals or of the public to the actions of health communicators, practitioners, and administrators. Taking responsibility for the health literacy exchange, health professionals are becoming more attentive to language, culture, structure, and content of our communication and program efforts. We are also becoming more aware of and starting to examine the norms, protocols, and structures of health systems that may constrain our most efficacious practices as well as erect barriers to the equitable access of the public. Health literacy studies are contributing to professional education, clinical practice, health education and promotion efforts, and the development of institutional policies. As the focus of attention in health literacy study and practice spans all the components/variables in the health literacy exchange, the potential to increase access and decrease inequities expands. Studies can more rigorously evaluate outcomes on multiple levels of change among individuals, in communities and workplaces, within institutions, and through policy and legislative action. As health literacy researchers recalibrate definitions and develop new measures for each of the component parts, we will be better prepared to understand and address the multilevel contributions to health disparities.

REFERENCES

Ancker, J. S., & Kaufman, D. (2007). Rethinking health numeracy: a multidisciplinary literature review. *Journal of the American Medical Informatics Association*, 14(6), 713–721. DOI 10.1197/jamia .M2464

Ancker, J. S., Senathirajah, Y., Rita Kukafka, R., & Starren, J. B. (2006). Design features of graphs in health risk communication: a systematic review, *Journal of the American Medical Informatics Association*, 13(6), 608–618.

Apter, A. J., Paasche-Orlow, M. K., Remillard, J. T., Bennett, I. M., Ben-Joseph, E. P., Batista, R. M., Hyde, J., & Rudd, R. E. (2008). Numeracy and communication with patients: they are counting on us. *Journal of General Internal Medicine*, 23(12), 2117–2124. DOI 10.1007/s11606-008-0803-x

Baur, C. (Ed.). (2010). U.S. Department of Health and Human Services. *National action plan to improve health literacy*. Washington DC: USDHHS. DOI 10.1177/1524839914538969

Baur, C., & Prue, C. (2014). The CDC clear communication index is a new evidence-based tool to prepare and review health information. *Health Promotion Practice, 15*, 629–637.

Berkman, N. D., Sheridan, S. L., Donahue, K. E., Halpern, D. J., & Crotty, K. (2011). Low health literacy and health outcomes: an updated systematic review. *Annals of Internal Medicine, 155*, 97–107.

Brach, C., Dreyer, B., Schyve, P., Hernandez, L. M., Baur, C., Lemerise, A. J., & Parker, R. (2012). *Attributes of a health literate organization.* Washington DC: National Academies of Science.

Cafiero, M. (2013). Nurse practitioners' knowledge, experience, and intention to use health literacy strategies in clinical practice. *Journal of Health Communication, 18*(Suppl 1), 70–81. DOI 10.1080/10810730.2013.825665

Coleman, C. (2011). Teaching health care professionals about health literacy: a review of the literature. *Nursing Outlook, 59*, 70–78.

Coleman, C. A., Hudson, S., & Maine, L. L. (2013). Health literacy practices and educational competencies for health professionals: a consensus study. *Journal of Health Communication, 4;18*(suppl 1), 82–102. DOI 10.1080/10810730.2013.829538

DeWalt, D. A., Callahan, L. F., Hawk, V. H., & et al. (2010). *Health literacy universal precautions toolkit. AHRQ Publication No. 10-0046-EF.* Rockville, MD: Agency for Healthcare Research and Quality.

Desjardins, R., Murray, T. S., & Tuijnman, A. C. (2005). *Learning a living: First results of the adult literacy and life skills survey.* Ottowa CA: Statistics Canada.

Doak, C. C., Doak, L. G., & Root, J. H. (1996). *Teaching patients with low literacy skills* (2nd ed.). Philadelphia, Pa: Lippincott-Raven Publishers. online at: www.hsph.harvard.edu/healthliteracy

Fagerlin, A., Zikmund-Fisher, B. J., & Ubel, P. A. (2011). Helping patients decide: ten steps to better risk communication, *JNCI: Journal of the National Cancer Institute, 103*(19), 1436–1443.

Fischhoff, B. (2013). The science of science communication. *Proceedings of the National Academy of Sciences of the United States of America, 110*(Suppl 3), 14033–14039.

Goto, A., Rudd, R. E., Alden, L. Y., & et al. (2014). Leveraging public health nurses for disaster risk communication in Fukushima City: a qualitative analysis of nurses' written records of parenting counseling and peer discussions. *BMC Health Services Research, 14*(1290), 1–9.

Goto, A., Rudd, R. E., Alden, L. Y., & Yoshida-Komiya, H. (2014). Health literacy training for public health nurses in Fukushima: a case study of program adaptation, implementation, and evaluation. *Japan Medical Association Journal, 57*(3), 146–143.

Green, J. A., Gonzaga, A. M., Cohen, E. D., & Spagnoletti, C. L. (2014). Addressing health literacy through clear health communication: a training program for internal medicine residents, *Patient Education and Counseling, 95* (1), 76–82.

Groene, R. O., & Rudd, R. E. (2011). Results of a feasibility study to assess the health literacy environment: Navigation, written, and oral communication in 10 hospitals in Catalonia, Spain. *Journal of Communication in Healthcare, 4*(4), 227–237. https://doi.org/10.1179/17538076 11Y.0000000005

Groene , R. O., Wills, J., Crichton, N., Rowlands, G., & Rudd, R. (2017). The health literacy dyad: the contribution of future G.P.s in England. *Education for Primary Care, 28*(5), 274–281.

Grosse, R. N., & Auffrey, C. (1989). Literacy and health status in developing countries. *Annual Review of Public Health, 10*(1), 281–297.

Health Literacy Toolshed. (2021) Online at http://www.healthliteracy.bu.edu. Retrieved 30 April 2021.

Hoover, A. G. (2019). Defining environmental health literacy. In Finn, S., O'Fallon, L. (eds.). *Environmental health literacy.* Springer.

Horowitz, A. M., Maybury, C., Kleinman, D. V., & et al. (2014). Health literacy environmental scans of community-based dental clinics in Maryland. *American Journal of Public Health, 104*(8), e85–e93.

Institute of Medicine. (2013). *Health literacy: Improving health, health systems, and health policy around the world: Workshop summary. Roundtable on Health Literacy.* Washington DC: National Academies of Science.

Johnson , T. V., Abbasi, A., Schoenberg, E. D., & et al. (2014). Numeracy among trainees: are we preparing physicians for evidence-based medicine. *Journal of Surgical Education, 71*(2), 211–215.

Karuranga , S., Sorensen, K., Coleman, C., & Mahmud, A. J. (2017). Health literacy competencies for European health care personnel. *Health Literacy Research and Practice, 1*(4) Published Online: October 05, 2017. https://doi.org/10.3928/24748307-20171005-01

Killian, L., & Coletti, M. (2017). The role of universal health literacy precautions in minimizing "medspeak" and promoting shared decision making. *AMA Journal of Ethics, 19*(3), 296–303. https://doi.org/10.1001/journalofethics.2017.19.3.pfor1-1703

Kindig, D. A., Panzer, A. M., & Nielsen-Bohlman, L. (Eds.). (2004). *Health literacy: A prescription to end confusion.* Washington DC: National Academies Press.

Kirsch , I. S. (1993). *Adult literacy in America: A first look at the results of the national adult literacy survey.* Washington DC: U.S. Government Printing Office, Superintendent of Documents (Stock No. 065-000-00588-3).

Kirsch, I. S. (2001). *The International Adult Literacy Survey (IALS): Understanding what was measured research report, education testing services, statistics and research division.* Princeton NJ: ETS Publication RR-01-25.

Kleinman, D. V., Baur, C. E., Rudd, R. E., Rubin, D. (2018). Health literacy. Issues briefs to inform development and implementation of healthy people 2030. Secretary's Advisory Committee for healthy people 2030. USDHHS. Online at: https://www.healthypeople.gov/2020/About-Healthy-People/Development-Healthy-People-2030.

Koh, H. K., Berwick, D. M., Clancy, C. M., Baur, C., Brach, C., Harris, L. M., Zerhusen, E. G. (2012). New federal policy initiatives to boost health literacy can help the nation move beyond the cycle of costly 'crisis care'. *Health Affairs,* 10–377. DOI 10.1377/hlthaff.2011.1169

Kutner, M., Greenberg, E., Jin, Y., & Paulsen, C. (2006). *The health literacy of America's adults: Results from the 2003 National Assessment of Adult Literacy (NCES 2006–483). U.S. Department of Education.* Washington, DC: National Center for Education Statistics.

Maybury , C., Horowitz, A. M., Yan, A. F., Green, K. M., Wang, M. Q. (2012). Maryland dentists' knowledge of oral cancer prevention and early detection. *Journal of the California Dental Association, 40*(4), 341–350.

McLaughlin , G. H. (1969). SMOG grading: a new readability formula. *Journal of Reading, 12,* 639–646.

Morello-Frosch, R., Varshavsky, J., Liboiron, M., Brown, P., Brody, J. G. (2015). Communicating results in post-Belmont era biomonitoring studies: lessons from genetics and neuroimaging research. *Environmental Research, 136,* 363–372. DOI: 10.1016/j.envres.2014.10.001

Mosenthal, P. B., & Kirsch, I. S. (1998). A new measure for assessing document complexity: the PMOSE/IKIRSCH document readability formula. *Journal of Adolescent & Adult Literacy, 41*(8), 638–657.

Murray, T. S., Rudd, R. E., Kirsch, I., Yamamoto, K., Grenier, S. (2007). *Health literacy in Canada. Initial results from the International Adult Literacy and Skills Survey.* Ottawa: Canadian Council on Learning.

National Center for Education Statistics. (2017). Program for the international assessment of adult competencies, U.S. State and County Estimates. Available online at https://nces.ed.gov/surveys/piaac/current_results.asp. Accessed May 2022.

Nutbeam, D. (1998). Health promotion glossary. *Health Promotion International, 13*(4), 349–364.

Nutbeam , D. (2008). The evolving concept of health literacy. *Social Science & Medicine, 67,* 2072–2078. DOI 10.1177/1359105313476978

OECD. (2013). OECD skills outlook 2013: first results from the survey of adult skills. Paris, France: OECD Publications. Available online: https://www.oecd.org/skills/piaac/

OECD PIAAC, (2017). OECD skills outlook 2017: skills and global value chains, Paris: OECD Publishing. Available online: https://www.oecd.org/skills/piaac/

OECD PIAAC, (2019). OECD skills outlook 2019: skills and global value chains, Paris: OECD Publishing. Available online: https://www.oecd.org/skills/piaac/

Oelschlegel, S., Graveel, K. L., Tester, E., Heidel, R. E., & Russomanno, J. (2018). Librarians promoting changes in the health care delivery system through systematic assessment. *Medical References Services Quarterly, 37*(2), 142–152.

Office of the Surgeon General (US); Office of Disease Prevention and Health Promotion (U.S.). (2006). *Proceedings of the Surgeon General's Workshop on Improving Health Literacy.* Rockville MD: Office of the Surgeon General (US). Available online from: https://www.ncbi.nlm.nih.gov/books/NBK44257/. Retrieved 1 May 2021.

Parnell, T. A. (2015). *Health literacy in nursing.* New York: Springer. ISBN-13: 978-0826161727.

Peters, E., Hibbard, J., Slovic, P., & Dieckmann, N. (2007). Numeracy skill and the communication, comprehension, and use of risk-benefit information. *Health Affairs, 26*(3), 741–748.

Purcell-Gates, V. E. (2007). *Cultural practices of literacy: Case studies of language, literacy, social practice, and power.* New York: Lawrence Erlbaum Associates Publishers.

Ramirez-Andreotta, M. D., Brody, J. G., Lothrop, N., Loh, M., Beamer, P. I., Brown, P. (2016). Reporting back environmental exposure data and free choice learning. *Environmental Health, 15*(1), 2. DOI 10.1186/s12940-015-0080-1

Roter, D. L. (2011). Oral literacy demand of health care communication: challenges and solutions. *Nursing Outlook, 59*(2), 79–84.

Rudd, R., & Baur C. (2020) Health literacy and early insights during a pandemic. *Journal of Communication in Healthcare, 13*(1), 13–16. https://doi.org/10.1080/17538068.2020.1760622

Rudd, R. E. (2003). *Health literacy objectives in U.S. Department of Health and Human Services, Office of Disease Prevention and Health Promotion. National Action Plan to Improve Health Literacy.* Washington DC: USDHHS.

Rudd, R. E. (2007). Health literacy skills of U.S. adults. *American Journal of Health Behavior, 31*(Suppl 1), S8–S18.

Rudd, R. E., The health literacy environment activity packet. Health literacy studies, Harvard T.H. Chan School of Public Health. Available online at: hsph.harvard.edu/healthliteracy/practice strategies and tools. Retrieved May 1, 2021.

Rudd, R. E. (2016). Numbers get in the way. Health literacy roundtable commentary. Washington DC: National Academy of Medicine. Available online at https://nam.edu/numbers-get-in-the -way. Retrieved 1 May 2021.

Rudd, R. E., Anderson, J. E. (2006). The health literacy environment of hospitals and health centers. Partners for action: making your healthcare facility literacy-friendly. Cambridge MA: National Center for the Study of Adult Learning and Literacy (NCSALL). online at: www.hsph.harvard. edu/healthliteracy/Practicestrategiesandtools. Retrieved 1 May 2021.

Rudd, R. E., & Baur, C. (2020). Health literacy and early insights during a pandemic. *Journal of Communication in Health Care, 13*(1), 13–16. https://doi.org/10.1080/17538068.2020.1760622

Rudd, R. E., Comings, J. P., & Hyde, J. (2003). Leave no one behind: Improving health and risk communication through attention to literacy. *Journal of Health Communication, 8*(Suppl 1), 104–115. DOI 10.1080/713851983

Rudd, R. E., McCray, A. T., & Nutbeam, D. (2012). Heath literacy and definitions of terms. Chapter 2. In *Health literacy in context: International perspectives* (pp. 13–32). Hauppauge: Nova Science Publishers.

Rudd, R. E., Oelschiegle, S., Grabeel, K. L., Tester, E., & Heidel, E. (2019). ERIC ED606503. Available online at: https://eric.ed.gov/?id=ED606503. Retrieved 1 May 2021.

Shoemaker, S. J., Wolf, M. S., & Brach, C. (2014). Development of the PatienE Materials Assessment Tool (PEMAT): a new measure of understandability and actionability for print and audiovisual patient information. *Patient Education and Counseling, 96*(3), 395–403.

Simonds, V. W., Margetts, M., & Rudd, R. E. (2019). Expanding environmental health literacy—a focus on water quality and tribal lands. *Journal of Health Communication, 24*(3), 236–243, DOI 10.1080/10810730.2019.1597948

Sorensen, K., Pelikan, J. M., Rothlin, F., Ganahl, K., Slonska, Z. l., Doyle, G., Fullam, J., Kondiis, B., Agrafiotis, D., Uiters, E., Falcon, M., Mensing, M., Tchamov, K., van den Broucke, S., & Brand, H. (2015). Health literacy in Europe: comparative results of the European health literacy survey (HLS-EU). *European Journal of Public Health*, http://dx/doi.org/10.1093/eurpub/ckO43

Tuijnman, A., Kirsch, I., Murray, S., & Jones, S. (1995). *Literacy, economy and society: Results of the first international adult literacy survey, 1994*. Ottowa CA: Statistics Canada.

van der Heide, I., Wang, J., Droomers, M., Spreeuwenberg, P., Rademakers, J., & Uiters, E. (2013). The relationship between health, education, and health literacy: results from the Dutch adult literacy and life skills survey. *Journal of Health Communication, 18*(supp1), 172–184. DOI: 10.1080/10810730.2013.825668

Wills, J. (2016). Where is health literacy in the education of health professionals?, in Proceedings of the 22nd IUHPE World Conference on Health Promotion, Curtiba, Brazil.

CHAPTER 8

Access to Healthcare

Latina M. Brooks and Jesse Honsky

LEARNING OBJECTIVES

⦿ Describe access to healthcare coverage and services in the United States.

⦿ Identify the unique needs of vulnerable populations in access to healthcare.

⦿ Identify barriers and facilitators for vulnerable populations when accessing healthcare.

⦿ Describe strategies to improve access to healthcare.

INTRODUCTION

While 87.8% of adults in the United States report having a usual place of healthcare, that number drops to 79.8% among those living in poverty (National Center for Health Statistics [NCHS], 2019). Of U.S. adults, only 65.3% report having a dental cleaning or examination in the last 12 months; in rural areas, 57.1% of the adult population report dental cleaning, compared with 66.6% of adults in large urban areas (NCHS, 2019). In 2019, 8.3% of adults report not receiving needed medical care due to cost; among adults living with a disability, that number increases to 14.8% (NCHS, 2019). Access to healthcare, including dental care, public health services, and mental and behavioral health services, is not equally distributed across the population. Differences in access to healthcare among populations are often related to social determinants of health and structural barriers such as employment, income, education and literacy levels, available services, location and transportation, race, ethnicity, gender, and age (Dickman et al., 2017).

The National Academy of Medicine (formerly the Institute of Medicine) defines access to care as "having the timely use of personal health services to achieve the best health outcomes" (Institute of Medicine [IOM], 1993, p. 4). This definition intentionally identifies both use of health services and health outcomes as standards for measuring access, because access to care is related to both utilization and quality of care (IOM, 1993). Limited access to healthcare does not have a single cause; rather, it is a complex issue that changes based on the population of people in need of care. There are several components of access to healthcare, and key among them are access to healthcare coverage, access to healthcare services, timeliness, and workforce (Agency for Healthcare Research & Quality [AHRQ], 2018; Office of Disease Prevention and Health Promotion (ODPHP), n.d.-a).

Coverage refers to health insurance coverage. Health insurance is important for people to enter the healthcare system and to reduce the burden of medical expenses. *Services* refers to the healthcare services available, such as primary care, preventive care, dental care, emergency medical services, and essential specialty care. *Timeliness* is the healthcare system's ability to provide appointments and care quickly when needed, which is closely linked to workforce—having healthcare providers who are "capable, qualified, [and] culturally competent" (AHRQ, 2018). Many vulnerable populations experience challenges to accessing healthcare related to lack of insurance coverage or difficulty obtaining services, and the barriers they face are often intertwined with other social determinants of health, such as safe housing, transportation, education, and job opportunities. This chapter provides further examples and context for the complex relationship between access to healthcare and social determinants of health as they relate to specific vulnerable populations, including those with disabilities and members of the LGBTQ+ population.

ACCESS TO HEALTHCARE COVERAGE

In the United States, 10.9% of the population between the ages of 0 and 64 years does not have health insurance (Tolbert et al., 2020). Across the United States, health insurance is closely tied to employment benefits: Of those insured, 49.6% of people have coverage through their employer. Despite this proportion, 73.2% of nonelderly adults who are uninsured work full time (Kaiser Family Foundation's [KFF's] State Health Facts, 2019; Tolbert et al., 2020), indicating that employer-sponsored plans do not provide sufficient coverage for all. There are multiple sources of private and government health insurance or services in the United States (Table 8.1). Another aspect of coverage is underinsurance, a condition in which an individual who has health insurance is still unable to afford care, whose plan does not cover the types of health services needed, and/or whose insurance plan has barriers to accessing services or plan benefits (Lavarreda et al., 2011). Examples of such barriers may include coverage limitations on when or where individuals can receive diagnostic testing or obtain medical devices or equipment.

Government programs such as Medicare, Medicaid, and CHIP help increase coverage rates for children under 18 and adults over 65, leaving adults ages 18 to 64 more likely to be uninsured (14.5% in the United States; NCHS, 2019). Lack of insurance is not always explained by work status or poverty—73.2% of nonelderly adults remain uninsured despite having a full-time worker in their family and just over half of the uninsured earn more than 200% of the federal poverty level (FLP; Tolbert et al., 2020). See Figure 8.1 for more detail. In addition to work status, income, and age, race and ethnicity are also linked to lack of coverage (see Figure 8.2). People who identify as Hispanic make up the largest percentage of uninsured adults in the United States (37.6%), despite Hispanic and Latino people making up only 18.5% of the total U.S. population (Tolbert et al., 2020; U.S. Census Bureau, 2019).

In recent history, the Affordable Care Act (ACA) has helped to significantly reduce the number of uninsured Americans. The law has three main goals: (a) to make health insurance affordable to more people, (b) to expand Medicaid to cover more low-income adults, and (c) to support innovation in medical care to lower healthcare costs (HealthCare.gov, n.d.). In 2010, when the ACA was signed into law, 17.8% of the U.S. population under age 65 was uninsured. In 2014, after most of the ACA provisions had taken effect, the uninsured rate dropped to 13.5%, and in 2019 the uninsured rate was 10.9% (Tolbert et al., 2020).

WHY IS COVERAGE IMPORTANT?

Individuals without health insurance are less likely to have a regular source of healthcare, less likely to use preventive services and screenings, more likely to delay or go without care due to cost, and report more problems getting care (Garfield et al., 2019). Uninsured individuals also have an increased risk of more serious health outcomes, such as chronic

TABLE 8.1 Types of Health Coverage in the United States

Type of Coverage	Population Covered	Description	Where to Find More Information
Private health insurance (healthinsurance.org, n.d.)	Available to all those who can afford it either through employment or directly purchasing from a health insurance company	Health insurance provided by private insurance companies	www.healthinsurance.org/glossary/private-health-insurance
Medicare (U.S. Centers for Medicare and Medicaid Services [CMS] n.d.-c)	People who are 65 or older, certain younger people with disabilities, and people with end-stage renal disease (ERSD)	Health insurance funded by the federal government	www.medicare.gov/
Medicaid (CMS, n.d.-b)	Required by federal law: Low-income families, qualified pregnant people and children, and individuals receiving Supplemental Security Income (SSI) States have additional options to provide coverage to low-income adults, children in foster care, or individuals receiving home or community services	Health insurance jointly funded by state and federal government Medicaid programs and eligibility differ from state to state	www.medicaid.gov/medicaid/index.html
Children's Health Insurance Program (CHIP; CMS, n.d.-a)	Children in families that earn too much to qualify for Medicaid. Some states offer CHIP coverage to pregnant people	Low-cost health insurance jointly funded by state and federal government CHIP programs differ by state and work closely with their respective state Medicaid programs	www.healthcare.gov/medicaid-chip/childrens-health-insurance-program
Military (Defense Health Agency, n.d.; U.S. Department of Veterans Affairs, 2021)	Members of the military and their families and military veterans	This includes both health insurance provided by the military (TRICARE) and the U.S. Department of Veterans Affairs (VA) healthcare system that provides direct healthcare to veterans. Funded by the federal government	www.tricare.mil www.va.gov/health-care
Indian Health Services (Indian Health Service, n.d.)	American Indian and Alaska Natives, from federally recognized tribes in the United States	Healthcare system funded by the federal government, not health insurance	www.ihs.gov

Note: This table provides general information about the most common forms of health insurance coverage and government health systems in the United States.

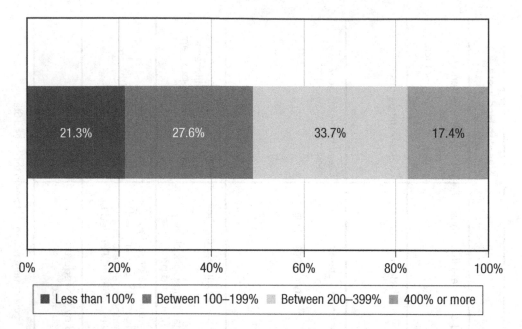

Figure 8.1 Rate of nonelderly uninsured and family income (federal poverty level [FPL] percentage), 2019.

Source: Data from KFF in Tolbert, J., Orgera, K., & Damico, A. (2020). *Key facts about the uninsured population.* www.kff.org/uninsured/issue-brief/key-facts-about-the-uninsured-population.

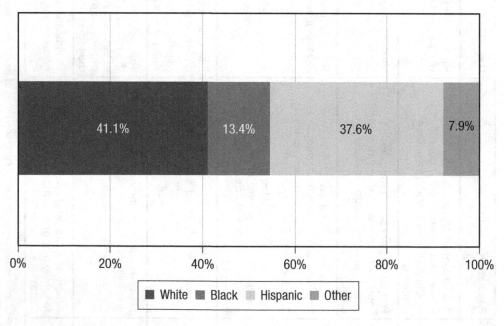

Figure 8.2 Rate of the nonelderly uninsured by race and ethnicity, 2019.

Source: Data from KFF in Tolbert, J., Orgera, K., & Damico, A. (2020). *Key facts about the uninsured population.* www.kff.org/uninsured/issue-brief/key-facts-about-the-uninsured-population.

illness, late-stage diagnosis of disease, and morbidity and mortality (Christopher et al., 2016; Garfield et al., 2019; Woolhandler & Himmelstein, 2017). Lack of health insurance is closely linked to other social determinants of health such as poverty, employment, race, ethnicity, and age; simply having health insurance cannot be viewed as a "silver bullet" to improve health disparities in the United States. While health insurance is linked to access and health outcomes, as well as reduced out-of-pocket expenses for healthcare and alleviated financial hardship related to medical bills, many insured individuals still report issues affording other essentials, taking on additional debt, and/or working additional hours or jobs because of medical bills (Dickman et al., 2017). Increasing coverage is only one strategy among many to decrease systemic barriers to healthcare and health. Understanding the specific needs of vulnerable populations who do not have health insurance coverage or who are underinsured will also help to identify solutions to address the barriers they face.

COVERAGE AND VULNERABLE POPULATIONS

People who do not have health insurance or are underinsured are vulnerable populations (American Hospital Association, 2016). Within this larger population there are subgroups of individuals who are at risk for disparate healthcare access and outcomes because of economic, cultural, ethnic, racial, or health characteristics. These subgroups may include patients who are racial or ethnic minorities, children, older adults, members of the LGBTQ+ population, people who are chronically ill or disabled, and those who are socioeconomically disadvantaged (Rice, 2019; Shi & Stevens, 2021). All healthcare providers should understand the challenges and the strengths of vulnerable populations in the communities where they work to best provide care. Many factors contribute to being uninsured or underinsured, and these factors can vary in different communities.

For example, one third of uninsured families are living at 200% to 399% of the FLP (see Figure 8.1; Tolbert et al., 2020). In most states, Medicaid is available to families and individuals with an income at 138% of the FLP, which was $21,960 for a family of three and $12,880 for a single adult in 2021 (KFF's State Health Facts, 2021). Only Washington, DC and Connecticut have higher limits, at 221% and 160%, respectively, and 14 states have set limits below the federal threshold of 138%. These cutoffs often leave gaps in coverage for people who make too much money to qualify for Medicaid, but who may not make enough to buy a private plan if they do not receive health insurance through their employer.

Undocumented Immigrants

Undocumented immigrants are another vulnerable population who are often uninsured. The estimate for the number of undocumented immigrants in the United States is between 10.5 and 12 million people (Kamarck & Stenglein, 2019). The most significant barrier many undocumented immigrants face in obtaining health insurance is living in poverty and being unable to afford insurance plans; additionally, most federal insurance plans are not available to this population (Beck et al., 2017). The only federal Medicaid available to undocumented immigrants is Emergency Medicaid, which covers individuals in active labor and acute medical emergencies, and which only covers services to stabilize patients. There is also federal funding for health insurance to cover pregnant people and children who are undocumented immigrants; however, the majority of undocumented immigrants are not eligible (Beck et al., 2017). Lack of insurance combined with poverty and fear of being deported often prevents many undocumented migrants from seeking care, making them more vulnerable to chronic conditions and serious disease outcomes because of delayed care.

People With Disabilities

People with disabilities are a large minority group and an often-overlooked vulnerable population who experience several disparities in healthcare regarding insurance coverage, finances, transportation, and poor coordination among healthcare providers (McClintock et al., 2016). This group encounters many financial, social, and physical/structural barriers, which can result in unmet needs and dissatisfaction with health care (Shandra, 2018). People with disabilities previously experienced lack of private health insurance due to pre-existing condition clauses that made obtaining adequate healthcare insurance difficult. Per the ACA, denial of health insurance due to pre-existing conditions by private insurers is no longer allowed (Krahn et al., 2015). Additionally, many people with disabilities are eligible for public health insurance; however, public health insurance does not cover all people with disabilities, nor all needed care. Therefore, members of this group are less likely to receive preventive care services and have unmet medical and dental needs (Mahmoudi & Meade, 2015).

CASE STUDY 8.1

Access to Care: Older, Developmentally Delayed Patient With Several Chronic Illnesses and New Onset of Perceived Hearing Loss

Ms. Renee Sharrod is 65 years old and developmentally delayed. Ms. Sharrod has always been considered high functioning although she is unable to read or write. In the past, Ms. Sharrod was able to respond to straightforward questions and follow direct instructions. However, as she has gotten older, she has developed hearing and speech difficulties as well as some mild cognitive decline. When Ms. Sharrod's mother passed away, Ms. Sharrod no longer had a direct caregiver to assist her with activities of daily living (ADLs) or with healthcare concerns. Shortly following the death of Ms. Sharrod's mother, Ms. Sharrod was moved into an apartment in an assisted-living facility.

The assisted-living facility does a marginal job of supporting Ms. Sharrod's ADLs, such as providing meals, assisting with bathing, and administering medications. However, when it comes to managing and facilitating treatment for Ms. Sharrod's many chronic health conditions, the facility falls short. The assisted living facility does not have well-trained or adequate caregiving staff to stay on top of healthcare visits, procedures, or equipment orders. Although Ms. Sharrod has adequate health insurance, she has no one to assist her with navigating the "red tape" involved, such as prior authorizations, and with understanding when and where she can seek services and how often. Additionally, Ms. Sharrod needs assistance with scheduling appointments, arranging transportation, and communicating with healthcare providers.

As mentioned previously, Ms. Sharrod has developed what is perceived as hearing loss. Ms. Sharrod's caseworker schedules an appointment for Ms. Sharrod to have her hearing checked. The assisted-living facility arranges the visit and sends an aide with Ms. Sharrod to the visit. Ms. Sharrod's hearing is evaluated at this visit, and it is determined that she has moderate hearing loss and needs hearing aids. Although this same healthcare facility also provides hearing aids, Ms. Sharrod's insurance will not cover the hearing aids from this health care facility; she can only receive hearing aids from a select few places. Ms. Sharrod goes home with an order for hearing aids but needs another appointment at a separate facility to be fitted for them. A few months go by, with the overworked caseworker attempting to find out from the insurance company where Ms. Sharrod can go to be fitted for hearing aids. A prior authorization is submitted and is finally obtained from Ms. Sharrod's insurance company. At this point, Ms. Sharrod is assigned a new caseworker, who is unaware of the prior authorization and the need to schedule an appointment to have Ms. Sharrod fitted for hearing aids, so several more weeks go by. Once Ms. Sharrod is finally scheduled and goes to be fitted for the hearing aids, she is informed that the hearing evaluation and order for hearing aids has expired. She now needs a new hearing evaluation and order for hearing aids. Although this current facility can perform hearing evaluations, Ms. Sharrod's insurance will not cover testing at this facility, only the hearing aids. Ms. Sharrod now needs another hearing test at yet another facility, essentially starting all over again.

This entire process has taken more than 9 months, and Ms. Sharrod still does not have hearing aids or any one person available to her to facilitate and connect the various steps it

(continued)

CASE STUDY 8.1 (*CONTINUED*)

takes to use her health insurance and access appropriate care. COVID-19 emerges about 2 months later and all efforts cease; there are not enough staff to address Ms. Sharrod's hearing loss issues. It has now been almost 2 years and Ms. Sharrod still does not have hearing aids; by all accounts her hearing has gotten significantly worse. Her speech is now being impacted by the hearing deficit. Of note, hearing loss is only one of Ms. Sharrod's health issues, which include diabetes, hypertension, and pulmonary hypertension. Although Ms. Sharrod has what would be considered adequate health insurance, her being older, developmentally delayed, and lacking a caregiver or advocate to coordinate her care means that she ultimately does not have adequate access to healthcare.

Discussion Questions

1. What other barriers might older persons or persons with disabilities face when trying to access healthcare?
2. What are steps you could take, both as an individual nurse and at the systems level, to improve access to care for older or developmentally delayed patients?
3. What could be done in situations where lack of advocacy resources and "red tape" restrict needed healthcare access?
4. Develop a policy that health professionals could create and implement to address the needs of individuals in assisted-living facilities. Provide a rationale for your proposed policy.

People Who Are Transgender or Gender Nonconforming

Transgender refers to a person whose gender identity differs from the sex assigned at birth (Safer & Tangpricha, 2019). Gender nonconformity refers to the degree to which an individual's appearance, behavior, interests, and subjective self-concept deviate from the conventional "norms" associated with male or female gender (Schoenbaum, 2020).

People who are transgender and gender nonconforming (TGNC) encounter barriers with health insurance (Kalma, 2016). Members of this group are less likely to have health insurance, particularly in the Midwest and South, when compared with people who are cisgender in accordance with "cultural norms" (Dickey et al., 2016). Furthermore, health insurance coverage for medically necessary transgender care is variable and does not always align with best practices and recommended care, despite federal rules prohibiting discrimination based on gender identity in healthcare (Ngaage et al., 2019; U.S. Department of Health and Human Services [DHHS], 2016). Other barriers TGNC people face include denial of coverage for gender-affirming surgery and hormone therapy, limited health insurance plan options to meet all health needs, and challenges with electronic health records (EHR) "linking registered sex with presumed organs and therefore making incorrect assumptions about needed interventions," leading to coverage denial of much-needed screenings or treatments (Learmonth et al., 2018, p. 273).

CASE STUDY 8.2

Access to Healthcare and the LGBTQ+ Patient Experience: Excerpts from an Interview with Ms. Rose Smart, Presented as a Commentary on Barriers to Access to Quality Care for Members of the LGBTQ+ Community

Ms. Rose Smart is a transgender woman who teaches and advocates for LGBTQ+ rights, access, and understanding in healthcare and in the community. Ms. Smart says that members of the

(*continued*)

CASE STUDY 8.2 (*CONTINUED*)

LGBTQ+ community experience access issues from the time they first check in for an appointment, where they might encounter hostility. The hostility can be overt, active hostility—for example, being told, "We don't serve your kind here"—or it could be more subtle, in the way of obliviousness. Ms. Smart says that the obliviousness comes up when people do not understand and do not want to understand. Many people working in healthcare may not be willing to take the time to learn, and so members of the LGBTQ+ community get mistreated. An example might be a same-sex couple who is treated as though one member is the patient and the other is the "ride," whereas a heterosexual couple sitting next to them is treated as a couple by the provider.

Ms. Smart notices that many members of the LGBTQ+ community are hesitant to talk about their social situation, family, friends, and dating, so things get missed when they seek healthcare. In her work, Ms. Smart educates providers on talking honestly about sex and sexuality and on how to ask the right questions. She explains that if providers are not asking the right questions about who someone is dating and what they do with that person, important things that are crucial to a person's health could be missed.

Transgender patients have their own challenges when it comes to healthcare. Ms. Smart describes "transgender broken arm syndrome," which is where "somebody gets hurt and they go to the doctor and the doctor says, 'Well, I don't know how to treat that [the actual problem] because you're trans.'" She tells the story of a transgender man she knew who had that exact experience during an emergency department visit. The man was cleaning the gutters on his house, and he fell off the ladder, injuring his shoulder and cutting his hand. The doctor stood at the foot of the gurney and said, "I don't know how to treat these things, I don't know about these things, I don't want to have to treat them." For the doctor, the "thing" was not the medical problem, the "thing" was the person who needed stitches in his hand and a shoulder immobilizer.

Although Ms. Smart is skilled at and experienced in advocating for herself and others, she still faces fear when navigating the healthcare system. She feels that although she can advocate for herself, she should not have to while in a vulnerable position. She also considers that if she must advocate for herself, she may not be receiving the best care—if the person treating her is overtly hostile or mostly passive aggressive, her care may not be adequate.

Ms. Smart believes that it is important for providers to become well-versed in caring for LGBTQ+ patients because, first and foremost, LGBTQ+ patients are people with *the same problems as everybody else*. Additionally, members of the LGBTQ+ community are part of an identifiable demographic that experiences health disparities. Ms. Smart states that when caring for LGBTQ+ patients, providers should acknowledge both those facts and then use appropriate language to ask questions in a way that creates openness, rather than closing a conversation. She reiterates that providers do not have to be experts, but having some knowledge is valuable.

To gain that knowledge, Ms. Smart suggests that providers can read current, accessible LGBTQ+ literature. She says that doing so does not necessarily require long courses or stacks of books; rather, just a few hours of reading, thinking, and paying attention to accessible material can change how LGBTQ+ patients perceive their providers.

Discussion Questions

1. How do healthcare professionals contribute to the patient's experience of their care?
2. How else might experiences described in this interview impact access to healthcare for people who are LGTBQ+?
3. What other barriers may people from the LGBTQ+ community face when trying to access healthcare?
4. What are steps you could take, both as an individual nurse and at the systems level, to improve access to care for LGBTQ+ people?

STRATEGIES TO IMPROVE HEALTH INSURANCE COVERAGE

Nurses and health professionals of all education levels and specialties can work to improve coverage for their patients and impact general coverage issues at both the individual and the systems level. An important step is to be knowledgeable about health insurance coverage, what types of coverage are available to the patient population, and what resources are available within the healthcare organization or community to help people find affordable insurance. All health professionals and advocates can screen individuals for social determinants of health to identify persons who are uninsured or underinsured, then refer them to appropriate resources (such as case managers or patient navigators) who can then help them with insurance and other barriers they may be experiencing (Cerisier, 2019). This process requires that nurses and all health professionals receive education about the importance of connecting the uninsured to care, what resources are available to the patients, and how to make referrals to those resources. In addition, the program needs to be structured in a way that it can easily be incorporated into existing workflow and take a minimal amount of time, so as to not overwhelm providers who are busy with other patient care responsibilities (Cerisier, 2019).

Nurses must also develop and work in programs with the interprofessional healthcare team designed to focus on uninsured individuals to help them obtain the health services they need. For example, a clinic in Arizona revised their cervical cancer screening process to increase the screening rates among their uninsured and underserved patients and to help connect them to a program that covers cancer screenings (Kiser & Butler, 2020). This change required nurses to engage the interprofessional healthcare team to get them on board, engage patients to educate them about cervical cancer screening, update the screening processes within the clinic, and set up a system to track the outcomes (Kiser & Butler, 2020). Doing so required skills in both understanding how to make change within the system of the clinic and how to educate patients about cervical cancer screenings. Additionally, all professionals involved in delivering health services, including those advocating for policy changes to support the program, must have employed a good understanding of the culture and needs of the population being served.

Systems level interventions to increase health insurance coverage include policy changes at the local, state, and federal levels. Nurses, along with other healthcare professionals, can advocate for policy changes within their communities and health systems to help better connect people to healthcare resources. Nurses can advocate at the state and national levels to increase the options for affordable health insurance. They can partner with health insurance companies to find ways to incentivize more comprehensive insurance plans that help reduce healthcare costs. The ACA was a starting point to reform healthcare and health insurance coverage in the United States. There is still much work to be done to improve coverage and access to care. Health providers are well positioned to move the goals of the ACA forward and beyond; through innovation, they can help reduce healthcare costs, improve quality, and increase access to care (Cleveland et al., 2019).

ACCESS TO HEALTHCARE SERVICES

Vulnerable populations often encounter difficulties accessing both basic and specialty health services. The types of health services needed for a specific population or community may vary based on need. However, offering a core of essential health services that are accessible to all members of the community is an important step in improving health equity. Essential health services include primary care, dental care, public health services, mental health and substance use treatment, emergency and observation services, transportation services, diagnostic services, home care, and a robust referral structure (American Hospital Association,

2016; ODPHP, n.d.-c; Robert Wood Johnson Foundation, n.d.). Services alone do not solve access to care issues, as these issues intersect with other access concerns. For example, services need to be available to patients, and the patients need to have transportation to get to service locations. Furthermore, patients often need health insurance to afford these services, and the services should be provided in a culturally competent manner that accounts for patient level of health or health status (Shi & Stevens, 2021).

Why Is Access to Services Important?

Primary care and transportation are examples of how access to services can impact healthcare and health outcomes. A key element of access to health services is having a usual source of care through a primary care provider (PCP). A PCP can be a nurse practitioner, physician, or physician assistant. In addition to PCPs, peer counselors, patient navigators, or advocates can be an effective part of the team to increase access to healthcare services. People who have a usual source of care are more likely to receive preventive care and screenings and have better health outcomes (ODPHP, n.d.-b).

Disparities in access can be observed when examining the unique needs of both rural and urban areas (see Chapter 17 for more details). In rural areas, transportation services play an important role in access to care. When patients have to travel long distances to access healthcare, and transportation is unavailable, time consuming, or expensive, then patients may delay or forego care altogether (Cromer et al., 2019). Access to specialty care is also a concern in some communities. A lack of specialty services such as mental and behavioral health, obstetrical, and surgical services in rural communities are often tied to financial constraints and the lack of healthcare providers in their communities. For example, many rural communities do not have a large enough population to sustain a specialty practice (Cyr et al., 2019). Additionally, the low reimbursement rate of Medicaid insurance dissuades many specialty providers from accepting individuals who rely on Medicaid for insurance coverage, making it difficult for those individuals to find and afford specialty care (Cyr et al., 2019).

Services and Vulnerable Populations

Rural communities face several health and social disparities. Namely, people in rural areas are older, more likely to experience poverty, and less likely to have health insurance. Rural populations also have higher rates of injury, smoking, suicide, and opioid misuse (AHRQ, 2017). There are fewer healthcare providers, including dentists, per capita in rural areas, particularly when it comes to specialty areas like neurology, anesthesia, and mental health (AHRQ, 2017; Cohen et al., 2021; Cyr et al., 2019). In addition, hospitals in rural communities have been closing, exacerbating access issues. In rural counties where hospitals have been closed, the median distance to travel to general inpatient services increased from 3.4 miles in 2012 to 23.9 miles in 2018; relatedly, the per capita number of advanced practice nurses, physicians, and physician assistants decreased (U.S. Government Accountability Office, 2020). Urban communities, on the other hand, are challenged by some of the same factors, but there are also differences.

Urban communities also face hospital closings, particularly hospitals located in low-income neighborhoods where most residents belong to racial or ethnic minority groups (Ko et al., 2014). These closings are often attributed to financial reasons, as hospitals in these neighborhoods typically serve people with Medicaid and Medicare health coverage, which does not reimburse providers as well as private health insurance. Furthermore, many patients at these hospitals are uninsured and cannot afford to pay for care themselves (Rau & Huetteman, 2020; Williams, 2019). Hospital closings have been linked to poor outcomes for people who live nearby, including access issues associated with increased transportation time, delays in receiving care, and decreased access to specialty care, as well as poorer overall health (Ko et al., 2014). The people who live in neighborhoods where urban hospitals are closing already experience higher levels of chronic illness and poverty, and closing local hospitals creates new barriers to accessing healthcare, potentially exacerbating existing health inequities (Rau & Huetteman, 2020; Williams, 2019).

In addition to the logistical barriers to services, some communities face additional challenges that compound the issues of access to healthcare. For example, Native Americans and Alaska Natives face the same issues with lack of providers and transportation experienced in both rural and urban areas (Cromer et al., 2019). Some Native Americans and Alaska Natives live in remote areas and must undergo extensive travel to reach clinics or hospitals. Others live in urban areas, but need to travel to Indian Health Services (IHS) facilities, which might be on reservations outside of the city, in order to access care. When Native American and Alaska Native people do access care, they tend to receive poor quality care because of insufficient funding of the IHS, understaffing, lack of medications, and cross-cultural difficulties (Cromer et al., 2019).

In the face of numerous challenges, steps are being taken to improve access for these communities. One provision of the ACA is to improve the quality of care and reduce health disparities among Native American and Alaska Native people by improving IHS infrastructure, increasing culturally appropriate programs, and recruiting culturally competent healthcare providers (Cromer et al., 2019; Patient Protection & Affordable Care Act, 2010). At both individual and community levels, healthcare providers can improve their cultural competence, support culturally appropriate interventions, and recognize how historical trauma in Native American and Alaskan Native communities may impact health today (Carron, 2020).

Strategies to Improve Access to Services

Improving access to services takes careful planning and coordination. One important step is to understand the health needs of a community or population to identify the health and social services that are most needed. Another provision of the ACA requires nonprofit hospitals to partner with local public health agencies to complete a Community Health Needs Assessments (CHNA) with the purpose of developing and implementing plans to improve the health of the people living in surrounding communities (American Hospital Association, n.d.). The CHNA can help identify the needs of a community and can help inform which healthcare services should be prioritized and how.

Another strategy for improving access to services is to bring the services to the people through programs like Mobile Health Clinics (MHC), School-Based Health Centers (SBHC), and Federally Qualified Health Centers (FQHC). MHCs are typically vehicles such as large vans or recreational vehicles that are outfitted with medical equipment and staff to provide healthcare services in different locations. These mobile clinics can serve both urban and rural areas that may not have access to services; such providers commonly offer primary care or preventive services such as screenings and create a needed link to help people access other services, such as prenatal care and chronic care (Yu et al., 2017). In addition to lowering the barriers to healthcare related to transportation, geography, or lack of health providers, the staff on MHCs have experience in providing culturally and linguistically competent care as well as patient-centered care, resulting in patients feeling more welcome and comfortable using MHCs compared to more traditional healthcare settings (Yu et al., 2017). SBHCs are clinics that provide medical, mental and behavioral health, dental, and/or vision and hearing care for students in schools, typically kindergarten through high school. SBHCs can be embedded within schools in urban, suburban, and rural communities and can serve as either a medical home for children and adolescents or an important link or supplement to existing healthcare (Arenson et al., 2019). SBHCs are linked to improved physical and mental health outcomes, particularly among children and adolescents, whose families face challenges accessing care due to issues like transportation, work schedules, or ability to pay for services (Arenson et al., 2019). FQHCs are community-based healthcare providers that receive funds from the Health Resources and Services Administration (HRSA) Health Center Program to provide primary care services in underserved areas (HRSA, 2017, para 1). These centers often integrate pharmacy, mental and behavioral health, and oral health services with primary care and efforts focused on medically underserved areas and populations. FQHCs accept all patients regardless of their ability to pay; when a patient must pay for services, they are billed on a sliding scale based on the patient's income. FQHCs also accept Medicaid, Medicare, and private insurance (HRSA, 2017). FQHCs help to improve access to healthcare by providing affordable health services in the locations with the highest need.

SBHCs, FQHCs, and larger healthcare systems also work to improve access to health services, by embedding multiple services in one location so that patients can get many of their health needs met in one place. For example, a patient can receive behavioral health counseling and primary care and retrieve prescriptions at the same clinical location, which saves time and reduces barriers to navigating the broader healthcare system.

Telehealth is another strategy for increasing access to services. Telehealth includes healthcare appointments conducted by video or phone, sending and receiving messages between patients and providers, and using remote monitoring so providers can track patient progress of vitals signs, blood glucose levels, or other health indicators (HRSA, 2021). Telehealth has long been used in rural areas as a way to provide access to specialty care and to fill in gaps if there are not enough providers in a particular area (Becevic et al., 2020). With the onset of the COVID-19 pandemic, telehealth use grew rapidly in 2020 as a means to provide care when in-person healthcare appointments were limited to prevent the spread of the SARS-CoV-2 virus. The expansion of telehealth during this time may have lasting effects on healthcare in the future; telehealth is now seen as a feasible solution to increase access to care (Doraiswamy et al., 2020). However, there is still more research needed to standardize and understand the impact of telehealth on health outcomes.

While the use of telehealth grew rapidly during the COVID-19 pandemic, there were still some patients who were unable to access care due to the digital divide (National Academies of Sciences, Engineering, and Medicine [NASEM], 2021). The digital divide creates economic, educational, and social inequalities between those who have computers and online access and those who do not (Van Dijk, 2020). The ability to provide telehealth from a clinic or hospital does not automatically translate to better access. Patients also must have necessary tools, such as home internet, computers, tablets, and phones, to access telehealth. Additionally, individuals must also learn how to use the technology, or else the technology simply becomes another barrier to access. Many vulnerable populations, including Black or Hispanic Americans; some Asian Americans, Native Americans, and Alaska Natives; and people living in rural and urban areas, have less access to home broadband internet and computers or other devices (Atske & Perrin, 2021; Vogels, 2021). While telehealth is a promising strategy to improve access to care, there is a possibility that it could perpetuate or exacerbate health and social disparities if the gap created by the digital divide is not closed as well (NASEM, 2021).

Workforce Issues and Access to Healthcare

The U.S. population is becoming more diverse, and minorities are expected to collectively make up the majority of the U.S. population by 2043 (U.S. Census Bureau, 2012). The lack of diversity in the healthcare workforce, particularly in nursing, medicine, and dentistry, remains persistent in the United States and has contributed to health disparities among minority populations. A 2004 report by the Sullivan Commission on Diversity in the Healthcare Workforce stated, "The fact that the nation's health professions have not kept pace with changing demographics may be an even greater cause of disparities in health access and outcomes than the persistent lack of health insurance for tens of millions of Americans. Today's physicians, nurses, and dentists have too little resemblance to the diverse populations they serve, leaving many Americans feeling excluded by a system that seems distant and uncaring." Although there have been some gains, the healthcare workforce continues to not represent the diversity of the U.S. population. In a recent study published in JAMA Network Open, using 2019 American Community Survey data, the authors found that across the 10 largest U.S. healthcare professions, Black, Hispanic, and Native Americans are underrepresented across all 10 (Salsberg et al., 2021). This holds true for advanced practice nurses (79.4% White), registered nurses (68.9% White), physicians (62.4% White), and dentists (68.7% White; Salsberg et al., 2021). In order to address current and future disparities in healthcare access, there must be intentional and strategic initiatives to increase the pipeline of underrepresented minorities in our schools of nursing, medicine, and dentistry.

COVID-19 Pandemic and Access to Healthcare

The COVID-19 pandemic has exacerbated access to healthcare issues for many people, especially vulnerable populations (Núñez et al., 2021). Reduction in healthcare services, diverting the healthcare workforce to COVID-19 care and prevention, and fear of exposure to the SARS-CoV-2 virus kept many people with chronic health conditions from receiving care in a timely manner and many healthy people from seeking preventive care (Núñez et al., 2021). High rates of unemployment early in the pandemic throughout the United States raised concerns about higher rates of uninsured people, due to reliance on employer-based health insurance plans across the country (Blumenthal et al., 2020). However, uninsured rates appear to be lower than prepandemic levels, possibly because of Medicaid expansion and the ability to purchase insurance through healthcare.gov or in state-based exchanges (McDermott et al., 2020; NCHS, 2021a). Box 8.1 summarizes some of the trends in access to care between 2019 and July 2021.

BOX 8.1: COVID-19 Pandemic and Access to Healthcare: Ages 18 and Older

Prepandemic Benchmarks (2019)*

9.1% reported delayed getting medical care due to cost

8.3% did not get needed medical care due to cost

14.5% were uninsured at the time of the interview

(NCHS, 2019)

Pandemic Trends

April 23–May 5, 2020

38.7% reported delayed medical care in the last 4 weeks due to the pandemic

31.7% reported not getting needed medical care in the last 4 weeks due to the pandemic

12.6% were uninsured at the time of the interview

June 23–July 5, 2021

14.6% reported delayed medical care in the last 4 weeks due to the pandemic

12.9% reported not getting needed medical care in the last 4 weeks due to the pandemic

11.0% were uninsured at the time of the interview

(NCHS, 2021a, NCHS, 2021b)

There is no direct prepandemic measure to compare the delay or not getting needed care. Cost is a common reason to delay or not get care but not the only reason. The data from 2020 do not specify exact reasons for reduced access to care, such as cancelations, cutbacks, transportation, avoiding burden on the healthcare system, or fear of exposure to the virus (NCHS, 2021a)

CONCLUSION

Access to care continues to be a major concern in the United States due to its complexity and is subject to influence by a variety of issues, including insurance, social determinants of health, and needs of vulnerable populations. Health professionals and policymakers can advocate within the government, their health systems, or other local organizations to allocate resources for services that may be lacking in their communities. Such individuals can contribute to finding solutions to access issues by researching and learning about issues associated with accessing services that impact healthcare costs, as well as by researching how to design healthcare services that provide quality care, increase access to care, and reduce overall healthcare costs.

REFERENCES

Agency for Healthcare Research and Quality. (2018, June). Elements of access to health care. https://www.ahrq.gov/research/findings/nhqrdr/chartbooks/access/elements.html

Agency of Healthcare Research and Quality. (2017). National healthcare quality and disparities report chartbook on rural health care (AHRQ Pub. No. 17(18)-0001-2-EF; p. 58). https://www.ahrq.gov/sites/default/files/wysiwyg/research/findings/nhqrdr/chartbooks/qdr-ruralhealthchartbook-update.pdf

American Hospital Association. (n.d.). Community health assessment toolkit. https://www.healthycommunities.org/resources/community-health-assessment-toolkit

American Hospital Association. (2016). Ensuring access in vulnerable communities—taskforce report and resources. American Hospital Association. https://www.aha.org/issue-landing-page/2016-11-16-ensuring-access-vulnerable-communities-taskforce-report-and-resources

Arenson, M., Hudson, P. J., Lee, N., & Lai, B. (2019). The evidence on school-based health centers: A review. Global Pediatric Health, 6, 2333794X19828745. https://doi.org/10.1177/2333794X19828745

Atske, S., & Perrin, R. (2021, July 16). Home broadband adoption, computer ownership vary by race, ethnicity in the U.S. Pew Research Center. https://www.pewresearch.org/fact-tank/2021/07/16/home-broadband-adoption-computer-ownership-vary-by-race-ethnicity-in-the-u-s/

Becevic, M., Sheets, L. R., Wallach, E., McEowen, A., Bass, A., Mutrux, E. R., & Edison, K. E. (2020). Telehealth and telemedicine in Missouri. Missouri Medicine, 117(3), 228–234.

Beck, T. L., Le, T.-K., Henry-Okafor, Q., & Shah, M. K. (2017). Medical care for undocumented immigrants: national and international issues. Primary Care, 44(1), e1–e13. https://doi.org/10.1016/j.pop.2016.09.005

Bernstein, R. (2012). U.S. Census Bureau projections show a slower growing, older, more diverse nation a half century from now. United States Census Bureau, Public Information Office. CB12-243. Available at https://www.census.gov/newsroom/releases/archives/population/cb12-243.html

Blumenthal, D., Fowler, E. J., Abrams, M., & Collins, S. R. (2020). Covid-19—Implications for the health care system. New England Journal of Medicine, 383(15), 1483–1488. https://doi.org/10.1056/NEJMsb2021088

Carron, R. (2020). Health disparities in American Indians/Alaska Natives: Implications for nurse practitioners. The Nurse Practitioner, 45(6), 26–32. https://doi.org/10.1097/01.NPR.0000666188.79797.a7

Cerisier, K. (2019). Connecting chronically ill, uninsured patients who use the emergency department as a medical home: A process improvement project. Journal of Emergency Nursing, 45(3), 249–253. https://doi.org/10.1016/j.jen.2018.08.011

Christopher, A. S., McCormick, D., Woolhandler, S., Himmelstein, D. U., Bor, D. H., & Wilper, A. P. (2016). Access to care and chronic disease outcomes among medicaid-insured persons versus the uninsured. American Journal of Public Health, 106(1), 63–69. https://doi.org/10.2105/AJPH.2015.302925

Cleveland, K. A., Motter, T., & Smith, Y. (2019). Affordable care: Harnessing the power of nurses. The Online Journal of Issues in Nursing, 24(2), Manuscript 2. https://doi.org/10.3912/OJIN.Vol24No02Man02

Cohen, C., Baird, M., Koirola, N., Kandrack, R., & Martsolf, G. (2021). The surgical and anesthesia workforce and provision of surgical services in rural communities: A mixed-methods examination. The Journal of Rural Health, 37(1), 45–54. https://doi.org/10.1111/jrh.12417

Cromer, K. J., Wofford, L., & Wyant, D. K. (2019). Barriers to healthcare access facing American Indian and Alaska natives in rural America. Journal of Community Health Nursing, 36(4), 165–187. https://doi.org/10.1080/07370016.2019.1665320

Cyr, M. E., Etchin, A. G., Guthrie, B. J., & Benneyan, J. C. (2019). Access to specialty healthcare in urban versus rural US populations: A systematic literature review. *BMC Health Services Research*, 19(1), 974. https://doi.org/10.1186/s12913-019-4815-5

Defense Health Agency. (n.d.). Tricare. Tricare.Mil.. https://www.tricare.mil/

Department of Health and Human Services, Office of the Secretary. (2016). Nondiscrimination in health programs and activities. *Federal Register*, 81(96), 31376–31473.

Dickey, L. M., Budge, S. L., Katz-Wise, S. L., & Garza, M. V. (2016). Health disparities in the transgender community: Exploring differences in insurance coverage. *Psychology of Sexual Orientation and Gender Diversity*, 3(3), 275. https://doi.org/10.1037/sgd0000169

Dickman, S. L., Himmelstein, D. U., & Woolhandler, S. (2017). Inequality and the health-care system in the USA. *The Lancet*, 389(10077), 1431–1441. https://doi.org/10.1016/S0140-6736(17)30398-7

Doraiswamy, S., Abraham, A., Mamtani, R., & Cheema, S. (2020). Use of telehealth during the COVID-19 pandemic: Scoping review. *Journal of Medical Internet Research*, 22(12), e24087. https://doi.org/10.2196/24087

Garfield, R., Orgera, K., & Damico, A. (2019). *The uninsured and the ACA: A primer–key facts about health insurance and the uninsured amidst changes to the affordable care act*. KFF. https://www.kff.org/report-section/the-uninsured-and-the-aca-a-primer-key-facts-about-health-insurance-and-the-uninsured-amidst-changes-to-the-affordable-care-act-introduction/

Health Resources & Services Administration. (2017, April 21). Federally qualified health centers. Official Web Site of the U.S. Health Resources and Services Administration. https://www.hrsa.gov/opa/eligibility-and-registration/health-centers/fqhc/index.html

Health Resources & Services Administration. (2021, August 16). What is telehealth? https://telehealth.hhs.gov/patients/understanding-telehealth/

HealthCare.gov. (n.d.). Affordable Care Act (ACA)—HealthCare.gov glossary. HealthCare.Gov. https://www.healthcare.gov/glossary/affordable-care-act/

healthinsurance.org. (n.d.). What is private health insurance? Healthinsurance.Org. https://www.healthinsurance.org/glossary/private-health-insurance/

Indian Health Service. (n.d.). Indian health service: The federal program for American Indians and Alaska natives>. Indian Health Service. https://www.ihs.gov/default/

Institute of Medicine. (1993). Access to health care in America. In M. Millman (Ed.), *Access to health care in America*. National Academies Press (US). https://www.ncbi.nlm.nih.gov/books/NBK235885/

Kalma, X. (2016). Mind your words. In Z. Sharman (Ed.), The remedy: Queer and trans voices on health and health care (pp. 128–130). Arsenal Pulp Press. https://zenasharman.com/the-remedy

Kamarck, E., & Stenglein, C. (2019, November 12). How many undocumented immigrants are in the United States and who are they? *Brookings*. https://www.brookings.edu/policy2020/votervital/how-many-undocumented-immigrants-are-in-the-united-states-and-who-are-they/

KFF's State Health Facts. (2019). Datasource: U.S. Census Bureau's American Community Survey (ACS). KFF. https://www.kff.org/other/state-indicator/total-population/

KFF's State Health Facts. (2021). Medicaid income eligibility limits for adults as a percent of the federal poverty level. KFF. https://www.kff.org/health-reform/state-indicator/medicaid-income-eligibility-limits-for-adults-as-a-percent-of-the-federal-poverty-level/

Kiser, L. H., & Butler, J. (2020). Improving equitable access to cervical cancer screening and management. *American Journal of Nursing*, 120(11), 58–67. https://doi.org/10.1097/01.NAJ.0000721944.67166.17

Ko, M., Needleman, J., Derose, K. P., Laugesen, M. J., & Ponce, N. A. (2014). Residential segregation and the survival of U.S. Urban Public Hospitals. *Medical Care Research and Review*, 71(3), 243–260. https://doi.org/10.1177/1077558713515079

Krahn, G. L., Walker, D. K., & Correa-De-Araujo, R. (2015). Persons with disabilities as an unrecognized health disparity population. *American Journal of Public Health*, 105(Suppl. 2), S198–S206. https://doi.org/10.2105/AJPH.2014.302182

Lavarreda, S. A., Brown, E. R., & Bolduc, C. D. (2011). Underinsurance in the United States: An interaction of costs to consumers, benefit design, and access to care. *Annual Review of Public Health*, 32(1), 471–482. https://doi.org/10.1146/annurev.publhealth.012809.103655

Learmonth, C., Viloria, R., Lambert, C., Goldhammer, H., & Keuroghlian, A. S. (2018). Barriers to insurance coverage for transgender patients. *American Journal of Obstetrics and Gynecology*, 219(3), 272.e1–272.e4. https://doi.org/10.1016/j.ajog.2018.04.046

Mahmoudi, E., & Meade, M. (2015). Disparities in access to health care among adults with physical disabilities: Analysis of a representative national sample for a ten-year period, *Disability and Health Journal*, 8(2), 182–190. https://doi.org/10.1016/j.dhjo.2014.08.007

McClintock, H., Barg, F., Katz, S., Stineman, M., Krueger, A., Colletti, P., Boellstorff, T., & Bogner, H. (2016). Health care experiences and perceptions among people with and without disabilities. *Disability and Health Journal*, 9(1), 74–82. https://doi.org/10.1016/j.dhjo.2015.08.007

McDermott, D., Cox, C., Rudowitz, R., & Garfield, R. (2020, December 9). *How has the pandemic affected health coverage in the U.S.?* KFF. https://www.kff.org/policy-watch/how-has-the-pandemic-affected-health-coverage-in-the-u-s/

National Academies of Sciences, Engineering, and Medicine. (2021). Population health in challenging times: Insights from key domains: proceedings of a workshop. National Academies Press. https://doi.org/10.17226/26143

National Center for Health Statistics. (2019). National health interview survey. Centers for Disease Control and Prevention. https://wwwn.cdc.gov/NHISDataQueryTool/SHS_adult/index.html

National Center for Health Statistics. (2021a, August 31). Reduced access to care—household pulse survey—COVID-19. https://www.cdc.gov/nchs/covid19/pulse/reduced-access-to-care.htm

National Center for Health Statistics. (2021b, October 6). Health insurance coverage—household pulse survey—COVID-19. https://www.cdc.gov/nchs/covid19/pulse/health-insurance-coverage.htm

Ngaage, L. M., Knighton, B. J., McGlone, K. L., Benzel, C. A., Rada, E. M., Bluebond-Langner, R., & Rasko, Y. M. (2019). Health insurance coverage of gender-affirming top surgery in the United States. *Plastic and Reconstructive Surgery, 144*(4), 824–833. https://doi.org/10.1097/PRS.0000000000006012

Núñez, A., Sreeganga, S. D., & Ramaprasad, A. (2021). Access to healthcare during COVID-19. *International Journal of Environmental Research and Public Health, 18*(6), 2980. https://doi.org/10.3390/ijerph18062980

Office of Disease Prevention and Health Promotion. (n.d.-a). Access to health services. Healthy People 2020. U.S Department of Health and Human Services. https://www.healthypeople.gov/2020/topics-objectives/topic/Access-to-Health-Services

Office of Disease Prevention and Health Promotion. (n.d.-b). Access to primary care. Healthy People 2020. U.S. Department of Health and Human Services. https://health.gov/healthypeople/objectives-and-data/social-determinants-health/literature-summaries/access-primary-care

Office of Disease Prevention and Health Promotion. (n.d.-c). Health care access and quality. Healthy People 2030. U.S. Department of Social Services. https://health.gov/healthypeople

Patient Protection and Affordable Care Act. (2010). Patient Protection and Affordable Care Act, 42 U.S.C. § 18001. (2010).

Rau, J., & Huetteman, E. (2020, September 15). Some urban hospitals face closure or cutbacks as the pandemic adds to fiscal woes. *NPR.* https://www.npr.org/sections/health-shots/2020/09/15/912866179/some-urban-hospitals-face-closure-or-cutbacks-as-the-pandemic-adds-to-fiscal-woe

Robert Wood Johnson Foundation. (n.d.). Access to care. RWJF. https://www.rwjf.org/en/cultureofhealth/taking-action/strengthening-services-and-systems/access-to-care.html

Rice, D. (2019). LGBTQ: The communities within a community. *Clinical Journal of Oncology Nursing, 23*(6).

Safer, J. D., & Tangpricha, V. (2019). Care of transgender persons. *New England Journal of Medicine, 381*(25), 2451–2460.

Salsberg, E., Richwine, C., Westergaard, S., Portela Martinez, M., Oyeyemi, T., Vichare, A., & Chen, C. P. (2021). Estimation and comparison of current and future racial/ethnic representation in the US health care workforce. *JAMA Network Open, 4*(3), e213789. https://doi.org/10.1001/jamanetworkopen.2021.3789

Schoenbaum, N. (2020). The new law of gender nonconformity. *Minnesota Law Review, 105*, 831.

Shandra, C. L. (2018). Disability as inequality: Social disparities, health disparities, and participation in daily activities. *Social Forces, 97*(1), 157–192.

Shi, L., & Stevens, G. D. (2021). *Vulnerable populations in the United States.* John Wiley and Sons.

Tolbert, J., Orgera, K., & Damico, A. (2020). *Key facts about the uninsured population.* KFF. https://www.kff.org/uninsured/issue-brief/key-facts-about-the-uninsured-population/

U. S. Government Accountability Office. (2020). Rural hospital closures: Affected residents had reduced access to health care services (GAO-21-93). https://www.gao.gov/products/gao-21-93

United States Census Bureau. (2019). U.S. Census Bureau quickfacts: United States, population estimates. Census.Gov. https://www.census.gov/quickfacts/fact/table/US/PST045219

U.S. Centers for Medicare and Medicaid Services. (n.d.-a). Children's Health Insurance Program (CHIP) eligibility requirements. HealthCare.Gov. https://www.healthcare.gov/medicaid-chip/childrens-health-insurance-program/

U.S. Centers for Medicare and Medicaid Services. (n.d.-b). Medicaid. Medicaid.Gov. https://www.medicaid.gov/medicaid/index.html

U.S. Centers for Medicare and Medicaid Services. (n.d.-c). Medicare.gov: The official U.S. government site for medicare. Medicare.Gov. https://www.medicare.gov/

U.S. Department of Veterans Affairs. (2021, March 15). VA health care. Veterans Affairs. https://www.va.gov/health-care/

Van Dijk, J. (2020). *The digital divide.* John Wiley and Sons.

Vogels, E. A. (2021, August 19). *Some digital divides persist between rural, urban and suburban America.* Pew Research Center. https://www.pewresearch.org/fact-tank/2021/08/19/some-digital-divides-persist-between-rural-urban-and-suburbanamerica/

Williams, J. P. (2019, July 10). Code red: The grim state of urban hospitals. *Us News and World Report.* www.usnews.com/news/healthiest-communities/articles/2019-07-10/poor-minorities-bear-the-brunt-as-urban-hospitals-close

Woolhandler, S., & Himmelstein, D. U. (2017). The relationship of health insurance and mortality: Is lack of insurance deadly? *Annals of Internal Medicine, 167*(6), 424–431. https://doi.org/10.7326/M17-1403

Yu, S. W. Y., Hill, C., Ricks, M. L., Bennet, J., & Oriol, N. E. (2017). The scope and impact of mobile health clinics in the United States: A literature review. *International Journal for Equity in Health, 16*(1), 178. https://doi.org/10.1186/s12939-017-0671-2

CHAPTER 9

Social-Ecological Approach to the Prevention and Mitigation of Child Maltreatment During a Time of Social Disruption

Linda A. Lewandowski and Linda C. Lewin

LEARNING OBJECTIVES

- Apply the social-ecological model to an analysis of risk and protective factors relating to child maltreatment, with an emphasis on the time of social disruption due to the COVID-19 pandemic.

- Identify physical, psychological, cognitive, and academic effects of child maltreatment and factors that may work to mitigate negative short- and long-term effects.

- Discuss the impact of social isolation; closure of schools, daycare facilities, and other community surveillance; and reduced availability of social and "safety net" resources on children, families, and communities, and implications for risk of child maltreatment.

- Discuss the impact of poverty, financial difficulty, job loss, racism, and other social determinants of health on individual, family, community, and societal risk and protective factors related to child maltreatment, and how these factors are highlighted during times of social disruption.

- Discuss the role of Child Protective Services (CPS) in relation to child maltreatment and service implications and modifications that occur during a time of social disruption and isolation such as that experienced by the whole of U.S. society in the COVID-19 pandemic.

- Use the social-ecological model to understand opportunities for proactive prevention of child maltreatment and to guide surveillance, recognition, and interventions in situations of child maltreatment at the individual, family, community, and societal levels.

This chapter describes a social-ecological approach to the prevention and mitigation of child maltreatment in the United States, focusing on the COVID-19 pandemic as a model of widespread social disruption. Recognizing the importance of identifying both risk and protective factors at each level of the model, this chapter explores the many influences on child maltreatment and the many opportunities for prevention and intervention at individual, relationship, community, and societal levels.

INTRODUCTION

The COVID-19 pandemic in 2020, 2021, and 2022 has provided a graphic example of an unexpected stressor that resulted in the disruption of many of our usual social systems and relationships. Children and families were isolated from many (perhaps most) of their usual social interactions and from community and societal connections and resources. The disruptions and isolation due to the pandemic occurred against the backdrop of long-standing, systemic racial inequities and injustices, many of which became startlingly evident in the aftermath of highly publicized police shootings and the resultant protests. All of this occurred in the context of a highly contentious and divisive presidential election and politicization of public health measures, which further contributed to a prevailing cultural aura of conflict, disruption, distrust, and high levels of stress (American Psychological Association [APA], 2020a). When these stressors were combined with risk factors such as poor social support systems, disrupted or nonexistent community resources, disrupted and/or substandard schools, and neighborhoods of disadvantage, the possibility of negative responses and outcomes was markedly increased.

One societal dynamic of continuing concern during the COVID-19 pandemic is that of child maltreatment. In any time, maltreatment is a very significant public health problem that affects approximately 1 billion children annually across the globe (Merrick & Latzman, 2014; Pinheiro, 2006; World Health Organization [WHO], 2020). However, during the COVID-19 pandemic, with disruptions in the usual supports and surveillance that occur in schools and communities, and little to no access to the usual social support from family, friends, daycare, or other community resources, concern among public health, child welfare, and healthcare professionals; educators; and other entities involved with the well-being and safety of children was heightened, and family violence increased (Usher et al., 2020).

Child maltreatment can be defined as "any act or series of acts of commission (abuse) or omission (neglect) by a parent or other caregiver that results in harm, potential for harm, or threat of harm to a child (Centers for Disease Control and Prevention [CDC], 2021; Leeb et al., 2008). Table 9.1 shows brief definitions of child maltreatment as identified by the CDC (2021).

In the past, child maltreatment was attributed solely to characteristics of parents. However, in 1993, Dubowitz and associates argued that an ecological model that includes the social context (i.e., family, community, society, and the broader culture, as well as socioeconomic factors) presented a more comprehensive and accurate picture of the circumstances that can lead to child maltreatment (Berube et al., 2020; Dubowitz et al., 1993). Ecosystem models are now identified as the most relevant models to provide an understanding of the phenomenon of child maltreatment and to suggest prevention and intervention approaches (Berube et al., 2020; Molnar et al., 2016; Shen et al., 2020; Tomison & Wise, 1999). Thus, we will use the social-ecological model developed by the CDC as a framework for this discussion (CDC, 2021).

The COVID-19 pandemic is an illustrative model of social disruption highlighting the multiple interrelationships of risk and protective factors that may contribute to the experience or perpetration of child maltreatment. Other types of widespread social disruption, such as natural disasters or war, may also result in similar negative outcomes (Catani et al., 2008; Olema et al., 2014).

TABLE 9.1 Brief CDC Definitions of Child Maltreatment Subtypes*

Subtype of Maltreatment	Definition
Physical abuse (PA)	Intentional use of physical force against a child that results in, or has the potential to result in, physical injury.
	Physical injuries to the anal or genital area or surrounding areas (e.g., anal or genital bruising or tearing; internal injuries resulting from penetration by a penis, hand, finger, or other object) that occur during attempted or completed sexual abuse (SA), or other physical injuries that result from attempted or completed SA (e.g., bruises due to restraint, hitting, pushing) are considered SA and do not constitute PA.
Sexual abuse (SA)	Any completed or attempted (noncompleted) sexual act, sexual contact with, or exploitation (i.e., noncontact sexual interaction) of a child by a caregiver.
Psychological abuse	Intentional caregiver behavior that conveys to a child that they are worthless, flawed, unloved, unwanted, endangered, or valued only in meeting another's needs.
Neglect	The failure to provide for a child's basic physical, emotional, or educational needs or to protect a child from harm or potential harm.
Failure to provide	Failure by a caregiver to meet a child's basic physical, emotional, medical/dental, or educational needs, or combination thereof.
Failure to supervise	Failure by the caregiver to ensure a child's safety within and outside the home given the child's emotional and developmental needs.

*For complete definitions, see Leeb et al., 2008.
Source: Centers for Disease Control and Prevention. (2021). *Child maltreatment: A public health overview and prevention considerations.* nursingworld.org

THE CDC SOCIAL-ECOLOGICAL MODEL

The four-level social-ecological model developed by the CDC (2021) provides a useful framework for understanding the factors that can lead to or prevent child maltreatment and that can guide potential prevention strategies. The overlapping rings in the model are nested within each other and influence each other in a reciprocal fashion. The CDC (2021) model is like Bronfenbrenner's well-established bioecological model (Bronfenbrenner, 1994), in which he posited that five interrelated systems, each nested within the next and influencing each other, played important roles in a child's development and well-being. The CDC social-ecological model demonstrates the "complex interplay between individual, relationship, community, and societal factors" (CDC, 2021) and is more streamlined and perhaps easier to apply than the Bronfenbrenner version. Each of the levels expresses a widening circle of influence: An adaptation of the CDC's (2021) description of each level is shown in Figure 9.1.

Individual Factors

The individual level focuses on the biological, personal history, and family factors that can increase the likelihood of becoming a victim or perpetrator of child maltreatment or other forms of violence. These include factors such as age, education, race, ethnicity, family income, and, in terms of possible perpetrators, substance use, psychopathology, or history of abuse.

Relationship Factors

The next level looks at the child's relationships that may increase the risk of experiencing violence as a victim or perpetrator or that may provide a protective "buffer." This includes relationships with family members, friends, and peers, as well as other types of relationships

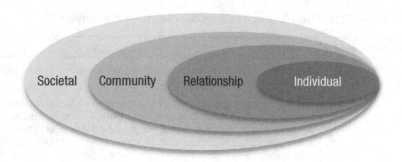

Figure 9.1 CDC Social-Ecological Model.

in the child's close social circle that may influence their behavior and contribute to their over-all experience. For example, parental stress related to many factors inherent in the COVID-19 pandemic, such as job loss, social isolation, death of a family member, financial difficulties, and problematic coping strategies such as alcohol or drug use, may affect the child-parent rela-tionship and lead to increased risk of child maltreatment (Griffith, 2020; Rodriguez et al., 2021).

Community Factors

This level encompasses the settings in which social relationships occur, such as schools, workplaces, faith-based institutions, and neighborhoods, and seeks to identify risk and protective factors that may prevent child maltreatment or, alternatively, further endanger children. The closure of schools and workplaces and "shelter in place" orders during the pandemic had many implications for children and families. The social determinants of health (U.S. Department of Health and Human Services [DHHS], 2020), especially poverty, housing instability, parental educational attainment, food insecurity, and lack of insurance have been found to be significantly associated with child maltreatment (Hunter & Flores, 2021). Child maltreatment has also been correlated with structural and neighborhood fac-tors such as community social organization: economic and family resources, residential instability, household and age structure, large numbers of children per adult resident, pop-ulation turnover, concentration of woman-headed families, and geographic proximity of neighborhoods to concentrated poverty (Coulton et al., 1995).

Societal Factors

The outer level of Figure 9.1 encompasses the broad societal factors that help to create a cli-mate in which child maltreatment and/or other types of violence or neglect are encouraged or inhibited These include social and cultural norms, beliefs, and customs as well as the broader health, economic, educational, and social policies that help to maintain economic or social inequalities between some groups in society.

Child maltreatment is thus a multidetermined phenomenon, with a combination of all of these factors—individual, relational, community, and societal—either contributing to or decreasing a child's level of risk. The model suggests that to prevent violence—in this case, child maltreatment—it is vital to intervene across multiple levels of the model at the same time. Intervening at multiple levels is more likely to have a greater influence on the effectiveness and sustainability of prevention efforts over time and to achieve a more widespread impact.

RISK AND PROTECTIVE FACTORS

In pioneering work, Garmezy (1971, 1981; Garmezy & Rutter, 1985; Masten & Garmezy, 1985) identified the concepts of risk, resilience, invulnerability, stress resistance, and risk and protective factors and launched a paradigm shift in how we understand children's responses to adverse events. Instead of focusing solely on the negative outcomes of adverse experiences such as maltreatment, resilience theory provides strong evidence that while some factors place children at increased risk, there are also "protective factors" that can help to decrease risk and help us understand more positive adaptations in the face of adversity (Rutter, 1985). More recent work on individuals' responses to adverse childhood experiences (ACEs), such as maltreatment, provide further understanding of the many factors involved in prevention of negative events and the mitigation of negative reactions to adverse events. A more in-depth discussion of ACEs is found in Chapter 22.

For the purposes of our discussion here, we return to the social-ecological model. Within each of the four levels in the CDC social-ecological model, various factors, called *risk factors*, can increase the likelihood of experiencing or perpetrating child maltreatment but may or may not be direct causes. A combination of individual, relational, community, and societal factors contribute to the risk of child abuse and neglect. Risk factors can also determine an individual's responses to the adverse events that they experience. They can be defined as "characteristics at the biological, psychological, family, community, or cultural level that precede and are associated with a higher likelihood of negative outcomes" (CDC, 2021).

Alternatively, other factors may lessen the likelihood of children being abused or neglected or of adults perpetrating violence. These *protective factors*—again, found in all levels of the model—may act as "buffers" or "positive countering events" (Substance Abuse and Mental Health Services Administration [SAMHSA], 2021) that help to prevent child maltreatment. The presence of protective factors also can reduce a risk factor's impact and lead to a lower likelihood of negative outcomes over time. Some risk and protective factors are fixed and do not change over time, while others are more dynamic and can be modified. Identifying and understanding protective factors are equally as important as researching risk factors. Effective prevention efforts focus on reducing those risk factors and strengthening protective factors that are most closely related to the problem being addressed—in this case, child maltreatment. Table 9.2 identifies protective factors at the individual, family, and community levels.

TABLE 9.2 Protective Factors for Child Abuse and Neglect

Individual Protective Factors	Family Protective Factors	Community Protective Factors
• Caregivers who create safe, positive relationships with children • Caregivers who practice nurturing parenting skills and provide emotional support • Caregivers who can meet basic needs of food, shelter, education, and health services • Caregivers who have a college degree or higher and have steady employment	• Families with strong social support networks and stable, positive relationships with the people around them • Families where caregivers are present and interested in the child • Families where caregivers enforce household rules and engage in child monitoring • Families with caring adults outside the family who can serve as role models or mentors	• Communities with access to safe, stable housing • Communities where families have access to high-quality preschool • Communities where families have access to nurturing and safe childcare • Communities where families have access to safe, engaging after-school programs and activities • Communities where families have access to medical care and mental health services • Communities where families have access to economic and financial help • Communities where adults have work opportunities with family-friendly policies

Source: Centers for Disease Control and Prevention. (2022). *Violence prevention.* www.cdc.gov/violenceprevention/childabuseandneglect/riskprotectivefactors.html.

TOXIC STRESS IN CHILDREN

When a stressful event, such as child maltreatment, occurs, an activation of the hypothalamic-pituitary-adrenal axis, the body's stress response system, is triggered (Herman et al., 2016). *Tolerable stress* occurs when a child is confronted with a severe, long-lasting, out-of-the-ordinary, event such as a natural disaster, a death of a family member, or child maltreatment, and the child is helped through the event by a supportive relationship with adults who help to "buffer" this experience and help the child adapt in a positive way. Buffering is the dynamics that parents engage in with their children that reduce the impact of stressors, such as emotional coaching, being available to openly discuss child worries, or maintaining household routines (Bate et al., 2021; Cohodes et al., 2021). When buffering occurs in the presence of other environmental and social protective factors, the activation of the stress response system is time-limited, and long-term effects are mitigated.

Toxic stress can occur when prolonged activation of the stress response system occurs due to the child experiencing stress that is strong, frequent, and/or prolonged, such as physical or emotional abuse, chronic neglect, caregiver substance abuse or mental illness, exposure to violence, and/or the burdens of chronic poverty. Toxic stress is not mitigated by protective, buffering social support (Condon et al., 2018; Reichel, 2019; Shonkoff et al., 2012). This kind of prolonged activation of the stress response system can lead to many long-term negative effects in the body and many chronic physical and mental health issues (Johnson et al., 2013). Preventing toxic stress is another goal of prevention and risk mitigation efforts.

SHORT- AND LONG-TERM EFFECTS OF CHILD MALTREATMENT ON THE CHILD

Physical Effects

Effects of or responses to maltreatment may occur right away or later in life and may impact multiple aspects of the individual's development and well-being: physical, cognitive, psychological, emotional, behavioral, spiritual (Merrick & Latzman, 2014).

Physical health effects may be directly due to the injuries suffered in the abuse such as bruises, fractures, burns, genital injuries, or sexually transmitted infections. Head trauma in infants and very young children may lead to death, visual impairment, motor impairment, and/or cognitive deficits (Parks et al., 2012). Numerous neurobiological and morphological brain changes have been identified in neuroimaging studies, and many of the long-term effects of these changes are still being studied (Teciher & Samson, 2016).

Physical and psychological effects may also be long-term and/or occur later in adulthood. The Adverse Childhood Experiences Study identified a strong relationship between childhood maltreatment and some of the leading risk factors for the top causes of death in adults, such as cancer, ischemic heart disease, depression, substance abuse, chronic lung disease, and liver disease. This study also noted that the greater the number of adverse events (such as multiple types of child maltreatment), the greater the number of negative health outcomes (Felitti et al., 1998; Merrick & Latzman, 2014).

Psychological Effects

Child maltreatment has been identified as "the most important preventable cause of psychopathology." It may account for about 45% of the population attributable risk for childhood-onset psychiatric disorders (Teicher & Samson, 2016). Children who have experienced child maltreatment are at risk of a myriad of mental health disorders (Merrick & Latazman, 2014) both internalizing (e.g., depression, anxiety) and externalizing (e.g., substance use, aggression) behaviors (Bolger & Patterson, 2001; Kaplow & Widom, 2007; Lippard & Nemeroff, 2020).

A number of studies and reviews of longitudinal and cross-sectional research have demonstrated the relationship between childhood maltreatment and subsequent oppositional defiant disorders, antisocial behaviors, and arrests for nonviolent and violent crime (NIkilona & Widow, 2019). However, higher verbal intelligence, reading ability, nonverbal reasoning, and cognitive flexibility were protective against arrests for violent crime, suggesting that interventions aimed at improving cognitive and neuropsychological functions may play an important role in reducing the risk of these negative behaviors (Nikilona & Widow, 2019).

Cognitive and Academic Difficulties

Deficits in cognition, difficulties in learning, and lower academic achievement are also outcomes associated with child maltreatment (Kerr et al., 2000). Maltreated children are often less attentive and engaged in school, have higher absenteeism, get lower grades, have lower test scores, and are more likely to drop out of school than children who are not maltreated (Langsford et al., 2007; Leiter, 2007). Children who experience child maltreatment are at greater risk than their peers for impaired executive functioning, such as working memory, inhibition, and processing speed (DePrince et al., 2009), and these functional deficits may continue into adulthood (Letkiewicz et al., 2021).

Still, some children who experience child maltreatment *do* achieve academically, demonstrating that individual characteristics of the child and of the social environment can serve as protective factors (Palmeri, 2021). For example, in one study (Coohey et al., 2011), children with higher intelligence and children with behavior problems showed higher math and reading scores. The investigators speculate that perhaps these two groups of children can attract more notice and attention, possibly leading to an increased likelihood of school personnel uncovering the maltreatment than might occur with children who are of average performance, are quiet, and do not bring attention to themselves via behavior problems. Children with high intelligence and those with behavior problems also were able to elicit more social support from adults, which could also be a positive protective factor (Coohey et al., 2011; Jaffe & Gallop, 2010).

The importance of identifying and implementing multilayered strategies of prevention is imperative as the consequences of child maltreatment may be profound, long-lasting, and multifaceted. Assessing for and augmenting family strengths and providing community resources may help to provide positive relationships that can buffer some of the negative effects of child maltreatment, thus working to prevent toxic stress.

IMPACT OF SOCIAL DISRUPTIONS DUE TO COVID-19 BY LEVELS IN THE SOCIAL-ECOLOGICAL MODEL

Impact on Reporting and Incidence

The actual effect of social disruption due to the COVID-19 pandemic on the occurrence of child maltreatment remains to be fully understood. Several investigative journalism commentaries (official reports in academic journals are not yet available) found that reports of suspected child abuse to child protection agencies from school personnel, daycare providers, healthcare providers, neighbors, and extended family members (the usual reporters of child abuse) decreased during the social isolation phases of the pandemic (Hager, 2020; Ho & Fassett, 2021; Schmidt & Natanson, 2020). An NBC news analysis of 43 states and Washington, DC conducted in April 2020 found a 40.6% decrease in each state relative to levels reported in April 2019 (Ingram, 2020).

In 2019, prior to the disruption of the pandemic, data from the U.S. DHHS showed that more than two thirds (68.6%) of all reports of alleged child abuse or neglect were made by professionals, with education professionals being the most common professional reporting group (DHHS, 2021). Thus, the closure of schools had a definite impact on the decreased number of suspected child maltreatment reports.

The impact that "fewer eyes on children and thus fewer reports" had on child maltreatment in the aggregate is hard to determine, particularly as most child abuse cases are not identified or prevented even in the best of times. A report from the Marshall Project noted that about 90% of children who are killed because of abuse or neglect did not have previous open child protective services (CPS) cases, indicating that the maltreatment of these children had never been identified or reported (Hager, 2020). Thus, most cases of child maltreatment remain unidentified and hidden in our society, with this situation even more of an issue during societal social disruption resulting in social isolation and disruption of social surveillance and resources.

Despite the decrease in reports to CPS, hospital emergency services reported sharp increases in the number and severity of inflicted child injuries and fatalities (Abramson, 2020). The CDC (Swedo et al., 2020) reported that while the actual number of emergency department visits related to child abuse and neglect remained stable, the percentage of emergency department visits related to child abuse and neglect that resulted in hospitalization significantly increased in 2020 among all age groups compared with 2019 (pre-pandemic).

Impact on Individual Factors

Child Factors

Certain individual characteristics of the child may place them at higher risk for child maltreatment, such as age (children younger than 4 years are at highest risk) or the presence of special needs that may increase caregiver burden, such as disabilities, special education needs, mental health issues, and/or acute or chronic physical illnesses (CDC, 2021). Children with disabilities may have been especially challenging during the pandemic if they could not understand the need for mask wearing and if their usual routines and supportive services were interrupted, placing more pressure and demand on their parents and primary caretakers (Fegert, 2020).

Parental/Perpetrator Factors

Parents with mental illness, single-parent families, and low-income families have higher risks of psychosocial problems due to such factors as partial resource closures or reduced mental health services, pressures to work from home while home schooling their children, fear of losing family members to illness, fear of unemployment and loss of health benefits, no co-parent, and no financial buffers (Fegert et al., 2020; Tso et al., 2020). The multiple, sometimes unrelenting, and seemingly unsolvable demands and stresses may place families at higher levels of stress and risk for child maltreatment (WHO, 2020).

A 2021 report from the DHHS (2021a) noted that in 2019, the 50 states, the District of Columbia, and Puerto Rico reported a total of 525,319 perpetrators of child maltreatment. In this analysis, each perpetrator was counted only once, regardless of the number of children or reports involved. More than three quarters of the perpetrators (77.5%) were parents of their victims, with slightly over half (53%) being women. More than four fifths (83%) were between the ages of 18 and 44 years. In terms of race or ethnicity, almost half of the perpetrators were White (48.9%), with African Americans comprising 21.1% and Hispanic Americans 19.7%. As noted , U.S. national data are not officially released for 2 years after any given calendar year, so any changes in these proportions during the pandemic years remain to be seen. Table 9.3 identifies additional risk factors for perpetration of child maltreatment at individual, family, and community levels (CDC, 2021).

TABLE 9.3 Risk Factors for Perpetration

Individual Risk Factors	Family Risk Factors	Community Risk Factors
◆ Caregivers with drug or alcohol issues ◆ Caregivers with mental health issues, including depression ◆ Caregivers who don't understand children's needs or development	◆ Families that have family members in jail or prison ◆ Families that are isolated from and not connected to other people (extended family, friends, neighbors) ◆ Family violence, including relationship violence	◆ Communities with high rates of violence and crime ◆ Communities with high rates of poverty and limited educational and economic opportunities ◆ Communities with high unemployment rates ◆ Communities with easy access to drugs and alcohol
◆ Caregivers who were abused or neglected as children ◆ Caregivers who are young or single parents or parents with many children Caregivers with low education or income ◆ Caregivers experiencing high levels of parenting stress and economic stress ◆ Caregivers who use spanking and other forms of corporal punishment for discipline ◆ Caregivers in the home who are not a biological parent ◆ Caregivers with attitudes accepting of or justifying violence or aggression	◆ Families with high conflict and negative communication styles	◆ Communities where neighbors don't know or look out for each other and there is low community involvement among residents ◆ Communities with few community activities for young people ◆ Communities with unstable housing and where residents move frequently ◆ Communities where families frequently experience food insecurity

Source: Centers for Disease Control and Prevention. (2022). *Violence prevention.* www.cdc.gov/violenceprevention/childabuseandneglect/riskprotectivefactors.html.

EFFECTS OF POVERTY, RACE, AND ETHNICITY ON CHILD MALTREATMENT

Poverty as a Major Factor

The experience of living in poverty places a myriad of stresses on families and this, along with many other factors as identified in our discussion of the ecological model, may increase the risk for child abuse and neglect. The rates of child abuse and neglect were five times higher for children in families with low socioeconomic status (SES) than for children in families with higher SES (CDC, 2021), even before the COVID-19 pandemic.

A comprehensive nationwide epidemiological study of child maltreatment in the United States found that poverty was the major determinant of prevalence. Kim & Drake (2018) found that with increasing county child poverty rates, the total and type-specific child maltreatment rates increased in all race/ethnicity groups. They noted that at similar poverty levels, the rates of reports for White families trended higher than those for Black families, while reports for Hispanic families trended lower. They concluded that "from a policy perspective, our data confirm emerging local findings showing that Black/White racial disproportionality in official maltreatment is almost certainly a reflection of economic issues, rather than bias in the child welfare systems" (Kim & Drake, 2018). The finding that

Hispanic Americans living in poverty situations had markedly lower rates of official child maltreatment once SES was controlled for may be due to social and cultural protective factors present in Hispanic culture, such as familism, religiosity, and strong social supports (Kim & Drake, 2018; Putnam-Hornstein et al., 2013).

Race and Racism Factors

Race and ethnicity often serve as markers for a complex interaction of economic, social, and environmental factors that influence the health of individuals, families, and communities (Putnam-Hornstein et al., 2013). Children of color are more likely to live in conditions of poverty than White children. The Kids Count data (Annie E. Casey Foundation, 2020) depict the percentage of children who live in families with incomes below the federal poverty level. Data from the past 10 years from the Kids Count Data Center show a consistent picture as illustrated by the 2019 data: Black or African American, 31%; American Indian, 30%; Hispanic or Latino, 23%; two or more races, 17%; Asian and Pacific Islander, 10%; and non-Hispanic White, 10%.

The role that systemic racism has played and continues to play in living conditions (individual, relational, community, and societal) that place children of color in more vulnerable positions is just beginning to be examined in our society. Concurrent with the COVID-19 pandemic, as noted earlier, high-profile incidents such as the deaths of Trayvon Martin, George Floyd, and others and the resultant Black Lives Matter movement (Turan, 2020) have awakened the nation's and the world's consciousness to long-standing systemic and cultural practices that place particularly African American families, but also other families of color, at a disadvantage compared to White families. A quote from the U.S. Conference of Catholic Bishops sums up the etiology of these disparities: "Today's continuing inequalities in education, housing, employment, wealth, and representation in leadership positions are rooted in our country's shameful history of slavery and systemic racism" (Koppleman, 2020).

Many social disruptions occurred in the 2020 to 2021 period. Protests and demonstrations took place in a highly contentious social and political climate during an election year already marked by high levels of distrust, perceived threat, and misinformation. The politicization of COVID-19 precautions and enforced public health measures served to increase confusion, discord, and risk to the public's health. These events occurring with a concurrent raging global pandemic of a potentially lethal illness led to extremely high levels of social disruption and stress that were especially difficult for those living in poverty and without adequate resources and support. Scenes of police brutality depicted in the media served as retraumatizing triggers, causing some African Americans to re-experience the trauma from confrontations they had experienced in the past.

Systemic racism has been defined as "the formalization of a set of institutional, historical, cultural and interpersonal practices within a society that more often than not puts one social or ethnic group in a better position to succeed, and at the same time disadvantages other groups in a consistent and constant manner that disparities develop between the groups over a period of time" (Koppleman, 2020).

As in every aspect of our society, systemic racism has been identified as operating in child protection decisions—certainly prior to, but also continuing during, the COVID-19 pandemic. The perceptions of disparities based on race must be teased out, however, by controlling for other known major risk factors. Derezotes et al. (2005) found that African American children were placed in foster care two to three times more often than White children. Others have found disparities in treatment and outcomes, such as multiple foster home changes, placements in group homes, and a decreased likelihood of return to the children's family of origin (Kokaliari, 2019). However, before concluding that these disproportionate numbers are due to racism in the system, more analysis is needed of co-occurring factors. Putnam-Hornstein et al. studied the full population of children born in California in

2002, linking birth records to CPS records to identify all child maltreatment referrals by age 5 years. They found that compared to White children, Black children were twice as likely to be referred for maltreatment, substantiated as victims, and entered into foster care by age 5 years. However, after controlling for socioeconomic and health factors associated with maltreatment, Black children had a lower risk of referral, substantiation, and foster care placement than socioeconomically similar White children.

Higher numbers of removals occur in low-income single parent African American families, who are more likely to live in unsafe neighborhoods with little choice in affordable housing (Kriz & Skivenes, 2011; Maguire-Jack et al., 2015).

A qualitative study by Kokaliari et al. (2019) provided a rich description of the complex, defeating experiences of African American families who encountered the child protection system during investigations and child removal. Themes included: child removal deemed as punishment for poverty by CPS, single parenthood, inflexibly strict CPS rules that made the families' situation more difficult, and unaddressed maternal trauma affecting parenting style. They also identified the many "system" expectations for multiple services for the child despite limited or no transportation options. Another theme was that of employers who were inflexible about scheduling time for the children's needs, placing the parents in untenable conflicts of unachievable expectations.

More Effects of Poverty and Low Income

Children living in poverty faced disproportional disruption, pandemic-related trauma, and economic instability during the COVID-19 pandemic. Poverty complicates parents' abilities to meet their children's needs. For example, food insecurity such as that experienced by increasing numbers of families during the pandemic has been shown in earlier studies to be associated with increased rates of psychological and physical aggression (Helton et al., 2019) and abuse (Yang, 2015), likely due to the myriad of other poverty-related stressors that are concomitant with food insecurity. School closures had a heavy impact on children living in poverty who rely most heavily on school-based services for nutritional, physical, and mental health needs in addition to their education (Masonbrink & Hurley, 2020). A survey conducted in April 2020 found that 35% of households with children younger than 18 years were food insecure, which was a twofold increase compared to 2018 (Wozniak et al., 2020), thus reflecting the economic impact of the pandemic on many families, especially those at the lower end of the SES spectrum.

Although some families experienced job loss, alternatively, many low-level jobs were deemed "essential" and parents were required to go to work, leaving their children in questionably safe childcare conditions and potentially vulnerable to child maltreatment. Because of the factors of enforced social isolation dictated by pandemic-related measures and less available resources and social supports, children from lower SES groups may also have been burdened with the care of siblings, grandparents, and other household members, some with physical and mental health disorders. Although these factors were present in low SES White families also, Black and Hispanic workers were overrepresented in the essential workforce, thus placing them at higher risk for COVID-19 exposure (Godoy & Wood, 2020; Shen et al., 2020). Thus, Black, Hispanic, and Native American families were disproportionally affected by COVID-19 illnesses and deaths of family members (CDC, 2020; Vasquez Reyes, 2020.)

Families of color are also more likely to live in neighborhoods with more structural factors that contribute to the development of chronic health conditions, such as neighborhood pollution leading to higher rates of asthma, thus making them more vulnerable to the respiratory effect of COVID-19 (Shen et al., 2020). Even prior to the COVID-19 pandemic, a report by WHO noted that "poor and unequal living conditions are the consequences of deeper structural conditions that together fashion the way societies are organized—poor social policies and programs, unfair economic arrangements, and bad politics." The toxic combination of these and other factors mentioned in this chapter led to the disproportionate impact of the pandemic. More illness, more deaths, and more losses mean more social disruption, which led to higher levels of stress at a time when social support was also difficult to access.

Attacks on Asian Americans

The pandemic and public health restrictions were used as pretext to attack minorities, particularly those of Asian descent, immigrants, and people with differing political views (European Union Agency for Fundamental Human Rights, 2021). Due to misinformation and false attributions that the virus was somehow the fault of Asian communities in the United States, Asian American families have been subjected to xenophobic remarks and actual physical attacks (Kambhampaty, 2020). Racial discrimination is associated with depression, anxiety, posttraumatic stress disorder, low self-esteem, and conduct problems in children as well as a higher risk for other mental and physical illnesses (Shonoff & Williams, 2020; Williams, 2018).

Effects of Economic Difficulties on Child Maltreatment

Multiple large prepandemic population-based surveillance studies of child maltreatment in the United States found that unemployed parents were approximately four times more likely to neglect their children and twice as likely to physically abuse them than employed parents (Sedlack et al., 2010). This was a directional finding replicated in large longitudinal studies that used parental self-report or official reports of child maltreatment (Slack et al., 2011).

In their annual Stress in America Study for 2020, the American Psychological Association (2020b) found that financial concern was a major source of stress. Nearly two out of three adults (63%) reported that money was a significant source of stress in their life (up from 46% in 2019), and around half of adults (52%) said they had experienced negative financial impacts due to the pandemic. Job stability was a source of stress for more than half of employed adults (56%). Those with lower incomes were disproportionately affected by the pandemic and other social changes in 2020. Almost three fourths (73%) of those with a household income of less than $50,000 reported that money was a significant source of stress, compared to 59% of those with a household income of more than $50,000. This disparity widened when looking at households that were at or below the federal poverty level (family of four = $26,200), with 79% expressing financial concerns versus 57% of those above the poverty level. Americans making less than $50,000 were also more likely to have been laid off (21%) compared with those making more than $50,000 (11%).

In this time of social disruption, many parents lost their jobs due to restrictive "stay-at-home" measures. Wong et al. (2021) found in their sample that parents experiencing income instability due to job loss and/or reduced income due to COVID 19 were two to three times as likely to physically maltreat their children compared with parents who did not experience income loss.

Rodriguez et al. (2021) found that mothers reported increased conflict with their children during the pandemic, including more yelling and physical and verbal aggression. Greater financial concern was associated with increased adverse pandemic-related parenting and higher child abuse risk scores. Their results were consistent with those found in other studies regarding the effects of economic strains and concerns on child maltreatment (Frioux et al., 2014; Slack et al., 2011). Sedlak et al. (2010) found that the risk of physical abuse was three times higher, and of neglect seven times higher, in families of low SES and/or with parental unemployment.

Interestingly, the Rodriguez et al. study (2021) found that the mother's subjective perception of financial duress was more predictive of higher abuse risk scores than actual employment disruption or job loss (Rodriquez et al., 2021). Thus, the subjective interpretation and evaluation of one's situation may be more of a determining factor of abusive behavior than the objective reality of the situation. These data demonstrate the interaction of system-level factors with individual and relational factors. Social isolation paired with the psychological and economic stressors accompanying the pandemic, as well as potential increases in negative coping mechanisms (e.g., excessive alcohol consumption), may have combined for some families to create a "perfect storm" to trigger an unprecedented wave of family violence (van Gelder et al., 2020).

However, positive coping strategies such as cognitive reframing can help to buffer the negative effects of even significant stressors. The stress and coping model of child maltreatment postulates that it is not the actual stressor, but the type of coping skills and strategies the family employs, that determine negative responses such as the risk of maltreatment (Hilson & Kuiper, 1994). Positive coping strategies can mitigate the effects of stress on parenting and child abuse (Lawson et al., 2020). Positive cognitive reframing is a type of coping strategy that emphasizes strength to overcome obstacles; stressors are reappraised, redefined, and made more manageable (Lazarus & Folkman, 1984; McCubbin et al., 1981). Parents are assisted in redefining a stressor as a more manageable dynamic, such as "with crisis comes opportunity" (Lawson et al., 2020). An example of positive cognitive reframing might be the parent who conceptualizes a recent job loss as incentive to look for new employment that has more flexibility to work from home or greater possibility for advancement than the old job. Positively reframing job loss helps to decrease negative effects and associated stress, which, in turn, reduces risk for physical abuse. These findings have important implications for prevention and intervention programs.

Impact on Relationship Factors

During the COVID-19 pandemic and in other periods of prolonged family stress, several risk factors related to prolonged proximity, fewer resources or supports, and/or problematic relationships can lead to increased rates of child maltreatment (Usher et al., 2020).

Parental Factors in Child Maltreatment

Two significant predictors of emotional and physical abuse during the COVID-19 pandemic were parental depression and a history of maltreating children (Lawson et al., 2020). Parental depression has long been recognized as a strong predictor of harsh parenting and as a key risk factor for child maltreatment (Cicchetti & Toth, 2005; Vreeland et al., 2019; Wolford et al., 2019). Also, parents were more likely to psychologically maltreat and physically abuse their children during the pandemic if they had a history of maltreating their children in the past. The odds of being psychologically maltreated and physically abused during the pandemic were 12 to 20 times higher, respectively, among children who were maltreated in the year before the pandemic (Lawson et al., 2020).

Balancing childcare and home-schooling responsibilities while simultaneously working from home with few to no outside supports is a dynamic that has contributed to "parental burnout," a type of stress that goes far beyond typical stress related to parenting and is defined as "a prolonged response to chronic and overwhelming parental stress" (Mikolajczak et al., 2019). Parental burnout is characterized by physical and mental exhaustion with physical symptoms such as somatic complaints and decreased sleep quality, emotional distancing from their children, a sense of incompetency in their role as a parent, and a feeling of being trapped in an uncomfortable situation with no way out (Hubert & Aujoulat, 2018; Mikolajczak et al., 2018). It can result when there is a mismatch between the demands of parenting and the resources available for parents to meet those demands, as occurred during the isolation phases of the COVID-19 pandemic. Research has shown that parents who experience burnout are more likely to engage in child maltreatment; thus, the need for supports for parents is evident (Griffith, 2020).

The tension within households during the COVID-19 pandemic was intensified by many factors, including school closures and the need for parents to assist and monitor their children's schooling, limited social contacts, reduced extended family contacts, unemployment/economic stress, potential for increased use of alcohol or other drugs by parents or older siblings, unemployment, prolonged financial strains, lack of access to stable internet connection, and issues related to food insecurity and possible loss of housing (Fegert et al., 2020; Seddighi et al., 2021). Stress also was intensified by the actual looming threat of a potentially fatal disease, actual stressful illness in family members or friends, need for quarantine arrangements in one's own home, and hospitalizations and deaths in situations where family members were not allowed to visit or to be with a dying family member.

Disruption of Social Networks

In previous studies of a different type of community disruption (i.e., a hurricane), one study found that in families who had previously experienced domestic violence, social factors such as decreased access to resources, increased stress due to job loss or strained finances, and disconnection from support systems led to higher rates of domestic violence and child abuse both during and in the aftermath of the hurricane (Serrata & Alvarado, 2019). Intimate partner (domestic) violence and child abuse often occur together (Wong et al., 2021). In a situation of forced isolation with family members in proximity for long periods without a break, an "escalating cycle of tension, power, and control" can occur, leading to abuse; especially when there are fewer options to flee to a family member or shelter or to implement a previous safety plan (Abramsom, 2020; Seddighi et al., 2021).

IMPACT ON COMMUNITY FACTORS

Importance of Schools and Daycare

Schools and daycare centers serve not only as a source of surveillance, but also as areas of socialization, peer and adult support, and free meals for children who need this resource. Already discussed is the stress that children and parents faced trying to keep up with school schedules, connection times, and online learning modalities. Particularly for younger school-age children, parents were expected to play a significant role in ensuring that their children were doing the online work and "tuning in" to the correct teacher or class at set times during the day and were assisting their children in the acquisition of knowledge in ways that are normally part of the teacher's role, not the parent's. These demands set up the dynamic for potential parent/child conflict, even in the most stable, advantaged families and neighborhoods, but so much more so in families with already high levels of competing demands, with more than one child, with parents trying to work at home and monitor "school," without reliable internet access or access to tablets or computers, and with low coping resources and high stress. As many as 10% to 30% of impoverished students experience high absenteeism from school related to lack of adequate home computer access, unreliable internet connection, and no parent availability to assist with online education, ultimately affecting reading levels and dropout and graduation rates (Goldstein et al., 2020).

Schools are also a critical mental health resource for children. Children who are from low-income households or have public insurance and children of color are more likely to receive mental health services exclusively from school settings. Thus, lack of access to these services may result in increased stress and behavioral issues for the child and the parent. The use of telehealth became more widespread during the pandemic, and some families were able to transition to this modality of continued counseling and support (APA, 2020b). Unfortunately, some children from low-income families who may have needed this resource the most were also more likely than their more advantaged peers to have issues of accessibility related to the electronic devices needed and/or consistent broadband internet access (Shen et al., 2020).

Importance of One's Zip Code

Where a family lives matters. Although past studies have identified individual and family factors as most important in determining child maltreatment and negative outcomes, many more recent studies have highlighted the important role of neighborhoods in affecting child, adolescent, and adult outcomes and well-being (Levanthal & Brooks-Gunn, 2000). Increasing evidence demonstrates the importance of one's zip code in determining health, well-being, and risk of child maltreatment (Molnar et al., 2016; Wallack & Thornburg, 2016). Put simply, "place matters" (Williams, 2013).

Several studies, including Molnar et al. (2016), found that neighborhood structural factors such as poverty, high levels of crime, housing stress, childcare burden, substance availability, and resident density can influence the number of a neighborhood's children who are victims of maltreatment. However, Molnar et al. (2016) extended this finding to include not only the impact of neighborhood structural factors but also the combined influence of neighborhood social processes on child maltreatment. The neighborhoods that had the highest child maltreatment rates were those that were "socially impoverished," in which needy families competed with other needy families for scarce resources (Garbarino & Sherman, 1980). Their combination approach included certain characteristics: (a) lower collective efficacy (i.e., a group's shared belief in their capabilities to succeed at certain tasks); (b) intergenerational closure (i.e., the extent to which parents know the neighborhood's children and the parents of their children's friends); (c) fewer social networks; and (d) higher levels of physical (e.g., graffiti, garbage, broken windows) and social (e.g., harassment on street, public intoxication, solicitation for sex workers) disorder.

Collective efficacy is an extension of Bandura's concept of self-efficacy (1995). It combines *social control* (i.e., neighbor's capacity to regulate the behavior of other residents according to desired goals) with *social cohesion* (i.e., mutual trust and solidarity among neighbors; Sampson et al., 1997). Mounting evidence from several studies suggests that collective efficacy has a protective influence over several different types of family and community violence (Molnar et al., 2016). Intergenerational closure functions as a protective factor by generating greater social support for children and shared norms about child rearing within the community (Carbonaro, 1999; Molar et al., 2016). A key element of the Strong Communities intervention, which lowered rates of child maltreatment, was to strengthen neighborhood social networks (Kimbrough-Melton & Melton, 2015). Physical and social disorder in a community fuels a breakdown of caring behavior and may erode social cohesion and social support for children and families, leading to situations of toxic stress (Gau et al., 2014).

Neighborhoods, communities, and generations with less resources (tangible as well as emotional) experience less buffering, have fewer protective factors, and thus are more vulnerable to negative outcomes.

Families who live in disadvantaged neighborhoods are more likely to be investigated by CPS, suggesting a potential reporting bias. One study found that the correlation between substantiated and unsubstantiated risks of child maltreatment was very high (a .8 correlation) and that these risks were higher in neighborhoods with low SES, more public disorder, and crime (Marco et al., 2020).

Child Protective Services During a Period of Virus Risk and Social Disruption

CPS agencies serve as part of the community response that includes assistance to families who are struggling to parent their children or to provide for their necessities, food, clothing, shelter, education, and healthcare. CPS caseworkers have at least an associate's or bachelor's degree in a human services field. Supervisors may have a master's degree in human services administration, although requirements may vary from state to state (Ohio Administrative Rule 5101-2-33-55, 2019). CPS staff have ongoing licensure and employee training requirements to support and update their skills and protocols (Ohio Child Welfare Training Program, n.d.) and that permit them to investigate if basic care and safety are being met in a household. If an investigation indicates neglect and/or abuse, the CPS agency may petition family court to remove the child for relative, foster, or group placement (DHHS, 2020).

Although many families may perceive CPS workers in an adversarial role with the threat of "they may take away my children" in their minds, CPS workers endeavor to keep families together by making referrals to other public and charitable organizations for services and resources such as food and clothing distribution, housing assistance, and crisis services to ensure that gaps in resources are being covered as much as possible. If CPS determines that children need to be removed from a home for their own safety, caseworkers prioritize placements with extended family members rather than foster care (Ohio 5101:2-39-01, 2016).

During long-term service disruptions, CPS must continue to provide all mandated services for at-risk families and yet keep their staff members safe from exposure to communicable infection themselves and ensure the safety (to the extent possible) of the families they serve. The COVID-19 pandemic presented several challenges for CPS staff in addition to their already very stressful and demanding jobs. Typically, investigators and service providers enter the households of families; however, to avoid the possibility of disease exposure, some case workers brought along folding chairs and held "home visit" meetings outdoors, socially distanced, or they held virtual meetings involving the family's use of phone or computer video cameras, if available. Investigators also used collateral information sources including neighbors, family members, and teachers in their investigations, and again, they had to be creative in their communication strategies to maintain protective measures against the virus. If in-home contacts were needed, staff members were tested for COVID-19 prior to visits and appropriate personal protective devices such as masks, shoe covers, and hand sanitizers were used (personal communication, March 2021).

The case study that follows describes an encounter that represents the efforts of CPS to transition to alternative protocols during the pandemic.

CASE STUDY 9.1

Kelsey was 16 years old when she became pregnant and was expelled from her parents' household. She dropped out of high school and moved into her 40-year-old boyfriend's trailer home located on a rural property. The infant girl was born without Kelsey having had any prenatal care, because she did not have health insurance and did not know how to apply for any assistance. The baby was healthy, although small for gestational age. Kelsey's boyfriend, Dale, tolerated the infant but did not co-parent and left baby care to Kelsey. During the pandemic, Dale lost his job and began drinking and smoking more heavily than usual. There was increasing tension and arguments, but Kelsey tried to appease Dale because she felt she had no other options without employment skills or baby care.

One day, Dale told Kelsey to walk to a convenience store to buy beer and cigarettes, leaving the baby behind under his supervision. When Kelsey returned, the trailer door was locked and she had to wait outside, knocking repeatedly until Dale answered. He was naked from the waist down, holding the baby. He explained he had begun to take a shower when he heard the baby crying and picked her up.

Later, when Kelsey changed her daughter's diaper, she was surprised to see bleeding on the baby's genitals and diaper. Kelsey took the baby to an urgent care center, who found a severe laceration that was highly suspicious of sexual assault and called CPS.

The baby's injury required surgical repair and a hospital stay. Kelsey returned to her boyfriend's trailer following the baby's surgery. It was determined that the baby's injury represented a level one emergency (the baby could not be returned home) and an emergency CPS worker was dispatched to the rural address. Upon arriving, the caseworker had

(continued)

CASE STUDY 9.1 (*CONTINUED*)

to sit outside on folding chairs as part of COVID social distancing protocol, reducing a full investigation of the trailer interior. Dale became hostile and threatened the caseworker for "trespassing." Kelsey agreed to take her baby and herself to a shelter that had masking and individual rooms, accompanied by the CPS emergency social worker.

Kelsey was referred to mental health counseling, long-term housing provisions, a supplemental nutritional program, a GED completion program, and job skills training coordinated through an ongoing CPS family caseworker to maintain mother/baby engagement. The CPS supervisor held a debriefing session with the emergency worker to express and process concerns about the potential for aggression by the alleged perpetrator in an isolated area.

Caring for the Caregivers

Investigating and intervening in possible or actual cases of child maltreatment can take a toll on the emotional and mental health of CPS workers. Thus, to prevent burnout and increase retention of staff, it is important to consider the mental health needs of the providers using a "caring for the caregivers" model. Intervening to support CPS workers serves to indirectly improve the experience of the children and families with whom they interact—a focus on the "Relationship" level of the social-ecological model. Possible supports include weekly "well-being" check-ins from supervisors, peer support, flexible hybrid home/office work schedules, making sure workers have functioning equipment (e.g., tablets for data collection), and creating a culture that supports venting and problem solving when staff are feeling anxious, troubled, or depressed and also provides opportunities to celebrate successes. Other strategies, such as weekly "town hall" meetings to jointly problem-solve issues that arise during social disruption, verbalizing appreciation, sending thank-you cards, or providing ongoing staff education and skill acquisition are also important (personal communications, March 2021; Posick et al., 2020).

IMPACT ON SOCIETAL FACTORS

Impact on Global Society

The introduction to a 2021 report issued by the European Union Agency for Fundamental Human Rights stated, "In 2020, the COVID-19 pandemic and the measures it prompted raised an unprecedented collective challenge to the fundamental and human rights of everyone living in the EU." It addressed the fact that this global health crisis was increasingly used as pretext for attacking "migrants, people with immigrant backgrounds, and fundamental rights"; that the Black Lives Matter movement had mobilized societies across the globe to address issues of racism, discrimination, and violence by law enforcement authorities; and that child abuse increased during this period of heightened stress and disruption (European Union Agency for Fundamental Human Rights, 2021). The impact of racial disparities and poverty were discussed earlier but are highlighted here as this report illustrates the truly global nature of the issues faced during this period of social disruption and the wider societal issues that impact children and families.

Economic Impact

During periods of economic downturn in the past, such as the Great Recession in 2007 to 2010, rates of child abuse and intimate partner violence both increased (Schneider et al., 2017). A similar correlation has been found between child maltreatment and the widespread financial difficulties associated with the COVID pandemic due to job losses, business closures, and other economic impacts due to the "stay-at-home" and shelter-in-place orders (Wong et al., 2021).

CHILD MALTREATMENT PREVENTION AND INTERVENTION

Proactive Versus Reactive Approaches

Experts have noted that the COVID-19 pandemic served to highlight the fact that the current system regarding child maltreatment is very "reactive," rather than being a system in which we have confidence that the infrastructure is in place to help support children and families and thus decrease the risk of child maltreatment during times of major social disruption (Ingram, 2020). A criticism of our current child welfare system and child protection systems is that they "are tasked with preventing, assessing, and resolving child maltreatment with few effective tools and little oversight" (Welch & Haskins, 2020). A report from the Brookings Institute (Welch & Haskins, 2020) notes that most of the families who come to the attention of child protection agencies are facing significant issues that contribute to, yet span beyond, child maltreatment such as poverty, continued economic uncertainty, substance abuse, homelessness, and many other factors included in our increasing understanding of the "social determinants of health."

As described in Chapter 7, social determinants of health are increasingly being recognized as major factors contributing to the health and well-being of children, families, and communities. Many pediatric practices and healthcare systems are now instituting social needs screening and in-person resource navigation services. Some studies show that this type of targeted intervention can decrease a family's report of social needs and improve children's overall health status (Gottlieb et al., 2016). More research is needed to identify the effectiveness of these types of approaches in decreasing child maltreatment.

In some cases of reported "neglect," the problem may be a lack of fundamental resources; perhaps not only in the family of concern, but also in the extended family and neighborhood, thus decreasing the chance of possible assistance from close others. In these cases, a lack of food, clothing, shelter, and healthy living conditions is due to poverty or financial crises. Taking a "public health approach" with referrals to food banks and other community resources is the most needed and effective approach to child maltreatment prevention.

Protective service agencies, United Way, and Departments of Health (e.g., Help Me Grow programs) can refer and advocate for parents who may be struggling with the activities necessary to get the help they need, such as filling out public housing applications, completing the Special Nutritional Women, Infants, and Children Program (WIC) application, finding baby and children's clothing, accessing school supplies, obtaining transportation vouchers for medical appointments, and applying to other programs for which they may qualify. Families who are bolstered by these efforts make greater progress toward improved parenting and building family management skills. Public community services may also align with religious (e.g., Catholic Social Services, Lutheran Social Services) and volunteer groups (e.g., Kiwanis Children's Fund) to enhance parental resource acquisition as their primary goal in building healthy families. Nevertheless, with families with fewer capabilities and resources, maintaining ongoing vigilance by helping relationships provides some buffering against neglect and opportunities for early intervention should it be necessary.

What is very clear is that a multilevel, proactive approach guided by the social-ecological model and designed to decrease or mitigate risk factors and increase protective factors has the greatest chance of success in preventing child maltreatment. Table 9.4 describes prevention strategies at each level of the social-ecological model.

The CDC has developed a "technical package" (Fortson et al., 2016) that is designed to provide professionals and communities with a select group of strategies based on the best available evidence to help prevent child abuse and neglect. The strategies included are strengthening economic supports to families; changing social norms to support parents and positive parenting; providing quality care and education early in life; enhancing parenting

TABLE 9.4 Prevention Strategies at Each Level of the Ecological Model

Level	Definition
Individual	Prevention strategies at this level promote attitudes, beliefs, and behaviors that prevent violence. Specific approaches may include conflict resolution and life skills training, social-emotional learning, and safe dating and healthy relationship skill programs.
Relationship	Prevention strategies at this level may include parenting or family-focused prevention programs and mentoring and peer programs designed to strengthen parent/child communication, promote positive peer norms, problem-solving skills, and promote healthy relationships.
Community	Prevention strategies at this level focus on improving the physical and social environment in these settings (e.g., by creating safe places where people live, learn, work, and play) and by addressing other conditions that give rise to violence in communities (e.g., neighborhood poverty, residential segregation, and instability, high density of alcohol outlets).
Societal	Prevention strategies at this level include efforts to promote societal norms that protect against violence as well as efforts to strengthen household financial security, education and employment opportunities, and other policies that affect the structural determinants of health.

Source: Centers for Disease Control and Prevention. (2021). *The social-ecological model: A framework for prevention*. Violence Prevention Injury Center, CDC.

skills to promote healthy child development; and intervening to lessen harms and prevent future risk. This resource is available in English and Spanish and can be used as a tool in efforts to impact individual behaviors, as well as family, community, and societal factors, that influence risk and protective factors for child abuse and neglect.

Community-Based Approaches

As noted previously, most child maltreatment prevention strategies in the past have focused on individual child, parent, and family factors. Less attention has been given to societal and community factors that impact the lives of children and families and may serve as risk or protective factors for child maltreatment. In the past decade or so, that focus has been slowly shifting.

Tomison and Wise (1999) note that efforts in the past to prevent child maltreatment "have been hampered by a failure to address the structural social forces and community-level factors that impact on children, families, and the propensity for child maltreatment" (p. 1). They highlight three major interventions that they perceive as key components of any child maltreatment prevention program at societal and community levels: (a) early intervention programs, (b) cross-sectoral collaboration, and (c) "whole of community" or comprehensive community initiatives. Other guidance for community-level developmental prevention approaches identifies three complementary initiatives to address the complex interactions of risk and protective factors, multilevel problems, and environmental influences. They are service integrations based on the enhancement of interagency communication and collaboration, cross-problem interventions that are comprehensive services that focus on separate problems that share common risk factors, and community-change interventions that address social attitudes, behaviors, and networks (Tomison & Wise, 1999).

A "Systems Level" Focus on Reducing Poverty

The Child Tax Credit plan that went into effect in the summer of 2021, called the "biggest anti-poverty program undertaken by the federal government in more than half a century"

(Stein, 2021), began disbursing monthly payments to most American parents with the intent of providing long-term support to lift families out of poverty and/or financial distress (The White House, 2021; Stein, 2021). This program is a significant "system level" intervention that may help to decrease "neglect" by giving families increased resources to provide necessities while also decreasing the risk of other forms of abuse that might otherwise be tied to parental stress regarding finances. A sustainable plan that will continue after the immediate pandemic period will be necessary to maintain long-term effects of decreasing poverty and the many risk factors that come with low socioeconomic resources.

CONCLUSIONS

Understanding and working to prevent the complex phenomenon of child maltreatment, especially during a time of social disruption such as the COVID-19 pandemic and the many other system level events that occurred concurrently, require a multilevel social-ecological model. An in-depth look at the risk factors at each level that place infants, children, and adolescents at risk for child maltreatment, as well as at the possible protective factors, using a strengths-based model is also necessary to guide prevention and treatment programs that will avert toxic stress and long-term negative consequences. To be truly effective in our prevention efforts, we must remedy the "socially toxic factors" that underpin child maltreatment and other family violence (Garbarino, 1995; Tomison & Wise, 1999), focusing on programs that promote positive social determinants of health.

One lesson learned from the significant social disruption of the COVID-19 pandemic, as well as other disasters and national crises, is that we must be prepared with proactive, intensive, and comprehensive multilayered services, especially for children and families who are most vulnerable. As we saw in this crisis, families and children who are already struggling will be the least resilient and most affected during emergencies. Services must be prospectively planned and in place so that we are not taken by surprise as we were to a large extent in the COVID-19 crisis. What can society do to help be more prepared, to move forward, to enhance our preparedness? First, we must develop a shared mindset in our culture that child well-being is a shared responsibility rather than maintaining a perspective that parents are the sole providers of all their children's needs (Berube et al., 2020).

We must develop targeted and comprehensive strategies to reduce systemic racism, social inequities, and disparities that place children of color, immigrants, children with disabilities, and other targeted groups in a position of disadvantage and risk compared with the rest of society. This will be a continued challenge given "the wariness of U.S. policy makers of supporting programs that are tailored to socially disadvantaged" people (Thompson, 1998). However, as one of the most highly developed democracies in the world, the United States should aim for the best social supports that provide for all children the opportunity to thrive, creating optimal situations for children to live, learn, and develop.

As members of professions that hold dear the ethical principles of social justice, beneficence, and dignity, we must be diligent in our communal voices in influencing policy that ensures advocacy for the best interest of the child, even, and perhaps especially, during times of social disruption and change.

ADDITIONAL RESOURCE

NIDA. (2020). Chapter 2: Risk and protective factors. https://www.drugabuse.gov/publications/principles-substance-abuse-prevention-earlychildhood/chapter-2-risk-protective-factorson

REFERENCES

Abramson, A. (2020). How COVID-19 may increase domestic violence and child abuse. American Psychological Association. http://www.apa.org/topics/covid-19/domestic-violence-child-abuse

Allison, M. L., Anne, L. W., Chinmayi, T., Michael, A. N., & Wendy, H. (2021). Cumulative childhood maltreatment and executive functioning in adulthood, *Journal of Aggression, Maltreatment & Trauma*, 30(4), 547–563. https://doi.org/10.1080/10926771.2020.1832171

American Psychological Association. (2020a). Psychology's understanding of the challenges related to the COVID-19 global pandemic in the United States. https://www.apa.org/about/policy/covid-statement.pdf

American Psychological Association. (2020b). *Stress in America 2020: A national mental health crisis*. https://www.apa.org/news/press/releases/stress/2020/report-october

Annie E. Casey Foundation. (2020). Children in poverty by race and ethnicity in the United States. Kids Count Data Center. https://datacenter.kidscount.org/data/tables/44-children-in-poverty-by-race-and-ethnicity#detailed/1/any/false/1729,37,871,870,573,869,36,868,867,133/10,11,9,12,1,185,13/324,323

Bate, J., Pham, P., & Borelli, J. (2021). Be my safe haven: Parent–child relationships and emotional health during COVID-19. *Journal of Pediatric Psychology*, 46(6), 624–634. https://doi.org/10.1093/jpepsy/jsab04

Bérubé, A., Clément, M. È., Lafantaisie, V., LeBlanc, A., Baron, M., Picher, G., Turgeon, J., Ruiz-Casares, M., & Lacharité, C. (2020). How societal responses to COVID-19 could contribute to child neglect. *Child Abuse & Neglect*, 104761. https://doi.org/10.1016/j.chiabu.2020.104761

Bolger, K. E., & Patterson, C. J. (2001). Children's internalizing problems and perceptions of control as functions of multiple types of maltreatment. *Development and Psychopathology*, 13, 913–940.

Bronfenbrenner, U., & Ceci, S. J. (1994). Nature-nurture reconceptualized: A bio-ecological model. *Psychological Review*, 10(4), 568–586. https://static1.squarespace.com/static/57309137ab48de6f423b3eec/t/59aea54d4c0dbfd7d6e43622/1504617811640/Bronfenbrenner%26Ce

Burke, N. J., Heilman, J. L., Scott, B. G., Weems, C. F., & Carrion, V. G. (2011). The impact of adverse childhood experience on an urban pediatric population. *Child Abuse and Neglect*, 35(6), 408–413.

Carbonaro, W. J. (1999). Opening the debate on closure and schooling outcomes: Comment on Morgan and Sørensen. *American Sociological Review*, 64(5), 682–686. https://doi.org/10.2307/2657369

Catani, C., Jacob, N., Schauer, E. et al. (2008). Family violence, war, and natural disasters: A study of the effect of extreme stress on children's mental health in Sri Lanka. *BMC Psychiatry*, 8, 33. https://doi.org/10.1186/1471-244X-8-33

Centers for Disease Control and Prevention. (2020, December 10). Disparities in deaths from COVID-19: Racial and ethnic health disparities. Disparities in COVID-19 Deaths (cdc.gov).

Center for Disease Control and Prevention. (2021, January 28). National center for injury prevention and control, division of violence prevention. The social-ecological model: A framework for prevention. Violence Prevention Injury Center CDC.

Center for Disease Control and Prevention. (2021, March 15). National center for injury prevention and control, division of violence prevention: Risk and protective factors. https://www.cdc.gov/violenceprevention/childabuseandneglect/riskprotectivefactors.html

Centers for Disease Control and Prevention. (2021, March 15). Preventing child abuse and neglect. Preventing Child Abuse & Neglect | Violence Prevention | Injury Center | CDC.

Chibnall, S., Dutch, N. M., Jones-Harden, B., Brown, A., Gourdine, R., Smith, J., Boone, A., & Snyder, S. (2003). Children of color in the child welfare system: Perspectives from the child welfare community. In U.S. Department of Health and Human Services, Children's Bureau, Administration for Children and Families. Children of Color in the Child Welfare System: Perspectives from the Child Welfare Community.

Chrisinger, B. W., Gustafson, J. A., King, A. C., & Winter S. J. (2019). Understanding where we are well: Neighborhood-level social and environmental correlates of well-being in the Stanford well for life study. *International Journal of Environmental Research and Public Health*.

Cicchetti, D., & Toth, S. L. (2005). Child maltreatment. *Annual Review of Clinical Psychology*, 1(1), 409–438. https://doi.org/10.1146/annurev.clinpsy.1.102803.144029

Cohodes, E. M., McCauley, S., & Gee, D. G. (2021). Parental buffering of stress in the time of COVID19: Family-level factors may moderate the association between pandemic-related stress and youth symptomatology. *Research on Child and Adolescent Psychopathology*, 49, 935–948. https://doi.org/10.1007/s10802-020-00732-6

Condon, E. M., Sadler, L. S., Mayes, L. C. 2018). Toxic stress and protective factors in multi-ethnic school age children: A research protocol. *Research in Nursing and Health*, 41, 97–106.

Coohey, C., Renner, L. M., Hua, L., Zhang, Y. J., & Whitney, S. D. (2011). Academic achievement despite child maltreatment: A longitudinal study. *Child Abuse and Neglect*, 35(9), 688–699. https://doi.org/10.1016/j.chiabu.2011.05.009

Coulton, C. J., Crampton, D. S., Irwin, M., Spilsbury, J. C., & Korbin, J. E. (2007). How neighborhoods influence maltreatment: A review of the literature and alternative pathways. *Child Abuse & Neglect*, 31(11–12), 1117–1142.

Coulton, C. J., Korbin, J. E., Su, M., & Chow, J. (1995). Community level factors and child maltreatment rates. *Child Development, 66*(5), 1262–1276. https://doi.org/10.1111/j.1467-8624.1995.tb00934.x

Dahlberg, L. L., & Krug, E. G. (2002). Violence—a global public health problem. In E. Krug, L. L. Dahlberg, J. A. Mercy, A. B. Zwi, & R. Lozano (Eds.). World report on violence child and health (pp. 1–21). World Health Organization.

DePrince, A. P., Weinzierl, K. M., & Combs, M. D. (2009). Executive function performance and trauma exposure in a community sample of children. *Child Abuse and Neglect, 33*, 353–361. https://doi/org/10.1016/j.chiabu.2008.08.002

Derezotes, D., Poertner, J., & Testa, M. (2005). Race matters in child welfare: The overrepresentation of African American children in the system. Washington, DC: CWLA Press.

Dubowitz, H., Black, N., Starr, R. H., & Zuravin, S. (1993). A conceptual definition of child neglect. *Criminal Justice and Behavior, 20*(1), 8–26.

European Union Agency for Fundamental Human Rights. (2021). The Coronavirus pandemic and fundamental rights: A year in review. https://fra.europa.eu/sites/default/files/fra_uploads/fra-2021-fundamental-rights-report-2021-focus_en.pdf

Fegert, J. et al. (2020). Challenges and burden of the Coronavirus 2019 (Covid-19) pandemic for child and adolescent mental health: A narrative review to highlight clinical and research needs in the acute phase and in the long return to normality. *Child and Adolescent Psychiatry and Mental Health, 14, 20.*

Felitti, V. J., Anda, R. F., Nordenberg, D., Williamson, D. F., Spit, A. M., Edwards, V., & Marks, J. S. (1998). Relationship of childhood abuse and household dysfunction to many of the leading causes of death in adults. The adverse childhood experiences (ACE) study. *American Journal of Preventive Medicine, 14*(4), 245–258.

Fortson, B. L., Klevens, J., Merrick, M. T., Gilbert, L. K., & Alexander, S. P. (2016). Preventing child abuse and neglect: A technical package for policy, norm, and programmatic activities. National Center for Injury Prevention and Control, Centers for Disease Control and Prevention. Preventing Child Abuse and Neglect: A Technical Package for Policy, Norm, and Programmatic Activities (cdc.gov)

Frioux, S., Wood, J. N., Fakeye, O., Luan, X., Localio, R., & Rubin, D. M. (2014). Longitudinal association of county-level economic indicators and child maltreatment incidents. *MaternalChild Health, 18*, 2202–2208.

Garbarino, J. (1995). *Raising children in a socially toxic environment.* Jossey Bass Publishers.

Garbarino, J., & Sherman, D. (1980). High-risk neighborhoods and high-risk families: The human ecology of child maltreatment. *Child Development, 51*(1), 188–198. https://doi.org/10.2307/1129606

Garmezy, N. (1971). Vulnerability research and the issue of primary prevention. *American Journal of Orthopsychiatry, 41*, 101–116.

Garmezy, N. (1981). Children under stress: Perspectives on antecedents and correlates of vulnerability and resistance to psychopathology.

Gau, J.M. (2014). Procedural justice and police legitimacy: A test of measurement and structure. *American Journal of Criminal Justice, 39*, 187–205. https://doi.org/10.1007/s12103-013-9220-8

Gau J. M., Corsaro, N. & Brunson, R. K. (2014). Revisiting broken windows theory: A test of the mediation impact of social mechanisms on the disorder—fear relationship. *Journal of Criminal Justice, 42*(6), 579–588.

Garmezy, N., & Rutter, M. (1985). Acute reactions to stress. In M. Rutter, & L. Hersov (Eds.), Child psychiatry: Modern approaches (2nd ed., pp. 152–176). Blackwell Scientific.

Godoy, M., & Wood, D. (2020, May 30). What do coronavirus racial disparities look like state by state? NPR. https://www.npr.org/sections/health-shots/2020/05/30/865413079/what-docoronavirus-racial-disparities-look-like-state-by-state

Goldstein, D., Popescu, A., & Hannah-Jones, N. (2020). *As school moves online, many students stay logged out.* The New York Times. https://www.nytimes.com/2020/04/06/us/coronavirus-schools-attendance-absent.html

Gottlieb, L. M., Hessler, D., Long, D., Laves, E., Burns, A. R., Amaya, A., Sweeny, P., Schudel, C., & Adler, N. (2016). Effects of social needs screening and in-person service navigation on child health: A randomized clinical trial. *JAMA Pediatrics, 170*(11), e162521.2521. https://doi/org/10:1001/jamapediatrics.2016.2521

Griffith, A. K. (2020). Parental burnout and child maltreatment during the COVID-19 pandemic. *Journal of Family Violence.* https://doi.org/10.1007/s10896-020-00172-2

Guy-Evans, O. (2020, November 9). Bronfenbrenner's ecological systems theory. *Simply Psychology.* https://www.simplypsychology.org/Bronfenbrenner.html

Hager, E. (2020, June 15). Is child abuse really rising during the pandemic? *The Marshall Project.* https://www.themarshallproject.org/2020/06/15/is-child-abuse-really-rising-during-thepandemichttps://www.simplypsychology.org/Bronfenbrenner.html

Helton, J. J., Jackson, D. B., Boutwell, B. B., & Vaughn, M. G. (2019). Household food insecurity and parent-to-child aggression. *Child Maltreatment, 24*(2), 213–221. https://doi.org/10.1177/1077559518819141

Herman, J. P., McKlveen, J. M., Ghosal, S., Kopp, B., Wulsin, A., Makinson, R., Scheimann, J., & Myers, B. (2016). Regulation of the hypothalamic-pituitary-adrenocortical stress response. *Comprehensive Physiology*, 6(2), 603–621. https://doi.org/10.1002/cphy.c150015

Hillson, J. M. C., & Kuiper, N. A. (1994). A stress and coping model of child maltreatment. *Clinical Psychology Review*, 14(4), 261–285. https://doi/org/10.1016/0272-7358(94)90025-6

Ho, S., & Fassett, C. (2021, March 29). Pandemic masks ongoing child abuse crisis as cases plummet. Associated Press. https://abcnews.go.com/Health/wireStory/ap-exclusive-pandemic-means-fewereyes-kids-welfare-76742073

Hubert, S., & Aujoulat, I. (2018). Parental burnout: When exhausted mothers open. *Frontiers in Psychology*, 9, 9. https://doi.org/10.3389/fpsyg.2018.01021

Hunter, A. A., Flores, G. (2021). Social determinants of health and child maltreatment: A systematic review. *Pediatric Research*, 89, 269–274. https://doi.org/10.1038/s41390-020-01175-x

Ingram, J. (2020, July 26). Has child abuse surged under COVID-19? Despite alarming stories from ERs, there's no answer. Nbcnews.com. https://www.nbcnews.com/health/kids-health/has-child-abusesurged-under-covid-19-despite-alarming-stories-n1234713

Jaffee, S. R., & Gallop, R. (2010). Social, emotional, and academic competence among children who have had contact with child protective services: Prevalence and stability estimates. *Journal of the American Academy of Child & Adolescent Psychiatry*, 46(6), 757–765. https://doi/org/10.1097/chi.0b013e318040b247

Johnson, S. B., Riley, A. W., Granger, D. A., & Riis, J. (2013). The science of early life toxic stress for pediatric practice and advocacy. *Pediatrics*, 131(2), 319–326.

Kambhampaty, A. P. (2020, June). *10 Asian Americans reflect on racism during the pandemic and the need for equality*. Time. https://time.com/5858649/racism-coronavirus/

Kaplow, J. B., & Widom, C. S. (2007). Age of onset of child maltreatment predicts long-term mental health outcomes. *Journal of Abnormal Psychology*, 116, 176–187. https://doi/org/10.1037/0021-843X.116.1.176

Kerr, M., Black, M. M., & Krishnakumar, A. (2000). Failure-to-thrive, maltreatment and the behavior and development of 6-year-old children from low-income urban families: A cumulative risk model. *Journal of Child Abuse & Neglect*, 24, 587–598. https://doi/org/10.1016/S0145-2134(00)00126-5

Kim, H., & Drake, B. (2018). Child maltreatment risk as a function of poverty and race/ethnicity in the USA. *International Journal of Epidemiology*, 47(3), 780–787. https://doi.org/10.1093/ije/dyx280

Kimbrough-Melton, R. J., & Melton, G. B. (2015). Someone will notice, and someone will care: How to build strong communities for children. *Child Abuse & Neglect*, 41, 67–78.

Kokaliari, E., Roy, A., & Taylor, J. (2019). African American perspectives on racial disparities in child removals. *Child Abuse & Neglect*, 139–148. https://doi/org/10.1016/j.chiabu.2018.12.023

Koppleman, A. (2020, September 23). What is systemic racism anyway? USA Today. https://www.usatoday.com/story/opinion/2020/09/23/systemic-racism-how-really-define-column/5845788002/

Križ, K., & Skivenes, M. (2011). How child welfare workers view their work with racial and ethnic minority families: The United States in contrast to England and Norway. *Children and Youth Services Review*, 33, 1866–1874. https://doi.org/10.1016/j.childyouth.2011.05.005

Langsford, J. E., Miller-Johnson, S., Berlin, L. J., Dodge, K. A., Bates, J. E., & Pettit, G. S. (2007). Early physical abuse and later violent delinquency: A prospective longitudinal study. *Child Maltreatment*, 12(3), 233–245. https://doi/org/10.1177/1077559507301841

Lawson, M., Piel, M. H., & Simon, M. (2020). Child maltreatment during the COVID-19 pandemic: Consequences of parental job loss on psychological and physical abuse towards children. *Child Abuse & Neglect*, 110(Pt 2), 104709. https://doi.org/10.1016/j.chiabu.2020.104709.

Lazarus R. S., Folkman S. (1984). Stress, Appraisal, and Coping. Springer Publishing Company.

Leeb, R. T., Paulozzi, L., Melanson, C., Simon, T., & Arias, I. (2008). Child maltreatment surveillance: Uniform definitions for public health and recommended data elements, Version 1.0. Centers for Disease Control and Prevention, National Center for Injury Prevention and Control. www.cdc.gov/violenceprevention/pdf/CM_Surveillance-a.pdf

Letkiewicz, A. M., Weldon, A. L., Tengshe, C., Niznikiewicz, M. A., & Heller, W. (2021). Cumulative childhood maltreatment and executive functioning in adulthood. *Journal of Aggression, Maltreatment & Trauma*, 30(4), 547–563. https://doi.org/10.1080/10926771.2020.1832171

Leiter, J. (2007). School performance trajectories after the advent of reported maltreatment. *Child and Youth Services Review*, 29, 363–382. https://doi.org/10.1016/j.childyouth.2006.09.002

Leventhal, T., & Brooks-Gunn, J. (2000). The neighborhoods they live in the effects of neighborhood residence on child and adolescent outcomes. *Psychological Bulletin*, 126(2), 309. https://courses.cit.cornell.edu/dea6610/leventhal.pdf

Lippard, E. T. C., & Nemeroff, C. B. (2020). The devastating clinical consequences of child abuse and neglect: Increased disease vulnerability and poor treatment response in mood disorders. *American Journal of Psychiatry*, 177(1), 20–36. https://doi.org/10.1176/appi.ajp.2019.19010020

Maguire-Jack, K., Lanier, P., Johnson-Motoyama, M., Welch, H., & Dineen, M. (2015). Research article: Geographic variation in racial disparities in child maltreatment: The influence of county poverty and population density. *Child Abuse & Neglect, 47*, 1–13. https://doi.org/10.1016/j.chiabu.2015.05.020

Marco, M., Maquire-Jack, K., Gracia, E., & Lopez-Quilez, A. (2020). Disadvantaged neighborhoods and the spatial overlap of substantiated and unsubstantiated child maltreatment referrals. *Child Abuse & Neglect, 104*, 104477. https://doi.org/10.1016/j.chiabu.2020.10477

Masonbrink, A. R., & Hurley, E. (2020). Advocating for children during the COVID-19 school closures. *Pediatrics, 146*(3), e20201440. https://pediatrics.aappublications.org/content/146/3/e20201440

Masten A. S., & Garmezy N. (1985). Risk, vulnerability, and protective factors in developmental psychopathology. In B.B. Lahey, & A.E. Kazdin (Eds.), Advances in clinical child psychology: Advances in clinical child psychology (vol. 8). Springer. https://doi.org/10.1007/978-1-4613-9820-2_1

McCubbin, H. L., Olson D., & Larsen, A. (1981). Family Crisis Oriented Personal Scales (F-COPES). In H. I. McCubbin, A.I. Thompson, M.A. McCubbin (Eds.), Family assessment: Resiliency, coping and adaptation-inventories for research and practice. University of Wisconsin System; pp. 455–507.

Merrick, M. T. & Latzman, N.E. (2014, January 31). Child maltreatment: A public health overview and prevention considerations. *OJIN: The Online Journal of Issues in Nursing, 19*(1), 2.

Mikolajczak, M., Gross, J. J., & Roskam, I. (2019). Parental burnout: What is it, and why does it matter? *Clinical Psychological Science, 7*(6), 1319–1329. https://doi.org/10.1177/2167702619858430

Molnar, E., George, R. M., Gilsanz, P., Hill, A. Subramanian, S. V., Holton, J. K., Duncan, D. T., Beatriz, E. D., & Beardslee, W. R. (2016). Neighborhood-level social processes and substantiated cases of child maltreatment. *Child Abuse & Neglect, 51*, 41–53.

Nikulina, V., & Widom, C. S. (2019). Higher levels of intelligence and executive functioning protect maltreated children against adult arrests: A prospective study. *Child Maltreatment, 24*(1), 3–16. https://doi.org/10.1177/1077559518808218.

Olema, D. K., Catani, C., Ertl, V., Saile, R., & Neuner, F. (2014). The hidden effects of child maltreatment in a war region: Correlates of psychopathology in two generations living in Northern Uganda. *Journal of Traumatic Stress, 27*(1), 35–41. https://doi.org/10.1002/jts.21892.

Palmeri, J. (2021). Child maltreatment and resilience in the academic environment. *Applied Psychology Opus.* https://wp.nyu.edu/steinhardt-appsych_opus/child-maltreatment-and-resilience-in-the-academic-environment/

Parks, S. E., Annest, J. L., Hill, H. A., & Karch, D. L. (2012). Pediatric abusive head trauma: Recommended definitions for public health surveillance and research. Centers for Disease Control and Prevention. www.cdc.gov/violenceprevention/pdf/pedheadtrauma-a.pdf

Pinheiro, P. S. (2006). *World report on violence against children.* United Nations. http://unviolencestudy.org/

Posick, C., Schueths, A. A., Christian, C., Grubb, J. A., & Christian, S. E. (2020). Child victim services in the time of COVID-19: New challenges and innovative solutions. *American Journal of Criminal Justice, 45*(4), 680–689. https://doi.org/10.1007/s12103-020-09543-3

Putnam-Hornstein, E., Needell, B., King, B., & Johnson-Motoyama, M. (2013). Racial and ethnic disparities: A population-based examination of risk factors for involvement with child protective services. *Child Abuse & Neglect, 37*, 33–46.

Rabin, A. I. J., Aronoff, J., Barclay, A. M., & Zucker, R. A. (eds.). (1981). *Further explorations in personality.* Wiley.

Reichel, C. (2019). Toxic stress in children has health effects that can last into adulthood. Harvard Kennedy School, Shore. https://journalistsresource.org/studies/society/public-health/aces-toxicstress-health-research/nstein Center on Media, Politics, and Public Policy

Rodriguez, C. M., Lee, S. J., Ward, K. P., & Pu, D. F. (2021). The perfect storm: Hidden risk of child maltreatment during the COVID-19 pandemic. *Child Maltreatment, 26*(2), 139–151. https://doi.org/10.1177/1077559520982066

Rutter, M. (1985). Resilience in the face of adversity: Protective factors and resistance to psychiatric disorder. *British Journal of Psychiatry, 147*, 598–611. https://doi.org/10.1192/bjp.147.6.598

SAMHSA. (2021). https://www.samhsa.gov/sites/default/files/20190718-samhsa-risk-protective-factors.pdf

Sampson, R. J., Raudenbush, S. W., & Earls, F. (1997). Neighborhoods and violent crime: A multilevel study of collective efficacy. *Science, 27*, 918–924.

Schenck-Fontaine, A., & Gassman-Pines, A. (2020). Income inequality and child maltreatment risk during economic recession. *Children and Youth Services Review, 112*, 104926.

Schmidt, S., & Natanson, H. (2020, April 30). With kids stuck at home, ER doctors see more severe cases of child abuse. Washington, D.C: The Washington Post.

Schneider, D., Harknett, K., & McLanahan, S. N. (2016). Intimate partner violence in the great recession. *Demography, 53*(2), 471–505. https://doi.org/10.1007/s13524-016-0462

Schneider, W., Waldfogel, J., & Brooks-Gunn, J. (2017). The great recession and risk for child abuse and neglect. *Children and Youth Services Review, 72,* 71–81. https://doi/org/10.1016/j.childyouth.2016.10.016. https://www.sciencedirect.com/science/article/abs/pii/S0190740916303395?via%3Dihub

Seddighi, H., Salmani. I., Javadi, M. H., & Seddighi, S. (2021). Child abuse in natural disasters and conflicts: A systematic review. *Trauma Violence Abuse, 22*(1), 176–185. https://doi/org/10.1177/1524838019835973

Sedlak, A. J., Mettenburg, J., Basena, M., Petta, I., McPherson, K., Green, A., & Li, S. (2010). *Fourth national incidence study of child abuse and neglect (NIS-4): Report to congress, executive summary.* http://www.acf.hhs.gov/sites/default/files/opre/nis4_report_congress_full_pdf_jan2010.pdf

Seratta, J. V., & Alvarado, M. G. H. (2019). Understanding the impact of Hurricane Harvey on family violence survivors in Texas and those who serve them. Texas Council on Family Violence. https://tcfv.org/wp-content/uploads/2019/08/Hurricane-Harvey-Report-FINAL-and-APPROVEDas-of-060619.pdf

Shen, J., Pecoraro, M., & Bellonci, M. (2020, September). Impact of the COVID-19 pandemic on children, youth and families. A brief produced by the Evidence-Based Policy Institute. Judge Baker Children's Center. https://jbcc.harvard.edu/sites/default/files/impact_of_the_covid19_pandemic_on_children_youth_and_families_.pdf

Shonkoff, J. P., Garner, A. S., Committee on Psychosocial Aspects of Child and Family Health, Committee on Early Childhood, Adoption, and Dependent Care, and Section on Developmental and Behavioral Pediatrics, Siegel, B. S., Dobbins, M. I., Earls, M. F., Garner, A. S., McGuinn, L., Pascoe, J., & Wood, D. L. (2012). The lifelong effects of early childhood adversity and toxic stress. *Pediatrics, 129*(1), e232–e246. https://doi.org/10.1542/peds.2011-2663

Shonkoff, J. P., & Williams, D. R. (2020). Thinking about racial disparities in COVID-19 impacts through a science-informed, early childhood lens. https://developingchild.harvard.edu/thinking-about-racial-disparities-in-covid-19-impactsthrough-ascience-informed-early-childhood-lens/

Slack, K. S., Berger, L. M., DuMont, K., Yang, M., Kim, B., Ehrhard-Dietzel, S., & Holl, J. L. (2011). Risk and protective factors for child neglect during early childhood: A cross-study comparison. *Children and Youth Services Review, 33,* 1354–1363.

Stein, J. (2021, July 15). IRS begins sending monthly checks to millions of American parents in crucial test for Biden.

Swedo, E., Idaikkadar, N., Leemis, R., Dias, T. Radhakrishnan, L., Stein, Z., Chen, M., Agathis, N., Holland, K. (2020, December 11). Trends in U.S. emergency department visits related to suspected or confirmed child abuse and neglect among children and adolescents aged,.18 years before and during the COVID-19 pandemic—United States, January 2019-September 2020. USDHHS, Centers for Disease Control and Prevention. *MMWR: Morbidity and Mortality Weekly Report, 69*(49).

Teicher, M. H. & Samson, J. A. (2016). Annual research review: Enduring neurological effects of childhood abuse and neglect. *Journal of Child Psychology and Psychiatry, 57*(3), 241–266. https://doi/org/10.1111/jcpp.12507

The White House. (2021). https://www.whitehouse.gov/child-tax-credit/

Thompson, P. J. (1998). Universalism and deconcentration: Why race still matters in poverty and economic development. *Politics and Society, 26*(2), 181–219.

Tomison, A., & Wise, S. (1999). Community-based approaches in preventing child maltreatment. Families in Australia survey. Australian institute of family studies (NCPC issues no. 11). *Child Maltreatment, 26*(2), 139–150.

Tso, W. W. Y., Wong, R. S., Tung, K. T. S., Rao, N., Fu, K. W., Yam, J. S. C., Chua, G. T., Chen, E. Y. H., Lee, T. M. C., Chan, S. K. W., Wong, W. H. S., Xiong, X., Chui, C. S., Li, X., Wong, K., Leung, C., Tsang, S. K. M., Chan, G. C. F., Tam, P. K. H., …, Ip, P. (2020, November 17). Vulnerability and resilience in children during the COVID-19te pandemic. *European Child and Adolescent Psychiatry.* https://doi.org/10.1007/s00787-020-01680-8

Turan, C. (2020, April 21). Black lives matter: A timeline of the movement. Cosmopolitan. https://www.cosmopolitan.com/uk/reports/a32728194/black-lives-matter-timeline-movement/

U.S. Department of Health and Human Services. (2021). Child maltreatment 2019: Summary of key findings. Administration for children and families, administration on children and families, *Children's Bureau.*

U.S. Department of Health and Human Services. (2020). Social determinants of health. *Healthy People 2030.* Office of Disease Prevention and Health Promotion. https://health.gov/healthypeople/objectives-and-data/social-determinants-health

Usher, K. Bhullar, N., Durkin, J., Gyamfi, N., & Jackson, D. (2020). Family violence and COVID-19: Increased vulnerability and reduced options for support. *International Journal of Mental Health Nursing.* https://doi.org/10.1111/inm.12735

Van Gelder, N., Peterman, A., Potts, A., O'Donnell, M., Thompson, K., Shah, N., & Oertelt-Prigione, S. (2020). COVID-19: Reducing the risk of infection might increase the risk of intimate partner violence. *EClinicalMedicine.* https://doi.org/10.1016/j.eclinm.2020.100348

Vasquez Reyes, M. (2020). The disproportional impact of COVID-19 on African Americans. *Health and Human Rights*, 22(2), 299–307.

Vreeland, A., Gruhn, M. A., Watson, K. H., Bettis, A. H., Compas, B. E., Forehand, R., & Sullivan, A. D. (2019). Parenting in context: Associations of parental depression and socioeconomic factors with parenting behaviors. *Journal of Child and Family Studies*, 28(4), 1124–1133. https://doi.org/10.1007/s10826-019-01338-3

Wallack, L., & Thornburg, K. (2016). Developmental origins, epigenetics, and equity: Moving upstream. *Maternal Child Health Journal*, 20, 935–940.

Welch, M., & Haskins, R. (2020). *What COVID-19 means for America's child welfare system*. https://www.brookings.edu/research/rebalancing-children-first/

William J. Carbonaro (1998). A little help from my friend's parents: Intergenerational closure and educational outcomes. *Sociology of Education*, 71(4), 295–313.

Williams, D. (2013, October 3). *Place matters: RWJF commission to build a healthier America. Place Matters Presentation*. Washington, DC: Place Matters Presentation by David Williams (slideshare.net).

Williams, D. R. (2018). Stress and the mental health of populations of color: Advancing our understanding of race-related stressors. *Journal of Health and Social Behavior*, 59(4), 466–485. https://doi.org/10.1177/0022146518814251

Williams, D. R., Costa, M. V., Odunlami, A. O., & Mohammed, S. A. (2008). Moving upstream: How interventions that address the social determinants of health can improve health and reduce disparities. *Journal of Public Health Management and Practice*, 14 (suppl), S8–S17. https://doi.org/10.1097/01.PHH.0000338382.36695.42

Wolford, S. N., Cooper, A. N., & McWey, L. M. (2019). Maternal depression, maltreatment history, and child outcomes: The role of harsh parenting. *American Journal of Orthopsychiatry*, 89(2), 181–191. https://doi.org/10.1037/ort0000365

Wong, J. Y., Wai, A. K., Wang, M. P., Lee, J. J., Li, M., Kwok, J. Y., Wong, C. K., & Choi, A. W. (2021). Impact of COVID-19 on Child maltreatment: income instability and parenting issues. *International Journal of Environmental Research and Public Health*, 18(4), 1501. https://doi.org/10.3390/ijerph18041501

World Health Organization Commission on the Social Determinants of Health. (2008). Closing the gap in a generation: Health equity through action on the social determinants of health (p. 1). World Health Organization.

World Health Organization. (2020, June 8). Fact Sheet: Violence against children. https://www.who.int/news-room/fact-sheets/detail/violence-against-children

Wozniak, A., Willey, J., Benz, J., & Hart, N. (2020). *COVID impact survey*. National Opinion Research Center.

Yang, M. (2015). The effect of material hardship on child protective service involvement. *Child Abuse & Neglect*, 41, 113–125. https://doi.org/10.1016/j.childyouth.2020.104926

CHAPTER 10

Mental Health as the Basis of All Health

Regina Bussing and Faye A. Gary

LEARNING OBJECTIVES

- Discuss the interconnection of general and mental health, and distinguish between mental health and mental illness.

- Integrate social determinants of health into the interplay of general and mental health.

- Explain the meaning of syndemics and apply to the COVID-19 pandemic and concurrent increases in mental disorders.

- Identify the mental-health related goals of Healthy People 2030.

- Connect the concept of adverse childhood experiences to the interplay between general and mental health.

- Identify hypothesized contributions toward reduced life expectancy in people affected by mental disorders.

- Explain wellness, self-care, and recovery practices that can improve mental health in persons with and without mental disorders.

INTRODUCTION: THE INTERCONNECTION OF GENERAL HEALTH AND MENTAL HEALTH

It is generally accepted that general health and mental health are intricately intertwined, and that mental health is important at all stages of life, from infancy through old age. For example, the World Health Organization (WHO) considers mental health an integral and essential component of health, and states in its constitution: "Health is a state of complete physical, mental, and social well-being and not merely the absence of disease or infirmity" (WHO, 2018). Furthermore, WHO describes mental health as a state of well-being in which an individual realizes their own abilities, can cope with the normal stresses of life, can work productively, and can contribute to their community. According to WHO, mental health is considered a fundamental and universal condition for human beings to think, emote, and interact with each other; earn a living; and enjoy life. WHO's viewpoint of mental health is further mirrored by the Centers for Disease Control and Prevention (CDC), who declare that "mental health includes our emotional, psychological, and social well-being. It affects how we think, feel, and act. It also helps determine how we handle stress, relate to others, and make healthy choices" (CDC, 2018). Furthermore, the CDC advises that it is important to distinguish between poor mental health and mental illness, as these terms are not interchangeable. Persons may experience poor mental health and yet not suffer from a specific diagnosable mental illness. For example, feelings of loneliness and hopelessness; poor sleep quality; unhealthy coping in the forms of increased alcohol use, binge television watching, and overeating have affected a large percentage of the U.S. population in response to the recent worldwide outbreak of a coronavirus-associated acute respiratory disease, referred to as coronavirus disease 19 (COVID-19). Yet symptoms only reach the intensity needed for formal diagnoses of new-onset mood or substance use disorders in a subset of those experiencing poor mental health. Conversely, a person with a severe mental disorder like chronic schizophrenia may be linked with a community-based care team that offers regular medication appointments enabling adherence to antipsychotic regimens that reduce psychosis symptoms, effective access to primary care to treat coexisting hypertension and reduce risk of early onset coronary disease, social engagement through a sober-living peer support group to reduce loneliness and despair, and family education about mental disorders to facilitate continued connections to the family of origin. In this example, the person with schizophrenia experiences extended periods of physical, mental, and social well-being, the ultimate goals of recovery, despite having a diagnosable mental illness.

There is also a reciprocal relationship between mental and physical health. Mental illnesses reduce expected life span; accelerate rates of aging (Wertz et al., 2021); and increase the risk for various chronic health conditions, including heart disease, diabetes, and stroke. Meanwhile, chronic medical conditions increase the risk of mental illness, especially depression (National Institute of Mental Health, 2021b). New insights about the interconnection between general and mental health continue to arise from studying the impacts of early trauma on health outcomes (Boyce et al., 2021). The interconnection is mediated through inflammation processes in childhood and adult years (Baumeister et al., 2016). The gut microbiome is considered a possible link in the puzzle (O'Mahony et al., 2017). This chapter addresses mental health, experienced as emotional, psychological, and social well-being, as the basis of all health, and examines disparities in mental health across populations, including those also affected by specific mental disorders, with a focus on the roots of disparities, historical phenomena, and solutions.

CASE STUDY 10.1: BECOMING THE HEAD OF THE HOUSE CAN BE DANGEROUS TO YOUR HEALTH

Rebecca is an outstanding and conscientious high school student. She celebrated her 14th birthday a few days before her high school adopted virtual instruction for the remainder of the year due to COVID-19. I was in contact with Rebecca and helped her to make the transition to virtual learning. She understood the need for the change and adapted well. She quickly organized her class schedule and study time to maximize her chances of earning As and staying on track to qualify for an academic scholarship. Her dream is to one day become a dentist and teach on a faculty at a university. However, a few weeks into virtual learning, things changed. Her mother, an essential worker, was required to work longer hours, and her grandmother moved into the home because she needed special care.

Rebecca had to assume the caregiving role for her two younger siblings and her grandmother, who has diabetes and hypertension. The two siblings were in elementary school and needed coaching with their school work; they had to share one computer. Rebecca became the "head of the house" while her mother worked long hours to support the family.

(continued)

CASE STUDY 10.1: BECOMING THE HEAD OF THE HOUSE CAN BE DANGEROUS TO YOUR HEALTH (*CONTINUED*)

She became highly cautious about touching and hugging her mother because of COVID-19 and the possibility of becoming ill. Rebecca would contact me, give me an update about her schoolwork, and share with pride all of the things she was accomplishing in the household to assist her family—she was proud but exhausted. Our conversations continued, and over time, there was a shift in Rebecca's tone, content, attitude, and behavior. Both of us began to be concerned. She abruptly shared a list of things that were starting to "make me feel like I am going crazy": Taking care of her grandmother's medications and checking "her sugar"; preparing breakfast and lunch for her grandmother and her two younger siblings; organizing and tutoring the siblings with homework—they were good students, too; cleaning the house and washing clothes; completing her homework and staying on task; helping her mother with other household demands and assuring everyone in the family that they would survive these hardships. Rebecca indicated that she could not sleep because of the racing thoughts in her head and the sense of feeling like she was "going crazy." She would tell herself not to go to sleep because "I might wake up crazy, and have to leave my family and go to one of those places where they lock you up." Rebecca knew something was wrong. Her capacity to care for her grandmother and siblings was waning; she was always tired and was beginning to be short and grumpy with everyone. But she was insightful enough to know that without a better "attitude," she could not help anyone. So she reached out for help. She phoned and said, "I am going crazy, I am going crazy, do you think I am crazy?" She received assistance immediately. Her mother and grandmother were also concerned about Rebecca and assisted with securing mental health services for her. Her mother dramatically decreased Rebecca's caregiving responsibilities and requested a change in her work schedule to accommodate her family's needs better. Today, Rebecca is doing well and remains in counseling. Her mother joins her in some of the sessions. Without mental health, there is no health—Rebecca and her family know that well. We hope others will learn from Rebecca and seek help when "life becomes tough and overwhelming."

SOCIAL DETERMINANTS OF HEALTH

Just as our understanding of the interconnectedness of general and mental health is increasing, so is our knowledge of the critical importance of social determinants of health (SDOH) in this interplay. As the United States moves toward value-based healthcare that incentivizes desirable outcomes over medical procedures, healthcare leaders are recognizing the importance of taking a holistic view, considering overall population health to improve care and achieve better health outcomes. WHO defines SDH as nonmedical factors that influence health outcomes, "the conditions in which people are born, grow, live, work and age, and the wider set of forces and systems shaping the conditions of daily life." There are various classification systems for SDH, and they generally include early life experiences and social and economic factors like income; education; employment; experiences of discrimination in its varied forms, like gender inequity and racial segregation; food insecurity; access to housing; neighborhood conditions, including crime rates and exposure to violence; transportation availability; and recreational opportunities, to name some examples (Bernardini et al., 2021; Hood et al., 2016; Magnan, 2017; Marmot & Bell, 2012). SDH exert an important influence on health inequities, and WHO points out that in countries at all levels of income, health and illness follow a social gradient, with lower socioeconomic position associated with worse health (WHO, 2021). As elaborated by Marmot & Bell, no country is immune from the social gradient, including countries with national healthcare services that provide free care at the point of delivery and that seek to enhance equitable access to healthcare (Marmot & Bell, 2012).

Achieving improved population health and enhanced patient experiences and outcomes, while reducing per capita cost of care, require addressing SDH and health equity, because they account for up to 80% of health outcomes (Hood et al., 2016). This is a rapidly moving field, and readers will benefit from accessing current information from such reputable sources as the National Institute of Minority Health and Health Disparities (NIMHD). In a recent workshop focusing on innovations in health disparities research (National Institute of Mental Health, 2020), the NIMHD deputy director, Dr. Webb-Hooper, identifies ongoing health disparities as the "wicked problem that is staring at all of us" and proposes "it's beyond time to accelerate meaningful progress and move into the third and fourth generation of health disparity science." She refers to first- and second-generation health disparities research as research that documented prevalence and contributing factors and mechanisms underlying health disparity risks, respectively. The third generation of health disparities research focuses on developing and testing specific interventions to reduce and eliminate disparities. The biggest gains will come from fourth-generation health disparities research that applies a "true health equity lens from the start of our efforts to their sustained completion" and pursues population-level interventions.

The NIMHD offers an evolving research framework to pursue these important goals; this framework integrates SDH among five domains of influence over the life course (biological, behavioral, physical/built environment, sociocultural environment, and healthcare system), and distinguishes four levels of influence and corresponding health outcomes; namely, individual health, family/organizational health, community health, and population health (NIMHD, 2018). Several adaptations illuminate how to use the NIMHD framework to reflect historic and sociocultural influences for unique populations. For example, the application to people from Puerto Rico identifies unique sociocultural environment influences in the form of English being taught as a second language, responses to discrimination linked to historical trauma and colonized mindset, an interpersonal network structure of extended families with women-headed households, and high levels of poverty and diaspora in the United States, among other unique influences (Lafarga Previdi & Velez Vega, 2020; Exhibit 10.1).

Syndemic Models of Health

The concept of "syndemics" adds further to our understanding of the cascading relationships between physical, mental, and social health. Syndemic theory addresses disease clustering, the aggregation of two or more diseases or health conditions in a population under conditions that exacerbate the negative health effects of any or all of the diseases involved. The disease conditions are made more deleterious by compromising social conditions like impoverishment (Islam et al., 2021; Singer et al., 2017). A syndemics-based approach goes beyond medical concepts of comorbidity and multimorbidity, and addresses the health consequences of identifiable disease interactions and the social, environmental, or economic factors that promote such interaction and worsen disease (Singer et al., 2017). As reviewed by Singer et al., the first reported syndemic was recognized during a research program focused on HIV risk prevention among drug users and described the clustering of substance abuse, violence, and AIDS (referred to as "SAVA"). They were in close conjunction with sets of other endemic conditions (e.g., other infectious diseases, infant mortality, drug abuse, suicide, homicide) and sustained by political/economic and social factors (e.g., unemployment, overcrowding, disrupted social networks). The results were evident in social marginalization, stigmatization, and limited resources in affected populations (Singer et al., 2017). Syndemics often involve adverse interactions among psychiatric and chronic diseases. For example, depression is a crucial element in the course and health outcomes of angina, arthritis, asthma, and diabetes (WHO, 2018), and is a component of the syndemics of violence, immigration, depression, type 2 diabetes, and abuse (termed VIDDA) affecting Mexican

EXHIBIT 10.1: National Institute on Minority Health and Health Disparities Research Framework

Lifecourse (↔, spanning all levels)

Domains of Influence	Individual	Interpersonal	Community	Societal
Biological	• Biological Vulnerability and Mechanisms	• Caregiver-Child Interaction • Family Microbiome	• Community Illness Exposure U.S. Navy presence in Vieques and Culebra Ashes from AES plant Hazardous waste sites • Herd Immunity	• Sanitation Water quality Immunization 85% in 35 mo (2014) • Pathogen Exposure Dengue, Chikungunya, Zika, Leptospirosis, STIs
Behavioral	• Health Behaviors • Coping Strategies Resilience Religion/Spirituality Communal bonds	• Family Functioning Extended family Women as heads of household • School/Work Functioning	• Community Functioning Solidarity Community councils	• Policies and Laws Puerto Rico Oversight, Management, and Economic Stability Act (PROMESA) Law Jones Act Civil Code
Physical/Built Environment	• Personal Environment	• Household Environment Deficient infrastructure Public housing Closed neighborhoods • School/Work Environment School closures Deficient infrastructure	• Community Environment Natural resources Social capital	• Societal Structure Almost 50% live in poverty Diaspora in the United States
Socio cultural Environment	• Socio-demographics 20% less than 18 years 20% 65 years or more 60% 18-64 years old • Limited English English taught as a second language • Cultural Identity Boricua/American citizens • Response to Discrimination Historical trauma Colonized mindset	• Social Networks Extended family Organized communities • Family/Peer Norms • Interpersonal Discrimination	• Community Resources Tourism Local businesses Local nongovernmental organizations • Community Norms • Local Structural Discrimination	• Societal Norms • Societal Structural Discrimination Racism Classism Sexism, Homophobia/Transphobia
Healthcare System	• Insurance Coverage Mi Salud program Private insurance Medicare/Medicaid • Health Literacy • Treatment Preferences Focus on remedial instead of prevention medicine	• Patient-Clinical Relationship • Medical Decision-Making	• Availability of Services Migration of physicians Private practices Difficulty receiving referrals Community health centers • Safety Net Services Community health centers	• Quality of Care Health professional shortage Poorly coordinated care Long wait times • Health Care Policies Department of Health Law (1912)
Health Outcomes	Individual Health	Family/Organizational Health	Community Health	Population Health

Levels of Influence spans the Individual, Interpersonal, Community, and Societal columns.

Source: Lafarga Previdi, I., & Vélez Vega, C. M. (2020). Health disparities research framework. Adaptation to reflect Puerto Rico's socio-cultural context. *International Journal of Environmental Research and Public Health, 17*(22), 8544. https://doi.org/10.3390/ijerph17228544.

immigrant women in the United States (Singer et al., 2017). More recently, the worldwide outbreak of COVID-19 unveiled a new syndemic of chronic disease: mortality related to COVID-19 and other causes, mental illness, substance use disorder, social vulnerability, and racial inequity (Singh et al., 2020). For example, in a recent U.S. study, after categorizing counties by social vulnerability/disadvantage, researchers examined incidence and mortality from COVID-19, together with prevalence of chronic diseases. Results showed a clustering of counties with high mortality, high chronic illness prevalence, and high social vulnerability. Counties in the most vulnerable group had twice the rates of COVID-19 cases and deaths compared with the least vulnerable group (Islam et al., 2021). In the United States, the disproportionally high rate of COVID-19 cases among racial/ethnic minorities can be linked to numerous social determinants of health, including access to health services and COVID testing, working in front-line jobs that do not allow social distancing or teleworking, and crowded living environments, to mention a few. As outlined by Bernardini et al. (2020), the mental health effects of the COVID-19 pandemic have been considerable and are anticipated to rise; they include serious stress associated with sleep problems, increased substance use, suicidality, depression, anxiety, and worsening of pre-existing mental disorders (Bernardini et al., 2021). For children and adolescents, similarly concerning findings have been reported (Singh et al., 2020).

Healthy People 2030 Goals

Considering the recent COVID-19 pandemic and syndemic impacts on population health, the U.S. Healthy People initiative is an especially relevant resource for communities and organizations seeking to improve health while eliminating health disparities (Healthy People, 2020a). From its origin as a 1979 landmark report by Surgeon General Julius Richmond, "Healthy People: The Surgeon General's Report on Health Promotion and Disease Prevention" (U.S. Department of Health, Education, and Welfare [DHEW], 1979), the current program, Healthy People 2030, represents the fifth iteration of this public health initiative. In a review of the genesis, history, context, and precedents of the U.S. Healthy People initiative, Green and Fielding point out several important phenomena, including its thematic consistency with WHO's *Health for All by 2000* declaration issued in 1978. There was a coincidental timing of the 1979 report with WHO's announcement of the virtual eradication of smallpox, and a conceptual consistency with a Canadian initiative, *A New Perspective on the Health of Canadians*, issued in 1974 by the Minister of Health of Canada (Green & Fielding, 2011). An important component of the latter was that it distinguished four areas of determinants of health, namely human biology, environment, lifestyle, and healthcare organizations, and emphasized to policymakers the scope of health outcome improvements that could be achieved from changes in environment and lifestyle. In subsequent decades, these four areas of health determinants continue to be recognized, but our understanding has been deepened beyond the original framework proposed (Laframboise, 1973). For example, eating behaviors were grouped under "lifestyle" variables and attributed to individual choices. However, we have become aware of the importance of sociocultural factors exemplified by food deserts or biological factors as expressed by microbiomes (Morar & Skorburg, 2020; Wiss et al., 2020). As suggested by Green and Fielding (2011), the inaugural U.S. Healthy People initiative was thus strongly influenced by three overlapping factors: the historical achievement of communicable disease control, an increasing focus on chronic diseases as leading causes of death, and concerns about the growing costs of healthcare. These factors are especially noteworthy because the fifth iteration of Healthy People faces a very different historical context. Communicable disease has moved to the forefront again, as demonstrated by the COVID-19 pandemic, and acute COVID-19 illness superimposed on chronic diseases became a leading cause of death. The worldwide pandemic has resulted in increased healthcare costs, and the economic effects of a shorter and less healthy life, estimated at $16 trillion or 90% of the annual gross domestic product for the United States (Cutler & Summers, 2020).

Assembled prior to the impact of the COVID-19 pandemic, and envisioning a society in which all people can achieve their full potential for health and well-being across the life span, the Healthy People, 2030 mission is to promote, strengthen, and evaluate the nation's efforts by identifying public health priorities/health indicators and offering tools to track progress (Healthy People, 2020b). Informed by the staggering fact that about half of all people in the United States will be diagnosed with a mental disorder at some point in their lifetime (Kessler et al., 2007), Healthy People 2030 places great emphasis on the prevention, screening, assessment, and treatment of mental disorders and behavioral conditions (Healthy People, 2020b). Hence, mental health is given a prominent role in the selection of leading health indicators for Healthy People 2030. Six of 23 high-priority indicators are mental health/substance related, namely drug overdose deaths, suicides, adolescents with major depression who receive treatment, current tobacco use among adolescents; adult binge drinking; and cigarette smoking in adults. These particular indicators are highly relevant in the context of the COVID-19 pandemic, because mental health effects include increased substance use and overdose deaths, as well as depression and suicidal acts (Bernardini et al., 2021). Healthy People 2030 is designed to encourage policymakers and health professionals in communities, states, and various organizations to select their own priorities, identify needs and set targets, find inspiration and practical tools, and then monitor progress using established benchmarks (Healthy People, 2020a; https://health .gov/healthypeople/tools-action/use-healthy-people-2030-your-work).

Adverse Child Events and Adverse Health Outcomes

Another important related concept undergirding the reciprocal relationship between mental and physical health involves early childhood traumatic experiences, clustering of risk factors, and subsequent health outcomes referred to as adverse child events (ACEs). The original ACE study is considered a "classic." It was conducted from 1995 to 1997 through a health maintenance organization (HMO), Kaiser Permanente, and it involved more than 17,000 HMO members. Results about the powerful associations between seven childhood ACEs (psychological or physical or sexual abuse; violence against mother; living with household members who were substance users, mentally ill, suicidal, or imprisoned) and adult disease, health status, and risk behavior were astounding: Persons who had experienced four or more categories of childhood exposure, compared with someone who had experienced none, had 4- to 12-fold increased health risks for alcoholism, drug abuse, depression, and suicide attempt; a 2- to 4-fold increase in smoking, poor self-rated health, 50 or more sexual intercourse partners, and sexually transmitted infection; and a 1.4- to 1.6-fold increase in physical inactivity and severe obesity (Felitti et al., 1998). Since the early study, research on ACEs has abounded, and the CDC developed intervention and education materials based on ACEs (www.cdc.gov/violenceprevention/aces/index. html accessed 2/28/2021). According to the CDC, ACEs are potentially traumatic events that occur in childhood and can include experiencing violence and abuse and growing up in a family with mental health or substance abuse problems. ACEs can exert toxic stress that may change brain development and subsequent physical and mental health. It is now well established that preventing ACEs in the first place can help lower the risk for chronic health conditions, including asthma, cancer, diabetes, and depression, and also reduce risky health behaviors such as smoking or heavy drinking (www.cdc.gov/vitalsigns/aces/pdf/ vs.-1105-aces-H.pdf; accessed 2/28/2021). Research is continuing because many states are collecting information about ACEs through the Behavioral Risk Factor Surveillance System (BRFSS). The BRFSS is an annual, state-based, random-digit-dial telephone survey that collects data from noninstitutionalized U.S. adults regarding health conditions and risk factors. Since 2009, 48 states plus the District of Columbia have included ACE questions for at least 1 year on their survey. The general findings continue to be similar to the original ACE study: Almost two thirds of surveyed adults report at least one ACE and over one quarter report three or more. Studies show a graded dose-response curve, such that risks for negative health outcomes increase with the number of ACEs. (See Chapter 22 for additional information on ACEs.)

Mental Disorder and Reduced Life Expectancy

Although socioeconomic factors are associated with significant health disparities, including reduced life expectancy, the largest health disparity is linked with having a severe mental illness (Colton & Manderscheid, 2006). Persons with mental disorders like schizophrenia, bipolar disorder, or depression die an average of 10 to 20 years younger than those without (Liu et al., 2017). Shortened life spans are not solely due to higher rates of suicide or unintentional injury in people with severe mental illness, but to acute or chronic medical illnesses, especially cardiovascular and metabolic disorders. A global review of mortality among people with mental disorders from 29 countries, including a meta-analysis of 203 cohort design studies, concluded that overall median years of life lost in persons with mental illness was 10.1 years, with 67% of deaths due to "natural causes" like acute or chronic illness, and 18% due to unintentional injury or suicide or "unnatural causes." Of note, in this international sample, no differences in mortality rates were found by geography, sample source, or diagnostic system, but mortality risk in all countries was nearly doubled by mental disorders for "natural causes" and increased 7-fold for "unnatural causes" (Walker et al., 2015). A recent U.S. study conducted in Medicaid populations found that patients with schizophrenia were 3.5 times more likely to die during the 7-year study period compared with the general population, and that estimated lost years of life were a staggering 28.5 years (Olfson et al., 2015). The five most common causes of death in people who were Medicaid beneficiaries and had a diagnosis of schizophrenia were ischemic or other heart disease (40%), accidents (14%), chronic obstructive pulmonary disease (11%), lung cancer (9%), and diabetes (7%; Olfson et al., 2015). Increased rates of these disorders have also been reported for patients with depression and bipolar disorder (Currier & Nemeroff, 2014; Gale et al., 2014; Roshanaei-Moghaddam & Katon, 2009; Rustad et al., 2011). Conversely, major depressive disorder has been found to co-occur at markedly higher rates among patients with various chronic health conditions, including over half of patients with Parkinson's disease and approximately one quarter of patients with cerebrovascular disease or with diabetes (National Center for Chronic Disease Prevention and Health Promotion, 2012; Box 10.1).

Further complicating the picture is "multimorbidity," or pairing of multiple chronic medical and mental disorders (Barnett et al., 2012) in the context of economic deprivation. In a health registry study of 314 medical practices in Scotland, health records of more than 1.7 million patients were examined for number and type of disorder comorbidities, gender, age, and socioeconomic status. Consistent with WHO reports of the social gradient of health, multimorbidity occurred 10 to 15 years earlier in people living in the most deprived areas compared with those in most affluent communities. Notably, socioeconomic deprivation was particularly associated with mental disorders (Barnett et al., 2012). The researchers advise that health systems need to evolve to address these multimorbidities and grow beyond disease-specific patient care models in medical education, clinical research, and hospital care (National Council for Behavioral Health, 2018). Intradisciplinary education, clinical practice, and research collaborations that are emerging in academic and health systems are projected to address these historical issues (Chhabra, 2021).

Finally, there are also compelling data from the Dunedin Multidisciplinary Health and Development Study that indicate that a history of psychopathology was associated with accelerated aging at midlife, years before the typical onset of age-related diseases (Wertz et al., 2021). The Dunedin study has followed the lives of 1,037 infants born between April 1972 and March 1973 at the Queen Mary Maternity Hospital in Dunedin, New Zealand, and is in its fifth decade of data collection, providing information across three generations of New Zealanders. Findings are enriched through specific substudies, including the Family Health History Study, which gathered information on first-degree relatives of the study cohort; the Parenting Study, which included cohort members who were now parenting a 3-year-old;

BOX 10.1: Severe Mental Disorders and Reduced Life Expectancy

Scope of premature mortality among people with severe mental disorders

- On average, a 10- to 25-year reduction in life expectancy
- Mortality risk ratio compared to general population
  - Psychosis 2.5 times
  - Mood disorder 1.9 times
  - Anxiety 1.4 times

Main proximal causes

- Chronic medical conditions
  - Cardiovascular disease and hypertension
  - Cancer
  - Respiratory illness
  - Infections
  - Diabetes
- Accidents and suicide

Contributing and preventable/mutable causes

- Individual factors
  - Genetics of general and mental health conditions
  - Mutable health behaviors (diet, tobacco and substance use, physical activity, risk behaviors
  - Mutable socioeconomics (unemployment, homelessness, low health literacy)

Health system

- Leadership (absent policies, guidelines, and financing for integrated care)
- Human resources
  - Inadequate integrated training for general healthcare of persons with severe mental disorders
  - Stigma within work force
- Service delivery
  - Fragmentation and lack of coordination
  - Nonevidence-based use of psychotropic medications (lack of metabolic monitoring, polypharmacy, lack of adherence-enhancing efforts)

Social and system determinants

- A pernicious challenge—higher mortality rates for people with severe mental disorders found world-wide, across various healthcare and health insurance systems
- Discriminatory insurance practices and carve-outs for mental health
- Limited investment in family, community, and neighborhood resources
- Sparse employment, housing, and social welfare supports for affected people

and the Next Generation Study, which focuses on 15-year-old teenagers whom the cohort members are parenting. The aging research findings on the original cohort members are based on a very carefully designed study that controlled for childhood factors and measured pace of aging as changes in 19 well-validated biomarkers. The study also documented changes in vision, hearing, balance, and motor and cognitive function through laboratory as well as self-report measures. The study accounted for health behaviors that could influence pace of aging, as well as for antipsychotic medications and the presence of physical disease.

Of note, accelerated aging was found across externalizing, internalizing, and thought disorders, and was not specific to a particular disorder group (Wertz et al., 2021).

Self-Care, Recovery, and Wellness

As outlined in the beginning of this chapter, mental health is an essential component of overall health, and self-care combined with effective self-advocacy play important roles in achieving the best health outcomes, including recovery. The importance of self-care has been acknowledged by the NIMH, describing self-care as "taking the time to do things that help you live well and improve both your physical health and mental health" (NIMH, 2021a). The NIMH offers five distinct wellness toolkits (focused on environments, feelings, physical fitness, relationships/social connections, and disease prevention), based on the realization that every person's "healthiest self" requires unique considerations. Self-care and effective advocacy, in the context of psychoeducation and stigma-busting, are at the heart of the National Alliance on Mental Illness (NAMI), the largest U.S.-based grassroots organization serving individuals and families affected by mental illness. Started in 1979 by family members of youths with severe mental disorders, NAMI has grown to an alliance with affiliates in every state (NAMI, 2021). NAMI offers various ways for individuals with mental disorders and their family members to get involved, through free education classes, support events, and organized advocacy initiatives. Families can learn about signs and symptoms of mental disorders, evidence-based treatments, and how to best support their affected family member—whether child, partner, or other relative—on their path to recovery. NAMI also offers well-received peer-to-peer education and support groups and stigma-reducing presentations in various community venues such as "Ending the Silence™" or "In Our Own Voice™."

An important example of an international community dedicated to improving the lives of those with severe mental illness is Clubhouse International (2021). Based on an underlying philosophy that people with mental illness can lead normal, productive lives when provided with a community that offers long-term relationships in a restorative environment, Clubhouse International is focused on obtaining employment, education, and housing. Initially founded in 1948 in New York, there are now over 300 Clubhouses in over 30 countries. Participation in Clubhouses is free of charge to members. Even though medical treatment is considered important, and Clubhouses may help members to locate and gain access to needed medical services, the focus is on being a social member and on social activities, rather than on being a patient in a medical treatment program. Clubhouses offer voluntary participation in work day programs, as well as educational and employment programs that connect members to paid jobs. Clubhouses follow International Standards for Clubhouse Programs™, which define the Clubhouse Model of rehabilitation and get reviewed every 2 years. The program reports impactful outcomes, including reductions in hospital stays and incarcerations, as well as increased employment rates, all of which translate into improved wellness and recovery goals.

Mental Health American (MHA) is another important U.S. organization designed to promote mental health as a vital component of overall wellness (MHA, 2021). It focuses on early identification and prompt treatment for individuals at risk, supports integrated care, and advocates for those needing assistance, with recovery as its primary goal. MHA local boards govern the organization through affiliates in more than 200 communities across the United States, with a national organization and its board of directors situated in Alexandria, Virginia. MHA was founded in 1906 by Clifford W. Beers (see the book, *The Mind that Found Itself*) and is a leading community-based organization that advocates for promoting mental health and addressing the comprehensive needs of individuals and families living with mental illness. Its mission includes promoting mental health and preventing disease through advocacy, education, research, and service. It highlights a Before Stage 4 (B4 Stage 4) approach to prevention and treatment: prevention; identify symptoms; develop a plan of action to stop or reverse disease progression; develop a pathway to overall health. Efforts in all affiliates include education and outreach, public policy, peer advocacy, social support, and services. Its associates work to protect the rights and dignity of individuals and families with mental illnesses and assist peers in their work by integrating their perspectives into all aspects of the organization.

CONCLUSIONS

General and mental health are intricately intertwined. Even though our genetic endowment plays a relevant role in our health outcomes, mutable experiences at the level of family, community, and society influence the expression and course of disease and, equally important, our experiences of well-being and resilience in the face of health challenges—be they general or mental health disorders, or, a frequent reality, a combination. Biomedical research over the past decade has provided us with compelling insights into what causes and perpetuates mental disorders, validating that these illnesses are not the result of faulty parenting or due to lack of character or weak willpower. Determinants of health and well-being are similar across the globe, as is an increasing desire to shed old stigmas that shorten the life expectancies and quality of life of those with mental disorders. The path is charted and the vision can be accomplished by using proven resources such as embodied by the Healthy People 2030 initiative (Healthy People, 2020b).

REFERENCES

Barnett, K., Mercer, S. W., Norbury, M., Watt, G., Wyke, S., & Guthrie, B. (2012). Epidemiology of multimorbidity and implications for health care, research, and medical education: A cross-sectional study. *Lancet*, *380*(9836), 37–43. https://doi.org/10.1016/S0140-6736(12)60240-2

Baumeister, D., Akhtar, R., Ciufolini, S., Pariante, C. M., & Montelli V., (2016). Childhood trauma and adulthood inflammation: A meta-analysis of peripheral C-reative protein, interleukin-6 and tumor necrosis factor-α. *Molecular Psychiatry*, *21*(5), 642–649. https://doi.org/10.1038/mp.2015.67

Bernardini, F., Attademo, L., Rotter, M., & Compton, M. T. (2021). Social determinants of mental health as mediators and moderators of the mental health impacts of the covid-19 pandemic. *Psychiatric Services*, appips202000393. https://doi.org/10.1176/appi.ps.202000393

Boyce, W. T., Levitt, P., Martinez, F. D., McEwen, B. S., & Shonkoff, J. P. (2021). Genes, environments, and time: The biology of adversity and resilience. *Pediatrics*, *147*(2). https://doi.org/10.1542/peds.2020-1651

Centers for Disease Control and Prevention. (2018, January 26, 2018). Learn about mental health. https://www.cdc.gov/mentalhealth/learn/index.htm

Chhabra, S. (2021). Challenges in health professionals' training and health care for wellness. *International Journal of Healthcare Management*, *14*(1), 230–235. https://doi.org/10.1080/20479700.2019.1641951

Clubhouse International. (2021). Clubhourse international-what we do. https://clubhouse-intl.org/what-we-do/overview/

Colton, C. W., & Manderscheid, R. W. (2006). Congruencies in increased mortality rates, years of potential life lost, and causes of death among public mental health clients in eight states. *Preventing Chronic Disease*, *3*(2), A42. https://www.ncbi.nlm.nih.gov/pubmed/16539783

Currier, M. B., & Nemeroff, C. B. (2014). Depression as a risk factor for cancer: From pathophysiological advances to treatment implications. *Annual Review of Medicine*, *65*, 203–221. https://doi.org/10.1146/annurev-med-061212-171507

Cutler, D. M., & Summers, L. H. (2020). The COVID-19 pandemic and the $16 trillion virus. *JAMA*, *324*(15), 1495–1496. https://doi.org/10.1001/jama.2020.19759

Felitti, V. J., Anda, R. F., Nordenberg, D., Williamson, D. F., Spitz, A. M., Edwards, V., … Marks, J. S. (1998). Relationship of childhood abuse and household dysfunction to many of the leading causes of death in adults. The adverse childhood experiences (ACE) study. *American Journal of Preventive Medicine*, *14*(4), 245–258. https://doi.org/10.1016/s0749-3797(98)00017-8

Gale, C. R., Batty, G. D., Osborn, D. P., Tynelius, P., & Rasmussen, F. (2014). Mental disorders across the adult life course and future coronary heart disease: Evidence for general susceptibility. *Circulation*, *129*(2), 186–193. https://doi.org/10.1161/CIRCULATIONAHA.113.002065

Green, L. W., & Fielding, J. (2011). The U.S. healthy people initiative: Its genesis and its sustainability. *Annual Review of Public Health, 32*, 451–470. https:/doi.org/10.1146/annurev-publhealth -031210-101148

Healthy People. (2020a). About healthy people 2030. https://health.gov/healthypeople/about

Healthy People. (2020b). Leading health indicators. https://health.gov/healthypeople/objectives -and-data/leading-health-indicators

Hood, C. M., Gennuso, K. P., Swain, G. R., & Catlin, B. B. (2016). County health rankings: Relationships between determinant factors and health outcomes. *American Journal of Preventive Medicine, 50*(2), 129–135. https:/doi.org/10.1016/j.amepre.2015.08.024

Islam, N., Lacey, B., Shabnam, S., Erzurumluoglu, A. M., Dambha-Miller, H., Chowell, G., Kawachi, I., & Marmot, M. (2021). Social inequality and the syndemic of chronic disease and COVID-19: County-level analysis in the USA. *Journal of Epidemiology and Community Health.* https://doi .org/10.1136/jech-2020-215626

Kessler, R. C., Angermeyer, M., Anthony, J. C., Graaf, Ron D. E., Demyttenaere, K., Gasquet, I., ... Ustun, T. B. (2007). Lifetime prevalence and age-of-onset distributions of mental disorders in the World Health Organization's World Mental Health Survey Initiative. *World Psychiatry, 6*(3), 168–176. https:// www.ncbi.nlm.nih.gov/pubmed/18188442

Lafarga Previdi, I., & Velez Vega, C. M. (2020). Health disparities research framework adaptation to reflect Puerto Rico's socio-cultural context. *International Journal of Environmental Research and Public Health, 17*(22). https:/doi.org/10.3390/ijerph17228544

Laframboise, H. L. (1973). Health policy: Breaking the problem down into more manageable segments. *Canadian Medical Association Journal, 108*(3), 388–391. https://www.ncbi.nlm.nih.gov/ pubmed/4691098

Liu, N. H., Daumit, G. L., Dua, T., Aquila, R., Charlson, F., Cuijpers, P., ... Saxena, S. (2017). Excess mortality in persons with severe mental disorders: A multilevel intervention framework and priorities for clinical practice, policy and research agendas. *World Psychiatry, 16*(1), 30–40. https:/ doi.org/10.1002/wps.20384

Magnan, S. (2017). Social determinants of health 101 for health care: Five plus five. *NAM Perspectives.* https://doi.org/10.31478/201710c

Marmot, M., & Bell, R. (2012). Fair society, healthy lives. *Public Health, 126*(suppl 1), S4–S10. https:/ doi.org/10.1016/j.puhe.2012.05.014

Mental Health America. (2021). Mental health America. https://www.mhanational.org/

Morar, N., & Skorburg, J. A. (2020). Why we never eat alone: The overlooked role of microbes and partners in obesity debates in bioethics. *Journal of Bioethical Inquiry, 17*(3), 435–448. https:/doi .org/10.1007/s11673-020-10047-2

National Alliance on Mental Illness. (2021). About NAMI. https://nami.org/About-NAMI

National Center for Chronic Disease Prevention and Health Promotion (Producer). (2012, 6/14/2021). Mental health and chronic disease. Issue brief. https://www.cdc.gov/ workplacehealthpromotion/tools-resources/pdfs/issue-brief-no-2-mental-health-and-chronic -disease.pdf

National Council for Behavioral Health. (2018, July 21, 2018). The largest health disparity gap in the nation: What you can do to close it. https://www.thenationalcouncil.org/BH365/2018/06/21/ the-largest-health-disparity-gap-in-the-nation-what-you-can-do-to-close-it/

National Institute of Mental Health (Producer). (2020, 5/23/2021). Identifying new directions in mental health disparities research: Innovations with a multidimensional lens - day one, part one. [Multimedia conference recording]. https://www.nimh.nih.gov/news/media/2020/identifying -new-directions-in-mental-health-disparities-research-innovations-with-a-multidimensional-lens -day-one-part-one

National Institute of Mental Health. (2021a). Caring for your mental health. https://www.nimh.nih .gov/health/topics/caring-for-your-mental-health/

National Institute of Mental Health. (2021b). Chronic illness and mental health: Recognizing and treating depression. https://www.nimh.nih.gov/health/publications/chronic-illness-mental-health/

National Institute on Minority Health and Health Disparities. (2018). National institute on minority health and health disparities research framework. https://nimhd.nih.gov/docs/research_ framework/research-framework-slide.pdf

O'Mahony, S. M., Clarke, G., Dinan, T. G., & Cryan, J. F. (2017). Early-life adversity and brain development: Is the microbiome a missing piece of the puzzle? *Neuroscience, 342*, 37–54. https:/doi .org/10.1016/j.neuroscience.2015.09.068

Olfson, M., Gerhard, T., Huang, C., Crystal, S., & Stroup, T. S. (2015). Premature mortality among adults with schizophrenia in the United States. *JAMA Psychiatry, 72*(12), 1172–1181. https:/doi .org/10.1001/jamapsychiatry.2015.1737

Roshanaei-Moghaddam, B., & Katon, W. (2009). Premature mortality from general medical illnesses among persons with bipolar disorder: A review. *Psychiatric Services, 60*(2), 147–156. https:/doi .org/10.1176/appi.ps.60.2.147 https://doi.org/10.1176/ps.2009.60.2.147

Rustad, J. K., Musselman, D. L., & Nemeroff, C. B. (2011). The relationship of depression and diabetes: Pathophysiological and treatment implications. *Psychoneuroendocrinology, 36*(9), 1276–1286. https://doi.org/10.1016/j.psyneuen.2011.03.005

Singer, M., Bulled, N., Ostrach, B., & Mendenhall, E. (2017). Syndemics and the biosocial conception of health. *Lancet, 389*(10072), 941–950. https://doi.org/10.1016/S0140-6736(17)30003-X

Singh, S., Roy, D., Sinha, K., Parveen, S., Sharma, G., & Joshi, G. (2020). Impact of COVID-19 and lockdown on mental health of children and adolescents: A narrative review with recommendations. *Psychiatry Research, 293*, 113429. https://doi.org/10.1016/j.psychres.2020.113429

U.S. Department of Health, Education, and Welfare. (1979). Healthy People: The surgeon general's report on health promotion and disease prevention. Washington, DC.

Walker, E. R., McGee, R. E., & Druss, B. G. (2015). Mortality in mental disorders and global disease burden implications: A systematic review and meta-analysis. *JAMA Psychiatry, 72*(4), 334–341. https://doi.org/10.1001/jamapsychiatry.2014.2502

Wertz, J., Caspi, A., Ambler, A., Broadbent, J., Hancox, R. J., Harrington, H., … Moffitt, T. E. (2021). Association of history of psychopathology with accelerated aging at midlife. *JAMA Psychiatry*. https://doi.org/10.1001/jamapsychiatry.2020.4626

Wiss, D. A., Avena, N., & Gold, M. (2020). Food addiction and psychosocial adversity: Biological embedding, contextual factors, and public health implications. *Nutrients, 12*(11). https://doi .org/10.3390/nu12113521

World Health Organization. (2018, March 30, 2018). Mental health: Strengthening our response. https://www.who.int/en/news-room/fact-sheets/detail/mental-health-strengthening -our-response

World Health Organization. (2021). Social determinants of health. https://www.who.int/health -topics/social-determinants-of-health#tab=tab_1

CHAPTER 11

Endemic Stress and Racism

Rachel Hardeman, Brittney N. Butler, Brigette A. Davis, Rebekah Israel Cross, Miamon Queeglay, and Eduardo M. Medina

LEARNING OBJECTIVES

- Define racism and understand how racism operates in various contexts.
- Explain the relationship among racism, health, and health inequalities.
- Understand how racism impacts health.
- Identify social determinants of health.
- Explain neighborhood effects on adverse health outcomes.
- Identify three current measures of racism in public health.

INTRODUCTION AND BACKGROUND

The term *racism* is rarely used in medical literature. Most clinicians in the United States are not explicitly racist and are committed to treating all patients equally; however, they operate in an inherently racist health system. Structural racism in the United States is entrenched (Figure 11.1), and a large and growing body of literature documents disparate outcomes for different races despite the best efforts of individual healthcare professionals. Endemic stress caused by racist systems is the root cause of health inequities. Researchers and clinicians have long used rhetoric implying that differences between races are intrinsic, inherited, or biological. Pre-Civil War physicians attributed poor health among enslaved people in America to their "biological inferiority" rather than to their conditions of servitude, and such beliefs persist today. Although several specific populations have been designated as "minority," including Asian Americans, Native Americans, and Latinx Americans, this chapter focuses on Black/African American people, given (a) the well-documented accounts of historical and contemporary racism in the literature, and (b) the fact that Black people in the United States are disproportionately burdened by numerous adverse health outcomes, and these disparities are often attributed to their race. This chapter identifies the varying dimensions of racism, highlights historical and contemporary examples of racism and its impact on current health behaviors and outcomes, and provides theories and measurements to

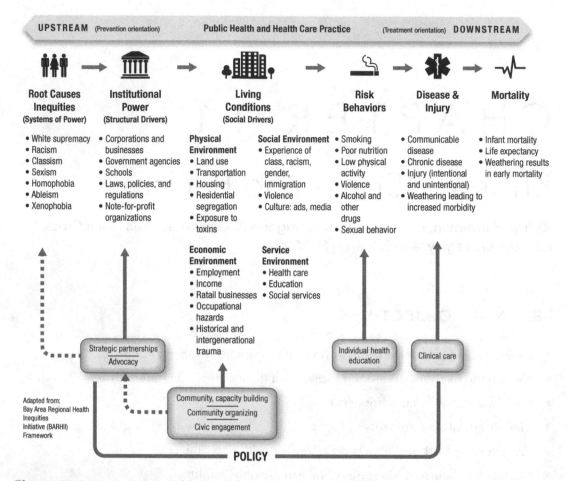

Figure 11.1 Inequities in Public Health and Healthcare Practice.

Note: Upstream refers to acknowledging and addressing the structural, societal, community and individual-level factors that influence health, whereas downstream refers to the dominant approach of treating individual-level factors and/or contributors without wholly addressing structural, societal, and community factors.

ground healthcare professionals interested in examining the relationship between racism and health. Table 11.1 provides terms and definitions related to dimensions of racism.

HOW RACISM IMPACTS HEALTH

Racism shapes health by creating and sustaining social contexts with inequitable risk exposures, differential access to health-promoting resources, and biological manifestations due to racialized stressors (Bailey et al., 2017; Williams et al., 2019). It intersects with various identities to shape and reinforce health inequities (Williams et al., 2019). Researchers have theorized and documented how racism across various sectors of society impacts health through behavioral, psychological, and physiological pathways (Williams et al., 2019). This section is a limited representation of the research.

Anti-Black Racism

Anti-Blackness is a confluence of institutions, culture, history, ideology, and codified practices that dehumanizes and marginalizes Black people. This is the common denominator of the health inequities that cut short the lives of Black people in the United States. Anti-Blackness is causing widespread suffering, not only for Black people and other communities

TABLE 11.1 Terms and Definitions

Term	Definition
Stereotypes	Beliefs and opinions about the characteristics, attributes, and behaviors of members of various groups (Routledge & CRC Press, 2021)
Prejudice	An attitude directed toward a person because they are a member of a particular racialized group (Routledge & CRC Press, 2021)
Discrimination	Treating a person differently from others based primarily on their membership (perceived or identified) in a marginalized group (Routledge & CRC Press, 2021)
Internalized Racism	When members of a racialized group internalize discriminatory group stereotypes and accept them to be true. The beliefs of these stereotypes may lead to them wanting to dissociate with characteristics and features of the group (Jones et al., 2020)
Interpersonal Racism	Individual-level discrimination based on prejudices and stereotypes of racialized groups developed by larger societal ideologies (Jones et al., 2000)
Institutional Racism	Legal and socially accepted practices that create racialized patterns of disproportionate and limited access to services, goods, wealth, knowledge, and opportunities. Due to its invisible nature, it does not require individual animus to reproduce itself; rather, it informs the customs or values of the dominant group, which is then used to continue the practice even when practices are outlawed (Jones et al., 2020); for example, in medical institutions like schools and hospitals
Structural Racism	The linkages across institutions where racism in one institution not only exacerbates experiences of racism in another institution, but also undergirds and maintains the existence of that linked institution (Bailey et al., 2017; Gee & Ford, 2011)
Obstetric Racism	An occurrence and analytic that best captures the unique experiences and conditions of Black mothers and birthing people's reproductive and perinatal care during pregnancy, labor, and birth at the intersections of obstetric violence and medical racism; a threat to positive birth outcomes (Davis, 2019)

of color, but also for society at large, and it is a threat to the physical, emotional, and social well-being of Black communities (Hardeman, 2016).

Anti-Blackness is a direct result of structural racism, which lies underneath, all around, and across society, and refers to the normalization and legitimization of an array of dynamics (historical, cultural, institutional, economic, and interpersonal) that routinely advantage other racial groups while producing cumulative and chronic adverse outcomes for Black people (Hardeman, 2016). Structural racism encompasses (a) history, which lies underneath the surface, providing the foundation for White supremacy in this country; (b) culture, which exists and influences our daily lives, providing the normalization and replication of anti-Black racism by all members of society; and (c) interconnected institutions and policies, the key relationships and rules across society providing the legitimacy and reinforcements to maintain and perpetuate anti-Black racism.

Health Behaviors

Much of the work exploring health inequities has focused on various individual-level health behaviors as ways to mitigate the burden of the disparities for Black families. However, research shows that anti-Black racism shapes health behaviors through the use of structural barriers that prohibit many Black families from engaging in behaviors that can improve health outcomes, such as accessing healthy foods, engaging in physical activity, accessing equitable educational opportunities, securing employment, and acquiring safe and stable housing, to name a few (Bailey et al., 2017; Chadha et al., 2020; Gee & Ford, 2011). Due to its omnipresence, it is often hard to disentangle individual behaviors from the structure that shapes them (Butler et al., 2020). For example, obesity has been identified as a key risk factor for numerous health outcomes (Dixon, 2010), with many interventions centered on weight loss (Dixon, 2010). However, this does not account for disparate zoning policies that create food deserts, with limited grocery stores and oversaturation of fast-food restaurants and corner stores leading to greater rates of consumption of unhealthy foods (Barker et al., 2012; Chen & Florax, 2010; Lovasi et al., 2009). Even when healthy foods are available, the affordability of those foods is a critical barrier further exacerbated by employment and wage disparities for Black families due to discrimination. Inequitable distribution of resources also leads to certain neighborhoods having fewer green spaces and outdated infrastructure, limiting the amounts of physical activity in which families are able to engage (Lovasi et al., 2009; Rigolon et al., 2018). Inequitable resources also limit access to jobs to those that are precarious and low-wage work, often limiting health insurance, reducing access to quality education that supports economic mobility, and restricting access to well-being. These policies and practices directly shape people's eating and physical activity patterns. Across all five domains of the social determinants of health, structural racism is hypothesized to be a root cause of the disproportionate burden for Black families (Yearby, 2020).

In addition to persistent structural barriers preventing health-promoting behaviors, racism in healthcare delivery and public health research persistently shapes the use of healthcare services for Black families (Hall et al., 2015; Lee et al., 2009). Stereotypes, racial beliefs, personal lived experiences, racial socialization, family, and upbringing all shape one's explicit and implicit biases. These biases then shape how people interact with others, as well as how they perceive themselves.

Personal experiences of inferior care, as well as historical experimentation on Black patients by hospital systems and research universities, have exacerbated mistrust in the healthcare system and deters engagement from this population (Washington, 2006). One notable example of experimentation on Black patients by the U.S. government was the U.S. Public Health Services Study of Untreated Syphilis. The study lasted from 1932 to 1972—40 years—and was begun to determine the natural course of untreated syphilis in Black men (Brandt, 1978). Even after a cure was widely available, the researchers purposely withheld and prevented participants from receiving treatment at other local healthcare facilities (Brandt, 1978). This study reinforced mistrust of healthcare systems and providers in Black communities, especially around clinical trials and vaccines (Alsan et al., 2020; Bajaj & Stanford, 2021; Scharff et al., 2010).

One timely example of the consequences of this historical racist medical injustice is the COVID-19 pandemic clinical trial participation and the hesitancy of Black people to be vaccinated. Despite being disproportionately impacted by the virus, many Black families are reluctant to get the vaccine, with only 14% of respondents saying they trusted the vaccine's safety, and only 18% saying they would get vaccinated (Bajaj & Stanford, 2021; Ogden, 2021). Knowledge of the syphilis study was also identified as a predictor of vaccine hesitancy in the sample (Ogden, 2021).

Discrimination in the healthcare system is a persistent and pervasive experience for Black families in the United Stated, and a byproduct of that discrimination is, for example, the myth that Black women are inherently predisposed to health conditions such as pre-eclampsia. For instance, the overall prevalence of pre-eclampsia is between 3% and 5%; however, the prevalence among Black birthing people is approximately 6.9%, and it is between 7% and 11% among Native American birthing people. Furthermore, while low-dose aspirin is recommended to prevent pre-eclampsia overall, a population-based study found that recurrent pre-eclampsia was reduced among Hispanic women, but there was no difference in the recurrent pre-eclampsia rate among non-Hispanic Black women

(Johnson & Louis, 2020), perhaps indicating anti-Black racism as a separate mechanism for this relationship (Johnson & Louis, 2020).

Another myth is that Black people feel less pain, with some healthcare providers internalizing these stereotypes and potentially providing inferior care, sometimes leading to the patient's death (Hoffman et al., 2016). An article published in the *New England Journal of Medicine* outlined the tragic example of Dr. Susan Moore. Dr. Moore was a family physician in Indianapolis and found herself hospitalized in November 2020 with COVID-19. An experienced clinician, Dr. Moore used social media to document her experience being undertreated and disrespected after being refused treatment when White physicians did not believe her pain levels. Her position: Anti-Black racism was the cause of her inferior medical care, a sentiment that a third of Black Americans share (Givens, 2021). One of the late Dr. Moore's final statements delivered via social media was prophetic: "This is how Black people get killed—when you send them home and they don't know how to fight for themselves" (Givens, 2021).

Often, people use coping behaviors that have adverse health impacts to overcome these experiences of discrimination (Corral & Landrine, 2012). For example, cigarette smoking is an identified risk factor for numerous adverse health outcomes, especially cancer and heart disease, which disproportionately affect Black people in the United States and cause mortality. However, research shows that among Black adults, there is a strong relationship between experiencing racial discrimination and smoking rates (Landrine & Klonoff, 2000). Additionally, the exposure to these maladaptive coping mechanisms, like smoking, is often exacerbated by segregation and limited access to resources (Landrine & Klonoff, 2000). The Centers for Disease Control and Prevention (CDC) notes that tobacco companies have used culturally tailored advertising images and messages to promote menthol cigarettes in predominantly Black neighborhoods. Research suggests that menthol cigarettes are more addictive than nonmentholated cigarettes, and the harmful chemicals are more easily absorbed as the cooling effect of menthol eases cigarette smoke inhalation (CDC, 2020). A larger proportion of Black smokers (63.4%) report attempting to quit, compared with White (56.2%) and Hispanic (53.5%) smokers. However, Black smokers report less success at quitting than both White and Hispanic smokers, likely due to less access to, and use of, effective cessation treatments, including medication and counseling. Research has shown that cigarettes are used as a significant coping tool for Black smokers to deal with stressful experiences of discrimination (Corral & Landrine, 2012; Parker et al., 2016). Additionally, Black families living in neighborhoods with concentrated poverty are exposed to more cigarette advertisements and are more likely to initiate smoking at earlier ages and make impulse purchases of cigarettes (Dauphinee et al., 2013; Robinson et al., 2018). Understanding the role that racism plays in shaping these health behaviors will aid in our ability to develop and implement equitable clinical recommendations, interventions, and policy solutions to address the root cause of these disparities.

Psychological Effects of Racial Discrimination

In addition to negatively impacting health behaviors, the emotional and mental outcomes of stressful experiences of racial discrimination have been well documented. Research shows that persistent and chronic stress, anxiety, and depression are associated with experiencing overt acts of discrimination and having to overcome structural barriers of racism, beginning in childhood (Brown et al., 2000). Chronic stress is one of the most understood risk factors for many diseases across populations, yet the role of racism as a source of this stress is often overlooked. The impacts of racism-related stress can occur before birth and persist over the life course (Jones et al., 2020) and have a direct impact on a myriad of health outcomes. Racism is also a source of trauma, either when it happens personally or when it happens to others who share the same racial identity. Current research illustrates that community-level trauma such as racialized police violence in communities can vicariously influence the health of Black people unrelated to those directly targeted. One such study found higher rates of adverse health conditions, such as high blood pressure, among Black people living in highly and inequitably policed areas, regardless of their individual contact with police. Another study found an association between fatal police violence in the community and unrelated pregnancy loss (Jahn et al., 2021), showing the spillover effect of living in these stressful environments, regardless of whether or not there are personal interactions with police.

Additionally, during a time when many acts of racism are caught on camera, Black people are consistently bombarded with images and videos of structural racism, sometimes having triggering effects and causing symptoms of posttraumatic stress disorder (Campbell & Valera, 2020). This is especially true for the impact of police killings of unarmed Black people on the mental health outcomes of Black families in the United States (Bor et al., 2018). Experiences of racism also impact sleep patterns, which has key implications for health outcomes (Hicken et al., 2013; Hoggard & Hill, 2018). One study found that there is a strong association between racial discrimination and poor sleep quality, and showed that the relationship was partially explained by ruminating tendencies over discriminatory experiences (Hoggard & Hill, 2018). Another found that among pregnant Black women, increases in experiences with racial discrimination were significantly associated with various measures of poor sleep quality (Francis et al., 2017). Racism-related poor sleep quality may be one possible explanation as to why Black women, across education levels and socioeconomic status, die of pregnancy-related causes at three to four times the rate of their non-Hispanic White counterparts.

Physiological Harms of Racism

Researchers have examined physiological harms of racism and have hypothesized a few key pathways for how external experiences of racism can be physiologically embodied (Green & Darity, 2010), including the allostatic load theory (McEwen & Stellar, 1993; McEwen, 2005). *Allostatic load* is described as the "wear and tear" on the body resulting from prolonged or chronic stress (McEwen & Stellar, 1993; McEwen, 2005). Allostasis is an adaptive process that maintains homeostasis in the body through production of hormones such as adrenaline and cortisol. These hormonal responses promote adaptation in the aftermath of acute stressors (McEwen, 2005). When these stressors become persistent, this regulatory process is disrupted and leads to disease (McEwen, 2005). As mentioned earlier, racism at every level serves as a stressor in the lives of Black people. This ongoing, racism-induced stress has been associated with higher allostatic load among Black adults (Ong et al., 2017).

Studies have demonstrated the importance of social environment on child and adolescent development (Trent et al., 2019). And while pediatricians are familiar with understanding and responding to environmental harms likely to influence child health and trajectory (such as child abuse and malnutrition), less attention has been paid to how to identify and disrupt the impact of racism on child health (Trent et al., 2019). As a field, there should be a concerted effort within pediatrics to understand how both personal and vicarious experiences with racism could adversely disrupt development of children, as well as a commitment to dismantling structural racism as a necessary component for positive youth development among Black children (Trent et al., 2019).

ANTI-BLACK RACISM IN THE HEALTH SCIENCES

Chattel Slavery and the Modern Concept of Race

Anti-Black racism can be traced to the transatlantic slave trade. The concept of biologically and socially distinct human groups was developed in Europe, particularly by the English, who propagated the idea that the Irish and other non-English Europeans were "less civilized" (Smedley & Smedley, 2012). The transatlantic slave trade was the first time in modern history that conquest and domination became primarily based on the idea of race. In other words, the concept of race developed to explain and justify the conquest and domination of populations that were phenotypically different from Europeans. In this context, it is helpful to think about race not as a characteristic of people, but as an ideology or worldview. According to Smedley and Smedley (2012), the racial worldview contends that racial groups are biologically distinct:

◆ Races are organized in a hierarchical ranking.
◆ Physical traits reflect internal traits (e.g., intelligence, morality).
◆ Traits are inherited.
◆ Races are created by God and/or nature and cannot be transcended.

These dimensions of the racial worldview are seen, to varying extents, in health sciences curricula, research methods, and health interventions. Race (the social interpretation of how one looks) is a social construct created to support racist ideas that upheld the enslavement of Black people and promulgated White supremacy. White supremacy is an ideology that characterizes White people, as well as their ideas and beliefs, as culturally and morally superior to non-White people, especially Black people. The imagery and language of white supremacy can be found (although it is not always obvious) across institutions and cultural iconography of predominantly White, colonized places such as in the United States (Williams et al., 2019). For instance, the depiction of important religious figures as White, the elevation of European features as globally attractive, and the omission and misrepresentation of harms done by early settler-colonialists are representative of this.

BRIEF HISTORY OF RACISM IN AMERICAN MEDICINE

The understanding of races as biologically different, the first component of the racial worldview, was embedded in the development and early practice of Western medicine. White physicians throughout what became the United States regularly treated Black people in ways that supported the notion of inherent difference. For example, Black people were used to test out new medical procedures. A well-known example is the physician credited as the "father of modern gynecology," James Marion Sims, who operated on enslaved women named Anarcha, Betsey, Lucy, and others without anesthetics. From these experiments, Sims developed the vaginal speculum and a technique to repair vesicovaginal fistula (Wailoo, 2018). The irony is that medical practitioners such as Sims believed that Black bodies were similar *enough* to White bodies to test out new medical tools on enslaved people before implementing them on their White patients. However, the underlying belief that Black people did not feel pain justified their refusal to use anesthesia (Washington, 2006). Furthermore, physicians tended to be more interested in the development of science through experimentation than they were in actually providing treatment.

Conversely, many physicians profited generously by marketing themselves as "Negro physicians" or experts on the Black body. The racism embedded in these specialized practices was not as blatant as the forced experiments, but they were harmful nonetheless. These physicians reinforced the idea that Black bodies "needed specialized, segregated care" (Hogarth, 2017, p. 163). With their help, segregated hospitals became the norm. Although the medical industry has largely condemned these acts of blatant and structural violence, there are vestiges of anti-Black racism embedded in health sciences today. For example, a recent study found that medical students believe that Black people feel less pain and *literally* have thicker skin and that Black people's blood coagulates faster (Hoffman et al., 2016). These false beliefs contribute to the vast racial disparities in pain management (Meghani et al., 2012).

RACISM AND MEDICAL SEGREGATION: CHANGE OVER TIME

To understand how racism is operating in a given moment, it is important to consider its inherently changing structure. One can look at the United States as an example to understand how racism has changed over time. Chattel slavery was once the racial structure in the United States, as was Jim Crow, an era when racial segregation was both legal and enforced, creating both separate and unequal worlds for Black and White citizens. Due to the Civil Rights movement, which was characterized by organizing, direct action, community mobilization, and ultimately lethal (e.g., Dr. King's assassination) and legal (e.g., *Brown v. Board of Education*) interventions, both structures were fundamentally altered. However, racial inequality has remained. Today, we are experiencing what some call the "new racism" (Bonilla-Silva, 2018). This new era is characterized by the cultural condemnation of overt racism (e.g., Ku Klux Klan) and the simultaneous perpetuation of covert or undercover racism. For example, few people will openly support racial segregation in schools; however, it is a common for parents of White children to politically oppose integration efforts for fear that integration will harm their children's educational prospects (Lipman, 2013; Shapiro, 2020). Racism is changing, but not necessarily in a direct, forward progression. We should understand how the mechanisms of racism are changing while acknowledging that race is still a "master category" of social inequality (Seamster & Ray, 2018). For example, consider segregation in medical settings—prior to the Civil Rights Act of 1968, segregated hospitals were the legal norm in the southern United States. Today, segregated hospitals are no longer codified in the law, but there is still a clear divide along racial lines regarding who does and does not have access to quality healthcare. First, healthcare access is correlated with racial residential segregation. Residents in majority-Black neighborhoods, for example, have fewer health-related organizations, including hospitals and community health centers (Freeman Anderson, 2017; Ko et al., 2014; Ko & Ponce, 2013). Second, racial inequities in healthcare coverage are also prevalent despite the "integration" of hospitals. Even the implementation of the Affordable Care Act did not reduce disparities as expected. The option for states to forego Medicaid expansion left many Black people—especially in the U.S. South—uninsured (Cross-Call, 2018). Research shows the decline in infant mortality rates among Black people residing in states that expanded Medicaid was twice that of Black infants born in states that did not expand Medicaid coverage (Bhatt & Beck-Saugé, 2018). This is vital, given that the majority of Black families in the United States reside in the South and that, as of 2021, many southern states still have not expanded Medicaid (Bhatt & Beck-Sagué, 2018). To date Alabama, Florida, Georgia, Mississippi, North Carolina, Oklahoma, South Dakota, South Carolina, Tennessee, Texas, Wisconsin, and Wyoming have yet to adopt the expansion.

The racial worldview (Smedley & Smedley, 2012) contends that racial groups are biologically distinct and hierarchically organized. In a U.S. context, Black people are placed at the bottom of the hierarchy. The consequences of this social ordering are evident in disparities across various domains in social life, including education, housing, employment, criminal justice, and health/healthcare systems. The following sections focus on tools to rigorously measure racism to understand its specific implications for population health.

THEORIES AND MEASUREMENTS FOR RESEARCHERS INTERESTED IN RACISM AND HEALTH

Theories guide all science by visualizing the complexities of our world (e.g., society, nature, behavior) and proposing relationships and mechanisms that explain these complexities (Krieger, 2011). The goal of science is to methodically examine the world through experiments, observations, and communications in order to better understand reality. Theory guides the scientific process through research decisions, such as which variables or relationships are important to explore, the methods chosen to test these relationships, and how to interpret any findings.

Researchers dedicated to understanding racism's influence on health are actively opposing long-held eugenics-based theories of racial disparities, which were used to argue that these differences are "natural" due to Black and Indigenous people's inherent genetic and cultural inferiority (Krieger, 2011). As far back as the 1899 publication of Dr. W.E.B. Du Bois's *The Philadelphia Negro,* alternative theories for racial health disparities have acknowledged how racism *determines* social environment and exposures to harm (Du Bois, 1899). Nevertheless, theories of genetic differences and cultural deficits of Black, Latinx, and Indigenous peoples are still used in studies to explain racial inequities in health—although none acknowledge the eugenics roots (Hardeman et al., 2020). Contemporary scientists studying racism's impact on health continue to propose alternative, inferiority-based theories about biology and lifestyle choices that predominate health research. Scientists have drawn from psychology, sociology, law, and other disciplines to develop theories on how *racism,* not race, influences health. The theories outlined in this section, and the measures and methods they generate, propose plausible, testable links between racism as a complexly structured, multilevel social phenomenon, and multiple mental and physical health outcomes.

Psychosocial Theories to Guide Racism Research and Practice

The earliest research on racism and health focused on interpersonal experiences of racism as a *psychosocial* stressor (Williams et al., 2019). The *psychosocial stress theory,* which posits that stress induces physiologic, behavioral, and mental health changes in individuals, serves well for biomedical and lifestyle theories of medicine and epidemiology. As such, the proposal that events of explicit, interpersonal racial discrimination—such as racial slurs and hate crimes—could be a specific stressor for Black people and a well-accepted mechanism for racial health disparities research.

In addition to discrimination itself being a psychosocial stressor, racial discrimination by institutions causes other psychosocial stressors, such as unemployment and housing instability (Williams et al., 2019). Together, discrimination by individuals and institutions is theorized to influence health through the physiologic and mind/body changes caused by stress. The physiologic processes of the sympathetic nervous system, which include cardiovascular changes (increased heart rate), hormonal changes (increased cortisol and adrenaline), and increased immune response, are actually useful when the stressor is acute. However, when prolonged, these changes increase blood pressure and inflammation and degrade body systems (Thompson et al., 2012).

Psychological theories have also guided research into *implicit* bias—unknown, unconscious bias that automatically influences the actions of perpetrators of racism. These theories draw on psychological and neurobiological frameworks of memory and cognition, and highlight how racist stereotypes, imagery, and language in a culture allow racist associations to persist unbeknownst to the actor. These psychological theories are also used to explain how racism becomes internalized by members of oppressed groups (Williams et al., 2019).

Theories of Social Patterns and Resource Inequality

The recognition that illness and health tend to follow socioeconomic status have generated theories that examine the role of social environment in racial disparities in health (Krieger, 2011). These theories are rooted in how access to income and wealth creates conditions that support health, when available, and degrade health, when unavailable (Williams et al., 2019). These theories connect access to safe environments, healthy foods, opportunities for physical activity, and safe working conditions to social class. These social resources, referred to as the *social determinants of health,* in addition to access to the highest quality healthcare, contribute to why socioeconomic class remains a strong predictor of morbidity and mortality, particularly in the United States. Social determinants of health, including economic stability, level of education, neighborhood and environment, and social relationships and interactions, are predisposing factors that influence health outcomes. The impact of social determinants of health is heightened for vulnerable populations and plays a crucial role in overall health outcomes; an example of this is found in maternal and infant health outcomes. The pathways between social determinants and birth outcomes have contributed to pervasive racial/ethnic disparities in maternal health and healthcare. For example, long-standing, complex sociodemographic and historical factors perpetuate the challenges Black women face in achieving positive birth outcomes (Kozhimannil et al., 2016).

Scholars of racism in health draw on these theories, highlighting how discrimination within institutional policies and by individual gatekeepers determines socioeconomic status by race (Williams et al., 2019), such that Black, Latinx, Native American, Asian, Pacific Islander, and many immigrant communities often occupy lower socioeconomic strata compared to their White counterparts. The consequences of discrimination in social resources create measurable disparities in social conditions, including the presence of racial residential segregation, rates of unemployment, the presence of food deserts, hyper-policing, and mass incarceration (Wildeman & Wang, 2017; Williams et al., 2019). (See Chapter 22 for information on redlining.)

Fundamental cause theory, introduced by sociologists Jo C. Phelan and Bruce G. Link in 1995, emphasizes the *persistence* of the relationship between health and social factors (Link & Phelan, 1995; Phelan & Link, 2013). Causes are considered "fundamental" because (a) the outcomes are not specific to a single disease, but rather multiple health outcomes; (b) health outcomes are caused by multiple risk factors; (c) the social causes involve access to resources; and (d) it is reproduced over time as the mechanisms are constantly changed and replaced as societal forces change around them. Racism is argued to be a fundamental cause of racial health disparities over time, due to its role in sorting people into neighborhoods (Williams & Collins, 2001) and socioeconomic classes (Phelan & Link, 2015).

Life course theories are often used by those studying racism and health, as they focus on the timing and accumulation of exposures over the life span. Life course theories posit that exposure to social conditions and stressors in certain life stages (e.g., in utero, early childhood, adolescence), due either to biological sensitivity or to the accumulation of exposures, help to explain racial health disparities (Gee et al., 2012).

Often missing from theories of social patterning are the actors that create and maintain these social conditions, such that some benefit as others, simultaneously, are harmed (Sewell, 2016). Indeed, structural racism persists precisely because those with power and resources are unmotivated to address the multiple root causes, as this would undermine the privileges obtained not through meritocracy, but through extraction and exploitation through land theft, slavery, racial terrorism, and racist policies such as the Jim Crow laws. *Critical race theory* (CRT) was developed in the context of legal studies, explicitly naming White supremacy and how it is ingrained across social systems toward the subordination of people of color. In 2010, Drs. Chandra Ford and Collins O. Airhihenbuwa introduced CRT to the public health community through their *Public Health Critical Race Praxis (PHCRP)*, to inform how racial disparities research be conducted, with an eye toward understanding how racial injustices are created through societal processes, and centering health disparities research itself within society, as a formal way to design rigorous science, evaluate methodology and approach, and, most importantly, implement strategies to undo the harms of racism on health (Ford & Airhihenbuwa, 2010). Key components of CRT also critical to PHCRP are race consciousness, which asks investigators to understand how racialization influences both the researcher and the research itself; understanding how racialization creates social positions or locations that may be replicated when the voices and goals of populations without privilege are further marginalized in research; and, finally, the reflexive nature of the work, meaning the ultimate goal is research for action and reconciliation, rather than for the sake of knowledge alone. Similarly, Nancy Krieger's *Ecosocial Theory of Disease Distribution* emphasizes how history, political economy, and other sociopolitical forces compose the ecology of society, determining how populations interact with each other and their environment over space and time and across the life course, to produce health and health disparities across and within populations (Krieger, 2011). Ecosocial theory further emphasizes *embodiment*, or how factors such as racism "get under the skin" through biological processes. Embodiment refers to how we physiologically incorporate the physical and social worlds in which we live. The theory has been used to highlight temporal and cumulative health effects of experiencing racism across the life course, across generations, and across time.

EXAMPLES OF MEASURES OF RACISM, GUIDED BY THEORY

Psychological and Psychosocial Measures

Measures of discrimination as a cause of psychosocial stress rely largely on self-reported experiences of discrimination, the most prominent being the Everyday Discrimination Scale (Williams et al., 1997) and the Major Experiences of Discrimination Scale (Williams et al., 2008), and the Experiences of Discrimination Scale (Krieger, 2020). Although discrimination measured in these ways is based on the respondent's perception of the experience, studies that have used these measures have shown robust relationships with physical, mental, and behavioral health outcomes (Lewis et al., 2015).

Arline Geronimus's "weathering hypothesis" draws on both psychosocial stress theory and life course theory to explain and measure racial health disparities (Geronimus, 1992). Geronimus posits that interpersonal racism across the life course leads to health wear and tear among Black populations, leading to a faster deterioration of the body, similar to aging. Studies examining the weathering hypothesis often compare the evidence of allostatic load across age groups and related health outcomes, including epigenetics (Geronimus et al., 2010).

Studies testing the cognitive association between race and racial stereotypes have also been used in health inequalities research. Implicit bias measures, such as the implicit association test (IAT) instrument, test how quickly individuals associate racial stereotypes (Krieger, 2020). IAT results have been used to measure cultural racism and health (Orchard & Price, 2017), although they are limited because people must "opt in" to take the test. Similar studies have found that White people and law enforcement officers of all races more quickly associate weapons with Black faces, as well as assume nonweapons are weapons when associated with Black faces, which potentially explains differences in racially influenced use of force by law enforcement. It is important to note that these studies do not necessarily distinguish between implicit and explicit prejudice but rather highlight the salience of racism within the culture (Mateo & Williams, 2020).

MEASURES FOR SOCIAL PATTERNING OF RESOURCES AND RACIST POLICIES

Racism in the allocation of social resources may be measured through experimental manipulation or through observing differences using administrative records, surveys, or census data. Audit studies are one type of experimental measure that manipulates race to elicit racism in decision-making or, similarly, through randomly assigned "vignettes" to measure differences in response to institutional gatekeepers, such as real estate agents, doctors, and teachers (Krieger, 2020). For instance, well-known audit studies have found that names associated with Black American ethnicity receive fewer job interview offers than names associated with White American ethnicity, even when the résumés are otherwise identical (Bertrand & Mullainathan, 2004). Similar studies have shown this is true for decisions to discipline children at school, influencing education (Okonofua & Eberhardt, 2015), and for prescribing opioids in medical treatment (Burgess et al., 2014).

Other studies may use medical records, disease registries (Davis et al., 2017), surveys, or other documentation to identify the racism in decision-making. For instance, the National Hospital Ambulatory Medical Care Survey, which collects information from hospitals about individual patient visits, has been used to measure discrimination in the provision of opioid medication for pain management (Benzing et al., 2020; Pletcher et al., 2008).

Methods aiming to measure structural processes are growing in health research but can be difficult, as they are multilevel and complex. Given the role of place in policy, many studies of structural racism use place-based measures, such as racial residential segregation (Groos et al., 2018), often as a fundamental cause. Other studies have examined spatial distribution and disparities of incarceration rates (Jahn et al., 2020), Black political representation, and disparities in mortgage loans, all of which can be derived from census or other administrative data (Gee, 2008; Mendez et al., 2014). The Index of Concentration at the Extremes (ICE) examines the spatial polarization of race, and race plus socioeconomic status, as evidence of racism (Chambers et al., 2018a, 2018b). Furthermore, novel measures may combine data across social determinants of health to create racism indices. One such example is Lukachko et al.'s measure of structural racism, which combines area-level measures of political participation (e.g., registration to vote, elected officials), judicial treatment (e.g., incarceration, death row), and employment (e.g., employment rates, occupational class) to create a composite measure of structural racism (Lukachko et al., 2014).

Finally, racism and health studies have aimed to look at the presence of racist *policies* as the indicator of racism. Studies have examined the change in health outcomes following the end of Jim Crow policies (Krieger et al., 2014) and the influence of the Civil Rights movement (Hahn et al., 2018). These studies leverage place (e.g., the states with Jim Crow laws), time, and race, and use novel statistical methods to explore theories outlined by critical race theory and ecosocial theory.

CASE STUDY 11.1: RACISM'S IMPACT ON THE HEALTH OF BLACK LIVES

Mrs. Cunningham is a 53-year-old Black woman with a history of hypertension, severe bilateral knee arthritis, posttraumatic stress disorder, generalized anxiety disorder, tobacco use, and prediabetes. She is cared for by her primary care provider, Dr. Martin.

Mrs. Cunningham is a small business owner and has stayed up to date with screening recommendations and regular annual visits. Due to the success of her small business, she does not qualify for state-sponsored public insurance. She pays for private insurance instead.

Mrs. Cunningham's severe knee arthritis is advanced and no longer responsive to intra-articular steroid injections, physical therapy, or palliation with NSAIDs. Mrs. Cunningham has been started on opioids as a temporizing measure to improve her ability to function until she can ultimately have her knees replaced. Mrs. Cunningham was initially very hesitant to start opioid medication because of her fears of becoming addicted.

Recently, her insurance premiums have increased, and she can no longer afford to pay them. Without insurance, she is unable to pay for her opioid medication. Mrs. Cunningham also stops seeing Dr. Martin because Dr. Martin's clinic only sees patients with insurance.

Mrs. Cunningham unfortunately cannot afford surgery and is now without any regular management of her chronic pain. Her function is deteriorating, and her ability to exercise is decreased, which worsens her hypertension and prediabetes.

Since she stopped seeing Dr. Martin regularly due to her lack of insurance, Mrs. Cunningham has had significant difficulty managing her severe chronic pain. She feels that she is often labeled as a "drug seeker" when she reports that her pain had been managed with opioids previously. She feels that she has to modulate her tone very carefully even

(continued)

CASE STUDY 11.1: RACISM'S IMPACT ON THE HEALTH OF BLACK LIVES (*CONTINUED*)

when she is in extreme pain. She understands that she needs knee surgery for definitive management of her end-stage osteoarthritis but cannot afford this surgery without health insurance. She spends a significant amount of time looking for insurance but can find only high-deductible plans that would not provide the coverage she needs.

Discussion Questions

There are many forms of racism that often work in concert to impact health and well-being. In this case study, can you identify the:

1. Internalized racism?
2. Interpersonal racism?
3. Institutional racism?
4. Structural racism?

CONCLUSION

Racism, ranging from historic, state-sanctioned denial of education, jobs, and housing, to their contemporary manifestations including state-sanctioned violence from law and immigration enforcement, mass incarceration, and housing discrimination, interact to design the sociocultural landscape in which all people in the United States reside. There is a widespread view that racism is perpetuated by "bad actors" and is relatively rare in contemporary American society. However, as scientists, clinicians, and others concerned about the persistently high risk for adverse health outcomes in the Black communities, it is important to understand, acknowledge, and combat the ordinariness of racism in the lives of Black people and the role it plays in perpetuating these inequities across various social determinants of health. This awareness can build a greater sense of equity as institutions begin transformative changes to address these disparities.

ADDITIONAL RESOURCES

Banks, K. H., Kohn-Wood, L. P., & Spencer, M. (2006). An examination of the African American experience of everyday discrimination and symptoms of psychological distress. *Community Mental Health Journal, 42*(6), 555–570.
Jim Crow Era-Timeline-Jim Crow Museum. (n.d.). Ferris State University. https://www.ferris.edu/htmls/news/jimcrow/timeline/jimcrow.htm
Whitley, Jr. B. E., & Kite, M. E. (2016). *Psychology of prejudice and discrimination*. Routledge.

REFERENCES

Alsan, M., Wanamaker, M., & Hardeman, R. R. (2020). The Tuskegee study of untreated syphilis: A case study in peripheral trauma with implications for health professionals. *Journal of General Internal Medicine, 35*(1), 322–325.
Bailey, Z. D., Krieger, N., Agénor, M., Graves, J., Linos, N., & Bassett, M. T. (2017). Structural racism and health inequities in the USA: Evidence and interventions. *The Lancet, 389*(10077), 1453–1463.
Bajaj, S. S., & Stanford, F. C. (2021). Beyond Tuskegee—vaccine distrust and everyday racism. *New England Journal of Medicine, 384*(5), e12.
Barker, C., Francois, A., Goodman, R., & Hussain, E. (2012). Unshared bounty: How structural racism contributes to the creation and persistence of food deserts. *Racial Justice Project*.
Benzing, A., Bell, C., Derazin, M., Mack, R., & MacIntosh, T. (2020). Disparities in opioid pain management for long bone fractures. *Journal of Racial and Ethnic Health Disparities, 7*, 740–745.

Bertrand, M., & Mullainathan, S. (2004). Are Emily and Greg more employable than Lakisha and Jamal? A field experiment on labor market discrimination. *American Economic Review*, 94(4), 991–1013.

Bhatt, C. B., & Beck-Sagué, C. M. (2018). Medicaid expansion and infant mortality in the United States. *American Journal of Public Health*, 108(4), 565–567. https://doi.org/10.2105/AJPH.2017.304218

Bhatt, C. B., & Beck-Sagué, C. M. (2018). Medicaid expansion and infant mortality in the United States. *American Journal of Public Health*, 108(4), 565–567.

Bonilla-Silva, E. (2018). Racism without racists: Color-blind racism and the persistence of racial inequality in America (5th ed.). Rowman & Littlefield.

Bor, J., Venkataramani, A. S., Williams, D. R., & Tsai, A. C. (2018). Police killings and their spillover effects on the mental health of black Americans: A population-based, quasi-experimental study. *The Lancet*, 392(10144), 302–310.

Brandt, A. M. (1978). Racism and research: The case of the Tuskegee syphilis study. *Hastings Center Report*, 21–29.

Brown, T. N., Williams, D. R., Jackson, J. S., Neighbors, H. W., Torres, M., Sellers, S. L., & Brown, K. T. (2000). "Being black and feeling blue": The mental health consequences of racial discrimination. *Race and Society*, 2(2), 117–131.

Burgess, D. J., Phelan, S., Workman, M., Hagel, E., Nelson, D. B., Fu, S. S. et al. (2014). The effect of cognitive load and patient race on physicians' decisions to prescribe opioids for chronic low back pain: A randomized trial. *Pain Medicine*, 15(6), 965–974.

Butler, B., Outrich, M., Roach, J., & James, A. (2020). Generational impacts of 1930s housing discrimination and the imperative need for the healthy start initiative to address structural racism. *Journal of Health Disparities Research and Practice*, 13(3), 4.

Campbell, F., & Valera, P. (2020). "The only thing new is the cameras": A study of U.S. college students' perceptions of police violence on social media. *Journal of Black Studies*, 51(7), 654–670.

Centers for Disease Control and Prevention. (2020, November 16). African Americans and tobacco use. Centers for Disease Control and Prevention. https://www.cdc.gov/tobacco/disparities/african-americans/index.htm

Chadha, N., Lim, B., Kane, M., & Rowland, B. (2020). Toward the abolition of biological race in medicine: Transforming clinical education. *Research, and Practice*. instituteforhealingandjustice.org.

Chambers, B. D., Baer, R. J., McLemore, M. R., & Jelliffe-Pawlowski, L. L. (2018a). Using index of concentration at the extremes as indicators of structural racism to evaluate the association with preterm birth and infant mortality—California, 2011–2012. *Journal of Urban Health*, 1–12.

Chambers, B. D., Erausquin, J. T., Tanner, A. E., Nichols, T. R., & Brown-Jeffy, S. (2018b). Testing the association between traditional and novel indicators of county-level structural racism and birth outcomes among black and white women. *Journal of Racial and Ethnic Health Disparities*, 5(5), 966–977.

Chen, S. E., & Florax, R. J. (2010). Zoning for health: The obesity epidemic and opportunities for local policy intervention. *The Journal of Nutrition*, 140(6), 1181S–1184S.

Corral, I., & Landrine, H. (2012). Racial discrimination and health-promoting vs. damaging behaviors among African-American adults. *Journal of Health Psychology*, 17(8), 1176–1182.

Cross-Call, J. (2018). Medicaid expansion continues to benefit state budgets, contrary to critics' claims. *Center on Budget and Policy Priorities*. https://www.cbpp.org/research/health/medicaid-expansion-continues-to-benefit-state-budgets-contrary-to-critics-claims

Dauphinee, A. L., Doxey, J. R., Schleicher, N. C., Fortmann, S. P., & Henriksen, L. (2013). Racial differences in cigarette brand recognition and impact on youth smoking. *BMC Public Health*, 13(1), 1–8.

Davis, B. A., Aminawung, J. A., Abu-Khalaf, M. M., Evans, S. B., Su, K., Mehta, R. et al. (2017). Racial and ethnic disparities in Oncotype DX test receipt in a statewide population-based study. *Journal of the National Comprehensive Cancer Network*, 15(3), 346–354.

Davis, D. (2019). "Obstetric racism: The racial politics of pregnancy, labor, and birthing." *Medical Anthropology, 38.7*(2019), 560–573.

Dixon, J. B. (2010). The effect of obesity on health outcomes. *Molecular and Cellular Endocrinology*, 316(2), 104–108.

Du Bois, W. E. B. (1899). The Philadelphia negro: A social study. Published for the University.

Ford, C. L., & Airhihenbuwa, C. O. (2010). Critical race theory, race equity, and public health: Toward antiracism praxis. *American Journal of Public Health*, 100(suppl 1), S30–S35. https://doi.org/10.2105/AJPH.2009.171058

Francis, B., Klebanoff, M., & Oza-Frank, R. (2017). Racial discrimination and perinatal sleep quality. *Sleep Health*, 3(4), 300–305.

Freeman Anderson, K. (2017). Racial residential segregation and the distribution of health-related organizations in urban neighborhoods. *Social Problems*, 64(2), 256–276.

Gee, G. C. (2008). A multilevel analysis of the relationship between institutional and individual racial discrimination and health status. *American Journal of Public Health, 98*(suppl 1), S48–S56.

Gee, G. C., & Ford, C. L. (2011). Structural racism and health inequities: Old issues, new directions. *Du Bois Review: Social Science Research on Race, 8*(1), 115–132.

Gee, G. C., Walsemann, K. M., & Brondolo, E. (2012). A life course perspective on how racism may be related to health inequities. *American Journal of Public Health, 102*(5), 967–974. https://doi. org/10.2105/AJPH.2012.300666

Geronimus, A. T. (1992). The weathering hypothesis and the health of African-American women and infants: Evidence and speculations. *Ethnicity & Disease, 2*(3), 207–221.

Geronimus, A. T., Hicken, M. T., Pearson, J. A., Seashols, S. J., Brown, K. L., & Cruz, T. D. (2010). Do US black women experience stress-related accelerated biological aging? *Human Nature, 21*(1), 19–38.

Givens, R. (2021). One of US. *New England Journal of Medicine.* https://doi.org/10.1056/ NEJMpv2100228

Green, T. L., & Darity, Jr. W. A. (2010). Under the skin: Using theories from biology and the social sciences to explore the mechanisms behind the black-white health gap. *American Journal of Public Health, 100*(S1), S36–S40.

Groos, M., Wallace, M., Hardeman, R., & Theall, K. P. (2018). Measuring inequity: A systemic review of methods used to quantify structural racism. *Journal of Health Disparities Research and Practice, 11*(2), 13.

Hahn, R. A., Truman, B. I., & Williams, D. R. (2018). Civil rights as determinants of public health and racial and ethnic health equity: Health care, education, employment, and housing in the United States. *SSM-Population Health, 4*, 17–24.

Hall, W. J., Chapman, M. V., Lee, K. M., Merino, Y. M., Thomas, T. W., Payne, B. K., & Coyne-Beasley, T. (2015). Implicit racial/ethnic bias among health care professionals and its influence on health care outcomes: A systematic review. *American Journal of Public Health, 105*(12), e60–e76.

Hardeman, R. R., Karbeah, J., & Kozhimannil, K. B. (2020). Applying a critical race lens to relationship-centered care in pregnancy and childbirth: An antidote to structural racism. *Birth: Issues in Perinatal Care, 47*(1):3–7. https://doi.org/10.1111/birt.12462

Hardeman, R. R., Medina, E., & Kozhimannil, K. B. (2016). Structural racsim and supporting black lives—the role of health care professionals. *New England Journal of Medicine, 375*, 2113–2115.

Hicken, M. T., Lee, H., Ailshire, J., Burgard, S. A., & Williams, D. R. (2013). "Every shut eye ain't sleep": The role of racism-related vigilance in racial/ethnic disparities in sleep difficulty. *Race and Social Problems, 5*(2), 100–112.

Hoffman, K. M., Trawalter, S., Axt, J. R., & Oliver, M. N. (2016). Racial bias in pain assessment and treatment recommendations, and false beliefs about biological differences between blacks and whites. *Proceedings of the National Academy of Sciences, 113*(16), 4296–4301. https://doi.org/10.1073/ pnas.1516047113

Hogarth, R. A. (2017). *Medicalizing blackness: Making racial difference in the Atlantic world, 1780–1840.* The University of North Carolina Press.

Hoggard, L. S., & Hill, L. K. (2018). Examining how racial discrimination impacts sleep quality in African Americans: Is perseveration the answer? *Behavioral Sleep Medicine, 16*(5), 471–481.

Jahn, J. L., Chen, J. T., Agénor, M., & Krieger, N. (2020). County-level jail incarceration and preterm birth among non-hispanic black and white US women, 1999–2015. *Social Science & Medicine, 250*, 112856.

Jahn, J. L., Krieger, N., Agénor, M., Leung, M., Davis, B. A., Weisskopf, M. G., & Chen, J. T. (2021). Gestational exposure to fatal police violence and pregnancy loss in US core based statistical areas, 2013–2015. *EClinicalMedicine, 36*, 100901.

Johnson, J. D., & Louis, J. M. (2020). Does race or ethnicity play a role in the origin, pathophysiology, and outcomes of preeclampsia? An expert review of the literature. *American Journal of Obstetrics and Gynecology, 24*, S0002-9378(20)30769-9. https://doi.org/10.1016/j.ajog.2020.07.038

Jones, S. C., Anderson, R. E., Gaskin-Wasson, A. L., Sawyer, B. A., Applewhite, K., & Metzger, I. W. (2020). From "crib to coffin": Navigating coping from racism-related stress throughout the lifespan of black Americans. *American Journal of Orthopsychiatry, 90*(2), 267.

Ko, M., & Ponce, N. A. (2013). Community residential segregation and the local supply of federally qualified health centers. *Health Services Research, 48*(1), 253–270.

Ko, M., Needleman, J., Derose, K. P., Laugesen, M. J., & Ponce, N. A. (2014). Residential segregation and the survival of U.S. Urban Public Hospitals. *Medical Care Research & Review, 71*(3), 243–260.

Kozhimannil, K. B., Vogelsang, C. A., Hardeman, R. R., & Prasad, S. (2016). Disrupting the pathways of social determinants of health: Doula support during pregnancy and childbirth. *Journal of the American Board of Family Medicine, 29*(3), 308–317. https://doi.org/10.3122/jabfm.2016.03.150300

Krieger, N. (2011). Epidemiology and the people's health: *Theory and context.* Oxford University Press.

Krieger, N. (2020). Measures of racism, sexism, heterosexism, and gender binarism for health equity research: From structural injustice to embodied harm—An ecosocial analysis. *Annual Review of Public Health, 41*, 37–62.

Krieger, N., Chen, J. T., Coull, B. A., Beckfield, J., Kiang, M. V., & Waterman, P. D. (2014). Jim Crow and premature mortality among the U.S. black and white population, 1960–2009: An age–period–cohort analysis. *Epidemiology (Cambridge, Mass.)*, 25(4), 494.

Landrine, H., & Klonoff, E. A. (2000). *Racial discrimination and cigarette smoking among blacks: Findings from two studies*. Ethnicity & Disease, 10(2), 195–202.

Landrine, H., & Klonoff, E. A. (2000). Racial segregation and cigarette smoking among blacks: Findings at the individual level. *Journal of Health Psychology*. https://doi.org/10.1177/135910530000500211

Lee, C., Ayers, S. L., & Kronenfeld, J. J. (2009). The association between perceived provider discrimination, health care utilization, and health status in racial and ethnic minorities. *Ethnicity & Disease*, 19(3), 330.

Lewis, T. T., Cogburn, C. D., & Williams, D. R. (2015). Self-reported experiences of discrimination and health: Scientific advances, ongoing controversies, and emerging issues. *Annual Review of Clinical Psychology*, 11, 407–440.

Link, B. G., & Phelan, J. (1995). Social conditions as fundamental causes of disease. *Journal of Health and Social Behavior*, 80–94.

Lipman, P. (2013). *The new political economy of urban education: Neoliberalism*, race, and the right to the city. Routledge.

Lovasi, G. S., Hutson, M. A., Guerra, M., & Neckerman, K. M. (2009). Built environments and obesity in disadvantaged populations. *Epidemiologic Reviews*, 31(1), 7–20.

Lukachko, A., Hatzenbuehler, M. L., & Keyes, K. M. (2014). Structural racism and myocardial infarction in the United States. *Social Science & Medicine*, 103, 42–50.

Mateo, C. M., & Williams, D. R. (2020). Addressing bias and reducing discrimination: The professional responsibility of health care providers. *Academic Medicine*, 95(12S), S5–S10. https://doi.org/10.1097/acm.0000000000003683

McEwen, B. S. (2005). Stressed or stressed out: What is the difference? *Journal of Psychiatry and Neuroscience*, 30(5), 315.

McEwen, B. S., & Stellar, E. (1993). Stress and the individual: Mechanisms leading to disease. *Archives of Internal Medicine*, 153(18), 2093–2101. https://doi.org/10.1001/ARCHINTE.1993.00410180039004

Meghani, S. H., Byun, E., & Gallagher, R. M. (2012). Time to take stock: A meta-analysis and systematic review of analgesic treatment disparities for pain in the United States. *Pain Medicine (Malden, Mass.)*, 13(2), 150–174. https://doi.org/10.1111/j.1526-4637.2011.01310.x

Mendez, D. D., Hogan, V. K., & Culhane, J. F. (2014). Institutional racism, neighborhood factors, stress, and preterm birth. *Ethnicity & Health*, 19(5), 479–499.

Ogden, A. (2021). COVID Collaborative survey: Coronavirus vaccination hesitancy in the Black and Latinx communities. https://www.covidcollaborative.us/content/vaccine-treatments/coronavirus-vaccine-hesitancy-in-black-and-latinx-communities

Okonofua, J. A., & Eberhardt, J. L. (2015). Two strikes: Race and the disciplining of young students. *Psychological Science*, 26(5), 617–624.

Ong, A. D., Williams, D. R., Nwizu, U., & Gruenewald, T. L. (2017). Everyday unfair treatment and multisystem biological dysregulation in African American adults. *Cultural Diversity and Ethnic Minority Psychology*, 23(1), 27.

Orchard, J., & Price, J. (2017). County-level racial prejudice and the black-white gap in infant health outcomes. *Social Science & Medicine*, 181, 191–198.

Parker, L. J., Kinlock, B. L., Chisolm, D., Furr-Holden, D., & Thorpe, Jr. R. J. (2016). Association between any major discrimination and current cigarette smoking among adult African American men. *Substance Use & Misuse*, 51(12), 1593–1599.

Phelan, J. C., & Link, B. G. (2013). Fundamental cause theory. In *Medical sociology on the move* (pp. 105–125). Springer.

Phelan, J. C., & Link, B. G. (2015). Is racism a fundamental cause of inequalities in health? *Annual Review of Sociology*, 41, 311–330.

Pletcher, M. J., Kertesz, S. G., Kohn, M. A., & Gonzales, R. (2008). Trends in opioid prescribing by race/ethnicity for patients seeking care in U.S. Emergency Departments. *JAMA*, 299(1), 70–78.

Racial Bias and Disparities in Proactive Policing. National Academies of Sciences, Engineering, and Medicine. (2018). Proactive policing: Effects on crime and communities. The National Academies Press. https://doi.org/10.17226/24928

Rigolon, A., Browning, M., & Jennings, V. (2018). Inequities in the quality of urban park systems: An environmental justice investigation of cities in the United States. *Landscape and Urban Planning*, 178, 156–169.

Robinson, C. D., Muench, C., Brede, E., Endrighi, R., Szeto, E. H., Sells, J. R., & Waters, A. J. (2018). Pro-tobacco advertisement exposure among African American smokers: An ecological momentary assessment study. *Addictive Behaviors*, 83, 142–147.

Routledge & CRC Press. (2021). *Psychology of prejudice and discrimination* (3rd ed.). https://www
.routledge.com/Psychology-of-Prejudice-and-Discrimination-3rd-Edition/Kite-Whitley-Jr/p/
book/9781138947542

Scharff, D. P., Mathews, K. J., Jackson, P., Hoffsuemmer, J., Martin, E., & Edwards, D. (2010). More
than Tuskegee: Understanding mistrust about research participation. *Journal of Health Care for the
Poor and Underserved*, 21(3), 879.

Seamster, L., & Ray, V. (2018). Against teleology in the study of race: Toward the abolition of the
progress paradigm. *Sociological Theory*, 36(4), 315–342. https://doi.org/10.1177/0735275118813614

Sewell, A. A. (2016). The racism-race reification process: A meso-level political economic framework
for understanding racial health disparities. *Sociology of Race and Ethnicity*, 2(4), 402–432.

Shapiro, E. (2020). How white progressives undermine school integration. The New York Times.
https://www.nytimes.com/2020/08/21/nyregion/school-integration-progressives.html

Smedley, A., & Smedley, B. D. (2012). Race in North America: Origin and evolution of a worldview
(4th ed.). Westview Press.

Thompson, R. S., Strong, P. V., & Fleshner, M. (2012). Physiological consequences of repeated
exposures to conditioned fear. *Behavioural Science (Basel)*, 2(2):57–78. https://doi.org/10.3390/
bs2020057

Trent, M., Dooley, D. G., & Dougé, J, (2019). The impact of racism on child and adolescent health.
Pediatrics, 144(2), e20191765. https://doi.org/10.1542/peds.2019-1765.

Wailoo, K. (2018). Historical aspects of race and medicine: The case of J. Marion Sims. *JAMA*, 320(15),
1529–1530. https://doi.org/10.1001/jama.2018.11944

Washington, H. A. (2006). Medical apartheid: The dark history of medical experimentation on Black
Americans from colonial times to the present. Doubleday Books.

Wildeman, C., & Wang, E. A. (2017). Mass incarceration, public health, and widening inequality in
the USA. *The Lancet*, 389(10077), 1464–1474.

Williams, D. R., Gonzalez, H. M., Williams, S., Mohammed, S. A., Moomal, H., & Stein, D. J. (2008).
Perceived discrimination, race and health in South Africa. *Social Science & Medicine*, 67(3), 441–452.

Williams, D. R., Yu, Y., Jackson, J. S., & Anderson, N. B. (1997). Racial differences in physical and
mental health: Socio-economic status, stress and discrimination. *Journal of Health Psychology*, 2(3),
335–351.

Williams, D. R., & Collins, C. (2001). Racial residential segregation: A fundamental cause of racial
disparities in health. *Public Health Reports*, 116(5), 404.

Williams, D. R., Lawrence, J. A., & Davis, B. A. (2019). Racism and health: Evidence and needed
research. *Annual Review of Public Health*.

Yearby, R. (2020). Structural racism and health disparities: Reconfiguring the social determinants of
health framework to include the root cause. *The Journal of Law, Medicine & Ethics*, 48(3), 518–526.

CHAPTER 12

Navigating the Ethical and Legal Challenges of Health Disparities

Olubukunola Mary Dwyer

LEARNING OBJECTIVES

◉ Discuss the areas where ethics and law overlap and at times conflict at the clinical bedside in the United States.

◉ Analyze the difficulties and challenges health disparities can bring to clinical decision-making for providers and patients.

◉ Review the best interest standard and harm principle.

◉ Analyze how shared decision-making can be used when considering nonbeneficial treatment.

◉ Explore the effects immigration and socioeconomic status can have in clinical situations.

◉ Examine the difficulties and challenges that arise when managing potential transplant recipient candidates.

INTRODUCTION

Law and ethics are distinct disciplines; however, there is recognition that the ethical characteristics of a society can have a major influence on the laws of that same society. Ethics is thought of as the discipline concerned with how a society determines what is morally good or bad, right or wrong. Simply put, what are the values of that society? Laws are created and written based upon these societal values, despite the possibility that these values may not be applied equally within a society. The extent of the influence ethics can have on a society's laws causes the disciplines to be thought of as intertwined and interdependent. In a clinical setting, the two disciplines are both called on to resolve difficult dilemmas, and both can be used to facilitate good medical practice and clinical decision-making. Despite this, depending on the dilemma at hand, the disciplines can be at odds because their focus and goals differ. When trying to resolve these dilemmas, providers must keep in mind that a legal recommendation may focus on reducing liability for the "client," meaning the institution or provider. Alternatively, an ethics recommendation tends to be focused on balancing the conflicting values of everyone involved, specifically the patient, their family, and the healthcare providers. This chapter explores some of the primary principles of clinical ethics and describes the interdependence and tensions that exist between ethics and law when striving to be a moral society by presenting three case studies of diverse populations that illustrate the decision-making processes when both legal and ethical principles are applied.

The Supreme Court case of *Obergefell v. Hodges* (2015) is an example of the interplay between the two disciplines and the effect the interplay can have on various health disparities in the clinical setting. This case legalized same-sex marriage across the United States in 2015. Prior to *Obergefell*, depending on the state in which a patient was receiving medical care, a same-sex spouse may not have had authority to act as a surrogate decision-maker. In the majority of states in the United States, the spouse is the default primary surrogate decision-maker for a patient when the patient loses decision-making capacity. States assume that a spouse is in the best position to know a patient's medical wishes and/or what is in the patient's best interest (Brudney, 2018). The discipline of ethics, specifically clinical ethics, has long recognized that it would be a moral good to have the person who knows the patient best make medical decisions for a patient, regardless of the gender or legal status of the potential surrogate (*Cruzan v. Missouri*, 1990). When *Obergefell* was decided, it brought parity and recognition that regardless of a surrogate decision-maker's gender, if the potential surrogate knows the patient's wishes, that person should be able to act on the patient's behalf. Specifically, if the potential surrogate is a same-sex spouse, they should be able to make medical decisions for the patient.

Health disparity related to sexual orientation and the matter of who has the right to act as a patient's surrogate decision-maker were not specifically argued before the Supreme Court. The court, however, did recognize in their opinion that marital status affects medical decision-making authority. In this example, the U.S. legal system caught up to what clinical ethics had already recognized, that a potential surrogate decision-maker's gender should not have any influence on who is involved in the medical decision-making for a patient. Instead, the relationship to the patient is the most important factor in the ethical justification for decisional authority.

This example illustrates not only the interaction between law and ethics, but also how a dilemma might be resolved differently depending on whether a healthcare provider chooses to follow the law or what is most ethically justifiable. Prior to *Obergefell*, there were a variety of legal mechanisms that dealt with status of same-sex marriage. For example, Ohio had a state constitutional amendment, passed in 2004, that made it unconstitutional for the state to recognize same-sex marriages or civil unions, including those performed out of state. Until 2015, a same-sex spouse in Ohio would not have the legal authority to act as the surrogate to make end-of-life medical decisions for a patient. Instead, that authority would have passed to the patient's blood relatives, such as an adult child or parents (Brudney, 2018). From an ethics standpoint, if the same-sex spouse had the most knowledge of the patient's values and medical wishes, that person would be determined to be the best surrogate decision-maker. In cases such as this, recognizing that the legal authority to act as the surrogate would lie with a parent or child, the same-sex spouse would be encouraged to work with the parent(s) and/or adult child(ren) to make medical decisions on the patient's behalf. This hopefully would ensure that both the law and ethics are satisfied when making a medical decision for the patient.

Differences in how law and ethics resolve dilemmas often put care providers in the proverbial "between a rock and a hard place"—do what is "right" or do what is legal? In general, providers tend to be very concerned about the potential legal ramifications of their actions but also want to do what is best for their patients. If a situation arises where a resolution could not satisfy both the law and ethics, there is a general belief that what is legal would presumptively determine the outcome of the dilemma to protect providers and health systems from lawsuits. Fortunately, that does not tend to be the case. Instead there is usually common ground that can be found between the two disciplines. If there is a direct statute or case law that would clearly conflict with what is ethical, a rarity indeed, there often is some reasonable way to interpret the applicable law that allows a provider to do what is ethical while not directly violating the law. Also, there are many legal "gray" areas where the law is "silent," meaning there is a lack of federal or state statutes and a lack of case law that provide clear guidance. In these areas, the recommendation that has the strongest ethical justification can be followed. Despite this and the delicate balance that exists between law and ethics, healthcare providers are still very concerned with the possibility of legal action, which leads to defensive medicine. Providers, which include nurses, physicians, midwives, and so on, must understand that filing a lawsuit occurs far more often than a patient or their family having a winning suit.

In this chapter, other examples of existing health disparities that have ethical or legal components are discussed in the context of clinical ethics cases. The different recommendations the two disciplines would give in these cases are also examined. How a court might actually resolve these cases is beyond the scope of this chapter and is not discussed. The discussion of these cases includes an exploration of the morally justifiable legal options available to the healthcare team to resolve these cases.

The field of medicine has evolved, becoming more inclusive in recognition of past and current mistakes that have been perpetrated against disadvantaged populations. These legal options are based on an emerging ethical standard proposed by the American Society for Bioethics and Humanities. A concluding recommendation that satisfies both disciplines is provided.

CLINICAL ETHICS CONSULTATION

The impetus for the creation of the field of clinical ethics resulted from a confluence of advancements in the fields of medicine and scientific research and a growing recognition that medicine is not always practiced in a moral manner. The history of clinical ethics goes back to antiquity, when the Hippocratic Oath was used as a guide of professional conduct for medical practitioners. The field became a major area of discourse within medicine with the revelations from the Nuremberg trials and the Tuskegee syphilis experiment. In the United States, the field further developed and drew closer to the bedside with the 1962 "God Committee" (Jonsen, 2007) and the legal cases of Karen Quinlan (In Re Quinlan, 1976) and Nancy Cruzan (*Cruzan v. Missouri*, 1990), both of which drew major national interest. These historical events illustrated to the field of medicine and to the public that there was a need for a consultative service that would assist healthcare professionals, patients, and their families in navigating the value-laden decisions that arise in healthcare. Figure 12.1 outlines the process of clinical ethics consultation, which has been adapted from the emerging standard for consultation from the American Society for Bioethics and Humanities (2011).

There are a variety of approaches for ethics consultation, which include authoritarian, consensus, and facilitation (Aulisio et al., 2000). For the cases that follow, the facilitation model is used. This approach has the ethics consultant elicit and elucidate the ethically relevant issues of the case. The ethicist also helps to improve the communication of those involved in the case by bringing together the relevant perspectives of those involved (American Society for Bioethics and Humanities, 2011; Shelton et al., 2016). There are a variety of approaches to ethics consultation, and the consults can be formal or informal. The cases that follow were all formal consults. Regardless of the approach used or the type of consult, generally all ethics consults follow the process standard outlined in Figure 12.1.

The vast majority of ethics consults start with a request by a member of the medical team, the patients, the family, or some other involved party, all of whom have access to an ethics consult. Once a request has been made, the consultant gathers the information relevant to the consult. Usually when gathering specific patient information, there is a review

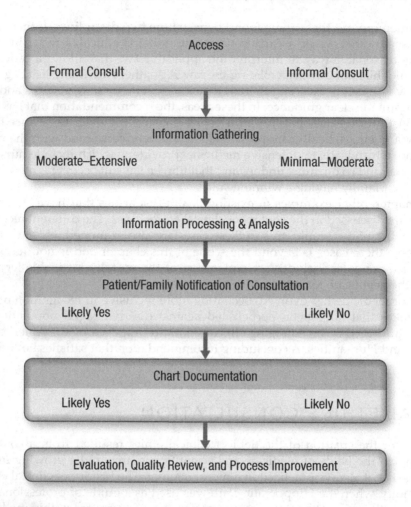

Figure 12.1 Ethics consultation process.

Source: From American Society for Bioethics and Humanities. (2011). *Core competencies for healthcare ethics consultation* (2nd ed.). American Society for Bioethics and Humanities.

of the patient's medical record, but also a meeting with the patient and any relevant family, friends, or support persons. This could occur during a one-on-one meeting between the patient/family and ethicist or during a medical team-family meeting. The amount of information gathering heavily depends on the type of ethical issue involved, the complexity of the consult, and the time pressures that may arise during the consult. The ethicist then turns their attention to processing and analyzing the information gathered by clarifying and determining the relevant ethical concepts, applicable policies including laws, medical and ethical standards, and institutional policies. During this step, the ethicist may be able to discern whether there are other applicable ethical issues that were not initially identified. The last part of this step involves identifying the range of ethically supportable options that could resolve the ethical conflicts. After processing and analyzing, the ethicist then determines whether the patient or family should be notified of the consult if they are not already aware of the consult from the initial request or from information gathering. The default standard is for the patient, family, and attending physician to be notified of the consult, but there are a limited number of instances where the patient or family would not be informed of the ethics consult. This usually arises for consults where the medical team is asking for general advice that is not patient specific, when there are conflicts between medical team members, when the patient or family have been overwhelmed by the volume and variety of medical team members, or when there are time constraints that do not allow for patient or family notification. The next step for an ethics consult is documentation of the consult. All ethics consults should be recorded in some manner—within an institutional database and/ or within a patient's medical record. Depending on the type of consult, the ethicist may or may not place a note in the patient's medical record. Generally, if there are ethics recommendations that will have a material impact on the patient's care, then an ethics consult note is placed. The last step of an ethics consult involves the evaluation and review of all ethics consults completed at the institution with the goal of improving the ethics consult service.

CASE STUDY 12.1

Jeremiah, a 7-year-old Amish boy, was in a car versus buggy accident in which he was ejected from the buggy. From the accident site, he was transported to the local hospital via an ambulance. While in transport to the local hospital and in the emergency department, his condition was stabilized, but it was determined that he had sustained a traumatic brain injury and injuries to his chest and abdomen. Providers at that facility met with Jeremiah's parents. It was recommended to them that he be transported via air ambulance to a level one pediatric trauma center. Transfer via an air ambulance was specifically recommended so that Jeremiah could receive time-sensitive interventions available at the trauma center. The center was located more than 2 hours away via ground transport. During the discussion of whether and how best to transport him, the risks and benefits of transfer and both methods of transport were discussed, including the cost of each mode of transport.

The providers in the emergency department were aware that members of the local Amish community often seek approval from the community's elders, who are traditionally men, before making important decisions. The community also typically participate in cost sharing for medical care and do not purchase insurance or participate in Medicare or Medicaid. Given this awareness, the providers at the local hospital were not surprised when Jeremiah's parents informed them that they needed to speak with their community's elders before making any decisions. The parents stated that they understood that they must decide whether Jeremiah should be transported and if so, how he would be transported. The providers at the pediatric trauma center were informed of this. The providers at the local hospital and pediatric trauma center requested a consult from the ethics team, based at the pediatric trauma center. Both Jeremiah's parents and the healthcare providers were concerned about how to transfer him to the trauma center and how choosing the less costly but longer transport time of ground transport would affect Jeremiah's outcomes. The ethics team was asked to help evaluate the values of everyone involved and the determination of best interests.

Amish and Rural Communities

In the United States, Amish communities are usually found in the northeast states of Indiana, Ohio, and Pennsylvania (Diebel, 2014). They are located in rural areas across these states and are thus affected by healthcare disparities attributable to their geographic location and isolation. Amish communities in and of themselves are insular due to their religious beliefs; they are reluctant to associate with and trust outsiders. This extends to their decision to not purchase or participate in insurance coverage. There is a strong sense of community accountability and some concerns that interaction with modern technology detracts from their religious lifestyle. Given these preferences and beliefs, the Amish tend to live in rural areas that enable them to perpetuate the lifestyle that supports their religious beliefs (Kraybill et al., 2013).

Rural communities, particularly Amish communities, are subject to disparities that include limited access to healthcare specialists and subspecialists and lower rates of insurance coverage (National Center for Health Statistics, 2019). In the case of Amish people, their choice to forego insurance coverage is attributable to their religious beliefs, but lack of access to routine primary and specialized care has significant effects on their health (Weyer et al., 2003). For example, Amish people in Lancaster county, Pennsylvania, have lower rates of diabetes, hypertension, and high cholesterol compared with other non-Hispanic White people in the United States. But Amish people in this county who do have these conditions are less likely to have their condition managed by medication, and there is a lack of awareness of or screening for these conditions (He et al., 2020). A number of factors have been suggested that contribute to inadequate diagnosis and management of chronic health conditions, including education gaps, lack of access to specialized services (e.g., endocrinologists, cardiologists), lack of insurance to pay for medications, and cultural reluctance to interact with those outside of their community (He et al., 2020; Kraybill et al., 2013; Weyer et al., 2003). Jeremiah's case illustrates how issues of access and the costs of care, in a complex situation that involves both cultural differences between patient and care team and pre-existing disparities in care, can impact medical decision-making. In Jeremiah's case, the decisions to be made have the potential to not only affect the patient and his parents, but also to have a financial impact on his wider community.

The Harm Principle and the Best Interest Standard

For medical providers and clinical ethicists, there are two ethical standards that could be used to determine whether pursuing state intervention, meaning asking for a court to appoint a decision-maker, is ethically justified to override parental decision-making. The two standards are the best interest standard and the harm principle. The best interest standard is more commonly known and has been used in law and medicine for several decades (Dolgin, 1996), while the harm principle is relatively new (Diekema, 2004); both standards have deficiencies. The harm principle was articulated by Douglas Diekema in response to the well-known challenges and shortcomings of the best interest standard. These challenges include its vagueness, that the values that arise with the notion of "best interest" can be influenced by the values of a judge, and whether the best interest of the child should be the sole consideration when making a treatment decision (Diekema, 2004; Dolgin, 1996). The harm principle proposes that state intervention is justified when parental decisions or actions are likely to cause harm to the patient/child or at least are more likely than other options to increase the likelihood of serious/substantial harm, suffering, or death to the child. Diekema has enumerated eight conditions (Box 12.1) that must be met before state intervention by the healthcare team should be pursued (Diekema, 2004). The harm principle and its conditions are not yet widely accepted due to its relative novelty. It is not used by the legal or medical fields but often is included in ethical analyses of pediatric cases. Given the limited acceptance of the harm principle, the more commonly used best interest standard is given a fuller discussion.

The disciplines of law and ethics have both explored the concept of "best interest." From a legal standpoint, the best interest standard is most commonly used in the area of American family law, specifically in regard to child custody issues. The U.S. legal system has enshrined this standard in case law, in which it is used to determine and protect the interests of children, even to the extent of limiting parental authority. In the 1944 case *Prince v. Massachusetts*, the Supreme Court recognized that parental authority is not absolute. In certain situations, it would be in the interest of the child for the state to act as a surrogate parent under the *parens patriae* doctrine. The state can act as the child's parent when it is determined that the parents are acting in a manner contrary to the best interest of the child. There is often reluctance in pursuing this action due to the potential emotional impact it could have on the child and the family. In the *Prince* case, parents were removing their

BOX 12.1: Conditions for Justified State Interference With Parental Decision-Making

By refusing to consent are the parents placing their child at significant risk of serious harm?

Is the harm imminent, requiring immediate action to prevent it?

Is the intervention that has been refused necessary to prevent the serious harm?

Is the intervention that has been refused of proven efficacy, and therefore likely to prevent the harm?

Does the intervention that has been refused by the parents not also place the child at significant risk of serious harm, and do its projected benefits outweigh its projected burdens significantly more favorably than the option chosen by the parents?

Would any other option prevent serious harm to the child in a way that is less intrusive to parental autonomy and more acceptable to the parents?

Can the state intervention be generalized to all other similar situations?

Would most parents agree that the state intervention was reasonable?

Source: Reproduced with permission from Diekema (2004). Parental refusals of medical treatment: The harm principle as threshold for state intervention. *Theoretical Medicine and Bioethics,* 25(4), 243–264. https://doi.org/10.1007/s11017-004-3146-6

children from school so they could distribute and sell religious literature, which was found to be in violation of child labor laws. The *Prince* case primarily focused on parental rights in the context of child labor and school attendance, and specifically prohibited using children as martyrs reflecting their parents' religious beliefs (*Prince v. Massachusetts*, 1944). The use of this standard has evolved and expanded to be used not only in these types of cases, but also in determining the adequacy and appropriateness of medical decisions made on the behalf of children (Kopelman, 1997).

Expansion of the use of the best interest standard has brought this legal standard to the bedside and outpatient clinic. It now also is used to determine whether parents' medical decision-making on behalf of their child—the patient—is in the best interest of the child. When this standard is applied at the bedside, it is used by the healthcare team to determine whether seeking state intervention is justified to prevent a decision that is not in the best interest of the child. In court, when the standard is applied, it can be used to limit parental rights by having the court-appointed decision-maker act as a surrogate parent for the child in question and make decisions. When the healthcare team and court are aligned in their determination of what is in the best interest of the child, the court-appointed decision-maker then has the authority to make medical decisions for the child.

When making the determination of whether it is ethically and legally justifiable for the healthcare team to pursue state intervention in order to protect the interest of the child, certain factors are taken into consideration. From an ethics standpoint, the team could determine whether the medical decisions of the parents would promote the maximal good for the child and/or which option would gain the child the highest net benefit from the available treatment options. Both require that the parents act in a way that is most favorable to the patient/child (Buchanan & Brock, 1990). Before pursuing legal action, the team may consider the feasibility, emotional impact, and time constraints of pursuing legal action in the context of time-sensitive interventions. It is sometimes more effective to present all acceptable options from which the parents can choose rather than having the healthcare team unilaterally identify and insist on the "ideal" option. In complex situations with practical constraints, this might best meet the goal of maximizing the good for the patient (Paris & Schreiber, 1996).

Recommendation

Given Jeremiah's stable condition at the local hospital and the specific injuries he sustained, the healthcare team and his parents have two decisions to consider: whether transfer should be pursued, and if so, which mode of transport? For both decisions, determining how best to maximize benefit must be the primary consideration. His condition has been stabilized, so his injuries are not imminently life-threatening. Nevertheless, despite his stable condition, further treatment is needed that is only available at the pediatric trauma center. Given the potential impact that foregoing transfer would have on his outcomes, it is unlikely that remaining at the local hospital could be seen as maximizing potential benefit to him. Therefore, refusing transfer would not be in Jeremiah's best interest, would not be ethically justifiable, and should not be pursued by the healthcare team or his parents.

Next, because the treatments Jeremiah would need are somewhat time sensitive, it would be prudent to get him to the trauma center sooner rather than later. However, the healthcare team could not say with certainty whether the time-sensitive interventions would be needed within the 2-hour window that it would take to transfer him by road. Given this, both modes of transfer are reasonable options, and both have the potential to maximize benefit to the patient. The choice of either air or ground transport would satisfy the ethical and legal best interest standard for Jeremiah.

Other Considerations

In the case outlined of Jeremiah, when applying the best interest standard to the parents' decision of which mode of transport to pursue, the team could also consider the rationale and values on which the parents based their decision-making. Are they considering how closely to adhere to their religious beliefs, and/or what is best for their community, such as which option has the lowest financial impact on the community? Or are they basing their decision only on what would bring about the maximal good and/or highest net benefit for their child? In general, both medical and legal assessments of theological consequences (i.e., consequences of violating religious tenets) are not used as a basis for determining best interest (Sher, 1983). Courts want children to have the opportunity to become adults who can choose their own religious beliefs. Thus, the team may likely recognize but discount this as a legitimate basis for justifying the parents' decisions. Also, interests of the patient generally outweigh interests of the community unless the case involves a threat to public health. If religious and community values are the primary motivators for the parents' decision and the decision is averse to Jeremiah's interest, then the healthcare team could file for state involvement. The healthcare team would be ethically and legally justified in pursuing state involvement. State involvement could span a variety of activities, such as having the court-appointed decision-maker participate in medical care plan meetings or having the court order evaluations of the child's home and access to the child's medical records. Note that respect for the unique values and beliefs of the parents and appreciation of the background disparities and economic consequences to the community do not justify agreeing with a parental decision that is clearly not in Jeremiah's interest, unlike the mode of transport decision, which does not have reasonably likely consequences for Jeremiah and thus can be left to the parents and community.

Without the time pressure involved in this case, there likely would have been a team family meeting held with Jeremiah's parents, their elders, the healthcare providers, and possibly the ethics consultant. This consultation was requested with the intent to advise the healthcare team, which provides the ethics consultant with room to determine whether it would be appropriate for them to attend the team family meeting. At the conclusion of this case, Jeremiah's parents chose to have him transported via air ambulance.

CASE STUDY 12.2

Mikel is a 37-year-old transgender male patient who is admitted for an unwitnessed fall at home. His medical history is significant for leukemia, chronic opiate use disorder, alcohol dependence, and an eating disorder. This is his fourth admission in the last 3 weeks. During the course of this admission, it is determined that his fall at home was caused by anemia and dehydration. Over the last month, he has needed several transfusions due to his anemia. He has become transfusion dependent, and continuation of his life is now dependent on repeated blood transfusions. When his cancer was first diagnosed, the healthcare team determined that his cancer was treatable. After this determination, the healthcare team had extensive discussions with Mikel explaining his condition, the recommended plan of care, and the various treatment options. The recommended treatment course included chemotherapy and possible radiation therapy to manage his leukemia. Outpatient psychiatric treatment was also recommended to manage his eating and addiction disorders.

Initially, Mikel was agreeable to the recommended plan of care and worked with the various members of the team to follow the care plan. He also met with social work staff to make arrangements for his outpatient care. Since his initial admission and diagnosis, however, Mikel has been unable to adhere to the healthcare team's treatment recommendations because he believes that issues with his diet are the underlying cause of his cancer. Over the course of his four admissions, he has met with the oncology and radiation oncology teams, nursing, social work, and nutrition services several times. The various team members have had discussions educating and re-educating Mikel about his condition and the plan of care that would be needed to manage his disease. During previous admissions, social work staff has worked with Mikel to find community resources that could help him with housing and outpatient psychiatric treatment. Unfortunately, Mikel has not followed up with any of these services, has missed outpatient appointments for his medical care and psychiatric needs, and has continued to have a restrictive caloric intake diet. During subsequent admissions, Mikel at times has refused medications and has refused to eat. Throughout these admissions, he has been able to demonstrate to the healthcare team that he has the capacity to understand his disease, but he continues to believe that certain behavioral and dietary changes will cure him. Due to an inability to appreciate the realities of his disease and to adhere to his treatment plan, his cancer has progressed.

Mikel informs his healthcare team that he currently lives in a motel with his 6-year-old son. Due to his financial issues, he does not have reliable transportation and cannot regularly attend his medical appointments. He has informed his team that he currently lacks social support because of his gender identity and his drug and alcohol use. He has provided the healthcare team with contact information for his mother and has given the team permission to contact her. The healthcare team has been very concerned about Mikel's prognosis. Given these concerns, the healthcare team has reached out to his mother to determine whether she could support Mikel while he is getting treatment by helping him get to appointments and assisting Mikel with following his plan of care. Some members of the team consider his condition to be terminal due to the progression of his disease, transfusion dependence, and ongoing drug and alcohol use. Team members recognize that his social constraints and financial situation have likely contributed to his inability to follow the treatment plan. There is also recognition that Mikel's ongoing poor understanding of his disease despite multiple conversations with various members of the healthcare team is also a contributing factor. The healthcare team considered whether it would be ethically appropriate to no longer offer curative medical treatment and to limit transfusions. There are also concerns about the welfare of Mikel's son and whether a referral to the local social service agency should be made. Details about Mikel's son are limited due to the medical team's focus on Mikel and the care he needs.

Transgender Health Disparities

Known and significant health disparities for transgender people exist in healthcare (Bradford et al., 2013). These disparities are understudied, but data have been collected from transgender individuals' self-reports. To date, the National Transgender Discrimination Survey is the largest study to collect data on the lives and experiences of transgender people. The survey found that, in addition to the limited access transgender people have to healthcare, they also face financial barriers such as lack of income and insurance, discrimination such as family rejection, and socioeconomic barriers, including lack of transportation, housing, and mental health resource access (Grant et al., 2011). These are just a few of the sources of disparity that transgender people face when they seek medical care.

When confronted with these barriers in addition to dealing with complex medical issues, transgender people are at risk for having poorer outcomes for survivable diseases. Mikel's case illustrates how these barriers impact a patient's decision-making and then in turn affect the medical treatments that are offered to the patient. It has the potential to create a vicious cycle of distrust and frustration by the healthcare team, who are trying to provide the best care available to their patient, and by the patient, who is trying to survive a serious illness and overcome the disparities he faces due to his social circumstances. For this case, when you add the additional layer of possible child endangerment, distrust and frustration can intensify.

Nonbeneficial Treatment

Medical providers and ethicists have struggled over how to define and identify nonbeneficial treatment. There has been some agreement that medical interventions that will not meet established physiological goals or treatments that would result in the patient not being able to survive outside of an acute care setting are nonbeneficial treatments (Kon et al., 2016). There is still much debate as to whether there is an ethical obligation to offer medical treatment that a provider has determined to be nonbeneficial (Bosslet et al., 2015). One of the prevailing arguments is based on the principle of autonomy, that providers have the autonomous right to refuse to provide treatment that is inconsistent with their professional judgment and the long-standing values of the profession. The principle of autonomy, simply put, is the right to be free of the excessive or coercive influence of others. This principle empowers agents (providers and patients) to be able to make their own informed decisions. However, autonomy does not empower agents to force or direct other autonomous agents to behave in a particular manner (Beauchamp & Childress, 2001). It does not prevent others from attempting to exert their influence, but it does place limits on an agent's coercive actions. For example, a provider cannot perform a medical procedure without a patient's consent and adherence, even if the provider has good reason to believe the procedure would benefit the patient. Likewise, providers have the right to refuse to provide treatments their patients are requesting or demanding if the requested treatment violates the provider's strongly held beliefs or values. This is specifically allowed and supported by various bodies and institutions, such as the American Association for Critical Care Nurses, the Society for Critical Care Medicine, and the American Thoracic Society (Bosslet et al., 2015).

Despite a recognition that providers are autonomous agents, there is a persistent belief that patients should have complete control over the direction of their medical care. To some, this right of control extends to being able to direct every aspect of their care, and if a provider refuses to supply certain treatments, this places limits on a patient's ability to control their medical care. An example would be patients who insist on the use of specific pain medication. The recent opioid epidemic illustrates some of the complications that arise when patients dictate their pain management and providers acquiesce to patient requests. In recognition of this viewpoint, shared decision-making between the patient and the provider is recommended, particularly in the context of life-sustaining nonbeneficial treatment. In this framework, the provider gives the patient facts about the disease condition and possible treatment options, while the patient supplies personal values such as being willing to undergo a long recovery process in a facility or valuing independence over a prolonged life. The patient's values are then used to evaluate the various options presented by the provider to make a decision (Brock, 1991). If the providers determine that certain treatments would likely result in an outcome that is contrary to an expressed patient value, that treatment option would not be pursued. This structure allows patients to remain in control of their care without binding providers to offering treatments that they determine would not be medically appropriate, would not be beneficial to the patient, and/or would conflict with the patient's expressed values. There are concerns that if providers were allowed to limit the treatment options they present to their patients, it would create the potential for providers to select treatment options based on inappropriate, nonmedical reasons. Studies have found that healthcare professionals are influenced by racial and ethnic biases, which have had an effect on the healthcare outcomes of their patients (Hall et al., 2015). Balancing the autonomous rights of patients and providers without allowing bias to play a role remains an ongoing struggle, but with recognition of these ongoing issues, progress can be made. Also, with the trend toward shared decision-making, there is not complete consensus among patients and professionals about the priority of patient autonomy when the patient demands a treatment the provider believes will not be effective.

There have been court cases and state statutes that protect and support provider autonomy when a provider recognizes that certain treatments are very likely to be nonbeneficial to a patient. States including California (California Probate Code § 4600-4806, 2011), Texas (Texas Advance Directives Act, 1999), and Virginia (Virginia Code §32.1-127; §54.1-2990) have statutes that provide protection to providers. A few other states have some protections available in physician orders for life-sustaining treatment–related statutes (e.g., Physician Orders for Life Sustaining Treatment). The strength of these protections varies, but they all have the potential to provide some protection to providers when they determine that the provision of requested treatments would be nonbeneficial and are contrary to their professional judgment. The vast majority of states in the United States and federal law are mostly silent on this issue. Some states prohibit the withdrawal of life-sustaining treatment without the agreement of the patient and/or family. The states that have this prohibition do not address whether a provider is obliged to offer or provide treatment that has not started. Given the variation of existing statutory protection across states and the variation of existing protections, there is a lack of clear legal guidance as to how to manage these cases.

This gap in the law also extends to court cases. Landmark cases regarding the withdrawal of treatment have been argued from the standpoint of the patient and/or their family refusing treatment or wanting the withdrawal of treatment that is currently being provided (In Re Quinlan, 1976). The only case law that comes close to the issue of withholding nonbeneficial treatment is the case of Baby K (In the Matter of Baby "K", 1993).This case was argued from the standpoint of a provider who wanted to limit ventilatory support for an infant who had been born with significant neurological deficit; her mother opposed treatment limitation. The child continually needed emergency ventilatory support on each hospital admission. The courts found that the Emergency Medical Treatment and Active Labor Act (EMTALA) stipulated that the provider is obligated to provide emergency treatment that would stabilize the child's condition and that the federal statute does not have an exception for futility (U.S. Court of Appeals, Fourth Circuit, 1994). This case regrettably does not provide insight as to what should happen when nonemergency treatment is being considered. Other cases that have dealt with the use of nonbeneficial treatment that a provider wants either to withhold (not offer) or to withdraw (if already begun) have involved patients who are dead by neurological criteria ("brain death"). These cases have also not been on point and have instead dealt with religious exceptions (Luce, 2015) or the legal criteria for determining death by neurological criteria (In Re Guardianship of Hailu, 2015). There has not yet been a case affirming or rejecting a provider's right to not offer a requested treatment that the provider has determined to be nonbeneficial.

Duty to Report (Mandated Reporting)

The duty to report arises in a variety of circumstances in the clinical setting. These include when elder abuse is suspected, if a patient poses an imminent risk to a third party, and specifically when child neglect or abuse is suspected. While providing medical care to a child or to an adult patient who has children, information could be disclosed to the healthcare team that causes the team to suspect child neglect has occurred or is occurring. Healthcare teams encounter this issue when providing care to patients with a substance use disorder who are also parents. Teachers, counselors, social workers, child care providers, and law enforcement officers, as well as healthcare providers, have a duty to report suspected child abuse and neglect that could occur when the parents have substance use disorder. The prevalence of the substance use problem in the United States is well known. An estimated 8.7 million children live with a parent or guardian with a substance use disorder (Lipari & Van Horn, 2017). Given how widespread this problem is, the healthcare team must carefully consider when their patient's substance use rises to the level that it endangers the welfare of a child. Generally, a report must be made if there is suspicion or a reason to believe that a child has been or is being abused or neglected (Child Welfare Information Gateway, 2019). In addition to determining whether to make a report, the team must weigh the ethical responsibility to keep their patient's medical information confidential against the ethical obligation to act in the child's best interest. Team members must also consider their professional duty as a mandated reporter of child abuse and neglect (*The Lancet*, 2019). Careful consideration of the specifics of each of these types of cases must occur. The team must also remain cognizant of their own biases given the disproportionate rates of reporting that occur when the patient is of a lower socioeconomic status, is an immigrant, or is member of a minority group or another marginalized community, such as transgender people (Chasnoff et al., 1990; Drake et al., 2011).

All states in the United States have statutes that involve mandated reporting. These statutes vary in their requirements for reporting, but they do have a commonality in requiring healthcare providers to report the abuse and neglect of children (Committee on Injury, Violence, and Poison Prevention, 2009). Usually when these situations arise, the child is also the patient, which allows for providers to have some direct knowledge about suspected abuse or neglect that has occurred. The vast majority of these statutes provide immunity to care providers who make reports in good faith out of concern for a child, even if it is later determined that no abuse or neglect has taken place. If, however, the provider fails to make a report and a child suffers harm as a result, providers are potentially subject to a variety of penalties (Child Welfare Information Gateway, 2019). When a parent's substance use endangers a child, a provider's duty to report remains. These situations are highly complex and must be handled delicately in order to not damage the patient/provider relationship. Also, it should be ensured that factors such as the parents' race, ethnicity, or socioeconomic status, as well as the provider's biases, are not playing a role in determining whether to report suspected abuse or neglect (Chasnoff et al., 1990; Luken et al., 2021).

Recommendation

When treatment limitation standards and shared decision-making are applied to Mikel's case, both the healthcare team and Mikel must engage in open and frank discussions. These discussions should not only explore Mikel's condition and prognosis, but also whether there is distrust and/or bias at play in the patient/provider relationship. To address these latter concerns, it could be helpful for Mikel to meet with the hospital's social worker. The purpose of this discussion would be to determine if Mikel has encountered incidents of discrimination, either in the past or presently, that have contributed to distrust of his medical team or that have created a barrier to his adherence to the recommended treatment plan. If specific concerns are identified, Mikel should be referred to a transgender support group, a clinic, or a psychologist who specializes in transgender issues. A provider from one of these services could provide support to Mikel and could also act as a bridge to help build trust between Mikel and his healthcare team while curative treatment is pursued. While working to address any concerns Mikel may have with trusting his healthcare team, the team must also determine whether any of their own biases may have played a role in medical decision-making. If any biases are found, they must be openly confronted and dealt with by removing their influence in determining Mikel's treatment options. If specific members of the healthcare team are identified to be problematic, they should be recused from Mikel's healthcare team. Once any issues of distrust and bias are handled and extra support for Mikel is in place, if there continue to be problems with Mikel adhering to the treatment plan, and his condition and prognosis continue to deteriorate, then plan of care discussions with Mikel can turn to changing the goals of care.

The healthcare team has expressed grave concerns about Mikel's condition and prognosis among themselves. They now have an obligation to present these concerns to Mikel along with the medical facts of his condition and prognosis. The medical facts of his condition would include available treatment options for him. These options range from continuing the current treatment course with curative intent to pursuing suboptimal treatment that might slow progression of his disease, to transitioning to a focus solely on comfort measures. Given the team's reluctance to pursue treatment with curative intent because Mikel's consistent inability to adhere to needed actions makes the treatments ineffective, they could explain to Mikel why the team is not recommending or offering this treatment option. Before informing Mikel that treatment with curative intent will not continue to be offered, Mikel and the team need to discuss what Mikel's treatment goals are. If his goal is to be completely cured of his leukemia, the team must gather and review all relevant clinical, psychological, and social data to definitively determine whether or not there is a reasonable likelihood that this treatment course could not meet Mikel's goal. If there is consensus among the team that treatment focused on cure is determined to be nonbeneficial, then the healthcare team would inform Mikel of this. Once informed of these medical facts, Mikel can then determine and express to the team what he values most in terms of his care and if he has any other treatment goals. If he continues to feel that behavior modification would help him, despite being informed otherwise by the team, he would be free to pursue this and he should consider transitioning his care to comfort measures. When assisting a patient who is transitioning to comfort measures, services like hospice and palliative care could be consulted to assist with the transition. Fully informed patients with decisional capacity have the right to make decisions that the healthcare team believes are poor or "bad" decisions. Alternatively, if Mikel wants his care to be shaped by his desire to spend more time with his son, in recognition of how far his disease has progressed, he could work with his team to find supportive treatment options, such as palliative care to manage his symptoms, to help him achieve this goal.

If Mikel expresses disagreement with the team's determination of his medical facts, he has the latitude to seek another opinion about his care or to pursue care elsewhere. The current team would have an obligation to facilitate this, particularly recognizing that he may have difficulty identifying other providers who are knowledgeable about the care of transgender persons. As described previously, Mikel has not yet expressed disagreement with the healthcare team, but he has voiced a belief as to the cause of his disease. If, because of this belief, he chooses to no longer engage with the team about his care, he should be fully informed of the consequences of his decision, the potential outcomes, and the choices available to him.

In addition to discussing the medical facts of his condition, the team should also discuss with Mikel their concerns about the welfare of his son and the team's responsibility to report these welfare concerns to child protective services. Social work staff should reassess with Mikel the community resources that could help him with housing and any other services and resources he may need. Given Mikel's prognosis, social situation, and lack of information about who cares for his son while he is hospitalized, the team could work with Mikel to find reasonable accommodations that would safeguard his son's welfare. A consult for the hospital's social work department could be made on this basis. If, however, Mikel has demonstrated that his drug and alcohol use has impaired his ability to care for his son to the extent of jeopardizing his son's safety, then a referral to the county's social services should be made on this basis. The healthcare team should ensure, if they are making a referral, that the basis of the referral is welfare concerns and not any provider biases. The welfare of Mikel's son should be the main concern for referral. The team should also limit information about Mikel's medical circumstances to only the amount absolutely needed to make the referral in order to keep Mikel's medical information confidential.

CASE STUDY 12.3

Jesse is a 31-year-old man with hypertension, diabetes, and end-stage renal disease. He is currently being evaluated as a potential kidney transplant recipient. He immigrated to the United States from Central America with his wife 8 years ago. Since then, he has been working with an immigration lawyer to pursue citizenship. He has no other family members in this country. Over the course of his care, Jesse has struggled with taking his prescribed medications and following the recommended diet. Jesse, his wife, and the healthcare team recognize that his struggles are due to his difficulty in understanding the instructions about when and how he should take the medications and which foods to eat, as well as his dislike of the prescribed diet, which excludes many of the foods traditional in his culture. Members of the team suspect that Jesse's low health literacy and language barrier are the underlying causes of his misunderstanding. As a result, his diabetes is not under control and he has a body mass index (BMI) of 32, meeting the threshold for obesity.

Jesse's healthcare team has been working with him and his wife over the past 5 months to optimize his medication adherence and to improve his diet. After his first evaluation for eligibility to be placed on the transplant list, the team met with Jesse and his wife to discuss methods to help him understand and follow the treatment plan the team recommended so that he would meet eligibility criteria. The methods included providing translated versions of his medication labels and prescriptions. Diet plans were created, along with diet education and consults with the transplant team dietician. During appointments, a translator was also used. Jesse's case has been discussed during two previous transplant team meetings. The team chose to list him as "status seven" instead of determining that he is not a transplant candidate. Potential transplant recipients listed as "status seven" are considered eligible but temporarily inactive; they cannot receive an available organ. The team elected to do this to give Jesse time to improve his treatment plan adherence, get his diabetes under better control, and lose weight, while facilitating an eventual change to active status. With a third recipient evaluation coming up, some members of the team are considering whether it would be appropriate to take Jesse off the list entirely if he has not made improvements. Jesse and his wife were informed of the team's concerns and that without better medication adherence, control of his diabetes, and a lower BMI, Jesse likely would not meet the criteria to become an active, listed potential recipient. The team as a whole are concerned with whether they have an obligation to supply more resources to Jesse to assist him with becoming a more suitable transplant candidate.

Immigrant Health Disparities in the United States

Health disparities and inequalities across racial and ethnic groups in the United States are pervasive and well-studied. A specific component of the study of the health of Americans focuses on the health of immigrants (Derose et al., 2007; Wallace et al., 2012). Research has provided consistent evidence of differences in health outcomes for ethnic groups (Bustamante et al., 2021; Coughlin, 2019; Engelman & Ye, 2019; Goldfarb et al., 2017; Singh et al., 2013). These disparities span a variety of ethnicities, including Hispanic people, foreign-born Asian people, and non-Hispanic African Americans, and also cuts across various age groups from birth to death. These studies have found existing disparities in the management of various aspects of health, including prenatal care (Goldfarb et al., 2017), diabetes (Engelman & Ye, 2019), and other chronic conditions (Singh et al., 2013). Attention has turned to not only identifying existing disparities but also examining the underlying factors that cause immigrants to be vulnerable when navigating the healthcare system. A study supported by the Robert Wood Johnson Foundation found that several factors affect immigrant health (Derose et al., 2007). They include socioeconomic background; immigration status; education and skill levels; English proficiency; federal and state laws; local policies; fear of authority; stigma; and marginalization. Due to these identified factors, immigrants have more barriers to accessing healthcare; have lower rates of health insurance coverage, which results in lower rates of healthcare usage; and receive lower-quality care than some members of the U.S.-born population (Derose et al., 2007; Wallace et al., 2012). Immigrants with end-stage renal disease often rely on emergency-only hemodialysis and as a result have worse health outcomes and quality of life due to their inability to afford and access private insurance and government insurance because of their legal status (Raghavan, 2018; Welles & Cervantes, 2019).

Immigration policy is a perpetual topic of heated debate in the United States. This topic and the ongoing issues with health policies in this country have raised awareness of exisiting immigrant health disparities (Edward, 2014; Gostin, 2019; Kline, 2019; Raghavan, 2018). Health professionals are now more aware of this disparity. As a result of its prominence, providers, healthcare institutions, the federal government, and some state governments have made efforts to address the causes of these disparities. Policies, discussed later in this chapter, have also been created to reduce the impact of these disparities and to improve immigrant health (Hall & Cuellar, 2016).

Justice and Resource Allocation

When the topic of organ transplantation is examined, the discussion often turns to the reality that organs are a very scarce resource and concern about how this resource is equitably distributed. From an ethics perspective, this issue is discussed in relation to the ethical principle of justice and equitable resource allocation. When analyzing how organs are distributed and whether the distribution of the organs is equitable, the focus tends to be on the organs themselves, specifically, the great imbalance between the demand and the supply of available organs, how to increase the supply, and how to evaluate possible recipients (Clarke et al., 1995; Freeman & Bernat, 2012). This has been a particularly persistent problem among communities of color. The causes for this disparity range from the belief that organ donation is a "White" issue, to mistrust of the healthcare system, to lack of education about organ donation (Callender & Miles, 2010; Morgan et al., 2013). Due to these causes, the rates of organ donation among minorities remain particularly low (Bratton et al., 2011). With these ongoing issues, rarely does the discussion turn to the resources that are used to assist a patient to become a transplant recipient candidate or to the equitable distribution of these resources. All potential transplant recipient candidates also are evaluated for their probable ability to care for and maintain this scarce resource. Providers recognize that they have an obligation to act as stewards for these scare resources. In doing so, not only must they equitably distribute this resource, but also they must discern who will be able to care for and maintain the resource (Sawinski & Locke, 2018). The following discussion focuses on the equitable access to resources needed by immigrants to assist them with becoming potential transplant candidates.

The ethical principle of justice requires that resources be equitably distributed; this is particularly true for the distribution of scarce resources (Beauchamp & Childress, 2001). This remains the primary principle discussed in the context of organ transplantation and is the reason why the principle of justice often arises when discussing organ transplantation. Similar to other areas of healthcare, all patients who need an organ transplant are confronted with issues around accessing and participating in the organ transplant system. But as noted, immigrants face unique challenges when accessing the healthcare system. These issues can affect an immigrant's ability to participate in the organ transplant system and can affect their candidacy. Although justice may dictate that immigrants have a right to equal access to the transplant system, justice does not necessarily require that more resources be provided to them to help make them eligible candidates for transplantation. For immigrants, as long as the same criteria are being used to evaluate all potential recipients, they are being given the same potential for access to organs unless the criteria themselves are flawed. Transplant selection criteria that exclude a patient from accessing the system include active substance use, severe cardiovascular disease, lack of insurance coverage or inability to cover the expenses of a transplant, inadequate social support, documented history of nonadherence with medical regimens or medications, morbid obesity, or uncontrolled psychiatric disorder that affects decision-making, such as depression (Chadban et al., 2020). There has been much criticism of these criteria and how they disproportionally limit access to transplantation for certain populations, such as those of lower socioeconomic status, certain immigrant populations, and those with disabilities. Specifically, the criterion of "adequate social support" has caused some concern for perpetuating disparities in access to organs (Chapman et al., 2013; Ladin et al., 2019). Despite the concern, this criterion has not been eliminated, justified by the need to limit distribution of this scarce resource to those who would benefit from the organ transplant and to maximize the benefit they would receive by being able to adequately care for the organ postoperatively. In most cases, this requires someone in the recipient's circle of family or friends who can assume responsibility for supporting and providing tangible assistance to the recipient as they recover.

Patient Bill of Rights and the Civil Rights Act

To provide effective care to patients, there must be a working collaboration between patients and their care providers. In an effort to support this collaboration, certain rights afforded to patients are guaranteed by federal law and various institutional policies, including the American Medical Association, the American Hospital Association, and the majority of healthcare facilities in the United States (Chen et al., 2007; Grubbs et al., 2006; Youdelman, 2008). These policies have existed since the early 1970s and have evolved and expanded to further empower patients so that they can have an active role in their health. Having an active role is especially dependent on the patient being able to make informed decisions and choices about their care. In order to do this, patients need to be able to understand the information provided to them. To meet this goal, having interpretation services available for all patients, including immigrant patients, has become a standard (Blanchfield et al., 2011; Ku & Flores, 2005). It is a component of the patient bill of rights and the Civil Rights Act of 1964. Title VI of the Act has been interpreted over time to require all health facilities that are federally funded to provide interpretation services to all patients who request it (Chen et al., 2007; Grubbs et al., 2006; Youdelman, 2008). Although it is possible that some patients are unaware of this law and thus are unable to take advantage of this service that should be available to them, it is more likely that a patient would be aware of what is guaranteed to them under the patient bill of rights.

There are multiple versions of the patient bill of rights. They provide certain universal protections that are already guaranteed under federal law. These protections include the rights of patients to obtain a copy of their medical records and to keep their health information private, and, very importantly, their right to informed consent. These rights are consistent across the many versions of the patient bill of rights that exist at healthcare facilities across the United States (Chen et al., 2007; Grubbs et al., 2006; 2007; Youdelman, 2008). Again, in order to support a patient's right to informed consent, interpretation services must be available to patients. In 2010, a version of the patient bill of rights was created when the Affordable Care Act (ACA) became law. Although the ACA dealt with patient protections when dealing with health insurance companies, it also ensured that healthcare facilities that accept federal dollars through Medicare provide protections for patients. As with most bills of rights, these protections include the requirement that patients learn about their treatment and health services in a language they can understand (The Patient Protection and Affordable Care Act, 2010). The Medicare Patient Bill of Rights also provides protection from discrimination, including discrimination based on race or national origin. It also allows for access to providers, specialists, and hospitals (Medicare, 2021). For Medicaid, all providers who receive federal funds must be in compliance with Title VI of the Civil Rights Act, and this includes the provision of language services (Medicaid, 2021). Despite these protections in place for all patients, including immigrants, the quality of healthcare that immigrants receive continues to be less than that of with patients born in the United States.

Recommendation

In Jesse's case, the transplant team has provided the standard support measures available to all potential transplant recipients. These measures include access to the transplant team and to dieticians for inclusion on the transplant list, dietary education, and the use of interpretation services. Given the fact that these measures have already been provided, as they would have been to any other patient who has need of these services, the question becomes how much more support should be provided and whether there is an obligation to "do more." Alternatively, would it be fair to provide more support than what is usually provided to other potential transplant patients? Knowing that immigrant patients have greater barriers to being able to access and use the healthcare services that exist for all patients, it could be ethically justified to provide a greater level of support than is normally provided to potential transplant patients. Some could argue that the protections available in the patient bill of rights and the measures that are already available to potential transplant patients exist in order to compensate for these barriers. However, as data have shown, this population of patients continues to have worse health outcomes despite the efforts and protections that exist to help them navigate the healthcare system (Bustamante et al., 2021; Coughlin, 2019; Engelman & Ye, 2019; Goldfarb et al., 2017; Khullar & Chokshi, 2019; Singh et al., 2013). Therefore, it would be ethically supportable to continue providing additional support to Jesse in order to assist him with becoming a potential transplant candidate.

Although it may be ethically supportable to provide him with this ongoing support to assist him with becoming a transplant candidate, this does not ensure that he will be listed as a potential recipient or that he will receive an organ. Given the ongoing scarcity of organs and the enduring need for potential recipients to demonstrate that they would maximize their benefit from receiving the organ, Jesse would still need to demonstrate that he can meet this requirement.

CONCLUSIONS

Managing the legal boundaries of providing ethically appropriate medical care has been an ongoing, daily struggle that care providers continue to negotiate with regularity. While there are laws, precedent, and guidance to help reduce the difficulty of doing so, data continue to show that health disparities for many populations persist. The cases in this chapter illustrate the ongoing existence of health disparities and how these disparities can impact the medical outcome of care in various populations. When providing care within existing legal and ethical standards in the United States, a provider still has to contend with existing societal shortcomings that a clinical provider cannot wholly address or find a solution for. Some of these shortcomings come in the form of cultural beliefs and practices; recognition and correction of provider biases; commodification of healthcare, which at times can prioritize profits; and seeing as many patients as possible over allocating time and resources to address a patient's ongoing clinical and unique social needs. The cases in this chapter illustrate how disparities affect the clinical care of patients and families of marginalized populations across the country who are dealing with a variety of health issues. With time, effort, and a rethinking of how healthcare should function in our society and country, the profound effect of these disparities may eventually be reduced to the point that all patients in the United States have better health outcomes.

DISCUSSION QUESTIONS

1. How is the principle of justice applied in clinical decision-making?
2. How do the Harm principle and the Best Interest principle differ?
3. The patient bill of rights specifies that the patient is entitled to the services of an interpreter, if requested. How have you seen this operationalized in your institution?
4. Do the criteria for organ recipient selection violate the ethical principle of justice? If so, how?
5. How would you balance the rights of Mikel with the need for safety for his son?

ADDITIONAL RESOURCES

Berger, J. T., DeRenzo, E. G., & Schwartz, J. (2008). Surrogate decision making: Reconciling ethical theory and clinical practice. *Annals of Internal Medicine, 149*(1), 48–53. https://doi.org/10.7326/0003-4819-149-1-200807010-00010

Brock, D. W. (1991). The ideal of shared decision making between physicians and patients. *Kennedy Institute of Ethics Journal, 1*(1), 28–47. https://doi.org/10.1353/ken.0.0084

Health Care Education and Reconciliation Act, Pub. L. No. 111-152, 124 Stat. 1029 (2010).

U.S. Department of Health and Human Services. (2016). *Children's bureau, penalties for failure to report and false reporting of child abuse and neglect.* https://www.childwelfare.gov/topics/systemwide/laws-policies/statutes/report/

REFERENCES

American Society for Bioethics and Humanities. (2011). Core competencies for healthcare ethics consultation (2nd ed.). American Society for Bioethics and Humanities.

Aulisio, M. P., Arnold, R. M., & Youngner, S. J. (2000). Health care ethics consultation: Nature, goals, and competencies. A position paper from the society for health and human values-society for bioethics consultation task force on standards for bioethics consultation. *Annals of Internal Medicine, 133*(1), 59–69. https://doi.org/10.7326/0003-4819-133-1-200007040-00012

Beauchamp, T. L., & Childress, J. F. (2001). Principles of biomedical ethics (5th ed.). Oxford University Press.

Blanchfield, B. B., Gazelle, G. S., Khaliif, M., Arocha, I. S., & Hacker, K. (2011). A framework to identify the costs of providing language interpretation services. *Journal of Health Care for the Poor and Underserved, 22*(2), 523–531. https://doi.org/10.1353/hpu.2011.0051

Bosslet, G. T., Pope, T. M., Rubenfeld, G. D., Lo, B., Truog, R. D., Rushton, C. H., Curtis, J. R., Ford, D. W., Osborne, M., Misak, C., Au, D. H., Azoulay, E., Brody, B., Fahy, B. G., Hall, J. B., Kesecioglu, J., Kon, A. A., Lindell, K. O., & White, D. B. (2015). An official ATS/AACN/ACCP/ESICM/SCCM policy statement: Responding to requests for potentially inappropriate treatments in intensive care units. *American Journal of Respiratory and Critical Care Medicine, 191*(11), 1318–1330. https://doi.org/10.1164/rccm.201505-0924st

Bradford, J., Reisner, S. L., Honnold, J. A., & Xavier, J. (2013). Experiences of transgender-related discrimination and implications for health: Results from the Virginia transgender health initiative study. *American Journal of Public Health, 103*(10), 1820–1829. https://doi.org/10.2105/ajph.2012.300796

Bratton, C., Chavin, K., & Baliga, P. (2011). Racial disparities in organ donation and why. *Current Opinion in Organ Transplantation, 16*(2), 243–249. https://doi.org/10.1097/MOT.0b013e3283447b1c

Brudney, D. (2018). The different moral bases of patient and surrogate decision-making. *Hastings Center Report, 48*(1), 37–41. https://doi.org/10.1002/hast.809

Buchanan & Brock. (1990). In Deciding for others (pp. 234–237), Essay. Cambridge University Press.

Bustamante, A. V., Chen, J., Félix Beltrán, L., & Ortega, A. N. (2021). Health policy challenges posed by shifting demographics and health trends among immigrants to the United States. *Health Affairs (Project Hope), 40*(7), 1028–1037. https://doi.org/10.1377/hlthaff.2021.00037

Callender, C. O., & Miles, P. V. (2010). Minority organ donation: The power of an educated community. *Journal of the American College of Surgeons, 210*(5), 708–717. https://doi.org/10.1016/j.jamcollsurg.2010.02.037

California Probate Code § 4600–§ 4806. (2011).

Chadban, S. J., Ahn, C., Axelrod, D. A., Foster, B. J., Kasiske, B. L., Kher, V., Kumar, D., Oberbauer, R., Pascual, J., Pilmore, H. L., Rodrigue, J. R., Segev, D. L., Sheerin, N. S., Tinckam, K. J., Wong, G., & Knoll, G. A. (2020). KDIGO clinical practice guideline on the evaluation and management of candidates for kidney transplantation. *Transplantation, 104*(4S1). https://doi.org/10.1097/tp.0000000000003136

Chapman, E. N., Kaatz, A., & Carnes, M. (2013). Physicians and implicit bias: How doctors may unwittingly perpetuate health care disparities. *Journal of General Internal Medicine, 28*(11), 1504–1510. https://doi.org/10.1007/s11606-013-2441-1

Chasnoff, I. J., Landress, H. J., & Barrett, M. E. (1990). The prevalence of illicit-drug or alcohol use during pregnancy and discrepancies in mandatory reporting in pinellas county, Florida. *New England Journal of Medicine, 322*(17), 1202–1206. https://doi.org/10.1056/nejm199004263221706

Chen, A. H., Youdelman, M. K., & Brooks, J. (2007). The legal framework for language access in healthcare settings: Title VI and beyond. *Journal of General Internal Medicine, 22*(suppl 2), 362–367. https://doi.org/10.1007/s11606-007-0366-2

Child Welfare Information Gateway. (2019). Major federal legislation concerned with child protection, child welfare, and adoption. https://www.childwelfare.gov/pubPDFs/manda.pdf

Clarke, O. W. (1995). Ethical considerations in the allocation of organs and other scarce medical resources among patients. *Archives of Internal Medicine, 155*(1), 29. https://doi.org/10.1001/archinte.1995.00430010033005

Code of Virginia, § 32.1-12. (2006). https://law.lis.virginia.gov/vacode/title32.1/chapter1/section32.1-12/

Committee on Injury, Violence, and Poison Prevention. (2009). Role of the pediatrician in youth violence prevention. *Pediatrics, 124*(1), 393–402. https://doi.org/10.1542/peds.2009-0943

Coughlin S. S. (2019). Social determinants of breast cancer risk, stage, and survival. *Breast Cancer Research and Treatment, 177*(3), 537–548. https://doi.org/10.1007/s10549-019-05340-7

Cruzan v. Missouri. (1990). Director, Missouri Department of Health, 497 U.S. 261. The Library of Congress. https://www.loc.gov/item/usrep497261/

Derose, K. P., Escarce, J. J., & Lurie, N. (2007). Immigrants and health care: Sources of vulnerability. *Health Affairs, 26*(5), 1258–1268. https://doi.org/10.1377/hlthaff.26.5.1258

Diebel, M. (2014, August 15). The Amish: 10 things you might not know. USA Today. https://www.usatoday.com/story/news/nation/2014/08/15/amish-ten-things-you-need-to-know/14111249/

Diekema, D. (2004). Parental refusals of medical treatment: The harm principle as threshold for state intervention. *Theoretical Medicine and Bioethics, 25*(4), 243–264. https://doi.org/10.1007/s11017-004-3146-6

Dolgin, J. L. (1996). Why has the best interest standard survived? The historic and social context. *Children's Legal Rights Journal, 16*(2). https://scholarlycommons.law.hofstra.edu/faculty_scholarship/433

Drake, B., Jolley, J. M., Lanier, P., Fluke, J., Barth, R. P., & Jonson-Reid, M. (2011). Racial bias in child protection? A comparison of competing explanations using national data. *Pediatrics, 127*(3), 471–478. https://doi.org/10.1542/peds.2010-1710

Edward, J. (2014). Undocumented immigrants and access to health care: Making a case for policy reform. *Policy, Politics & Nursing Practice, 15*(1–2), 5–14. https://doi.org/10.1177/1527154414532694

Engelman, M., & Ye, L. Z. (2019). The immigrant health differential in the context of racial and ethnic disparities: The case of diabetes. *Advances in Medical Sociology, 19*, 147–171. https://doi.org/10.1108/S1057-629020190000019008

Freeman, R. B., & Bernat, J. L. (2012). Ethical issues in organ transplantation. *Progress in Cardiovascular Diseases, 55*(3), 282–289. https://doi.org/10.1016/j.pcad.2012.08.005

Goldfarb, S. S., Smith, W., Epstein, A. E., Burrows, S., & Wingate, M. (2017). Disparities in prenatal care utilization among U.S. versus foreign-born women with chronic conditions. *Journal of Immigrant and Minority Health, 19*(6), 1263–1270. https://doi.org/10.1007/s10903-016-0435-x

Gostin L. O. (2019). Is affording undocumented immigrants health coverage a radical proposal? *JAMA, 322*(15), 1438–1439. https://doi.org/10.1001/jama.2019.15806

Grant, J. M., Mottet, L. A., Tanis, J., Harrison, J., Herman, J. L., & Keisling, M. (2011, February 3). *Injustice at every turn: A report of the national transgender discrimination survey.* National Center for Transgender Equality and National Gay and Lesbian Task Force. https://transequality.org/sites/default/files/docs/usts/USTS-Full-Report-Dec17.pdf

Grubbs, V., Chen, A. H., Bindman, A. B., Vittinghoff, E., & Fernandez, A. (2006). Effect of awareness of language law on language access in the health care setting. *Journal of General Internal Medicine, 21*(7), 683–688. https://doi.org/10.1111/j.1525-1497.2006.00492.x

Hall, E., & Cuellar, N. G. (2016). Immigrant health in the United States. *Journal of Transcultural Nursing, 27*(6), 611–626. https://doi.org/10.1177/1043659616672534

Hall, W. J., Chapman, M. V., Lee, K. M., Merino, Y. M., Thomas, T. W., Payne, B. K., Eng, E., Day, S. H., & Coyne-Beasley, T. (2015). Implicit racial/ethnic bias among health care professionals and its influence on health care outcomes: A systematic review. *American Journal of Public Health, 105*(12), e60–e76. https://doi.org/10.2105/AJPH.2015.302903

He, S., Ryan, K. A., Streeten, E. A., McArdle, P. F., Daue, M., Trubiano, D., Rohrer, Y., Donnelly, P., Drolet, M., Newcomer, S., Shaub, S., Weitzel, N., Shuldiner, A. R., Pollin, T. I., & Mitchell, B. D. (2020). Prevalence, control, and treatment of diabetes, hypertension, and high cholesterol in the Amish. *BMJ Open Diabetes Research & Care, 8*(1), e000912. https://doi.org/10.1136/bmjdrc-2019-000912

National Center for Health Statistics. (2019). Health United States-2019-Table 49-CDC. https://www.cdc.gov/nchs/hus/contents2019.htm

Jonsen, A. R. (2007). The god squad and the origins of transplantation ethics and policy. *The Journal of law, Medicine & Ethics: a Journal of the American Society of Law, Medicine & Ethics, 35*(2), 238–240. https://doi.org/10.1111/j.1748-720X.2007.00131.x

In Re Guardianship of Hailu. (2015). In Re Guardianship of Hailu, 2015 NV 89. The Supreme Court of the State of Nevada. https://law.justia.com/cases/nevada/supreme-court/2015/68531.html

In Re Quinlan. (1976). In Re Quinlan, 70 N.J. 10, 355 A.2d 647. The Supreme Court of New Jersey. https://law.justia.com/cases/new-jersey/supreme-court/1976/70-n-j-10-0.html

In the Matter of Baby "K". (1993). In the Matter of Baby "K", 832 F. Supp. 1022, (E.D. Va. 1993).

Khullar, D., & Chokshi, D. A. (2019). Challenges for immigrant health in the USA-the road to crisis. *Lancet (London, England), 393*(10186), 2168–2174. https://doi.org/10.1016/S0140-6736(19)30035-2

Kline N. (2019). When deservingness policies converge: US immigration enforcement, health reform and patient dumping. *Anthropology & Medicine, 26*(3), 280–295. https://doi.org/10.1080/13648470.2018.1507101

Kon, A. A., Shepard, E. K., Sederstrom, N. O., Swoboda, S. M., Marshall, M. F., Birriel, B., & Rincon, F. (2016). Defining futile and potentially inappropriate interventions. *Critical Care Medicine, 44*(9), 1769–1774. https://doi.org/10.1097/ccm.0000000000001965

Kopelman, L. M. (1997). The best-interests standard as threshold, ideal, and standard of reasonableness. *Journal of Medicine and Philosophy, 22*(3), 271–289. https://doi.org/10.1093/jmp/22.3.271

Kraybill, D. B., Johnson-Weiner, K., & Nolt, S. M. (2013). *The Amish.* Johns Hopkins University Press.

Ku, L., & Flores, G. (2005). Pay now or pay later: Providing interpreter services in health care. *Health Affairs, 24*(2), 435–444. https://doi.org/10.1377/hlthaff.24.2.435

Ladin, K., Emerson, J., Berry, K., Butt, Z., Gordon, E. J., Daniels, N., Lavelle, T. A., & Hanto, D. W. (2019). Excluding patients from transplant due to social support: Results from a national survey of transplant providers. *American Journal of Transplantation, 19*(1), 193–203. https://doi.org/10.1111/ajt.14962

Lipari, R. N., & Van Horn, S. L. (2017). Children living with parents who have a substance use disorder. In *The CBHSQ Report* (pp. 1–7). Substance Abuse and Mental Health Services Administration (US).

Luce, J. M. (2015). The uncommon case of Jahi McMath. *Chest, 147*(4), 1144–1151. https://doi.org/10.1378/chest.14-2227

Luken, A., Nair, R., & Fix, R. L. (2021). On racial disparities in child abuse reports: Exploratory mapping the 2018 NCANDS. *Child Maltreatment, 26*(3), 267–281. https://doi.org/10.1177/10775595211001926

Morgan, M., Kenten, C., Deedat, S., & Donate Programme Team (2013). Attitudes to deceased organ donation and registration as a donor among minority ethnic groups in North America and the U.K.: A synthesis of quantitative and qualitative research. *Ethnicity & Health*, *18*(4), 367–390. https://doi.org/10.1080/13557858.2012.752073

Obergefell v. Hodges. (2015). Obergefell et al. v. Hodges, Director, Ohio Department of Health, et al., 576 U.S. 644. The Supreme Court of the United States. https://www.supremecourt.gov/opinions/14pdf/14-556_3204.pdf

Paris, J. J., & Schreiber, M. D. (1996). Parental discretion in refusal of treatment for newborns. *Clinics in Perinatology*, *23*(3), 573–581. https://doi.org/10.1016/s0095-5108(18)30229-x

Patient Protection and Affordable Care Act. (2010). Patient Protection and Affordable Care Act of 2010, Pub. L. No. 111–148, 124 Stat. 119.

Prince v. Massachusetts. (1944). Prince v. Massachusetts, 321 U.S. 158. The Library of Congress. https://www.loc.gov/item/usrep321158/

Raghavan, R. (2018). Caring for undocumented immigrants with kidney disease. *American Journal of Kidney Diseases: The Official Journal of the National Kidney Foundation*, *71*(4), 488–494. https://doi.org/10.1053/j.ajkd.2017.09.011

Medicare. (2021). Rights & protections for everyone with Medicare. https://www.medicare.gov/claims-appeals/your-medicare-rights/rights-protections-for-everyone-with-medicare

Sawinski, D., & Locke, J. E. (2018). Evaluation of kidney donors: Core curriculum 2018. *American Journal of Kidney Diseases*, *71*(5), 737–747. https://doi.org/10.1053/j.ajkd.2017.10.018

Shelton, W., Geppert, C., & Jankowski, J. (2016). The role of communication and interpersonal skills in clinical ethics consultation: The need for a competency in advanced ethics facilitation. *The Journal of Clinical Ethics*, *27*(1), 28–38.

Sher, E. J. (1983). Choosing for children: Adjudicating medical disputes between parents and the state. *New York University Law Review*, *58(1)*, 157–206.

Singh, G. K., Azuine, R. E., Siahpush, M., & Kogan, M. D. (2013). All-cause and cause-specific mortality among US youth: Socioeconomic and rural–urban disparities and international patterns. *Journal of Urban Health*, *90*(3), 388–405. https://doi.org/10.1007/s11524-012-9744-0

Texas Advance Directives Act. (1999). Texas Advance Directives Act of 1999, § 166.001–§ 166.166. https://statutes.capitol.texas.gov/Docs/HS/htm/HS.166.htm

The Lancet. (2019). Under the influence: Dealing with impaired carers of children. *The Lancet*, *394*(10214), 2040. https://doi.org/10.1016/s0140-6736(19)33050-8

Medicaid. (2021). Translation and interpretation services. https://www.medicaid.gov/medicaid/financial-management/medicaid-administrative-claiming/translation-and-interpretation-services/index.html

U.S. Court of Appeals, Fourth Circuit. (1994). In re Baby K. *The Federal Reporter*, *16*, 590–599.

Virginia Code, § 54.1-2990. (2014). https://law.justia.com/codes/virginia/2014/title-54.1/section-54.1-2990

Wallace, S. P., Torres, J., Sadegh-Nobari, T., Pourat, N., & Brown, E. R. (2012). Undocumented Immigrants and Health Care Reform. UCLA Center for Health Policy Research. https://healthpolicy.ucla.edu/publications/Documents/PDF/undocumentedreport-aug2013.pdf

Welles, C. C., & Cervantes, L. (2019). Hemodialysis care for undocumented immigrants with end-stage renal disease in the United States. *Current Opinion in Nephrology and Hypertension*, *28*(6), 615–620. https://doi.org/10.1097/MNH.0000000000000543

Weyer, S. M., Hustey, V. R., Rathbun, L., Armstrong, V. L., Anna, S. R., Ronyak, J., & Savrin, C. (2003). A look into the Amish culture: What should we learn? *Journal of Transcultural Nursing*, *14*(2), 139–145. https://doi.org/10.1177/1043659602250639

Youdelman, M. K. (2008). The medical tongue: U.S. laws and policies on language access. *Health Affairs (Project Hope)*, *27*(2), 424–433. https://doi.org/10.1377/hlthaff.27.2.424

CHAPTER 13

Race, Ethnicity, and Population Health

Derek M. Griffith

LEARNING OBJECTIVES

● Explain the distinction between race and ethnicity.

● Discuss how race and ethnicity are determinants of socioeconomic status.

● Apply race and ethnicity accurately to population health research questions.

INTRODUCTION

One of the largest and most fundamental challenges to understanding the heterogeneity among population health is how we define and use the terms "race" and "ethnicity" (Bonham et al., 2018; Ford & Kelly, 2005). While population health has continued to grow as a field, the question of why race and ethnicity have such epidemiological and clinical significance remains an important issue (Geronimus et al., 2016; Krieger, 2003). The frequency of including race and ethnicity as variables would suggest there is some consensus on the conceptualization and appropriate uses of each term, but that is not the case (Ford & Harawa, 2010; Ford & Kelly, 2005; LaVeist, 1995; Smedley & Smedley, 2005). There is little consensus on what race means, although it is one of the most commonly reported variables in health research (Griffith, 2020; LaVeist, 1994, 1995). Race is often confused with ethnicity, family history, ancestry, genotype, human biological variation, socioeconomic status, unmeasured social factors, and environmental context, and it is not always clear how and why people use these constructs in their research (Griffith & Griffith, 2008; Griffith et al., 2006; LaVeist, 1995). In addition, the relationship between self-identified race and ethnicity and observable (e.g., skin color, eye shape), biological (e.g., gene frequency, gene expression), psychosocial (e.g., racial identity, ethnic identity, social class, economic position, sexual orientation) and cultural (e.g., religion, country of origin) characteristics is unclear (Ford & Harawa, 2010; Griffith, 2016; Griffith & Griffith, 2008). This lack of clarity limits our ability to understand the epidemiological, clinical, or population health relevance of groups organized by race and ethnicity.

In some areas of biomedical and public health research and practice, there is a tendency to rely on the demographic boxes that people check as a proxy for their risks, resources, and potential resilience (LaVeist, 1994, 1995). While these factors have demonstrated how they are defined by others, demographic labels do not capture the complexity of how people identify and define themselves or what their risk is for disease morbidity and mortality (Griffith, 2016, 2020; Idossa et al., 2018). Historically, race, ethnicity, and other demographic and psychosocial boxes that people check have been the markers of marginalization (LaVeist, 1994; Morning, 2015; Smedley & Smedley, 2005) and the markers of who is most likely to experience racism (Ford et al., 2019a; Jenkins et al., 2019; Patrinos, 2004). When and why should you use race, and when and why should you use ethnicity? This chapter includes an overview of the definitions, origins, challenges, and benefits of using race and ethnicity in population health research and offers suggestions for how to use these terms to advance the field with the goal of helping to inform strategies to achieve population health equity.

BACKGROUND

Researchers often offer their perspectives on the appropriate use of race and ethnicity, but there continues to be considerable heterogeneity across disciplines, healthcare settings, states, and other units about how information on race and ethnicity should be incorporated, studied, and interpreted (Bonham et al., 2019). Race is a construct determined largely by political and social forces (LaVeist, 1995), and ethnicity refers to self-defined groups of people who have common cultural traits (e.g., traditions, language, sense of history, country of origin; Smedley & Smedley, 2005). The significance and meaning of race and ethnicity vary by country, and these concepts are contingent upon economic, legal, political, social, and cultural practices (Idossa et al., 2018). Racial classification is not stable, nor is it permanent; people can be a member of one race in one country and another race in a different country (Prewitt, 2005). For example, in the United States, someone who has one parent who identifies as White and another parent who identifies as Native American would be asked to self-identify as White or Native American or to choose more than one racial category. In Brazil, this same individual would have the opportunity to choose Caboclo, a category that specifically recognizes someone who is White and indigenous to that country.

In addition to the heterogeneity in the concept of race, every generation has sought scientific justification for the way their social and political arrangements are organized by race and ethnicity (Byrd & Clayton, 2000; Frank, 2007). The global burden of disease morbidity and mortality is concentrated in people who self-identify as members of population groups that are smaller in number, lower in social status, indigenous to their setting, of African descent, or immigrants to a particular area (Ford et al., 2019a; Ford et al., 2019b; Griffith et al., 2011). Race continues to be a social category that precisely captures the impact of racism and differential access to power, social, and economic resources, and other desired resources in society rather than a biological construct that reflects innate differences (Jones, 2019; LaVeist, 2000).

RACE

There is no single concept of race. Race may be defined as a subjective social construct based on skin color, hair texture, and other observed or ascribed characteristics that have acquired socially significant meaning (LaVeist, 1994, 1995, 2000). It is important to recognize that part of the reason the notions of race have such power across so many aspects of life and all sectors of society is because they represent a viable, not a valid, frame (Brown et al., 2006; Griffith, 2018). Frame viability describes the extent to which an explanation for a pattern of health is culturally and politically salient, regardless of its accuracy, and frame validity describes the extent to which an explanation is empirically true (Brown et al., 2006; Griffith, 2018). Notions of race are particularly powerful because at times, the cultural and scientific notions of race were both viable and valid, and efforts to separate cultural and political ideals from the "objectivity" of science seem best understood through a historical lens.

A Brief History of Race as a Construct

The history of race as a construct is complex and contentious. For a full treatment of this topic, please see books like Byrd and Clayton's *An American Health Dilemma* (2000), or Kendi's *Stamped from the Beginning* (2016). The concept of race emerged in the 16th century (Kendi, 2016; Smedley & Smedley, 2005). The 500-year history of the concept of race can be organized into three periods: the period of racial lineage, the period of racial type, and the sociocultural period, which together stretch from the dawn of science in the 16th century to the present day (Byrd & Clayton, 2000).

The period of racial lineage stretches from the 16th century to the beginning of the 19th century. During this period, the focus of scholarship on race was principally on the notion of lineage, or linking animals, including humans, by common descent or origin. Most scientific efforts on race were driven by efforts to divide human beings into lines of descent from primitive ancestors (Byrd & Clayton, 2000). This lineage, and the racial hierarchy it spawned, was permanent, unchangeable, and presumed to have existed since the Creation, to be consistent with Judeo-Christian traditions and Biblical stories that connected skin color and other physical and moral standards and characteristics (e.g., black skin was a mark of being cursed). This notion of racial lineage was one of the key foundations of the anchors of our racial hierarchy, with people of African descent at the bottom and people of European descent at the top. The notion of racial lineage connected people of African descent and the idea that "black" represented unclean, inferior, ugly, and cursed. This idea also linked the notion of being of European descent with purity, superiority, beauty, and other positive characteristics (e.g., White European males representing the pinnacle of human evolution; Byrd & Clayton, 2000).

The period of racial type emerged in the 17th and 18th centuries and persisted throughout the 19th century. During this time, the natural sciences and racial thought began debating the taxonomy of race, and quantification, statistical methods, and taxonomic advances assumed important roles (Byrd & Clayton, 2000). The idea of assessing and classifying people based on skin color, hair length, hair texture, and other physical features became important criteria and proxies for other factors. Quantitative measures of facial angles, cranial capacities, skull contours and dimensions, and other physical features were supposed to correlate with and even predict such factors as intelligence and character traits, but they did not. Despite these efforts, these pseudoscientific measures of biological differences could not be empirically validated as markers of human potential (Byrd & Clayton, 2000).

The third period in the history of the concept of race is the sociocultural period (Byrd & Clayton, 2000). This relatively brief and most recent period reflects the scholarship of the latter part of the 20th century and into the 21st century. The 20th century brought about the notion of the social construction of race and the focus on the sociopolitical factors that underlie the creation and utilization of racial categories. These factors reflect the growing appreciation for the multidimensional nature of a person's identity and the need to capture and distinguish among the factors often confused with race, like genetics (Bonham et al., 2018). The current era also is consistent with the notion of self-identified race.

The idea that race is about self-definiton is a relatively recent notion. Until 1960, race was not identified by the individual in the U.S. decennial census or by the patient in the context of the U.S. healthcare system (Prewitt, 2005). Prior to 1960, race was assigned by U.S. census enumerators or intake staff in healthcare settings, whose judgment in such matters was constrained by social and political realities in each era and setting (Prewitt, 2005). In our current era, how people self-identify as being a member of a particular race can be distinguished by three aspects of racial identity: internal, external, and expressed. Internal racial identity is what one believes about their race, given the historical, social, and political context in which they grew up and live. External racial identity is what their physical features suggest their race to be, or what racial group others typically assume that individual to be. And expressed racial identity is how one explicitly describes or defines their race to others (Harris & Sim, 2002).

Why We Should Stop Using "Caucasian" in Population Health and Elsewhere

One of the few terms, if not the only term, that remains in common use since it was coined during the racial type period is "Caucasian." It is critical to recognize the history and meaning of the term and why this term is problematic given what we understand about the science of race (Bhopal & Donaldson, 1998; Freeman, 2003; Painter, 2010). This term provides an important cautionary tale about making sure that we understand the history and meaning of terms that are common in society and in population health.

Craniometry (the study of cranial capacity) and phrenology (the study of the shape and texture [bumps] of the skull) became the leading criteria for distinguishing among races during the racial type era of the 17th to 19th centuries (Byrd & Clayton, 2000). This and other pseudoscientific methods were used to support the notion that cranial measurements and dimensions were useful proxies for intelligence and beauty (i.e., human beauty was considered a scientifically certified racial trait; Painter, 2010). Johann Friedrich Blumenbach, a German scientist, believed that the Georgians from the region of the Caucasus mountains were the most beautiful race of human beings. In the Caucasus mountains of Russia, Blumenbach found a more "beautiful" skull with a larger cranial capacity than those found elsewhere in the world (Freeman, 2003; Painter, 2010). Based on this finding, Blumenbach then coined the term "Caucasian" and concluded that this group must be the most intelligent and beautiful of all racial groups (Bhopal & Donaldson, 1998; Freeman, 2003; Painter, 2010).

Attributes such as beauty and intelligence (and other cognitive abilities such as the ability to learn) were used to explain the heritability of such complex constructs as criminality and intelligence (Byrd & Clayton, 2000). Blumenbach also used craniometry and phrenology to argue that Caucasians "must" be the highest in the racial hierarchy and Mongolians (later Asians) and Ethiopians (African Blacks) were considered "degenerate forms of the Caucasian ideal" (Byrd & Clayton, 2000, p. 97). These "scientific" findings were considered "natural and irrefutable" and provided the scientific justification for U.S. federal and state policies such as chattel slavery of Black Americans (Byrd & Clayton, 2000; Painter, 2010). Because Caucasian is scientifically inaccurate and rooted in fundamentally flawed scholarship and reflects a legacy of scientific racism, its use should be eliminated from all languages, and particularly from use in medicine, nursing, and other population health-related contexts.

Race and Genetics

While there is no debating that the phenotypic characteristics associated with race—such as skin color and hair form—are certainly influenced by genes, we do not know how many genes exist that are associated with socially and historically constructed races, much less how they affect health (Bonham et al., 2018; Goodman, 2000). Leading scholars studying race and genetics have argued that race should be removed from genetics research, including Francis Collins, the Director of the National Institutes of Health (Collins, 2004); Vence Bonham, the Director of the National Human Genome Research Institute (Bonham et al., 2018); and others (Yudell et al., 2016). They argue that the imprecise use of racial and ethnic data as population descriptors in genomics research can miscommunicate the complex relationships among social identity, ancestry, socioeconomic status, and health, and perpetuate the myth that discrete genetic groups exist (Bonham et al., 2018). The use of existing racial and ethnic categories as surrogates for global genomic variation has critical limitations for health promotion, disease prevention, disease treatment, and population health research (Bonham et al., 2018).

The concept of race emerged after people from different continents came in contact with one another (e.g., Europeans "discovering" North America and the Indigenous peoples residing on what has become the United States; Smedley & Smedley, 2005). Nevertheless, researchers noted that the main genetic clusters occur because of a history of human migration out of Africa to various continents across the globe (Guo et al., 2014). Because of these patterns of migration, the main genetic clusters of focus in research on genetics and ancestry are clusters that occur among those from Europe/Middle East, sub-Saharan Africa, or Asia, the Pacific Islands, or Indigenous peoples (Guo et al., 2014). These groups represent the root categories of the majority of the human subpopulations, yet these categories can be further subdivided by genetic markers within these classifications (Guo et al., 2014).

The goal of genetics is to identify the specific genes and gene variants that influence the risk of disease, a health outcome of interest, or a response to a particular drug (Risch et al., 2002). Genetic categorization can occur at the level of the individual, irrespective of the individual's race, ethnicity, or geographic origins (Risch et al., 2002). Self-reported racial categories remain a poor proxy for the presence of health-relevant genetic variants that differ across race groups, and genes are almost always a minor and insufficient cause for disease (Diez Roux, 2012). If genes are good ways to identity someone's risk for a particular health issue, it is important to distinguish that risk from their self-reported race and ethnicity because those factors are also highly correlated with social determinants of health that vary markedly across racial and ethnic groups (Diez Roux, 2012).

The Challenge of Connecting Race, Genetics, and Health

Krieger (2010, 2019) argues that the major changes in rates of disease in the most recent century can be explained only by changes in gene expression, not gene frequency. For more than 60 years, science has demonstrated that race is an invalid biological concept (Byrd & Clayton, 2000; Diez Roux, 2012; Goodman, 2000; Kaplan & Bennett, 2003). This is not to say that there are no genetic differences between races, but very few have been found that directly relate to health (Diez Roux, 2012; Goodman, 2000). Some diseases that have a genetic basis appear to fall in ways that are consistent with U.S. racial categories (e.g., sickle cell disease), but these diseases actually reflect other factors that do not fall only along U.S. racial categories (e.g., sickle cell disease occurs more often among people from parts of the world where malaria is or was common, such as sub-Saharan Africa and the Mediterranean). Science has yet to identify a set of genes that correspond with social conceptions of race, and there remains no evidence that the units of interest for medical genetics correspond to what we call races (Bonham et al., 2018; Cooper & Kaufman, 1998; Cooper et al., 2003; Diez Roux, 2012; Smedley & Smedley, 2005). The notion that self-identified racial groups are genetically discrete fails in three key areas: The racial groups are not genetically distinct; the racial categories are not reliably measured; and the racial differences by genes are not meaningful for understanding health differences (Smedley & Smedley, 2005). Overwhelmingly, data have shown that there is greater genetic variability within racial groups as opposed to between groups. While some traits vary by race, the inference does not follow that genetic variation falls into racial categories (Bonham et al., 2018; Callier, 2019; Cooper & Kaufman, 1998; Cooper et al., 2003). The "science" of ascribing racial differences in health to fixed biological traits has long been discredited, and it remains a gross oversimplification to assume that differences in genetic susceptibility could explain observed racial differences in health outcomes because genes are rarely expressed without some environmental context (Diez Roux, 2012).

ETHNICITY

Ethnicity encompasses aspects of culture, social life, and personal identity that socially defined groups tend to share (Ford & Harawa, 2010). Ethnic groups consist of people who share a common language, geographic locale, place of origin, religion, sense of history, traditions, values, or dietary habits. Because these attributes are learned, they can be transmissible to others, such as through the adoption of clothing, folklore, foods, or language (Smedley & Smedley, 2005). Typically, people self-identify with their ethnic group, which is particularly useful for understanding personal identity and social or cultural characteristics (Ford & Harawa, 2010). It is inaccurate to include physical traits (e.g., skin color, hair texture) in a definition of ethnic identity (Smedley & Smedley, 2005). At its roots, cultural traits and human behaviors are viewed as socially acquired traditions and patterns that distinguish population groups from one another (Smedley & Smedley, 2005).

Ethnicity comprises two dimensions: the attributional and the relational. The attributional dimension describes the unique sociocultural characteristics (e.g., culture, diet) of groups, and the relational dimension captures characteristics of the relationship between an ethnically defined group and the society in which it is situated (Ford & Harawa, 2010). In the context of population health, the attributional dimension is useful for understanding how people define their ideals and expectations of others and how these factors are expected to be defined across the life course. While people may understand Western hegemonic ideals that are largely set by Western, Educated, Industrialized, Rich, and Democratic (WEIRD) cultures in a particular time and place, they also may ascribe to subgroup ideals that are specific to ethnic groups (Jones, 2010).

The relational dimension highlights how ethnicity is a useful proxy for where people live and the likelihood of exposure to health-harming environments and substances, social disadvantages, or health-promoting resources (Ford & Harawa, 2010; LaVeist, 2000). People who have physical features that identify them as Black or some other marginalized racial group are likely to face discrimination based on those physical characteristics (LeBrón & Viruell-Fuentes, 2019). For example, someone whose physical characteristics are often interpreted by others as indicating that they are of African descent (Black) is likely to have worse health outcomes that someone who does not share the same physical characteristics, regardless of their ethnic identification (LaVeist et al., 2012).

Race and Ethnicity in the United States and Globally

In the United States, the federal Office of Management and Budget (OMB) established and maintains standards for classifying and counting the race and ethnicity of the U.S. population (Blank et al., 2004). The OMB explicitly indicates and emphasizes that their classifications of race and ethnicity are neither anthropologically nor scientifically based. The goals of the OMB race and ethnicity categories are to collect data on broad population groups in the United States and to facilitate monitoring, adherence to, and enforcement of civil rights laws, but these categories are not used consistently across states, locales, and settings in the United States (Griffith et al., 2006; Mays et al., 2003). Scholars have noted that there remains a need to use OMB categories in biomedical research, particularly to monitor the inclusion of racial and ethnic groups that have historically been underrepresented in research (Mays et al., 2003).

The racial and ethnic categories used in health and medical settings tend to be congruent with local, state, and national conceptions and standards. It is important to note that this is often done for good reason. For example, in Dearborn, Michigan—which has the largest and most diverse community of Arab Americans in the United States—hospitals and other units in the area may subdivide the White population in the city to distinguish Arab Americans from other White Americans, and further subdivide Arab Americans by country of origin, primary language spoken, religion, and other factors. These efforts to expand beyond OMB categories may be important in Dearborn because it can facilitate the ability of healthcare systems and other units to build the capacity of these organizations and institutions to better serve their patients and other customers. The key, however, is that these categories should be able to be reaggregated into OMB categories to facilitate population health research and practice.

The first U.S. decennial census was conducted in 1790 (Idossa et al., 2018; Mays et al., 2003). Since this census, the race categories have changed almost every census (Blank et al.,

2004). The 2000 census was the first opportunity U.S. residents have had to self-identify as more than one race. This modification reflects the changing perceptions of race and ethnicity in the United States., but it also poses significant problems for monitoring and evaluating data collected by race and ethnicity (Harris & Sim, 2002).

In the U.S. decennial census, the race category where there has been the most change is in who is considered White (Blank et al., 2004; Borak et al., 2004). In the early 20th century, Italian, Irish, Jewish, and other southern and eastern European immigrants were classified as "non-White" to distinguish them from the earlier Anglo-Saxon Protestant settlers (Borak et al., 2004). In response to changing social and political attitudes and needs, over the following decades many of these groups were included in the "White" category, diminishing the focus on ethnic differences and immigrant status and demonstrating how social and political factors influence racial categories.

In the United States, race and ethnicity often erroneously are operationalized as though they are similar enough concepts that they can be measured together. In the United States identifying race—Black, White, Asian, Native American, or Native Hawaiian/Pacific Islander—should be done separately from asking someone to indicate their ethnicity (e.g., Hispanic/Latinx). Often, however, questions of race and ethnicity are combined in ways that cannot be disaggregated to allow for race to be analyzed separately from ethnicity. Treating race and ethnic categories as synonyms hinders analysis of race and ethnicity by OMB categories. Lack of clarity in distinguishing race from ethnicity racializes ethnic groups (e.g., Latinx in the United States), or treats ethnic groups as though their social, behavioral, and cultural characteristics and attributes have deeper meaning and implications than what is assumed of ethnic groups (LeBrón & Viruell-Fuentes, 2019).

Black Americans and the "One-Drop Rule"

In the United States, Black or African American is a category of "hypodescent": the automatic cultural expectation that a child will be identified as a member of the subordinate group when the child has parents who were of two different races. In the United States, this is known as the "one-drop rule," and it applies only to Black people (Freeman, 2003). If someone has one ancestor who was considered Black, that person was also considered Black regardless of physical appearance or how many generations had passed between that person and the individual of interest (Freeman, 2003; Idossa et al., 2018). For example, the descendants of the union of Thomas Jefferson and Sally Hemmings have been classified as Black, and were subject to chattel slavery, Jim Crow segregation, and other policies despite being as equally related to a "founding father" of the United States as they were to Ms. Hemmings.

The Origin of the Term "Hispanic"

In 1978, the OMB created the Statistical Policy Directive that coined the current use of the term "Hispanic" (Borak et al., 2004). Though originally used to describe people of Iberian (ancient Spanish) ancestry, "Hispanic" became a category to fulfill the ideological and political function of capturing the wave of Spanish-speaking immigrants from Latin American and Caribbean countries during the last two decades of the 20th century. "Hispanic" identifies neither an ethnic group nor a minority group, but a set of diverse populations and cultures that share a common language (Borak et al., 2004). This category has been identified as the primary ethnic category in federal government documents, and Hispanic Americans have been one of the largest groups to check "other" for their race. Because Hispanic was a common term in the eastern United States and Latino was more common in the West, the terms are often used together as Hispanic/Latino.

Race and Ethnicity Outside the United States

The idea of being able to identify with more than one race is consistent with the strategies many countries use across the globe (Morning, 2015). For example, in Brazil there are a number of terms for proxies of race, and they tend to map onto skin color, heritage, and socioeconomic status (Carvalho et al., 2004). Similar to the United States, those of European descent are at the top of the racial hierarchy and those of African descent or descendants of indigenous peoples are at the bottom. Census enumerators ask people to identify themselves as black (*preto*, of African descent), white (*branco*, of European descent), yellow (*amarelo*, of East Asian descent), indigenous (*indígena*, of Amerindian descent), or as someone who is multiracial (*pardo*). Among those who identify with more than one race or ethnicity, Brazilians may also identify as Mulatto (Black and White), Cafuzo (Black and Amerindian), Caboclo (White and Amerindian), Jucara (Black, Amerindian, and White), or Ainoco (White and East Asian; Carvalho et al., 2004).

In a review of national census ethnicity and race categories (Morning, 2015), it was common for countries that experienced European colonialism (e.g., Brazil) to include a category for indigenous status (Morning, 2015). Often the goal of including these categories is to distinguish those who are of European ancestry or who inhabited the land prior to European settlement from those who came after colonization and slavery (Morning, 2015). Interestingly, in this global study of national censuses, indigenous status was not found on any European or Asian censuses (Morning, 2015).

RACE/ETHNICITY OR RACISM?

Historically, public health, medicine, nursing, and the social sciences have focused on defining and addressing race, not racism. "In so doing, it has helped to reify the notion of race and obscure the underlying role of racism in producing the patterns of health inequities that persist in our society" (Jenkins et al., 2019). Jenkins et al. (2019) argue, "The problem in America is not race. The problem is not that people look different from each other. The problem is that people are treated differently because of the way they look. The problem is racism" (p. 35). It is because of racism that race and ethnicity are markers of factors that influence social class, economic position, and other social determinants of health (Kawachi et al., 2005; LeBrón & Viruell-Fuentes, 2019; Phelan & Link, 2015; Smedley, 2019).

Racism is a term that describes an analytic tool to explain power systems, patterns, and outcomes that vary by population groups and that are broader than the explicit decisions and practices of individuals, organizations, or institutions. While cultural narratives and media coverage often present it as reflecting aberrant views of a minority of people, racism often is aligned with the normative culture of particular eras, geographic contexts, and locales (Came & Griffith, 2018; Griffith & Semlow, 2020).

Racism is a useful frame for characterizing the policies and practices that create underlying social conditions that lead to disease concentration, clustering, and interaction. Racism is a system, not an individual characteristic or a personal moral failing (Griffith & Semlow, 2020; Griffith et al., 2007). Racism is *a system of power* whose mechanisms are in the structures, policies, practices, norms, and values of our decision-making (Jones, 2019). Focusing on prejudicial attitudes and discriminatory behavior ignores the historical, social, and political aspects of the system of oppression and focuses the issue on race-contingent behavior or actions ("disparate treatment"), rather than identifying how decisions not seemingly affected by race can still produce differential outcomes ("disparate impact"; Came & Griffith, 2018). Racism unfairly disadvantages some individuals and communities, unfairly advantages others, and saps the strength of the whole society through the waste of human resources (Jones, 2019).

Although historically, racism has been used to describe discrimination based on race, *racialization* provides a framework for understanding how the social and historical context makes ethnic groups, religious minorities, and others subject to racism and xenophobia similar to racial groups (LeBrón & Viruell-Fuentes, 2019; Samari et al., 2019). In contrast to groups being able to define themselves, racialization describes a process by which others define a group and ascribe to it characteristics associated with where the group comes from, what it believes in, or how it organizes itself socially and culturally (Samari et al., 2019). In addition to these external definitions, groups can elect to racialize themselves as a political strategy, an act of resistance, and a demonstration of power rooted in a positive racialized identity. For example, Latinx peoples have come together in the United States to celebrate their heterogeneity and the commonalities of their experience in this country.

CONCLUSION

This chapter provides context, definitions, and distinctions between two of the most commonly reported variables in population health—race and ethnicity—and highlights the role that racism plays in characterizing the relevance of race and ethnicity in terms of population health and the creation and maintenance of health disparities. While biology and behavior certainly put people at risk, so does their position in the social hierarchy, which is strongly influenced by their race or ethnicity (Phelan & Link, 2015). There is a need to push scholars to continue to refine how they use race and ethnic categories in health research (Bonham et al., 2018, 2019; Kaplan & Bennett, 2003). Population health research should begin to consistently capture self-identified race and ethnicity data, social and cultural identity, family background, and ancestry data derived from genomic analyses (Bonham et al., 2018).

Race and ethnicity should be used in ways that reflect the multidimensional nature of people's identities and other biopsychosocial factors (Bonham et al., 2018), and these terms should be used when researchers can specify and scientifically justify their relevance to the findings. Before the study is conducted, researchers should be able to justify and articulate these and other questions:

1. Why (or why not) they are including race and ethnicity in their study?
2. What racial or ethnic groups are they comparing, and why?
3. Are they using OMB categories or some other categories, and why?
4. What are they using race and ethnicity as proxies for (e.g., shared social experience, racialized stress exposure, cultural beliefs)? How do they understand what racial or ethnic differences reflect?
5. Do they hypothesize that there will be racial or ethnic differences?
6. If there are or if there are not racial or ethnic differences, what does that mean for the initial research questions and for the larger field?
7. What are the strengths and limitations of the ways they use race and ethnicity in the study (Bonham et al., 2018; Kaplan & Bennett, 2003)?

In sum, normalizing the practice of being more explicit and precise in what we mean when we use terms like race and ethnicity will help improve population health research and practice. These areas will improve because we will be able to be more precise and thoughtful about what differences matter, why they matter, and what differences mean. Also, it will help population health researchers and practitioners understand what similarities exist and what differences do not matter for population health and well-being.

Despite it being a social construct, race should be used when the aim of the research is to explore how racial stratification influences health. Ethnicity should be used to explore how aspects of social life and personal identity affect health or how social stratification and exposures to stress, racism, or discrimination are racialized and vary by ethnicity (Ford & Harawa, 2010). While each country has distinct frameworks for categorizing race, ethnicity, and other socially meaningful categories, it will be important for leaders in the field of population health to harmonize the ways that race, ethnicity, and ancestry data are ascertained, categorized, and applied. Having racial and ethnic categories that meaningfully cross geographic and disciplinary boundaries will advance population health and help achieve population health equity for all people.

REFERENCES

Bhopal, R., & Donaldson, L. (1998). White, European, Western, Caucasian, or what? Inappropriate labeling in research on race, ethnicity, and health. *American Journal of Public Health, 88*(9), 1303–1307.

Blank, R. M., Dabady, M., & Citro, C. F. (Eds.). (2004). *Measuring racial discrimination.* Washington, DC: National Academies Press.

Bonham, V. L., Green, E. D., & Pérez-Stable, E. J. (2018). Examining how race, ethnicity, and ancestry data are used in biomedical research. *JAMA, 320*(15), 1533–1534.

Bonham, V. L., Green, E. D., & Pérez-Stable, E. J. (2019). Race and ethnicity data in research—reply. *JAMA, 321*(12), 1218.

Borak, J., Fiellin, M., & Chemerynski, S. (2004). Who is hispanic? Implications for epidemiologic research in the United States. *Epidemiology, 15*(2), 240–244.

Brown, P., McCormick, S., Mayer, B., Zavestoski, S., Morello-Frosch, R., Altman R. G. et al. (2006). "A lab of our own" environmental causation of breast cancer and challenges to the dominant epidemiological paradigm. *Science, Technology & Human Values, 31*(5), 499–536.

Byrd, W. M., & Clayton, L. A. (2000). *An American health dilemma.* Routledge.

Callier, S. L. (2019). The use of racial categories in precision medicine research. *Ethnicity & Disease, 29*(supp), 651–658.

Came, H., & Griffith, D. (2018). Tackling racism as a "wicked" public health problem: Enabling allies in anti-racism praxis. *Social Science & Medicine, 199*, 181–188.

Carvalho, J. A. M. D., Wood, C. H., & Andrade, F. C. D. (2004). Estimating the stability of census-based racial/ethnic classifications: The case of Brazil. *Population Studies, 58*(3), 331–343.

Coates, T.-N. (2015). *Between the world and me.* Text publishing.

Collins, F. S. (2004). What we do and don't know about 'race', 'ethnicity', genetics and health at the dawn of the genome era. *Nature Genetics, 36*(11), S13–S15.

Cooper, R. S., Kaufman, J. S., & Ward, R. (2003). Race and genomics. *New England Journal of Medicine, 348*(12), 1166–1170.

Cooper, R. S., & Kaufman, J. S. (1998). Race and hypertension: Science and nescience. *Hypertension, 32*(5), 813–816.

Diez Roux, A. V. (2012). Conceptual approaches to the study of health disparities. *Annual Review of Public Health, 33*, 41–58.

Ford, C. L., Griffith, D. M., Bruce, M. A., & Gilbert, K. L. (2019a). Introduction. In C. L. Ford, D. M. Griffith, M. A. Bruce, & K. L. Gilbert (Eds.), *Racism: Science and tools for the public health professional* (pp. 1–8). APHA Press.

Ford, C. L., Griffith, D. M., Bruce, M. A., & Gilbert, K. L. (2019b). Preface. In C. L. Ford, D. M. Griffith, M. A. Bruce, & K. L. Gilbert (Eds.), *Racism: Science and tools for the public health professional* (pp. xxv–xxvii). APHA Press.

Ford, C. L., & Harawa, N. T. (2010). A new conceptualization of ethnicity for social epidemiologic and health equity research. *Social Science and Medicine, 71*(2), 251–258.

Ford, M. E., & Kelly, P. A. (2005). Conceptualizing and categorizing race and ethnicity in health services research. *Health Services Research, 40*(5 pt 2), 1658–1675.

Frank, R. (2007). What to make of it? The (re) emergence of a biological conceptualization of race in health disparities research. *Social Science & Medicine, 64*(10), 1977–1983.

Freeman, H. P. (2003). Commentary on the meaning of race in science and society. *Cancer Epidemiology, Biomarkers & Prevention, 12*(3), 232s–236s.

Geronimus, A. T., James, S. A., Destin, M., Graham, L. F., Hatzenbuehler, M. L., Murphy, M. C. et al. (2016). Jedi public health: Co-creating an identity-safe culture to promote health equity. *SSM-Population Health, 2*, 105–116.

Goodman, A. H. (2000). Why genes don't count (for racial differences in health). *American Journal of Public Health, 90*(11), 1699.

Griffith, D. M., & Griffith, P. A. (2008). Commentary on "perspective on race and ethnicity in Alzheimer's disease research". *Alzheimer's & Dementia, 4*(4), 239–241.

Griffith, D. M., Mason, M., Yonas, M., Eng, E., Jeffries, V., Plihcik, S. et al. (2007). Dismantling institutional racism: Theory and action. *American Journal of Community Psychology, 39*(3–4), 381–392.

Griffith, D. M., Metzl, J. M., & Gunter, K. (2011). Considering intersections of race and gender in interventions that address U.S. men's health disparities. *Public Health, 125*(7), 417–423.

Griffith, D. M., Moy, E., Reischl, T. M., & Dayton, E. (2006). National data for monitoring and evaluating racial and ethnic health inequities: Where do we go from here? *Health Education & Behavior, 33*(4), 470–487.

Griffith, D. M., & Semlow, A. R. (2020). Art, anti-racism and health equity: "Don't ask me why, ask me how!" *Ethnicity & Disease, 30*(3), 373–380.

Griffith, D. M. (2018). "Centering the margins": Moving equity to the center of men's health research. *American Journal of Men's Health*, 1557988318773973.

Griffith, D. M. (2016). Biopsychosocial approaches to men's health disparities research and policy. *Behavioral Medicine*, 42(3), 211–215.

Griffith, D. M. (2020). Preface: Precision medicine approaches to health disparities research. *Ethnicity & Disease*, 30(suppl 1).

Guo, G., Fu, Y., Lee, H., Cai, T., Mullan Harris, K., & Li, Y. (2014). Genetic bio-ancestry and social construction of racial classification in social surveys in the contemporary United States. *Demography*, 51(1), 141–172.

Harris, D. R., & Sim, J. J. (2002). Who is multiracial? Assessing the complexity of lived race. *American Sociological Review*, 614–627.

Idossa, D., Duma, N., Chekhovskiy, K., Go, R., & Ailawadhi, S. (2018). Commentary: Race and ethnicity in biomedical research—classifications, challenges, and future directions. *Ethnicity & Disease*, 28(4), 561.

Jenkins, W. C., Schoenbach, V. C., Rowley, D. L., & Ford, C. L. (2019). Chapter 1: Overcoming the impact of racism on the health of communities: What we have learned and what we have not. In C. L. Ford, D. M. Griffith, M. A. Bruce, & K. L. Gilbert (Eds.), *Racism: Science & tools for the public health professional* (pp. 15–45).Washington, DC: APHA Press.

Jones, C. P. (2019). Chapter 11: Action and allegories. In C. L. Ford, D. M. Griffith, M. A. Bruce, & K. L. Gilbert (Eds.), *Racism: Science & tools for the public health professional*. Washington, DC: APHA Press.

Jones, D. (2010). A WEIRD view of human nature skews psychologists' studies. *Science*, 328(5986), 1627.

Kaplan, J. B., & Bennett, T. (2003). Use of race and ethnicity in biomedical publication. *JAMA*, 289(20), 2709–2716.

Kawachi, I., Daniels, N., & Robinson, D. E. (2005). Health disparities by race and class: Why both matter. *Health Affairs*, 24(2), 343–352.

Kendi, I. X. (2016). *Stamped from the beginning: The definitive history of racist ideas in America*. Hachette UK.

Krieger, N. (2010). Chapter 11: The science and epidemiology of racism and health: Racial/ethnic categories, biological expressions of racism, and the embodiment of inequality—an ecosocial perspective. *What's the use of Race?* 225.

Krieger, N. (2019). Chapter 12: Epidemiology—Why epidemiologists must reckon with racism. In C. L. Ford, D. M. Griffith, M. A. Bruce, & K. L. Gilbert (Eds.), Racism: Science & tools for the public health professional. Washington, DC: APHA Press.

Krieger, N. (2003). Does racism harm health? Did child abuse exist before 1962? On explicit questions, critical science, and current controversies: An ecosocial perspective. *American Journal of Public Health*, 93(2), 194–199.

LaVeist, T. A. (1994). Beyond dummy variables and sample selection: What health services researchers ought to know about race as a variable. *Health Services Research*, 29(1), 1–16.

LaVeist, T. A. (1995). Why we should continue to study race … but do a better job: An essay on race, racism and health. *Ethnicity & Disease*, 6(1–2), 21–29.

LaVeist, T. A. (2000). On the study of race, racism, and health: A shift from description to explanation. *International Journal of Health Services*, 30(1), 217–219.

LaVeist-Ramos, T. A., Galarraga, J., Thorpe, R. J., Bell, C. N., & Austin, C. J. (2012). Are black hispanics black or hispanic? Exploring disparities at the intersection of race and ethnicity. *Journal of Epidemiology and Community Health*, 66(7), e21.

LeBrón, A. M. W., & Viruell-Fuentes, E. A. (2019). Chapter 21: Racism and the health of latina/latino communities. In C. L. Ford, D. M. Griffith, M. A. Bruce, & K. L. Gilbert (Eds.), *Racism: Science & tools for the public health professional* (pp. 413–428). Washington, DC: APHA Press.

Mays, V. M., Ponce, N. A., Washington, D. L., & Cochran, S. D. (2003). Classification of race and ethnicity: Implications for public health. *Annual Review of Public Health*, 24, 83.

Morning, A. (2015). Ethnic classification in global perspective: A cross-national survey of the 2000 census round. Social Statistics and Ethnic Diversity (pp. 17–37). Springer.

Painter, N. I. (2010). John Friedrich Blumbach names white people "Caucasian". In The History of White People (pp. 72–91). WW Norton & Company.

Patrinos, A. (2004). 'Race' and the human genome. *Nature Genetics*, 36(11), S1–S2.

Phelan, J. C., & Link, B. G. (2015). Is racism a fundamental cause of inequalities in health? *Annual Review of Sociology*, 41, 311–330.

Prewitt, K. (2005). Racial classification in America: Where do we go from here? *Daedalus*, 134(1), 5–17.

Risch, N., Burchard, E., Ziv, E., & Tang, H. (2002). Categorization of humans in biomedical research: Genes, race and disease. *Genome Biology*, 3(7).

Samari, G., Alcalá, H. E., & Sharif, M. Z. (2019). Chapter 23: Racialization of religious minorities. In C. L. Ford, D. M. Griffith, M. A. Bruce, & K. L. Gilbert (Eds.). *Racism: Science & tools for the public health professional.* Washington, DC: APHA Press.

Smedley, B. D. (2019). Chapter 24: Toward a comprehensive understanding of racism and health inequities: A multilevel approach. In C. L. Ford, D. M. Griffith, M. A. Bruce, & K. L. Gilbert (Eds.). *Racism: science & tools for the public health professional* (pp. 469–478).Washington, DC: APHA Press.

Smedley, A., & Smedley, B. D. (2005). Race as biology is fiction, racism as a social problem is real: Anthropological and historical perspectives on the social construction of race. *American Psychologist, 60*(1), 16–26.

Yudell, M., Roberts, D., DeSalle, R., & Tishkoff, S. (2016). Taking race out of human genetics. *Science, 351*(6273), 564–565.

CHAPTER 14

Marginalized Populations: Examining Vulnerability and Health Inequities Through the Framework of Caste

Michelle DeCoux Hampton, Noelene Moonsamy, Ningning Guo, and Ena Arce

LEARNING OBJECTIVES

- Identify three systemic barriers to healthcare for vulnerable populations in the United States.

- Compare and contrast the social and economic conditions that influence health and illness to the advantage of dominant and the disadvantage of nondominant group members.

- State the impact of intersectional identity on health outcomes.

- Develop an individual-level plan of action to address health disparities in your clinical practice.

- Identify systems-level interventions to implement change that addresses health inequities for vulnerable populations in the community.

INTRODUCTION

Vulnerable populations are at risk for poor health outcomes related to unmet physical, psychological, or social needs. Individuals accumulate risk due to health status (individual, family, and community), exposure to health hazards, and resource availability (Aday, 2001; Mechanic & Tanner, 2007). A systematic review ($n = 337$) examined health outcomes in vulnerable individuals who were homeless, engaged in sex work, diagnosed with substance use disorders, or imprisoned, and results revealed excessive mortality rates, with many deaths associated with injuries or other external causes. However, there was also a high burden of infectious, mental, cardiovascular, and respiratory disease (Aldridge et al., 2018). The higher morbidity and mortality rates identified in this study are examples of health inequities. These disparate outcomes affect vulnerable populations disproportionately compared with members of groups with lower cumulative risk.

The World Health Organization (WHO) defines health inequities as "differences in health status or ... the distribution of health resources between different population groups, arising from social conditions in which people are born, grow, live, work and age" (WHO, 2018). Rather than an individual's preferences or behaviors, health inequities result from systemic barriers and discrimination that affect social, economic, and environmental policy at local, state, and national levels (Institute of Medicine [IOM], 2003; National Academics of Sciences, Engineering, and Medicine [NASEM], 2017). Positive and adverse health effects accrue depending on healthcare access, housing, education, and employment resources (social determinants of health). Individuals with the fewest resources experience a heavier disease burden and premature mortality (Marmot et al., 2010).

In *Caste: The Origins of Our Discontents,* a Pulitzer Prize–winning and *New York Times* best-selling book, Wilkerson (2020) explored the experience of Black citizens in the United States through the lens of caste. The Human Genome Project, initiated in 1990, mapped the location and sequence of human DNA and produced linkage maps that can track inherited traits from generation to generation (National Institutes of Health [NIH], 2021). One of the significant findings was no discernable genetic variation between individuals who identify as Black, White, or other races (Collins, 2004). As a result, scholars define race as a social–political and social–psychological construct that influences health, housing, education, and employment outcomes as a function of the environment rather than of biology (Ford & Kelly, 2005). Caste is also defined as "an artificial construction, a fixed and embedded ranking of human value that sets the presumed supremacy of one group against the presumed inferiority of other groups based on ancestry and often immutable traits" (Wilkerson, 2020, p. 17). India's caste system in Southeast Asia preceded that of the United States' by thousands of years, and the U.S. system influenced race law in Germany before World War II (Dirks, 2011; Wilkerson, 2020). According to Whitman (2017), "Nazis engaged in a detailed study of American immigration law, American second-class citizenship law, and American anti-miscegenation and mongrelization law ...[and the] attraction in the system of Jim Crow segregation" (Whitman, 2017, p. 135). Hitler commissioned a team of more than 40 lawyers to travel to the United States to study the application of Jim Crow laws and the legal justification for subjugating Black, Native American, Puerto Rican, Filipino, and Chinese populations in the United States to advance his eugenics agenda in Germany beginning in the 1930s (Little, 2021; Whitman, 2017). Officials in the Nazi party used this information to normalize the practice of race discrimination policy within the general population of Germany (Gellately, 2001).

In the United States, segregation and discrimination that advantaged White Americans and disadvantaged Black Americans, Native Americans, and Alaska Natives in housing, education, employment, and voting were sanctioned by law until the passage of the Civil Rights Acts of 1964 and 1968 (Georgetown University Law Library, 2021a), but even though legislation technically outlawed "discrimination based on race, color, religion, sex, or national origin," inequities persisted. In surveys of Black Americans between 1968 and 2000, perceptions of the success of the Civil Rights Movement and legislation ranged from approximately 53% to 65% (Santoro, 2015). The highest percentage was recorded in 1980, but by 1984, it dropped to 53%, coinciding with reduced income, residential migration to high-poverty neighborhoods, and increased unemployment within Black communities during the Reagan Administration (Santoro, 2015). In a Pew Research Center study of more than 10,000 U.S. adults following several highly publicized police brutality incidents, including the murder of George Floyd and the subsequent protests and public outcry, 86% of Black respondents compared with 39% of White respondents stated that the United States has not made sufficient progress on racial equality for Black people. Also, 76% of Black respondents and 26% of White respondents said Black people are treated less fairly when seeking medical care (Horowitz et al., 2020).

This chapter aims to examine the relationship between these economic disparities and social structures created by the U.S. caste system and how they contribute to inequities and disparities in health and education, which negatively impact the overall well-being of individuals and communities. Wilkerson's eight pillars of caste are applied to examine systemic factors that contribute to health inequities within vulnerable groups. The eight pillars are (a) divine will and the laws of nature, (b) heritability, (c) endogamy and control of marriage, (d) purity versus pollution, (e) occupational hierarchy, (f) dehumanization and stigma, (g) terror as enforcement, and (h) inherent superiority versus inherent inferiority (Wilkerson, 2020; Table 14.1). The pillars of caste address the impact of individual acts of discrimination, such as experiencing racial slurs or physical assault. Further, Wilkerson (2020) addresses the function of systems that uphold and reinforce the dominant caste's power and privilege.

Contrary to individual acts of discrimination, systemic bias and discrimination are self-sustaining and permeate every aspect of U.S. life, including but not limited to education,

TABLE 14.1 Eight Pillars of Caste: Description and Historical Examples

Pillar	Description	Examples from an era of enslavement or Jim Crow segregation
Divine will and the laws of nature	Elevated or subordinate status of one group over another is justified based on religious dogma or false beliefs in inherent differences	Rationalized Black enslavement with the story of Ham, a biblical character with black skin, who was cursed by Noah
Heritability	Confinement of a person to the caste assigned at birth	Belief in the genetic inferiority of Black people. Children of Black enslaved women and White enslavers were also enslaved
Endogamy and control of marriage	Restricts marriage to persons of the same caste only	Legislation that prohibited marriage or sexual relations between Black and White persons (violations by wealthy and powerful White men were often overlooked)
Purity versus pollution	Protects perceived "purity" of the dominant caste from "contamination" by others	Black people were prohibited from using swimming pools, drinking fountains, lunch counters, public schools, universities, and so forth, that were intended for use by White people
Occupational hierarchy	Limits career opportunities to those that align with predetermined, caste-dictated, roles	After slavery, the majority of Black men and women continued to work in agricultural or domestic service of White persons
Dehumanization and stigma	Denies basic human rights and dignity or associates a group of people with negative characteristics to normalize exploitation and abuse	Enslaved persons were prohibited from crying and forced to sing when separated from family members who were sold
Terror as enforcement	Suppresses nondominant group resistance with the use of physical and psychological violence	Use of lynching to punish minor social code violations such as eye contact with a White person
Inherent superiority versus inherent inferiority	Internalized beliefs reinforce supremacy of the dominant group and inferiority of others	Black bus riders sitting or standing behind White riders

Source: Data from Wilkerson, I. (2020). Caste: The origins of our discontents. Penguin Random House.

employment, housing, accumulation of wealth, and healthcare. This chapter focuses primarily on healthcare systems, health professional education, and health policy with examples from research literature and news media that illustrate the impact of caste on vulnerable populations. Nondominant groups represented in this chapter include Black, Indigenous, Native American, Alaska Native, Latinx, LGBTQ+ (lesbian, gay, bisexual, transgender, queer+), and immigrant populations with limited English proficiency. However, the framework can be applied to any group negatively affected by systemic inequities that result in disparate social, economic, educational, or health outcomes.

EIGHT PILLARS OF CASTE

Divine Will and the Laws of Nature

The roots of the Black inferiority myth, and its influence on poor health outcomes in Black Americans, originated in slavery with the full endorsement of the medical establishment. In an extensive review of research about the history of Black health, Byrd and Clayton (1992) reported that medical professionals' endorsement of false beliefs that Black persons were "subhuman" and inferior to Whites justified the massive overwork and inadequate nutrition, clothing, and sanitation to which enslaved African people were subjected. False beliefs that Black people, compared with White people, were less intelligent, more tolerant of heat and pain, or more prone to certain illnesses were published in professional journals and taught in medical schools across the country (Cartwright, 1851; Interlandi, 2019; Figure 14.1). For example, the term "drapetomania" was invented to describe a "disease" characterized by attempting to run away from enslavement (Coard, 2019). Marion Sims was a gynecologist who developed a procedure to treat obstetric fistula by operating on a group of nine enslaved women and girls repeatedly, without anesthesia, to perfect the process. One

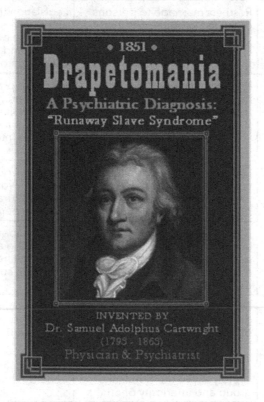

Figure 14.1 Medical journals perpetuated myths of Black inferiority and disease.

17-year-old girl named Anarcha underwent the procedure 29 times over 4 years (Cronin, 2020). As a result of such beliefs and practices, the healthcare system was more likely to exacerbate health inequities than to meet the needs of Black people (Byrd & Clayton, 1992). Throughout slavery and its immediate aftermath, many Black Americans received either no treatment or care that was inferior to that of White Americans; if care was accessible at all, it was provided in overpopulated and underresourced care settings (Byrd & Clayton, 1992).

The results of the Human Genome Project revealed that, genetically, there is no way to distinguish one race from another (Collins, 2004; Human Genome Program, 2008). The lack of a physiologic distinction among racial groups might resolve the debate about race-based differences regarding intellectual ability, health, or physical characteristics in science-driven, health professional fields; however, 16 years after the Human Genome Project's completion, 73% of laypersons (n = 92) and 50% of medical students and residents (n = 222), reported that at least one false belief about Black people was possibly, probably, or definitely true (i.e., "Blacks experience less pain," "Whites have larger brains than Blacks," or "Blacks have nerve endings that are less sensitive than Whites"; Hoffman et al., 2016). Further, medical students and residents who believed more false statements were more likely to select inaccurate diagnoses and treatment recommendations for Black patients.

Similarly, in a systematic review, 35 of 42 studies found that nurses, physicians, and other healthcare workers had equal rates of implicit bias compared with the general population. Among studies that analyzed correlations, higher levels of implicit bias were associated with a lower quality of care that resulted in inappropriate diagnosis, tests ordered, and treatment decisions, as well as poor communication (FitzGerald & Hurst, 2017). This finding illustrates the detrimental effect of unconscious beliefs on individual clinical encounters with Black patients. It further supports findings that stereotypes, bias, and clinical uncertainty may negatively influence a healthcare provider's ability to provide equal treatment and affects access to critical services to preserve life and reduce morbidity and mortality (Burgess et al., 2008; Epstein et al., 2000; Graham et al., 2018; IOM, 2003; Hoffman et al., 2016; Sabin & Greenwald, 2012).

However, health professionals can also impact outcomes at the community or national level. Recently, for example, a physician and state senator appointed to lead the Ohio State Senate Health Committee implied that disproportionate rates of coronavirus in the Black community might be explained by a failure to adhere to hand hygiene, mask, or social distancing recommendations (Amiri, 2021). When pressured to resign by community members, the senator refused and touted "a long record of providing healthcare to minority neighborhoods and … multiple mission trips at his own expense to treat those from disadvantaged countries." The implication that COVID-19–related health inequities resulted from individual attitudes and behaviors ignores the impact of systemic factors that contribute significantly to human health and illness. Health professionals and health policymakers who serve in Congress and in federal, state, and local organizations wield substantial power in the lives and health of their constituents. If they view health inequities as a personal failure rather than the result of systemic factors, they are unlikely to enact effective health policies. Policies that affect social determinants of health are necessary to improve health and reduce illness in vulnerable communities (Marmot, 2017; Perez-Stable & Sayre, 2019; Thornton et al., 2016).

Heritability

Heritability refers to a person's perpetual disposition to the caste assigned at birth, regardless of socioeconomic status or education (Wilkerson, 2020). For example, Serena Williams is an accomplished American athlete known for her achievements in tennis, as well as for her history of life-threatening blood clots, and she is a Black woman. In 2011, Ms. Williams was diagnosed and treated for multiple pulmonary emboli. In 2018, she experienced shortness of breath after a cesarean section and immediately notified a nurse. She asked for "a CT.[computerized tomography] scan and a blood thinner," and the nurse, rather than investigating further, dismissed her concerns as confusion due to pain medication (Salam, 2018). Ms. Williams's world-renowned fame, informed health literacy, and wealth failed to provide her the power or privilege that a White celebrity, or likely any White woman, could wield in that situation. She was forced to advocate for herself and fortunately survived. Still, her experience illustrates that racism is likely a contributing factor in high maternal mortality rates among Black women due to conditions that are, most of the time, preventable (Centers for Disease Control and Prevention [CDC], 2019; Figure 14.2).

While both White and Black adults report discrimination in healthcare, White adults report it less frequently and perceive more extraordinary privilege with even modest gains in income and education (Stepanikova & Oates, 2017). However, the reverse is true for Black adults, who report that exposure to discrimination increases at higher education and income levels (Bleich et al., 2019; Colen et al., 2018). Therefore, even though education and higher socioeconomic status might confer a degree of economic privilege, it does not equate to power or privilege when engaged with dominant group members in healthcare settings. In general, Black (or potentially other marginalized) people who are poor, lack health insurance, or have knowledge of the healthcare system, have even less capital to advocate for themselves successfully (Box 14.1).

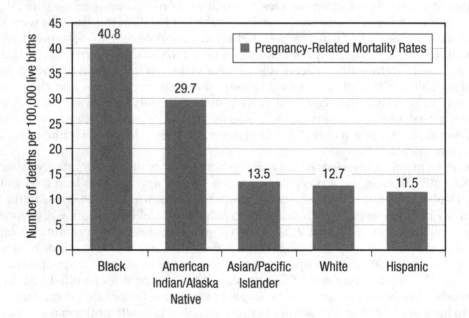

Figure 14.2 Pregnancy-related mortality by race.

Source: Adapted from Centers for Disease Control and Prevention. (2019). Racial and ethnic disparities continue in pregnancy-related deaths: Black, American Indian/Alaska Native women most affected. Centers for Disease Control. https://www.cdc.gov/media/releases/2019/p0905-racial-ethnic-disparities-pregnancy-deaths.html.

BOX 14.1: Pillar 2

A Black physician contracted coronavirus and went to the emergency department for treatment of severe pain and shortness of breath. A White physician, assigned to her case, knew she was a physician, but dismissed her symptoms and planned her discharge. She endured pain for hours before any medication was administered and felt she was treated like a "drug addict" because she was Black. She died 2 weeks later due to COVID-19 complications (Eligon, 2020).

Endogamy and Control of Marriage

The first case tried before the U.S. Supreme Court regarding same-sex marriage was in 1970. Over the following 45 years, various state laws were passed to legalize or ban it, but in 2015, same-sex marriage was legalized in all 50 states (Georgetown University Law Library, 2021b; *Obergefell et al. v. Hodges*, 2015). Though available research indicates that legally married LGBTQ+ persons and unmarried same-sex partners in long-term partnerships have similar physical health indicators, legally married partners report a better quality of life associated with more significant social and economic resources (Goldsen et al., 2017). Further, compared with same-sex couples involved in civil partnerships or informal cohabitation relationships, married partners reported increased subjective well-being, possibly due to decreased stigma (Boertien & Vignoli, 2019). Marriage also yielded an indirect health benefit: employer-sponsored health insurance. In studies of health insurance coverage of same-sex couples, partners who were not married were more likely to report being uninsured, with reports of improved insurance rates after same-sex marriage was legalized (Downing & Cha, 2020; Gonzales, 2017). In a review of studies regarding the impact of the Affordable Care Act (ACA), increased rates of insurance among the poor and underserved resulted in improved access, lower costs, and increased use of ambulatory services, which are critical for the prevention of illness and the maintenance of health (Kominski et al., 2017).

Purity Versus Pollution

Medicaid Expansion

The ACA became law in 2010. Despite its potential to increase the number of insured U.S. residents, legislative and public opposition undermined its implementation. Medicare and Medicaid are both public, federally funded insurance programs. According to the Kaiser Family Foundation (KFF), 77% of more than 1,800 survey respondents (who self-identified as Hispanic 29.3%; Black 20.0%; Asian/Native Hawaiian/Pacific Islander 4.3%; and Native American/Alaska Native 1.1%) considered Medicare an essential government program, but favorability rates for Medicaid and its expansion were inconsistent. Black and White respondents were among those with the most remarkable difference in favorability ratings, with 80% of Black respondents in support of Medicaid expansion, in contrast with only 46% of White respondents, even though White Americans were the most frequent beneficiaries of Medicaid (41.1%; KFF, 2019, 2021; Figure 14.3).

The discrepancy might be explained by Medicaid's association with healthcare for poor and underserved populations. According to Metzl (2019), even after Kentucky successfully implemented the ACA and demonstrated improved health outcomes, many White residents in neighboring Tennessee remained opposed. It is possible that Kentucky's use of an alternative name (other than the ACA) reduced opposition. Still, in Tennessee-based focus groups, even uninsured participants diagnosed with severe, life-threatening illnesses remained opposed to government intrusion in their personal lives or their "tax dollars paying for Mexicans or welfare queens" (p. 3). The stigma of health insurance for all and its association with low socioeconomic status or foreign "others" rendered it unacceptable to many who could also benefit (Metzl, 2019). This narrative, sustained in political debates since 2010, inspired Supreme Court challenges to the ACA, which threatened but failed to overturn the law in 2012, 2015, and 2021 (Liptak, 2021).

Appropriate Use of Interpreter Services

Undocumented immigrant populations, who are often at the center of debates about expanded coverage, face multiple barriers to healthcare access, including delays or avoidance of care due to inability to pay, lack of transportation, or the requirement to supply citizenship or legal residency documentation. Individuals who fear deportation are forced

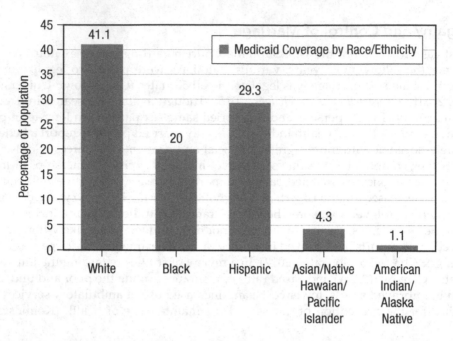

Figure 14.3 Medicaid insurance coverage by race and ethnicity in the United States.

Source: Adapted from Kaiser Family Foundation. (2019). *Distribution of the nonelderly with Medicaid by race/ethnicity.* https://www.kff.org/medicaid/state-indicator/medicaid-distribution-nonelderly-by-raceethnicity/?currentTimeframe=0&selectedRows=%7B%22wrapups%22:%7B%22united-states%22: %7B%7D%7D%7D&sortModel=%7B%22colId%22:%22Location%22,%22sort%22:%22asc%22%7D.

BOX 14.2: Pillar 4

A woman living in Washington, D.C., has a son with asthma. Because she lacks a green card, she fears divulging her contact information to the provider, and fears police detainment if stopped by police in transit to the appointment. She stated, "Now I feel scared to even go to a new doctor because you don't know what can happen. You have to give all the information—give your address and personal information—and if I don't know somebody, I don't go" (Adams, 2018). This avoidance of primary care is known to contribute to costly urgent and emergency care when routine health screenings and services for the management of common and chronic conditions are underused.

to choose between healthcare and family security (Doshi et al., 2020; Hacker et al., 2015; Kennedy, 2018; Box 14.2).

The inability to communicate in English and the lack of interpreter services are additional risk factors that limit access, quality, and effectiveness of care. Although interpreter service use is supported by evidence and required by law, its use is inconsistent in healthcare settings. In a study of 354 emergency department providers, most used nonprofessional interpreters, including other department staff, family members, or friends (65%). Most were unaware of language assistance policies (67%) and denied that they received prior training regarding interpreter service use (81%; Taira et al., 2020). A study that used two national surveys as source data found that 25.3% of hospitals with a moderate to high need for language services and 34.6% of those with low demand failed to offer them (Schiaffino et al., 2016). In a study of malpractice claims in four states, 32 of 35 were associated with the failure to use professional interpreters, despite the legal requirement to do so. In these cases, the use of children, spouses, or no interpreter resulted in misdiagnosis, missed allergies, adverse medication or treatment reactions, delays in care, and miscommunication of informed consent and discharge instructions. These errors resulted in death or serious injuries such as infection, limb loss, organ failure, and brain damage (Quan, 2013).

In California, 28.8% of the state's population in 2018 spoke Spanish as the primary language at home (Statistical Atlas, 2018). These data could explain disparities in health screening. For example, only an estimated 55% of California's Latinx adults receive colorectal cancer screening tests, a rate lower than that of White (77.5%) and Black adults (77.3%; Steele et al., 2013). Similar to the inability to follow discharge instructions provided only in English, non-English speakers are also less likely to receive recommended preventive healthcare such as screenings for cancer (Sentell et al., 2013).

Health Services Access for Native American and Alaska Native Populations

Native American and Alaska Native populations are also affected by insufficient healthcare access. Federal and state healthcare agencies that serve this population are underfunded and underresourced. The federal government must finance healthcare for all Native American and Alaska Native persons through Indian Health Services (IHS; 2021), but geographical and policy barriers limit access to the service. Data from the 5-year American Community Survey revealed that a majority (68%) of IHS-covered Native American and Alaska Native respondents lived on tribal lands. Further, IHS coverage was more frequently reported by respondents with higher incomes, possibly because they had the means and resources to travel to healthcare sites (Bhaskar & O'Hara, 2017). A study of more than 1,000,000 Medicare beneficiaries found that Native American or Alaska Native participants were most likely to live in rural areas and had difficulty accessing needed care (Martino et al., 2020; Box 14.3). Problems with scheduling appointments and the burden and expense of traveling from rural areas to IHS centers present significant obstacles to access (Kaiser Health News, 2016). A listing of U.S. IHS locations included 161 sites, primarily located in New Mexico, Arizona, and South Dakota. Fifteen of the 25 state listings had only one or two sites (IHS, 2021), with the remaining 25 states reporting no available IHS sites (Figure 14.4). Even Native American

BOX 14.3: Pillar 5

After 25 Sioux tribe members of a South Dakota reservation died of COVID-19, a woman sheltered in place with her mother to avoid infection. After her mother's fall and a broken hip, the woman was forced to take her to the hospital, risking exposure to the virus. As she feared, both became infected, and her mother died 2 weeks later (Siegler, 2021).

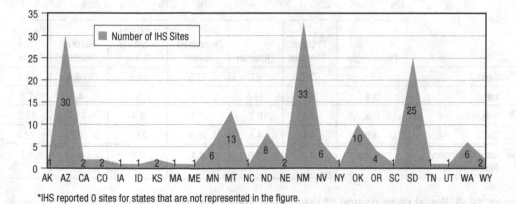

*IHS reported 0 sites for states that are not represented in the figure.

Figure 14.4 Number of Indian Health Service sites by state.

Source: Adapted from Indian Health Service. (2021). *Indian Health Service: The federal health program for American Indians and Alaska Natives.* IHS Headquarters. https://www.ihs.gov/locations/

persons who lived in urban areas, while closer to providers and care settings, could not access all services (such as no-cost prescriptions) if the site was not affiliated with the IHS (Kaiser Health News, 2016). As evidenced by the gaps in the care system for vulnerable populations, it is possible that universal health coverage could be a means to improve U.S. health outcomes. Still, to overcome political opposition, the image of public health insurance might require rehabilitation and a paradigm shift.

Occupational Hierarchy

The occupational hierarchy ensures that dominant caste members assume the most prestigious and highly compensated positions. At the same time, the nondominant group takes positions with lower pay or less desirable work conditions (Wilkerson, 2020). Throughout the COVID-19 pandemic, essential workers were among the lowest paid and the most exposed to risk. Essential workers continued to work in food service, healthcare support, cleaning services, and transportation despite public health advisories for most of the population to work from home (when possible) to avoid infection. Because more essential workers were Black and Latinx, they also experienced higher death rates from COVID-19 (Rogers et al., 2020).

In healthcare, Black and Latinx healthcare workers were more commonly represented among nursing assistants and licensed vocational nurses, with comparatively lower representation among physicians, psychologists, physical therapists, and registered nurses (Figure 14.5). This discrepancy affects income inequality and perpetuates health inequities by preventing Black, Indigenous, and other people of color (BIPOC) from entering health profession fields. According to the Health Resources and Services Administration (HRSA, 2006), BIPOC are more likely to practice in underserved communities. In the highest paid health professional roles, White practitioners were most prevalent (83.5% of psychologists,

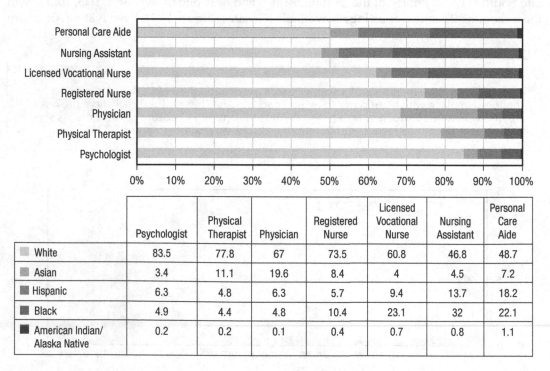

	Psychologist	Physical Therapist	Physician	Registered Nurse	Licensed Vocational Nurse	Nursing Assistant	Personal Care Aide
White	83.5	77.8	67	73.5	60.8	46.8	48.7
Asian	3.4	11.1	19.6	8.4	4	4.5	7.2
Hispanic	6.3	4.8	6.3	5.7	9.4	13.7	18.2
Black	4.9	4.4	4.8	10.4	23.1	32	22.1
American Indian/ Alaska Native	0.2	0.2	0.1	0.4	0.7	0.8	1.1

Figure 14.5 Racial composition of the United States' healthcare workforce.

Source: Adapted from Health Resources and Services Administration & National Center for Health Workforce Analysis. (2017). *Sex, race, and ethnic diversity of U.S. health occupations (2011–2015).* U.S. Department of Health and Human Services. https://bhw.hrsa.gov/sites/default/files/bureau-health-work force/data-research/diversity-us-health-occupations.pdf.

77.8% of physical therapists, 67.0% of physicians, and 73.5% of registered nurses; HRSA, 2017). The discrepancy in nursing is unlikely related to a lack of interest, as 32.0% of certified nursing assistants and 23.1% of licensed vocational nurses are Black (HRSA, 2017), a higher representation than Black residents in the general population (13.4%; U.S. Census Bureau, 2021). However, several studies suggest that limited mentoring and support could present obstacles. A systematic review of 18 studies identified multiple barriers to mentorship program sustainability, including lack of funding, burdensome time commitments for mentors, and minimal institutional support (Beech et al., 2013). Health professional education admission policies could also present barriers.

BIPOC representation among registered nurses is disproportionate to overall representation in the U.S. population, with the most significant discrepancy in southern states (Hampton et al., 2022; Xue & Brewer, 2014). A study of associate and bachelor's degree nursing programs that examined admission criteria identified potential barriers for underrepresented students in the South compared with other U.S. regions. Southern nursing programs were significantly more likely to require a majority of academic metric criteria, such as multiple grade point average requirements, standardized tests, and strict limits regarding prerequisite course repetition. They were also significantly less likely to require references, essays, or volunteer work, components of holistic admissions review (HAR; Hampton et al., 2022).

Studies regarding the implementation and effectiveness of HAR are limited, but of the available studies, the evidence supports its use. HAR effectively increased underrepresented students in a medical program from approximately 11% to 20% (Witzburg & Sondheimer, 2013) and from 11% to 16% in a nursing program (Wros & Noone, 2018). A third program evaluation reported that 28% of non-White or first-generation students would not have been admitted with the last academic metric-only admission criteria (Wagner et al., 2020). In a study of dental education programs, Black student enrollment remained virtually unchanged, increasing from 5.3% to 5.8% between 2010 and 2019, despite setting goals to increase diversity (Nalliah et al., 2021). Further, 10 of 66 dental programs admitted no Black students, despite receiving 236 applications. In addition to admission criteria, inequities in school funding, family wealth, and health disparities in majority Black, Hispanic, and other marginalized communities (Ladson-Billings, 2007) can affect students' academic performance and preparedness to compete for limited opportunities in health professional education programs (see Narrative 14.1). The lack of a diverse faculty might also be a deterrent.

NARRATIVE 14.1: UNEQUAL OPPORTUNITIES IN EDUCATION

Sandra (she/her/hers), a 22-year old college graduate, loved reading as a child, and attended a predominantly Black, Catholic school. She was an enthusiastic student until third grade, when her teacher was abruptly terminated mid-year. A substitute replaced her and administered frequent, timed multiplication tests. The tests were anxiety-provoking because Sandra was unable to complete all the test items in the time allowed. When her mother approached the teacher to request reassurance for Sandra, the teacher responded with silence and a stare, so Sandra's mother tutored her in the evenings. Although her anxiety grew, Sandra's grade performance remained above average.

In fourth grade, Sandra went to a new school. There were many non-White, but very few Black, students. Her teacher noticed that anxiety influenced Sandra's math test performance and sat with her at a table during test time, and Sandra continued to perform well. In fifth grade, her teacher exclaimed in a parent–teacher conference, "I couldn't tell by looking at [Sandra] that she was such an academic!" In sixth grade, Sandra received her first C grades in math and science, and she relayed messages from her teachers that included comments such as, "A 'C' is average and it's what *most* of us should be getting," and "Some

(continued)

NARRATIVE 14.1: UNEQUAL OPPORTUNITIES IN EDUCATION (*CONTINUED*)

kids are good students and others are good at sports." Sandra's mother spoke to Sandra's three junior high school teachers at the first parent–teacher conference to discuss her sudden decline in grade performance. Again, she was met with stares and silence, so she hired tutors. Despite the decline in grade performance, Sandra's performance on annual standardized tests remained above average in all content areas. Similarly, she performed well on the high school placement exam. In the required high school reference letter, Sandra's math teacher wrote that she "was placed in a slow learners math group," a detail that was never discussed in 3 years of parent–teacher conferences. Despite this negative evaluation, Sandra was admitted to her high school of choice. In her first physics exam, she was devastated when a teacher wrote "Duh" next to an incorrect response and feared that she would embarrass herself or that other students—who frequently compared grade performance—would learn about her low marks. Throughout the year, Sandra found it difficult to get out of bed in the morning for school, and her despair deepened after the deaths of her grandmother and uncle due to cancer. She ended the year with three Ds and changed schools.

Although her grade performance improved immediately, Sandra's withdrawn demeanor led to intermittent reports of disrespectful behavior in the classroom. A high point of her junior year was working with a young, Black teacher who committed herself to helping Sandra work through her math anxiety. She finished the year with an A in the class and the highest statistics advanced placement (AP) test score in the class. The AP statistics class started in mid-August of the following year, and by mid-September, Sandra's teacher sent an email to report that she was failing the class. To avoid further impact to her grade point average, Sandra's mother worked to assist Sandra in dropping the class. The request was met with resistance and hostility by the school's administration, despite the fact that it was only 4 weeks into the class and college applications were pending. With limited support by the counseling staff, Sandra submitted applications to only four California public universities. Despite a strong standardized test score and consistently above-average performance in junior and senior years, Sandra was declined admission to all of the public institutions. She accepted an offer to play basketball at a private university on the East Coast and decided to apply to the nursing program.

The application required high school transcripts, standardized test scores, a background check, and a report from the high school counselor. Sandra was declined admission to the nursing program. Alternatively, she studied film and excelled academically without tutoring, accommodations, or support of any kind. Her grade point average earned her a position on the Dean's list several semesters, and prior to graduating with her bachelor's degree, she was accepted into a graduate program at a private university. Although pleased with her achievements and resilience, Sandra wondered how the requirement for such resilience altered her academic trajectory.

Dehumanization and Stigma

Between 2009 and 2021, U.S. presidential administrations enacted, rescinded, and re-enacted transgender protections three times. Initial protections banned discrimination in public school districts, education programs, and school-based activities. When the protections were revoked, schools and businesses were allowed to exclude transgender people from single-sex homeless shelters and from military service, use of single-sex restrooms, and participation in sports activities (Cameron, 2020; Cooper & Shear, 2021). These exclusions were similar to state-sanctioned segregation before the passage of the Civil Rights Act in 1964. The vacillating policies surrounding transgender rights coincided with the increasing violent killings of transgender people in the United States. The Human Rights Campaign

(2021) tracked these data, and approximately 20 to 30 deaths due to violence were reported per year between 2013 and 2019. There was a spike to 44 in 2020, with higher rates of death among Black (n = 23) and Latinx (n = 9) persons (Human Rights Campaign, 2020). As of early 2021, there were 21 violent deaths (Human Rights Campaign, 2021). Like lynching in the Jim Crow South (Wilkerson, 2020), the denial of humanity presents a danger to the health and safety of transgender people.

Concerning healthcare, 31% of transgender individuals reported they were uninsured (Harvard School of Public Health et al., 2017). Further, they frequently faced discrimination (Harvard School of Public Health et al., 2017). Two national surveys documented that transgender individuals experienced acts of discrimination associated with transgender bias that impacted their quality of life. Acts included bullying, physical or sexual assault, homelessness, job loss, incarceration, unemployment, and housing discrimination (Grant et al., 2011; James et al., 2016). BIPOC participants reported experiencing the highest rates of unemployment (e.g., 28% for Black respondents vs. 14% for respondents overall) and housing discrimination (e.g., 47% for Native American respondents and 38% for Black respondents vs. 19% for respondents overall; Grant et al., 2011). Both surveys also found that several participants reported that they were often unable to pay for or were denied medical care altogether for transition-related and routine services. They also reportedly received poorer quality care, such as postponements of health services due to discrimination or verbal harassment by providers. Transgender people who were Black, were immigrants, or traded sex for money or goods were at exceptionally high risk for poor treatment (Grant et al., 2011; James et al., 2016). A follow-up to the U.S. Transgender Survey was scheduled in 2020, but funding and logistic challenges due to the COVID-19 pandemic forced the investigators to delay its administration (Sosin, 2020).

Even for people with health insurance, gender-affirming therapy might be excluded from coverage in healthcare policies (Stroumsa, 2014). A comprehensive report of HealthCare.gov marketplace insurance plans found that in 2021, 7% of available programs (n = 1,386) included transgender-specific exclusions, an increase of 4% from 2020 (Out2Enroll, 2021). The plans with exclusions limited access to hormone therapy, mental health treatment, and surgical procedures necessary to treat gender dysphoria. Transgender individuals may be subjected to hostile environments in nearly every aspect of life. They face challenges in accessing care due to economic barriers, national and state legislation, and individual-level bias and discrimination, resulting in increased risk for poor health outcomes.

Further, transgender people with intersectional identities, such as BIPOC or homeless individuals, are at increased risk (Grant et al., 2011; James et al., 2016). Local and national policies are needed to restore their fundamental human rights and protections and address their unmet healthcare needs (see Case Study 14.1). The University of California—San Francisco's Center of Excellence for Transgender Health published primary care guidelines that can be used to inform and guide gender-affirming and immediate healthcare needs. The guidelines include information about creating a safe environment, approaches to physical examination, and hormone therapy initiation (Deutsch, 2016).

CASE STUDY 14.1: INPATIENT PSYCHIATRIC ADMISSION

Victoria (pronouns she/her/hers), 17 years old, was admitted to an inpatient psychiatric unit after an overdose. After a recent sexual assault and beating, Victoria moved in with her grandmother and lived there for 3 months prior to admission. Her grandmother is tolerant of her desire to transition, but does not approve of her "lifestyle choice," praying that "Jesus will forgive her." Victoria began gender-affirming hormone therapy 6 months ago, but after her mother lost her job due to the COVID-19 pandemic, she also lost her health insurance. With no insurance, she was no longer able to afford gender-affirming therapy and

(continued)

CASE STUDY 14.1: INPATIENT PSYCHIATRIC ADMISSION (*CONTINUED*)

overdosed on amitriptyline (prescribed for anxiety and depression), but survived. When admitted, Victoria surrendered her estradiol supply, per facility policy, and later asked the charge nurse for her daily dose. First, the staff ignored her. Then, when they responded, they used her dead name, Derek, and refused to call the physician to obtain an order for the medication. The physician, who met with Victoria the following day, told her that the therapy was not safe for adolescents and encouraged her to follow up with her primary care provider after discharge.

Discussion Questions

1. What could you do immediately to advocate for Victoria?
2. What intervention would you recommend for the health professional staff to increase awareness and reduce personal biases?
3. What organizational policies would help to prevent or reduce future discrimination or inequitable treatment of transgender patients admitted to the unit?
4. What health-related concerns are important to consider for Victoria as a transgender adolescent?
5. Script a statement to advocate for Victoria's ongoing gender-affirming therapy based on clinical practice guidelines (Deutsch, 2016).

Terror as Enforcement

In April 2018, the federal government adopted a "zero-tolerance policy" prohibiting border crossing from Mexico into the United States (Domonoske & Gonzales, 2018). The policy included a cruel provision that separated children from parents and detained them in cells. In September 2020, a whistleblower and several detained immigrants filed a complaint against a detention center in Georgia (Project South et al., 2020; Treisman, 2020). The complaint described multiple cases of abuse, including forced hysterectomies, unsanitary conditions, and refusal to test and treat detainees for coronavirus. Similar to severe beatings intended to deter enslaved persons from running away, the cruel and inhumane conditions in detention centers were designed to instill a sense of fear to prevent future immigration attempts. As a result, survivors could experience significant psychological trauma for years to come. In a study of 425 children who were screened for symptoms of posttraumatic stress disorder after being held in detention centers, 17% met the criteria for the diagnosis, and 44% demonstrated at least one symptom in the domains of re-experiencing, avoidance, cognitive or mood change, and increased arousal (MacLean et al., 2019). In a study of 1,500 adults, those who experienced more adverse childhood or traumatic events had a higher likelihood of alcohol use as adults and chronic disease, depression, and posttraumatic stress disorder (Chang et al., 2019).

Inherent Superiority Versus Inherent Inferiority

Racism is internalized when persons within a marginalized group accept the negative assumptions about their racial group and themselves, their abilities, and their self-worth (Jones, 2000). It is associated with higher anxiety levels and symptoms of stress (Graham et al., 2016). While stress is physiologically beneficial to the body in appropriate doses, excessive or chronic stress, also known as allostatic load, can overwhelm homeostatic mechanisms and damage a person's health. Outcomes might include increased incidence of chronic disease and the experience of disability, pain, or earlier mortality (Guidi et al., 2021; Schneiderman et al., 2005). In a systematic review of 267 studies regarding the allostatic load, the following criteria were used to measure the concept: (a) the presence of a significant source of distress (e.g., chronic stress, a significant life event) or (b) stress associated with symptoms such as insomnia, anxiety, changes in energy, social or occupational functioning, or coping with daily life demands (Guidi et al., 2021). High allostatic load levels are associated with poor physical and mental health outcomes, such as cardiovascular disease, diabetes, stroke, anxiety and depression, and obesity (Beckie, 2012; Brody et al., 2014; Seeman et al., 2001).

Geronimus et al. (2006) identified the connection between race and allostatic load, noting that Black subjects' allostatic load scores were higher than those of White subjects in all age groups. Black women's scores exceed those of Black men. In a 2016 study ($n = 176$), the allostatic load was also significantly higher in Black women and was associated with discrimination, resultant negative affect, and impaired sleep (Tomfohr et al., 2016). Studies within Indigenous Canadian and Hispanic populations also identified elevated allostatic load levels. They were associated with discrimination, country of birth, and duration of residency in the United States/Canada (Currie et al., 2020; Salazar et al., 2016).

IMPLICATIONS

While not all vulnerable populations could be explicitly addressed here, this chapter provides a guide for examining vulnerability and risk for poor health using the framework of caste. Although much of the language regarding discrimination or bias pertains to race, White is not the only dominant group identity. Male sex, heterosexual identity, Christian religious affiliation, higher socioeconomic status, or nondisabled status afford dominant group members similar positions of power and privilege in U.S. society (Black & Stone, 2005; Minarik, 2017).

As the research literature on health disparities grows, investigators are beginning to address racism at the systemic level. Gee et al. (2009) used the analogy of discrimination as an iceberg. The observable part of the iceberg is visible above the water. It includes individual discriminatory acts and hate crimes, but the more substantial components of discrimination lie below the water's surface. These include implicit biases that are sometimes unconscious to the person who holds them and structural policies that support ongoing segregation and systems that advantage the dominant group and disadvantage non dominant group members (Gee et al., 2009). The Robert Wood Johnson Foundation proposed a health equity model that emphasizes individualizing health care delivery according to need (see also Figure 5.1).

Bowen Matthew (2015, p. 189) proposed antidiscrimination legislation reform as a potential remedy, stating that changes in laws "will impact social norms and incentivize longlasting protective interventions by institutional healthcare providers." Jones (2018), a leading expert in social determinants of health and antiracist activism, proposed a public health antiracism campaign. Jones identified three actions that individuals and organizations can take to begin the work of dismantling institutional, personally mediated, or internalized racism: (a) name racism and acknowledge its impact, (b) ask "How is racism operating here?" to identify the structures that sustain it, and (c) organize to take action (Jones, 2018). While both Jones and Bowen Matthew acknowledge that antibias training should accompany initiatives to address personally mediated racism and health disparities, meaningful change cannot occur without direct action at the institutional level—notably, actions involving health legislation, organizational policy, expanding access to health professional education, and healthcare funding.

CONCLUSION

Health inequities arise from multiple intersecting causes and require multifaceted approaches to reduce their occurrence and impact. Suggestions for improvement include, but are not limited to, the expansion of the ACA or the adoption of universal health care in the United States, reinstating affirmative action policies in organizations to allow for proportional representation of BIPOC in employment and educational settings, and expanding diversity and inclusion policies, such as widespread integration of holistic hiring practices or admissions review in higher education institutions. Such actions have the potential to reduce or eliminate the economic and educational disparities that negatively impact the health of BIPOC and other marginalized communities.

DISCUSSION QUESTIONS

1. What parallels can you draw among the pillars of caste and marginalized populations not represented in this chapter?
2. Are you aware of additional issues that influence racism or bias in healthcare or health professional education systems?
3. Identify individual and institutional actions (i.e., legislation, policies, practices) that might be implemented to improve health equity in your community.
4. What have you done to assess and monitor your bias in your daily activities and during the clinical encounter?
5. Discuss five activities that you could implement to improve your sensitivity to people who are members of minority and marginalized groups, including immigrants, migrants, and other displaced people.
6. Discuss the history of your particular racial/ethnic group in the context of being integrated into American culture.

REFERENCES

Adams, R. (2018, January 25). Immigration crackdown raises fears of seeking health care: Enforcement under the Trump administration sends the sick into the shadows. *Roll Call*. https://www.rollcall.com/2018/01/25/immigration-crackdown-raises-fears-of-seeking-health-care/

Aday, L. (2001). *At risk in America: The health and health care needs of vulnerable populations in the United States* (2nd ed.). Jossey-Bass Inc.

Aldridge, R.W., Story, A., Hwang, S.W., Nordentoft, M., Luchenski, S.A., Hartwell, G., Tweed, E.J., Lewer, D., Katkireddi, S.V., & Hayward, A.C. (2018). Morbidity and mortality in homeless individuals, prisoners, sex workers, and individuals with substance use disorders in high-income countries: A systematic review and meta-analysis. *Lancet, 391*, 241–250. https://doi.org/10.1016/S0140-6736(17)31869-X

Amiri, F. (2021, January 22). Legislator who questioned Black hygiene to lead health panel. Associated Press. https://apnews.com/article/health-ohio-coronavirus-pandemic-0dd121777081707b4c061ed8e4649df6

Beckie, T. M. (2012). A systematic review of allostatic load, health, and health disparities. *Biological Research for Nursing, 14*(4), 311–346. https://doi.org/10.1177/1099800412455688

Beech, B.M., Calles-Escandon, J., Hairston, K.G., Langdon, S.E., Latham-Sadler, B.A., & Bell, R.A. (2013). Mentoring programs for underrepresented minority faculty in academic medical centers: A systematic review of the literature. *Academic Medicine, 88*(4), 541–549. https://doi.org/10.1097/ACM.0b013e31828589e3

Bhaskar, R. & O'Hara, B. J. (2017). Indian health service coverage among American Indians and Alaska Natives in federal tribal lands. *Jorunal of Health Care Poor Underserved, 28*(4), 1361–1375. https://doi.org/10.1353/hpu.2017.0120

Black, L. L. & Stone, D. (2005). Expanding the definition of privilege: The concept of social privilege. *Journal of Multicultural Counseling and Development, 33*, 243–255. https://doi.org/10.1002/j.2161-1912.2005.tb00020.x

Bleich, S. N., Findling, M. G., Casey, L. S., Blendon, R. J., Benson, J. M., SteelFisher, G. K., Sayde, J. M., & Miller, C. (2019). Discrimination in the United States: Experiences of black Americans. *Health Services Research, 54*(suppl 2),1399–1408. https://doi.org/10.1111/1475-6773.13220

Boertien, D., & Vignoli, D. (2019). Legalizing same-sex marriage matters for the subjective well-being of individuals in same-sex unions. *Demography, 56*, 2109–2121. https://doi.org/10.1007/s13524-019-00822-1

Bowen Matthew, D. (2015). Just medicine: A cure for racial inequality in American health care. New York University Press.

Brody, G. H., Lei, M. K., Chae, D. H., Yu, T., Kogan, S. M., & Beach, S. R. H. (2014). Perceived discrimination among African American adolescents and allostatic load: A longitudinal analysis with buffering effects. *Child Development*, 85(3), 989–1002. https://doi.org/10.1111/cdev.12213

Burgess, D. J., Crowley-Matoka, M., Phelan, S., Dovidio, J. F., Kerns, R., Roth, C., Saha, S., & van Ryn, M. (2008). Patient race and physicians' decisions to prescribe opioids for chronic low back pain. *Social Science and Medicine*, 67(11), 1852–1860. https://doi.org/10.1016/j.socscimed.2008.09.009

Byrd, W. M. & Clayton, L. A. (1992). An American health dilemma: A history of blacks in the health system. *Journal of the National Medical Association*, 84(2) 189–200.

Cameron, C. (2020, July 24). Trump presses limits on transgender rights over supreme court ruling. The New York Times. https://www.nytimes.com/2020/07/24/us/politics/trump-transgender-rights-homeless.html

Cartwright, S. (1851). Diseases and peculiarities of the negro race. De Bow's Southern and Western Review, *IV*, 331–336. https://www.google.com/books/edition/Debow_s_Review/3K9IAAAAYAAJ?q=Negro+Cartwrig%20%20%20ht&gbpv=0#f=false

Centers for Disease Control. (2019). Racial and ethnic disparities continue in pregnancy-related deaths: Black, American Indian/Alaska Native women most affected. Centers for Disease Control. https://www.cdc.gov/media/releases/2019/p0905-racial-ethnic-disparities-pregnancy-deaths.html

Chang, X., Jiang, X., Mkandarwire, T., & Shen, M. (2019). Associations between adverse childhood experiences and health outcomes in adults aged 18–59. *PLoS ONE*, 14(2), e0211850. https://link.gale.com/apps/doc/A573035302/HWRC?u=csusj&sid=bookmark-HWRC&xid=dbac9631

Coard, M. (2019, March 15). Drapetomania: Compliant blacks sane, resistant blacks insane. The Philadelphia Tribune. https://www.phillytrib.com/commentary/drapetomania-compliant-blacks-sane-resisting-blacks-insane/article_0087a2d0-1acb-5364-870c-1205212e0a13.html

Colen, C. G., Ramey, D. M., Cooksey, E. C., & Williams, D. R. (2018). Racial disparities in health among nonpoor African Americans and Hispanics: The role of acute and chronic discrimination. *Social Science and Medicine*, 199, 167–180. https://doi.org/10.1016/j.socscimed.2017.04.051

Collins, C. F. (2004). What we do and don't know about 'race', 'ethnicity', genetics and health at the dawn of the genome era. *Nature Genetics*, 36(11), S13–S15. https://doi.org/10.1038/ng1436

Cooper, H., & Shear, M. (2021, January 25). Biden ends military's transgender ban, part of broad discrimination fight. The New York Times. https://www.nytimes.com/2021/01/25/us/politics/biden-military-transgender.html

Cronin, M. (2020). Anarcha, Betsey, Lucy, and the women whose names were not recorded: The legacy of J Marion Sims. *Anaesthesia and Intensive Care*, 48(S3), 6–13. https://doi.org/10.1177/0310057X20966606

Currie, C. L., Copeland, J. L., Metz, G. A., Moon-Riley, K. C., & Davies, C. M. (2020). Past-year racial discrimination and allostatic load among indigenous adults in Canada: The role of cultural continuity. *Psychosomatic Medicine*, 82(1), 99–107. https://doi.org/10.1097/PSY.0000000000000754

Deutsch, M. B. (2016). Guidelines for the primary and gender-affirming care of transgender and gender nonbinary people. Center of Excellence for Transgender Health. https://transcare.ucsf.edu/sites/transcare.ucsf.edu/files/Transgender-PGACG-6-17-16.pdf

Dirks, N. B. (2011). Castes of mind: Colonialism and the making of modern India. Princeton University Press.

Domonoske, C., & Gonzales, R. (2018, June 19). What we know: Family separation and "zero tolerance" at the border. National Public Radio. https://www.npr.org/2018/06/19/621065383/what-we-know-family-separation-and-zero-tolerance-at-the-border

Doshi, M., Lopez, W. D., Mesa, H., Bryce, R., Rabinowitz, E., Rion, R. et al. (2020). Barriers & facilitators to healthcare and social services among undocumented Latino(a)/Latinx immigrant clients: Perspectives from frontline service providers in Southeast Michigan. *PLoS One*, 15(6), e0233839. https://doi.org/10.1371/journal.pone.0233839

Downing, J., & Cha, P. (2020). Same-sex marriage and gains in employer-sponsored insurance for U.S. adults 2008–2017. *American Journal of Public Health*, 110(4), 537–539. https://doi.org/10.2105/AJPH.2019.305510

Eligon, J. (2020, December 25). Black doctor dies of COVID-19 after complaining of racist treatment. The New York Times. https://www.nytimes.com/2020/12/23/us/susan-moore-black-doctor-indiana.html

Epstein, A. M., Ayanian, J. Z., Keogh, J. H., Noonan, S. J., Armistead, N., Cleary, P. D., Weissman, J. S., David-Kasdan, J. A., Carlson, D., Fuller, J., Marsh, D., & Conti, R. M. (2000). Racial disparities in access to renal transplantation—clinically appropriate or due to underuse or overuse? *New England Journal of Medicine*, 343(21), 1537–1544. https://doi.org/10.1056/nejm200011233432106

FitzGerald, C., & Hurst, S. (2017). Implicit bias in healthcare professionals: A systematic review. *BMC Medical Ethics*, 18(1), 19. https://doi.org/10.1186/s12910-017-0179-8

Ford, M. E. & Kelly, P. A. (2005). Conceptualizing and categorizing race and ethnicity in health services research. *Health Services Research, 40*(5), 1658–1675. https://doi.org/10.1111/j.1475-6773.2005.00449.x

Gee, G. C., Ro, A., Shariff-Marco, S., & Chae, D. (2009). Racial discrimination and health among Asian Americans: Evidence, assessment, and directions for future research. *Epidemiologic Reviews, 31*, 130–151. https://doi.org/10.1093/epirev/mxp009

Gellately, R. (2001). Backing Hitler: Consent and Coercion in Nazi Germany. Oxford University Press.

Georgetown University Law Library. (2021a, January 27). A brief history of the civil rights movement in the United States. https://guides.ll.georgetown.edu/c.php?g=592919&p=4172702

Georgetown University Law Library. (2021b, April 21). A timeline of the legalization of same-sex marriage in the U.S. https://guides.ll.georgetown.edu/c.php?g=592919&p=4182201

Geronimus, A. T., Hicken, M., Keene, D., & Bound, J. (2006). "Weathering" and age patterns of allostatic load scores among blacks and whites in the United States. *American Journal of Public Health, 96*(5), 826–833. https://doi.org/10.2105/AJPH.2004.060749

Goldsen, J., Bryan, A. E. B., Kim, H.-J., Muraco, A., Jen, S., & Fredriksen-Goldsen, K. I. (2017). Who says I do: The changing context of marriage and health and quality of life for LGBT older adults. *Gerontologist, 57*(S1), S50–S62. https://doi.org/10.1093/geront/gnw174

Gonzales, G. (2017). Health insurance coverage among Puerto Rican adults in same-sex relationships. *Jorunal of Health Care Poor Underserved, 28*(3), 915–930. https://doi.org/10.1353/hpu.2017.0088

Graham, G. N., Jones, P. G., Chan, P. S., Arnold, S. V., Krumholz, H. M., & Spertus, J. A. (2018). Racial disparities in patient characteristics and survival after acute myocardial infarction. *JAMA Network Open, 1*(7), e184240. https://doi.org/10.1001/jamanetworkopen.2018.4240

Graham, J. R., West, L. M., Martinez, J., & Roemer, L. (2016). The mediating role of internalized racism in the relationship between racist experiences and anxiety symptoms in a black American sample. *Culturl Divers and Ethnic Minor Psychology, 22*(3), 369–376. https://doi.org/10.1037/hea0000251

Grant, J., Mottet, L., Tanis, J., Harrison, J., Herman, J., & Keisling, M. (2011). Injustice at every turn: A report of the national transgender discrimination survey. https://www.transequality.org/sites/default/files/docs/resources/NTDS_Report.pdf

Guidi, J., Lucent, M., Sonino, N., & Fava, G.A. (2021). Allostatic load and its impact on health: A systematic review. *Psychotherapy and Psychosomatics, 90*, 11–21. https://doi.org/10.1159/000510696

Hacker, K., Anies, M., Folb, B. L., & Zallman, L. (2015). Barriers to health care for undocumented immigrants: a literature review. *Risk Management and Healthcare Policy, 8*, 175–183. https://doi.org/10.2147/RMHP.S70173

Hampton, M., Dawkins, D., Rickman Patrick, S., O'Leary-Kelley, C., Onglengco, R., & Stobbe, B. (2022). Nursing program admission barriers in the United States: Considerations for increasing black student enrollment. *Nurse Educator, 47*(1).

Harvard School of Public Health, Robert Wood Johnson Foundation, & National Public Radio. (2017, November 21). Poll finds a majority of LGBTQ Americans report violence, threats, or sexual harassment related to sexual orientation or gender identity; one-third report bathroom harassment. https://www.hsph.harvard.edu/news/press-releases/poll-lgbtq-americans-discrimination/

Health Resources and Services Administration. (2006). The rationale for diversity in the health professions: A review of the evidence. In U.S. Department of Health and Human Services. https://www.semanticscholar.org/paper/The-Rationale-for-Diversity-in-the-Health-%3A-A-of-Saha-Shipman/6df3f71b73df07800b82250c2bf87ce594bbf667

Health Resources and Services Administration & National Center for Health Workforce Analysis. (2017). Sex, race, and ethnic diversity of U.S. health occupations (2011–2015). In U.S. Department of Health and Human Services. https://bhw.hrsa.gov/sites/default/files/bureau-health-workforce/data-research/diversity-us-health-occupations.pdf

Hoffman, K. M., Trawalter, S., Axt, J. R., & Oliver, M. N. (2016). Racial bias in pain assessment and treatment recommendations, and false beliefs about biological differences between blacks and whites. *Proceedings of the National Academy of Sciences of the United States of America, 113*(16), 4296–4301. https://doi.org/10.1073/pnas.1516047113

Horowitz, J. M., Parker, K., Brown, A., & Cox, K. (2020, October 6). Amid national reckoning, Americans divided on whether increased focus on race will lead to major policy change: More Black adults now say the country has work to do to address racial inequality; attitudes of White adults largely unchanged since 2019. Pew Research Center. https://www.pewresearch.org/social-trends/2020/10/06/amid-national-reckoning-americans-divided-on-whether-increased-focus-on-race-will-lead-to-major-policy-change/

Human Genome Program, U.S. Department of Energy. (2008). Genomics and its impact on science and society: A 2008 primer. https://web.ornl.gov/sci/techresources/Human_Genome/publicat/primer2001/

Human Rights Campaign. (2021). Fatal violence against the transgender and gender non-conforming community in 2021. https://www.hrc.org/resources/fatal-violence-against-the-transgender-and-gender-non-conforming-community-in-2021

Human Rights Campaign. (2020). Fatal violence against the transgender and gender non-conforming community in 2020. https://www.hrc.org/resources/violence-against-the-trans-and-gender-non-conforming-community-in-2020

Indian Health Service. (2021, March 13). Indian Health Service: The federal health program for American Indians and Alaska Natives. IHS Headquarters. https://www.ihs.gov/locations/

Institute of Medicine. (2003). Unequal treatment: Confronting racial and ethnic disparities in healthcare. https://www.nap.edu/catalog/12875/unequal-treatment-confronting-racial-and-ethnic-disparities-in-health-care

Interlandi, J. (2019). Why doesn't the United States have universal health care? The answer begins with policies enacted after the Civil War. In N. Jones (Ed.), *The 1619 Project*. New York Times. https://www.nytimes.com/interactive/2019/08/14/magazine/1619-america-slavery.html

James, S. E., Herman, J. L., Rankin, S., Keisling, M., Mottet, L., & Anafi, M. (2016). The report of the 2015 U.S. Transgender Survey. National Center for Transgender Equality. https://transequality.org/sites/default/files/docs/usts/USTS-Full-Report-Dec17.pdf

Jones, C. (2018). Toward the science and practice of antiracism: Launching a national campaign against racism. *Ethnicity & Disease, 28*(suppl 1), 231–234. https://doi.org/10.18865/ed.28.S1.231

Jones, C. (2000). Levels of racism: A theoretic framework and a Gardener's tale. *American Journal of Public Health, 90*, 1212–1215. https://doi.org/10.2105/ajph.90.8.1212

Kaiser Family Foundation. (2019). Distribution of the nonelderly with Medicaid by race/ethnicity. https://www.kff.org/medicaid/state-indicator/medicaid-distribution-nonelderly-by-raceethnicity/?currentTimeframe=0&selectedRows=%7B%22wrapups%22:%7B%22united-states%22:%7B%7D%7D%7D&sortModel=%7B%22colId%22:%22Location%22,%22sort%22:%22asc%22%7D

Kaiser Family Foundation. (2021, March 3). KFF health tracking poll: The public's views on the ACA. https://www.kff.org/interactive/kff-health-tracking-poll-the-publics-views-on-the-aca/#?response=Favorable--Unfavorable&aRange=twoYear

Kaiser Health News. (2016, April 14). Underfunding and access barriers to healthcare for Native Americans, especially on the reservation. https://www.healthcarefinancenews.com/news/underfunding-and-access-are-barriers-healthcare-native-americans-especially-reservation

Kennedy, K. (2018, January 21). Deportation fears have legal immigrants avoiding health care. Associated Press. https://apnews.com/article/9f893855e49143baad9c96816ec8f731

Kominski, G. F., Nonzee, N. J., & Sorensen, A. (2017). The affordable care act's impacts on access to insurance and health care for low-income populations. *Annual Review of Public Health, 38*, 489–505. https://doi.org/10.1146/annurev-publhealth-031816-044555

Ladson-Billings, G. (2007). Pushing past the achievement gap: An essay on the language of deficit. *Journal of Negro Education, 76*(3), 316–323. https://www.jstor.org/stable/40034574

Liptak, A. (2021, June 17). Affordable Care Act survives latest Supreme Court Challenge. New York Times. https://www.nytimes.com/2021/06/17/us/obamacare-supreme-court.html

Little, B. (2021). How the Nazis were inspired by Jim Crow: To craft legal discrimination, the Third Reich studies the United States. A&E Television Networks, LLC. https://www.history.com/news/how-the-nazis-were-inspired-by-jim-crow

Marmot, M. (2017). Social justice, epidemiology and health inequalities. *European Journal of Epidemiology, 32*, 537–546. https://doi.org/10.1007/s10654-017-0286-3

Marmot, M., Allen, J., Goldblatt, P., Boyce, T., McNeish, D. et al. (2010). Fair society, healthy lives – the marmot review: strategic review of health inequities in England post-2010. The Marmot Review. http://www.instituteofhealthequity.org/resources-reports/fair-society-healthy-lives-the-marmot-review/fair-society-healthy-lives-full-report-pdf.pdf

Martino, S. C., Elliott, M. N., Hambarsoomian, K., Garcia, A. N., Wilson-Frederick, S., Gaillot, S., Weech-Maldonado, R., & Haviland, A. M. (2020). Disparities in care experienced by American Indian and Alaska Native medicare beneficiaries. *Med Care, 58* 981–987. https://doi.org/10.1097/MLR.0000000000001392

MacLean, S. A., Agyeman, P. O., Walther, J., Singer, E. K., Baranowski, K. A., & Katz, C. L. (2019). Mental health of children held at a United States immigration detention center. *Social Science and Medicine, 230*, 303–308.

Mechanic, D., & Tanner, J. (2007). Vulnerable people, groups, and populations: Societal view. *Health Aff (Millwood), 26*(5), 1220–1230. https://doi.org/10.1377/hlthaff.26.5.1220

Metzl, J. (2019). *Dying of whiteness: How the politics of racial resentment is killing America's Heartland*. Basic Books.

Minarik, J. D. (2017). Privilege as privileging: Making the dynamic and complex nature of privilege and marginalization accessible. *Journal of Social Work Education, 53*(1), 52–65. https://doi.org/10.1080/10437797.2016.1237913

Nalliah, R. P., Timothé, P., & Reddy, M. S. (2021). Diversity, equity, and inclusion interventions to support admissions have had little benefit to black students over past 20 years. *Journal of Dental Education, 85*(4), 448–455. https://doi.org/10.1002/jdd.12611

National Academies of Sciences, Engineering, and Medicine. (2017). Communities in Action: Pathways to equity. The National Academies Press. https://www.ncbi.nlm.nih.gov/books/NBK425848/pdf/Bookshelf_NBK425848.pdf

National Institutes of Health. (2021). What is the Human Genome Project? https://www.genome.gov/human-genome-project/What

Obergefell et al. v. Hodges. (2015). Certiorari to the United States court of appeals for the sixth circuit. https://www.supremecourt.gov/opinions/14pdf/14-556_3204.pdf

Out2Enroll. (2021). Summary of findings: 2021 marketplace plan compliance with section 1557. https://out2enroll.org/out2enroll/wp-content/uploads/2020/11/Report-on-Trans-Exclusions-in-2021-Marketplace-Plans.pdf

Perez-Stable, E. J. & Sayre, M. H. (2019). Reducing health disparities to promote health equity through policy research. *Ethnicity & Disease, 29*(S2), 321–322. https://doi.org/10.18865/ed.29.S2.321

Project South, Georgia Detention Watch, Georgia Latino Alliance for Human Rights, & South Georgia Immigrant Support Network. (2020). Institute for the elimination of poverty and suicide. https://projectsouth.org/wp-content/uploads/2020/09/OIG-ICDC-Complaint-1.pdf

Quan, K. (2013). The high costs of language barriers in medical malpractice. In S. L. Spector & M. Youdelman (Eds.). University of California, Berkeley, School of Public Health. National Health Law Program. https://healthlaw.org/resource/the-high-costs-of-language-barriers-in-medical-malpractice/

Rogers, T. N., Rogers, C. R., VanSant-Webb, E., Gu, L. Y., Yan, B., & Qeadan, F. (2020). Racial disparities in COVID-19 Mortality among essential workers in the United States. *World Medical & Health Policy.* https://doi.org/10.1002/wmh3.358

Sabin, J. A., & Greenwald, A. G. (2012). The influence of implicit bias on treatment recommendations for 4 common pediatric conditions: Pain, urinary tract infection, attention deficit hyperactivity disorder, and asthma. *American Journal of Public Health, 102,* 988–995. https://doi.org/10.2105/AJPH.2011.300621

Salam, M. (2018, January 11). For Serena Williams, childbirth was a harrowing ordeal. She's not alone. The New York Times. https://www.nytimes.com/2018/01/11/sports/tennis/serena-williams-baby-vogue.html

Salazar, C. R., Strizich, G., Seeman, T. E., Isasi, C. R., Gallo, L. C., Aviles-Santa, L. M., Cai, J., Penedo, F. J., Arguelles, W., Sanders, A. E., Lipton, R. B., & Kaplan, R. C. (2016). Nativity differences in allostatic load by age, sex, and Hispanic background from the Hispanic Community Health Study/Study of Latinos. *SSM Popul Health, 2,* 416–424. https://doi.org/10.1016/j.ssmph.2016.05.003

Santoro, W. A. (2015). Was the civil rights movement successful? Tracking and understanding black views. *Sociological Forum, 30*(S1), 627–647. http://www.jstor.org/stable/43654410

Schneiderman, N., Ironson, G., & Siegel, S. D. (2005). Stress and health: Psychological, behavioral, and biological determinants. *Annual Review of Clinical Psychology, 1,* 607–628. https://doi.org/10.1146/annurev.clinpsy.1.102803.144141

Schiaffino, M. K., Nara, A., & Mao, L. (2016). Language services in hospitals vary by ownership and location. *Health Affairs (Project Hope), 35*(8), 1399–1403. https://doi.org/10.1377/hlthaff.2015.0955

Seeman, T. E., McEwen, B. S., Rowe, J. W., & Singer, B. H. (2001). Allostatic load as a marker of cumulative biological risk: MacArthur studies of successful aging. *Proceedings of the National Academy of Sciences of the United States of America, 98*(8), 4770–4775. https://doi.org/10.1073/pnas.081072698

Sentell, T., Braun, K. L., Davis, J., & Dsavis, T. (2013). Colorectal cancer screening: Low health literacy and limited English proficiency among Asians and Whites in California. *Journal of Health Commununication, 18*(suppl 1), 242–251. https://doi.org/10.1080/10810730.2013.825669

Siegler, K. (2021, February 19). Why native Americans are getting COVID-19 vaccines faster. *National Public Radio.* https://www.npr.org/2021/02/19/969046248/why-native-americans-are-getting-the-covid-19-vaccines-faster

Sosin, K. (2020, August 25). The only comprehensive study on transgender people is not coming out as planned: The U.S. Trans Survey offers some of the only data on trans life in America, but a nonprofit's shortfalls and the pandemic threaten its future. The 19th. https://19thnews.org/2020/08/the-only-comprehensive-study-on-transgender-people-is-not-coming-out-as-planned/

Statistical Atlas. (2018, January 27). Languages in California. https://statisticalatlas.com/state/California/Languages

Steele, C., Rim, S., Joseph, D., King, J., & Seeff, L. (2013). Colorectal cancer incidence and screening – United States, 2008 and 2010. *Morbidity and Mortality Weekly Report, 62*(3), 53–60.

Stepanikova, I., & Oates, G. (2017). Perceived discrimination and privilege in health care: The role of socioeconomic status and race. *American Journal of Preventive Medicine, 52*(suppl 1), S86–S94. https://doi.org/10.1016/j.amepre.2016.09.024.

Stroumsa, D. (2014). The state of transgender health care: policy, law, and medical frameworks. *American Journal of Public Health, 104*(3), e31–e38. https://doi.org/10.2105/AJPH.2013.301789

Taira, B. R., Torres, J., Nguyen, A., Guo, R., & Samra, S. (2020). Language assistance for the care of limited English proficiency (LEP) patients in the emergency department: A survey of providers and staff. *Journal of Immigrant and Minority Health*, 22, 439–447. https://doi.org/10.1007/s10903-019-00964-9

Thornton, R. L. J., Glover, C. M., Cene, C. W., Glik, D. C., Henderson, J. A., & Williams, D. R. (2016). Evaluating strategies for reducing health disparities by addressing the social determinants of health. *Health Affairs (Millwood)*, 35(8), 1416–1423. https://doi.org/10.1377/hlthaff.2015.1357

Tomfohr, L. M., Pung, M. A., & Dimsdale, J. E. (2016). Mediators of the relationship between race and allostatic load in African and White Americans. *Health Psychology*, 35(4), 322–332. https://doi.org/10.1037/hea0000251

Treisman, R. (2020, September 16). Whistleblower alleges 'medical neglect,' questionable hysterectomies of ICE detainees. *National Public Radio*. https://www.npr.org/about-npr/177066727/visit-npr

United States Census Bureau. (2021). Quick facts. United States Department of Commerce. https://www.census.gov/quickfacts/fact/table/US/RHI225219

Wagner, R., Maddox, K. R., Glazer, G., & Hittle, B. M. (2020). Maximizing effectiveness of the holistic admission process: Implementing the multiple mini interview model. *Nurse Educator*, 45(2), 73–77. https://doi.org/10.1097/NNE.0000000000000702

Whitman, J. Q. (2017). Hitler's American model: The United States and the making of Nazi race law . Princeton University Press.

Wilkerson, I. (2020). *Caste: The origins of our discontents*. Random House.

Witzburg, R. A., & Sondheimer, H. M. (2013). Holistic review—shaping the medical profession one applicant at a time. *New England Journal of Medicine*, 368(17), 1565–1567. https://doi.org/10.1056/NEJMp1300411

World Health Organization. (2019, August 23). Lead poisoning and health. World Health Organization. https://www.who.int/news-room/fact-sheets/detail/lead-poisoning-and-health

World Health Organization. (2018, February 22). Health inequities and their causes. World Health Organization. https://www.who.int/news-room/facts-in-pictures/detail/health-inequities-and-their-causes#:~:text=Health%20inequities%20are%20differences%20in,right%20mix%20of%20government%20policies

Wros, P., & Noone, J. (2018). Holistic admissions in undergraduate nursing: One school's journey and lessons learned. *Journal of Professional Nursing*, 34, 211–216. https://doi.org/10.1016/j.profnurs.2017.08.005

Xue, Y., & Brewer, C. (2014). Racial and ethnic diversity of the U.S. national nurse workforce 1988-2013. *Policy, Politics & Nursing Practice*, 15(3–4), 102–110. https://doi.org/10.1177/1527154414560291

SECTION III
Exemplars of Health Disparities

CHAPTER 15

Self-Care Management of Individuals With Diabetes in Vulnerable Populations

Mary Beth Modic

LEARNING OBJECTIVES

- Describe the epidemiology, diagnosis, and treatment of diabetes.

- Explore the factors, including the social determinants of health (SDH), that impact the successful management of diabetes.

- Discuss the impact that health literacy and numeracy have on diabetes self-care practices.

- Understand the use of technology such as insulin pumps and external glucose monitors in managing diabetes.

- Examine communication strategies that foster relationships between patients and their healthcare providers.

- Describe the seven key focus areas for diabetes management espoused by the Association of Diabetes Care and Education Specialists (ADCES).

INTRODUCTION

Diabetes is now the most expensive chronic disease in the United States. It is a global concern with an estimated global cost projected to exceed $760 billion (International Diabetes Federation [IDF], 2019). This chapter (a) reviews the epidemiology, diagnosis, and treatment of diabetes; (b) explores the environmental, socioeconomic, and physiological factors, including the social determinants of health, that impact the development of type 2 diabetes mellitus (T2DM); (c) discusses technological and programmatic resources to help persons with diabetes; (d) discusses the impact of health literacy and numeracy on diabetes self-care practices; (e) examines communication models and mnemonics that foster relationships between patients and providers; and (f) describes the seven key focus areas for diabetes management espoused by the Association of Diabetes Care and Education Specialists (ADCES).

The Epidemiology, Diagnosis, and Treatment of Diabetes

Diabetes is an international health concern. The IDF purports that 537 million adults (age 20–79 years) are living with diabetes across the globe. This number includes individuals living with both type 1 diabetes mellitus (T1DM) and T2DM, and represents an increase of 74 million individuals (16%) since 2019 (IDF, 2021). The top 10 countries with the most significant prevalence of diabetes spans continents. See Table 15.1 for global diabetes prevalence by region. China has the greatest number of people living with diabetes (IDF, 2019). In 2019, the World Health Organization [WHO] attributed 1.5 million deaths to diabetes globally (Fang et al., 2021; IDF, 2019).

The prevalence of diabetes has increased from less than 1% of the population in the United States in 1958 to more than 10.5% in 2020 due to changes in physical activity and the increased consumption of processed food (Centers for Disease Control and Prevention [CDC], 2020a). The economic costs of diabetes have escalated by 28% from 2012 to 2017. Approximately one out of every four healthcare dollars in the United States is spent on diabetes, with 61% being spent on individuals 65 years and older (American Diabetes Association [ADA], 2018a). Individuals diagnosed with diabetes have medical costs that average $9,600 a year (ADA, 2018a). The CDC reported in 2020 that 34.2 million people have diabetes, and 88 million have prediabetes.

Diabetes is the seventh leading cause of death in the United States. Of all healthcare expenses associated with diabetes, only 14% is expended on treating the disease itself, while 86% is spent on managing diabetes complications (Statista.com, 2021). Of the $3.6 trillion spent annually on healthcare in the United States, only 3% or $108 billion is spent on health promotion and disease prevention (Trust for America's Health, 2021).

TABLE 15.1 Diabetes Prevalence Across the World (2021)

Regions	2021 Diabetes Prevalence	2045 Diabetes Prevalence	Number Undiagnosed (in millions)	Deaths in 2021	Diabetes Expenditures (U.S. dollars)
World	536.6 million	783.2 million	239.7 (1 in 2 people)	6.7 million	$966 billion
Africa	24 million	55 million	12.7 (1 in 2 people)	406.000	No data reported
Europe	61 million	69 million	21.9 (1 in 3 people)	1.1 million	$189 billion
Middle East and North Africa	73 million	136 million	27.3 (1 in 3 people)	796,000	No data reported
North America and Caribbean	51 million	63 million	12.2 (1 in 4 people)	931,000	$415 billion
South and Central America	32 million	49 million	10.7 (1 in 3 people)	410,000	$65 billion
Southeast Asia	90 million	151 million	46.2 (1 in 2 people)	747,000	$10 billion
Western Pacific	206 million	260 million	108.7 (1 in 2 people)	2.3 million	$24 billion

Source: International Diabetes Federation. (2021). *IDF diabetes atlas (10th ed.).* International Diabetes Foundation. https://diabetesatlas.org/

Diabetes mellitus occurs when there is a disruption of beta cell function in the pancreas. The beta cells become incapable of maintaining adequate insulin secretion to prevent hyperglycemia. Classifications of different types of diabetes have evolved over the years as knowledge has advanced. Terms have changed from juvenile- and adult-onset diabetes to insulin-dependent and noninsulin-dependent diabetes and, most recently, type 1 (T1DM) and type 2 (T2DM). The change in name was necessary to clarify two important concepts. Firstly, children as young as 3 years old are being diagnosed with T2DM (Yafi, 2015), which contradicts the "adult-onset" label. This rise in T2DM in children is being attributed to the growing number of children who are either overweight or obese. The increased incidence of obesity and being overweight in children have resulted from physical inactivity, overeating, an unhealthy diet due to living in food deserts or familial food practices, and stress (Buttermore et al., 2021). Some studies have suggested that children of women with gestational diabetes may be at greater risk of developing T2DM later in life due to an adverse intrauterine environment (Buttermore et al., 2021). The second factor that led to renaming diabetes types is that adults diagnosed with diabetes may require insulin to manage their blood glucose negating the label of non insulin-dependent (Buttermore et al., 2021). In addition to T1DM and T2DM, there are several other types of diabetes, including gestational diabetes, latent diabetes of adulthood (LADA), mature onset diabetes of youth (MODY), neonatal diabetes, Flatbush/Wolfram Syndrome, and steroid-induced diabetes, which preclude examination in this chapter (Cornell et al., 2020).

T1DM accounts for approximately 5% to 10% of diabetes diagnoses. It is characterized by absolute insulin deficiency. While the exact etiology is not known, it is posited that there is an environmental trigger, such as a virus, coupled with genetic susceptibility, which causes an autoimmune response that attacks the beta cells resulting in their destruction (ADA, 2018b). It occurs primarily in children and adolescents and is one of the most frequently diagnosed chronic conditions. T1DM is not preventable (IDF, 2019). The classic symptoms of weight loss, polyuria (excessive urination), polydipsia (excessive thirst), polyphagia (extreme hunger), and high glucose are often exhibited at the time of diagnosis (ADA, 2020). Exogenous insulin is necessary to sustain life because the beta cells of the pancreas no longer produce insulin. Without insulin, a person with T1DM will die.

T2DM is a complex metabolic disorder with many genetic and environmental causes. The precise cause of T2DM is not entirely understood (ADA, 2020). There is an association with genetic predisposition, obesity, physical inactivity, and aging. Tremendous efforts are being directed to uncover the genetic determinants of the disease. It is predicted that future research will discover that the etiology of diabetes will be the interaction of genes with the environment (IDF, 2021). T2DM usually begins with insulin resistance. This occurs when glucose uptake is impaired in the liver, skeletal muscle, and adipose tissue, and the body cannot use the insulin that is secreted. Individuals often experience no symptoms before their diagnosis. As a result, there may be an extended period before a diagnosis of diabetes is rendered, where microvascular and macrovascular changes may have already occurred (ADA, 2020).

T2DM is initially treated by lifestyle modifications that include recommendations or consultations to other health professionals on how to increase physical activity, eat more healthfully, maintain a healthy weight, and increase the hours of restful sleep to prevent beta-cell apoptosis. Oral glucose-lowering medications, noninsulin injectables, and insulin may be necessary to manage T2DM in addition to lifestyle changes (IDF, 2021). Approximately 90% to 95% of all diabetes cases are attributed to T2DM (ADA, 2021). See Table 15.2 for a comparison of T1DM and T2DM. Prediabetes is a precursor to the development of T2DM. It is a condition where glucose is higher than normal but does not meet the diagnostic threshold for diabetes. Individuals with an A1C between 5.7% (glucose value of 117 mg/dL) and 6.4% (glucose value of 137 mg/dL) are considered to have prediabetes. The A1C test is also known as the glycated hemoglobin test; it measures the percentage of glucose attached to the hemoglobin in red blood cells and assesses a person's average blood glucose level over the previous 3 months (ADA, 2018c).

TABLE 15.2 Comparison of Type 1 and Type 2 Diabetes

Descriptor	Type 1 Diabetes	Type 2 Diabetes
Prevalence	◆ Found in 5%–10% of diabetics	◆ Found in 90%–95% of diabetics
Symptoms and diagnosis	◆ Usually diagnosed before the age of 30 ◆ Characterized by the absence of insulin production ◆ Sudden onset of symptoms ◆ Symptoms include excessive thirst, urination, weight loss, and high serum glucose levels ◆ Cause is unknown although an infection causing an autoimmune response attacking the pancreas and the beta cells is possible ◆ Weak family history ◆ More common in Caucasians	◆ Usually diagnosed after the age of 40 but has been in found in children ◆ Characterized by insulin resistance ◆ Slow onset of symptoms ◆ Symptoms include excessive thirst and urination, weight loss and high serum glucose levels ◆ Risk factors include lifestyle issues such as obesity ◆ Strong family history ◆ More common in Black and Hispanic individuals. Most common in Native Americans
Treatment	Endogenous Insulin necessary for survival	May be treated with lifestyle changes alone or in combination with oral drugs, noninsulin injectables, or insulin

Source: Data from Cornell, S., Halstenson, C., & Miller, D. (Eds.) (2020). *The art and science of diabetes care* (5th ed.). Association of Diabetes Care and Education Specialists.

People with prediabetes tend to be overweight or obese and have impaired fasting glucose (IFG) between 100 and 125 mg/dL and impaired glucose tolerance (IGT) (CDC, 2020b). Recall that individuals with prediabetes may not even know they have it and are at risk of developing T2DM (Cornell et al., 2020). Individuals with prediabetes are encouraged to lose weight, increase physical activity, and change their daily consumption of foods high in calories and low in nutritional value.

While losing weight often seems daunting to a person with more than 50 pounds to lose, healthcare professionals can encourage individuals to set realistic and achievable goals. The Diabetes Prevention Program (DPP) outcomes support achievable goal setting. The DPP was a 27-center randomized clinical trial that examined the results of diabetes prevention strategies in 1,079 racially and ethnically diverse individuals at high risk for developing T2DM. The study demonstrated that participants who lost 7% of their body weight and increased their daily physical activity to 150 minutes per week, resulting in a 700-calorie expenditure increase per day, reduced their risk of developing T2DM by 58% (DPP Research Group, 2002). A follow-up study examining the impact of the DPP revealed that the effects of the lifestyle interventions and use of metformin (an oral glucose-lowering agent) were sustained for 15 years, although there was some reduced efficacy. There was a substantive reduction in the rate of developing T2DM in the intervention group compared to the placebo group (Kriska et al., 2021).

The U.S. Preventive Services Task Force (2021) recommends that screening for prediabetes be considered for all nonpregnant adults ranging in age from 35 to 70 years who are overweight with a body mass index (BMI) of 25 kg/m² or are obese with a BMI of 30 kg/m². Screening should be offered at a younger age to an individual from a population with a high prevalence of diabetes, including American Indian/Alaska Native, Black, Hawaiian/Pacific

TABLE 15.3 Diabetes by Race/Ethnicity

American Indian/Alaskan Native	14.5%
Black/non-Hispanic	12.1%
Hispanic	11.8%
Asian American	9.5%
White/non-Hispanic	7.4%

Source: American Diabetes Association. (2022). Statistics about diabetes. https://diabetes.org/about-us/statistics/about-diabetes

Islander, Hispanic/Latinos populations. People of Asian descent with a BMI of 23 kg/m^2 should also be screened. The lower BMI criteria for Asian individuals is due to the association of fat distribution in the abdomen and increased risk of diabetes at a lower BMI (Hsu et al., 2015).

Diabetes can contribute to developing heart disease, kidney disease, adult-onset blindness, and nontraumatic amputations (CDC, 2020a). Of all the racial and ethnic groups in the United States, American Indians and Alaskan Natives have the highest prevalence of diabetes among individuals in the five racial and ethnic classifications. Diabetes is also more prevalent in Hispanics and African Americans than White individuals (ADA, 2018c; Table 15.3). While there is no empirical evidence to explain why these groups of individuals are at higher risk than other races or ethnicities, various biological, behavioral, environmental, and socioeconomic factors affect the development of diabetes in these groups. It is conjectured that African Americans and Latinos have increased insulin resistance and more significant insulin secretion/hyperinsulinemia (Spanakis & Golden, 2013). This means that since insulin cannot get into muscle, fat, and the liver, the body compensates by making more insulin resulting in hyperinsulinemia (Buttermore et al., 2021).

Factors Influencing the Development of Diabetes

Obesity

Obesity represents one of the most decisive factors in the development of T2DM.

BMI is a screening tool for determining underweight, normal/average weight, overweight, and obesity. Being overweight equals a BMI between 25 and 30 kg/m^2. The diagnosis of obesity is assigned to an individual with a BMI greater than 30 kg/m^2. In addition to the frequently cited explanations for the obesity epidemic—increase in sedentary lifestyles and overconsumption of calorically dense food—the nutritional landscape is different. How food is grown, raised, processed, cooked, and prepared has changed over the last four decades affecting its nutritional value (Popkin et al., 2012). Home economic classes have been eliminated from high school curricula, processed and prepared foods have become commonplace, and the frequency of eating away from home has become more routine since the 1970s (Nelson, 2013). In the 1970s, the portion of the "average" American budget allocated to dining out was 25%, in 1985 the percentage increased to 35%, by 1996, it was 40%, and in 2018, 44% of all food dollars was spent on eating away from home (Critser, 2003; Paulis, 2020). Finally, portion size, particularly in restaurants, has risen significantly over the five decades resulting in increased calorie consumption for the same food item. Today an average hamburger weighs approximately 12 ounces, and in the 1950s, it averaged 2.8 ounces.

While weight and BMI are indices of general health, where an individual carries excess adipose tissue is also of clinical significance. Fat accumulated in the lower body, hips, thigh, and buttocks is described as a pear shape body habitus. The fat is subcutaneous and is often more challenging to lose. An excess of fat in the abdomen is "visceral fat" or "intra-abdominal fat." Individuals with an abundance of visceral fat may be described as having central adiposity. Their abdomen protrudes significantly, and they are considered to have a body habitus that is apple-shaped. Visceral fat is correlated with higher total cholesterol, low-density lipoproteins (LDL) referred to as "bad cholesterol," and lower high-density lipoproteins (HDL) known as "good cholesterol" (Cornell et al., 2020).

Social Determinants of Health

The SDH are the nonphysiological conditions that influence the health and well-being of individuals, including the development of diabetes. They are the conditions in which people are born, live, grow, learn, play, pray, and work (Hill-Briggs et al., 2021). Neighborhood factors, such as food insecurity, inhabitable housing, and community safety, have been associated with glucose management (Walker et al., 2016). Healthcare providers need to be skilled in assessing the impact SDH have on an individual's ability to self-manage their diabetes. A comprehensive discussion of SDHs is presented in Chapter 8 and throughout the book. The discussion of SDH in this chapter is limited to the physical environment and its effect on diabetes management.

ZIP Codes

Poverty is a powerful predictor of health outcomes. A study examining the differences in opportunities for growth and development of children in the 100 largest metropolitan areas in the United States where children reside revealed that 76% of African American children and 69% of Latino children live under worse conditions than the "worst-off" White children (Williams et al., 2010). A potential public health measure in optimizing preventive efforts could be the U.S. postal ZIP code, which has been identified as the hidden vital sign, suggesting that an individual's overall health and well-being is predicated in part on where the person lives (Herrick et al., 2016; Ideastream Public Media, 2017; Williams et al., 2010). The variables in ZIP codes that influence an individual's overall health include neighborhood safety, stable and safe housing, employment opportunities, air quality, access to transportation, fresh food, quality education, and healthcare (Herrick et al., 2016; Ideastream Public Media, 2017; Williams et al., 2010).

Ecological diabetes studies have revealed a geographically distinct area comprised of 644 counties in the southern United States known as the "Diabetes Belt." The Diabetes Belt is part of the country characterized by persistent poverty, with 40% of its citizens living below the poverty level compared to 10% of counties outside the region. Approximately 30% of the people living in the Diabetes Belt are obese, physically inactive, and uninsured (Myers et al., 2017).

The Diabetes Belt is characterized by a diabetes prevalence of 11% or greater of the adult population. Not all the states in the Diabetes Belt have similar rates of diabetes distribution. Ohio and Texas have just a few counties with high diabetes prevalence, while every county in Mississippi exceeds 11% (Myers et al., 2017). Concomitantly, Mississippi has the fewest physicians per capita in the United States, and the fewest number of diabetes care and education specialists to provide diabetes education.

The Diabetes Belt is populated by two medically disadvantaged groups: low-income White individuals in Appalachia and Black individuals in the rural South. The researchers' findings revealed that before the adoption of the Afordable Care Act, 39% of the population living in the Diabetes Belt was uninsured compared to 34% in the non-Belt areas. In states where Medicaid was expanded, uninsured rates decreased rapidly to 13% in the Diabetes Belt and 15% in non-Belt counties (Lobo et al., 2019). The study investigators suggested that the Medicaid expansion may have helped to increase access to preventive health services in the Diabetes Belt.

These findings reinforce the importance of education about preventive services, including health promotion and disease prevention programs that are accessible to the poor and uninsured (Butler, 2017). Continued research is necessary to determine the contribution of race/ethnicity and the SDHs on access and quality of care, and impact on diabetes outcomes, most notably in the South, where the prevalence of diabetes is high (Walker et al., 2016).

Environment

Living in underserved communities and prolonged exposure to environmental stressors can negatively impact one's physiologic well-being and lead to high "allostatic load." Allostatic load is defined as the "cumulative effect of chronic stress and life events" (Guidi et al., 2021). The chronic wear and tear on an individual's physiology can lead to the release of proinflammatory cytokines and cortisol, which can accelerate the development and progression of T2DM (Dendup et al., 2018; Hill-Briggs et al., 2021). The concept of the allostatic load has been the subject of a myriad of research studies examining its link to poor health outcomes and chronic illness, including heart disease, cancer, and depression. In studies examining allostatic load and people with diabetes, researchers noted a disruption of multisystem responses to stress, as indicated by elevated blood pressure, heart rate, total cholesterol, salivary cortisol, and plasma IL-6 levels (Guidi et al., 2021). This suggests that chronic stress is likely to be a factor in the difficulty of achieving good glycemic control in populations living in poverty.

Researchers examining the quality of the environment and diabetes prevalence in the United States concluded that counties with poor sociodemographic environments have a greater prevalence of diabetes (Jagai et al., 2020). The research team used the Environmental Quality Index (EQI), a county-level measurement of the cumulative environmental exposures occurring in the United States. The EQI assesses the quality of the following domains: air, water, land, built environment, and sociodemographic across the rural/urban continuum. Upon analysis of all county data, higher diabetes prevalence rates were associated with poorer air quality, poorer sociodemographic factors, and worse built environment factors. The quality of air a person breathes has a significant influence on the development of T2DM. Poorer individuals and people of color are among those who face higher exposures to pollutants.

It is well known that living in urban areas reduces spending time in nature. Green spaces, forests, fields, trees, shrubs, and flowers can play a role in preventing noncommunicable diseases. Trees contribute to health by reducing the amount of sunlight hitting buildings and pavement, thus cooling the air (Hill-Briggs et al., 2021).

Sleep

Poor quality and duration of sleep is a public health concern, so much so that it has been included as a national health priority in Healthy People 2030 (Office of Disease Prevention and Health Promotion, 2021). Sleep disorders include irregular sleep timing, difficulty falling asleep, staying asleep, and sleeping too long. Several studies have identified that sleeping less than 7 hours or more than 9 hours is associated with an increased risk of diabetes and impaired glucose tolerance (Ogilvie & Patel, 2018; Laposky et al., 2016). Sleep is considered essential to body restoration, thermoregulation, and tissue renewal. It is also critical for cognitive functioning, particularly alertness, attention, and vigilance (Walker, 2017). Impaired alertness and vigilance can be especially dangerous to a person requiring insulin who might inadvertently overdose themselves with too much rapid-acting insulin.

People who get less sleep tend to be heavier than those who get the recommended amount of sleep and who are well rested. Sleep loss triggers changes in the autonomic nervous system which can lead to an increase in blood pressure and cortisol secretion and contribute to insulin resistance. Fretful, interrupted, or insufficient hours of sleep contribute to a myriad of conditions and behaviors that impact an individual's overall health. Socioeconomic status (SES) has been associated with sleep quality and duration. Employment status, income, education, healthcare coverage, and food security are all related to sleep health (Laposky et al., 2016). Findings of the survey investigating race and ethnicity and sleep duration reveal that Black/African Americans were nearly 2.7 times as likely to be "very short sleepers" and nearly two times as likely to be "short sleepers" compared with non-Hispanic Whites. They also found that non-Mexican Hispanics/Latinos were approximately 2.7 times as likely to be very short sleepers. In addition, Asians and others were four times as likely to be very short sleepers and twice as likely to be short sleepers (Whinnery et al., 2014).

The physical environment also affects the quality of sleep. An individual may live in an unsafe community or be exposed to environmental noise caused by traffic sounds, which prevent sound sleep. Urban light pollution has also been associated with more significant sleep/wake variability contributing to increased daytime sleepiness and shorter sleep duration (Ohayon & Milesi, 2016). Agricultural workers also experience poor sleep quality due to a lack of windows that open and extreme heat due to lack of air conditioning (Sandberg et al., 2014).

Workers on nonstandard hours are also at risk for sleep disorders. Nonstandard schedules are those scheduled outside of Monday through Friday, 6:00 a.m. to 6:00 p.m. These schedules are more prevalent among low-wage workers. Working during the night is associated with an array of chronic conditions, including cancer, cardiovascular disease, metabolic syndrome, obesity, and T2DM due to circadian rhythm disruption (Ohayon & Milesi, 2016). Technology may also contribute to sleep deprivation. The use of digital devices exposes the retinas to blue light, which affects sleep quality by suppressing melatonin, a hormone that contributes to the sleep/wake cycle (Wahl et al., 2019).

Food Insecurity

Struggling with food insecurity affects 13.8 million households, with 2.2 million living in rural food insecure areas (Walker et al., 2020). The U.S. Department of Agriculture (USDA) defines food insecurity "a household-level economic and social condition of limited or uncertain access to adequate food." The defining characteristic of very low food security is that "food intake of household members is reduced and their normal eating patterns are disrupted because the household lacks money and other resources for food" (USDA Economic Research Service, 2022). Living in a food desert is often described as living in a location where purchasing affordable, nutritious food is challenging. Households with children who are living in a single parent household and households with incomes at or below the federal poverty level are also vulnerable (Hill-Briggs et al., 2021; U.S. Department of Health and Human Services [DHHS], 2021). Older adults with diabetes may also live below the poverty level and experience food insecurity. Individuals who live in rural communities are also food insecure, with 15.4% living below the federal poverty level.

The USDA details the responses of people who reported very low food security on its website, with 94% of people stating they could not consume a balanced diet and 69% indicating that they went hungry due to an inability to purchase food (USDA, 2020). The ability to access nutritious, adequate, and safe food affects not only an individual's well-being but also the ability to manage chronic health conditions, such as diabetes. When people find it difficult to access healthy food, it becomes even more challenging to follow the recommended meal plan for diabetes. They are confronted with accessing and preparing food and coordinating the meal with medication times to prevent hyper- or hypoglycemia. Food insecurity is associated with a higher A1C and poorer overall health outcomes, among many other conditions (Berkowitz et al., 2018; Martino et al., 2017).

An intervention directed at food insecure individuals diagnosed with diabetes with an A1C of 8.0% (183 mg/dL) is the Fresh Food Farmacy. Patients living in central Pennsylvania were referred to a program that provided nutrition education, wellness classes, a mobile app, and access to an interprofessional team consisting of a dietitian, pharmacist, community health worker, pantry clerk, and registered nurse health manager. A dietician prescribes fresh fruits, vegetables, lean proteins, and whole grains that provide two meals a day for 5days per week for a family of four. Patients are also offered weekly menus and recipes for each meal (Geisinger Health, 2021). After 18 months, there was a 2-point reduction in A1C values, a 31.3% improvement in glucose measurements, and a reduction of diabetes complications in 40% of patients participating in the program. The cost of the program is approximately $2,400 per patient, reflecting a cost savings of $16,000 to $24,000 per patient to the healthcare system (National Academies of Sciences, Engineering, and Medicine, 2019).

Farmers' markets are another intervention that provides nutritious food to low-income, rural, people of color, and food insecure individuals. Farmers' markets not only provide healthy fresh food options, but they also promote a sense of community. The relationship between health and social interactions suggests that farmers' markets offer essential public health benefits. One crucial outcome of farmers' markets is the unique opportunity for market patrons to learn about food from the growers. A novel program in Oregon educates children by giving them $2 to spend on fresh produce every time they visit the farmers' markets. They are helped to create a log of what they purchase with their $2 at each visit, and their choices are reviewed by program volunteers (Lohr, 2017). Outcomes from this program resulted in the development of the "Market Kids Sprout Club," which extends into community centers and daycare centers (Lohr, 2017). While they provide nutritious options, farmers' markets also have limitations due to their seasonal availability and limited weekly hours. Collaborating with existing grocery stores and healthcare organizations can improve the availability and quality of fruits and vegetables for those living in food-insecure neighborhoods (Donahue et al., 2021). Community gardens are a recent and powerful concept as well. Residents can grow food and teach the youth about science and nutrition simultaneously.

Medication Affordability and Acceptance

The famed U.S. Surgeon General C. Everett Koop once remarked, "Drugs don't work in people who do not take them" (Lindenfield & Jessup, 2017). Since 2009, the cost of insulin has increased more than 1,000% (Rajkumar, 2019). A vial of insulin lispro (Humalog®) cost $21 in 1999 but in 2021 cost $274 (Lilly Pharmaceutical Company, 2021). The primary reason identified for the increase in cost is the demand, as insulin is a lifesaving drug. Other factors include a virtual monopoly by pharmaceutical companies as only three pharmaceutical companies manufacture insulin, barriers to biosimilar entry into the market, lobbying efforts of insulin manufacturers, and pharmacy benefit managers who gain financially from higher prices (Rajkumar, 2019). There are no government-established cost limits on medications in the United States. The newer formulations of insulins, known as insulin analogues, are preferable for glucose management as they more closely mimic normal physiology (Isaacs, 2019). Examples of insulin analogues include insulin glargine (Lantus), insulin determir (Levemir), insulin deguldec (Tresiba), insulin lispro (Humalog), insulin aspart (Novolog), and insulin glulisine (Apidra).

The older varieties of insulin, including Regular and Neutral Protamine Hagedorn (NPH) insulin, are available at Walmart Pharmacies for $25.00 for a 10 mL vial containing 1,000 units of insulin. An open vial of insulin must be discarded after 28 days due to the stability of the insulin. Patients with T1DM may require 2 to 3 vials of insulin a month; patients with T2DM may require six or more vials.

Critical to a person's ability to self-manage diabetes is the ability to afford the treatment. A few states have passed insulin affordability legislation that caps copays at $35 per vial, yet insulin access for the uninsured and underinsured in other states remains problematic. Healthcare professionals need to collaborate with policymakers, pharmaceutical companies, and payers to advocate for affordable insulin and educate patients about available resources to help them access insulin (Isaacs, 2019).

Most individuals with diabetes will require more than one diabetes medication to manage their glucose. However, insulin is not always included as part of the medication plan in people with T2DM. Cultural beliefs and values, perceptions of safety, social factors, and health literacy influence the willingness to take insulin. Insulin usage among Whites is higher than in ethnic minority populations (Rebolledo & Arellano, 2016). Many people with T2DM have expressed hesitation to initiate insulin because of fear. African Americans associate insulin with organ damage. Hispanics/Latinos worry that a need to take insulin results from their inability to control their diabetes, and people from Asian cultures may be anxious that insulin may interfere with religious practices (Rebolledo & Arellano, 2016). American Indians often express dread and perceive insulin as a last resort, leading to complications and death (Carson et al., 2015). Most individuals who require insulin express an aversion to needles. Tools and techniques to mitigate the fear of injections and facilitate successful initiation of insulin therapy include a comprehensive assessment of the person's fears, guided practice with feedback, relaxation techniques, and follow-up monitoring (Kruger et al., 2015).

Role of Health Literacy

Diabetes requires that people actively and accurately engage in behaviors that contribute to their health, promote their well-being, and reduce the risk of complications (Association of Diabetic Educators, 2020). This is known as self-management in the world of diabetes care and education. Daily diabetes care depends on people having adequate health literacy and numeracy skills. Health literacy is defined as "the degree to which individuals have the capacity to obtain, process and understand basic health information and services needed to make appropriate health decisions" (Ratzan & Parker, 2000). See Chapter Eight for an in-depth discussion about health literacy. Numeracy, also known as quantitative skill, is "the ability to understand and use numbers in daily life" (Osborn et al., 2009). Individuals who struggle with health literacy and numeracy experience frequent hospitalizations, higher healthcare costs, increased emergency department (ED) visits, poor or suboptimal treatment decisions, and higher death rates. It is suggested that 15% to 40% of people with diabetes have trouble understanding, remembering, and following health recommendations (Aaby et al., 2017; Cavanaugh, 2011). For those who struggle with math concepts, visual images are helpful when determining portion size (Figure 15.1).

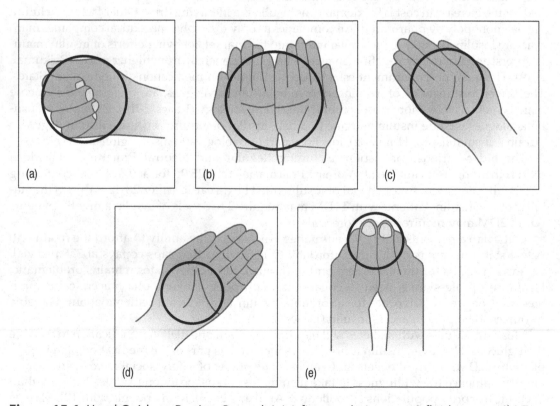

Figure 15.1 Hand Guide to Portion Control. (a) A fist equals 1 cup or 8 fluid ounces. (b) Two cupped hands equal 1 cup. (c) A cupped hand equals ½ cup. (d) The palm of the hand equals 3 ounces. (e) From the knuckle to the tip of the thumb equals 1 tablespoon.

In 2021, researchers surveyed 4,397 adults with diabetes from four southern states and Washington, DC, about three health literacy tasks important to diabetes care. The three tasks examined were getting access to health information, understanding the health information presented verbally by healthcare providers, and understanding written health information (Rafferty et al., 2021). The findings revealed that 5.9% of the subjects had difficulty obtaining information, 10.7% found it challenging to comprehend the information provided by their healthcare provider, and 12.0% found it difficult to grasp the written health information. Individuals who struggled with understanding both verbal and written communication had never attended a diabetes self-management education class (Rafferty et al., 2021).

Storytelling is a powerful educational tool that promotes learning and remembering. Stories offer insights into life, show how characters make choices, and help convey essential information to guide future actions. Stories are remembered more frequently than facts and can be used with low-health literacy individuals (CDC, n.d.-b; Day, 2009). Stories offer encouragement and have been successfully used with immigrant and refugee adults with diabetes, those living in rural and underserved communities who have diabetes, and American Indian children with T2DM (Andrae et al., 2020, Gucciardi et al., 2019; Reusch, 2019; Satterfield et al., 2014; Wieland et al., 2017). Stories are revered in the American Indian/Alaskan Native communities. The stories, known as *Eagle Books,* were written by Georgia Perez and Terry Lofton and are beautifully illustrated to resonate with the young reader. The *Eagle Books* contain four overarching themes: follow traditions, make wise choices, eat healthy foods, and be active (Satterfield et al., 2014). The books are free from the CDC website.

People living with diabetes need to make complex decisions daily that require sophisticated math skills (Table 15.4). Low numeracy skills are prevalent in vulnerable populations and other groups and are significant contributors to poor glycemic outcomes

TABLE 15.4 Numeracy Skills and Diabetes Self-Care Activities

Numeracy Skills	Diabetes Self-Care Activities*
Addition	Reading food labels
Subtraction	Determining serving size from food label
Multiplication	Planning meals
Division	Calculating the amount of carbohydrates from food label
Fractions	Measuring portion size
Decimals	Interpreting blood glucose (BG) values
Multiple steps	Evaluating glucose trends/patterns over time
Counting	Making insulin adjustments based on glucose patterns
Number hierarchy	Reading and interpreting medication directions
Time	Calculating the amount of correctional insulin if needed
	Determining bolus/prandial doses based on carbohydrate consumption and BG values
	Treating hypoglycemia accurately
	Correlating A1C measure with BG values
	Applying carbohydrate to insulin ratios (ICR) if wearing insulin pump
	Anticipating needs for refills of medications and equipment

*List is not organized by priority of skills or completeness of all self-care diabetes behaviors.

Source: R.O., Wolff, K., Cavanaugh, K., & Rothman, R. (2010). Addressing health literacy and numeracy to improve diabetes care. *Diabetes Spectrum, 23*(4), 238–243.

(Cavanaugh et al., 2008). Researchers in Tennessee conducted an electronic survey of 151 individuals with T2DM assessing their literacy, numeracy skills, and medication adherence. Patients enrolled in the study had been diagnosed with diabetes for an average of 9 years and had an average A1C value of 8% (glucose value of 183 mg/dL). Patients who had not completed high school and earned less than $40,000 a year had lower health literacy and numeracy skills. They also had difficulty following their medication plan, resulting in sub-optimal glucose management (Nandyala et al., 2017).

Two valid and reliable versions of the Diabetes Numeracy Test (DNT) were created to assess numeracy quickly in the clinical setting. The DNT-15 contains 15 items and the DNT-5 includes 5 questions that help to identify specific gaps in an individual's mathematic competency (Zaugg et al., 2014). The questions require multiple mathematical steps. Questions in both modified instruments assess a person's ability to calculate carbohydrate servings, evaluate glucose values, and determine insulin dose based upon glucose value and total carbohydrates consumed.

Support for the Management of Diabetes

Technology

Insulin pumps and continuous glucose monitoring devices provide alternatives to multiple daily injections and finger sticks. Insulin pumps are worn externally and are about the size of a deck of cards. Insulin pumps are computerized devices powered by an external battery. The pump has a reservoir that is filled with insulin. The insulin infuses subcutaneously through a thin plastic catheter called an insulin set. The pump is worn 24 hours a day and continuously delivers preprogrammed amounts of insulin. It is preprogrammed to calculate and deliver the precise amount of insulin for meals after the individual enters the number of carbohydrates consumed. The insertion site is changed every 72 hours. The average cost of an insulin pump ranges from $4,500 to $5,600. If an individual qualifies for Medicaid services, the insulin pump, insulin, and supplies will often be covered. However, it should be noted that racial disparities remain in the use of diabetes technology, with White children being prescribed insulin pumps twice as often as Black children and 1.5 times more than Hispanics/Latino children (Agarwal et al., 2021). The disparity can be attributed to the implicit bias of health professionals believing that people of color do not possess the skills to manage the technology safely (Agarwal et al., 2021).

Continuous glucose monitors (CGMs) constantly monitor and record fluid glucose levels. Patients and families may refer to this as "sensor therapy." CGM systems use a tiny sensor inserted under the skin to assess glucose in the interstitial fluid. The sensor stays in place for several days to 2 weeks and then is replaced. A nondisposable transmitter is connected to the sensor and sends glucose levels via radio waves from the transmitter to a pager-like wireless monitor. A prescription is required for CGMs and insulin pumps. CGMs can range from $160 to $500 a month without health insurance, making this technology inaccessible for many.

Programs to Assist Individuals and Families

Several pharmaceutical companies have collaborated with social services search engines that connect people who need assistance. The search engines link people seeking help with verified free or low-cost services within their ZIP code. The variety of services includes healthcare, food delivery, transportation, and job training. Examples of assistance under the "food" category may consist of food pantries, neighborhood community gardens, emergency food, food delivery, payment for meals, and nutrition assistance.

"Aunt Bertha" is an example of an online database that connects human services, government agencies, places of worship, and charities to serve every zip code in the United States. The organization's mission is to make relevant information accessible to people within their own ZIP code. The site pulls in all the services,nationally, regionally, and locally, and then provides the specific requested services available in the user's neighborhood. Aunt Bertha has collaborated with the United Way in many states to request assistance if internet services are not available. In addition, data analytics are available so that social service agencies and policymakers can review the benefits that consumers have requested and address the services for which there are no resources. The resources are free to the end-user (Gray, 2014). Since its introduction in 2010, Aunt Bertha has served 4 million people (Aunt Bertha, 2020).

Lists of resources may be distributed during diabetic education classes, as patient handouts at the time of diabetes diagnosis or accessed on the web.

Lack of social support has been associated with suboptimal outcomes in people with diabetes (Hill-Briggs et al., 2021). Linking members in the community, such as family members, lay leaders, peer supporters, and community healthcare workers, to people living with diabetes is receiving increasing attention from the American Medical Association and the Agency for Healthcare Research and Quality (ADA, 2021). The Future of Nursing 2020 to 2030 Report released by the National Academy of Medicine (NAM) articulates the nursing profession's vision: to reduce health disparities and improve the health and well-being of the nation in collaboration with other healthcare professionals and policymakers (NAM, 2021).

Models for Diabetic Education

Mnemonic for Teaching the Interpretation of Blood Glucose Values

Interpreting blood glucose values is an essential skill for people living with diabetes. It requires the individual to know the "target range" for blood glucose, take the glucose value obtained from the meter, and plot the number on the worksheet, which is provided to them in class, and then decide if the number is low, high, or in the target range. This skill is most often learned in diabetes self-management education and suppor (tDSMES) classes. Participants are provided with a visual image of where their glucose has been trending. After reviewing with the class facilitator, they are asked to share their glucose patterns and "key points" from the previous week. The facilitator validates the amount of glucose in the target range, and inquires about possible reasons for the highs and lows outside the target range. People who take insulin need to be able to trend their glucose values and decide how to prevent hypo- and hyperglycemic events.

Participants provide support to their classmates and offer ideas on preventing a craving or locating a food pantry if they live with food insecurity. In addition to learning the mechanics of plotting out blood glucose values and knowing when the values are in range or too low or high, participants also receive instruction on adjusting their insulin dose to prevent glucose values that are out of range. They are instructed to avoid low values first, then examine values associated with meals and determine what actions can be taken and then strategies to correct the fasting blood glucose values. The mnemonic to remember the process is:

◆ **Halt the Hypos** (means preventing low blood glucose events).
◆ **Pare the Prandial** (requires adjusting the mealtime dose or making changes to the meal plan).
◆ **Fix the Fasting** (includes adjusting the basal insulin dose). Hypoglycemia needs to be corrected first, as low glucose values can lead to neuroglycopenic symptoms of confusion, seizures, coma, and possibly death.

Relationship-Centered Communication

The R.E.D.E. Model

Humans are social beings who require connection, a need for feeling acknowledged and validated. (Windover et al., 2014). There are a variety of communication models available to enhance relationships between caregivers and clinicians. The R.E.D.E. model (pronounced "ready") is offered in this chapter for its ease of use in various clinical settings. R.E.D.E. provides a framework to optimize personal connections through three phases of a therapeutic relationship: establishment, development, and engagement (Windover et al., 2014). All caregivers must exhibit value and respect when meeting and greeting patients through words and actions. The first phase of the R.E.D.E. model, identified as establishment, concentrates on caregiver behaviors that foster connection. The second phase of R.E.D.E. is developing the relationship. This phase focuses on learning about the patient and gathering the person's narrative about living with a sudden illness or chronic condition. The final phase of the R.E.D.E. model is known as engagement. The focus of this phase is determining the patient's understanding of what was discussed and identifying any potential barriers. A patient may not remember all the self-care management recommendations discussed. Still, human interactions, which include rapport, expressions of care, support, validation, and acknowledgment of emotions, tend to be more memorable. Learning how to express empathy is essential. The R.E.D.E. model offers specific conversational strategies that help caregivers build relationships with their patients. It promotes the use of empathy as a relational skill. The framework allows patients to voice their concerns early, feel comfortable sharing their personal stories, and create an emotionally safe environment. The R.E.D.E. model has been demonstrated to improve measures of patient satisfaction, reduce physician burnout, improve physician empathy and self-efficacy, and support the ongoing refinement of communication skills training (Boissy et al., 2016).

Person-Centered, Strength-Based Language

In 2017, the ADA and the American Association of Diabetes Educators, who changed their name to the Association of Diabetes Care and Education Specialists (ADCES), published an important paper on the use of language in diabetes care (Dickinson et al., 2017). The authors embraced the concept of person-centered language, first advocated by the American Psychological Association in 1992 (Granello & Gibbs, 2016). Person-centered language is defined as the "use of words that acknowledges the individuality and uniqueness of a person, rather than referring to an individual as a disease, disability or illness" (Dickinson et al., 2017).

The concept of person-centered language is essential because people do not live in the role of their disease, except when there is a health crisis associated with their condition. Otherwise, they go about living life loving their families, participating in meaningful work, and contributing to their communities. They do not live life as a "patient." It has been suggested that people with diabetes spend fewer than 6 hours per year interacting with caregivers and functioning in the patient role (Holt & Speight, 2017). Dickinson et al. (2017) posited that describing individuals by a diagnosis, "diabetic" or "uncontrolled," or by a behavior, "unmotivated" or "disinterested," may be perceived as hurtful and disrespectful. Person-centered care fosters respect, trust, and choice to optimize a person's participation in shared decision-making about their diabetes care (Dickinson et al., 2017).

Person-centered language has been described in the literature for decades. The "language movement" began in 1974, when those living and caring for people with disabilities held the first self-advocacy conference (Crocker & Smith, 2019). They followed this with the Handicapped Children Act, now called the Individuals with Disabilities Act (IDEA), that required all children to receive "free and appropriate education." That was followed by the Federal Developmentally Disabled Assistance and Bill of Rights Act that mandated that all states develop advocacy programs to receive federal monies (94th Congress, 1975). In 1984, AIDS activists created the "Denver Principles," declaring their autonomy, individuality, and humanity. They called on the healthcare community to refer to them as "people with AIDS," not "AIDS victims" (Kapitan, 2017). Broom and Whittaker (2004) interviewed 119 individuals diagnosed with diabetes. Many participants verbalized the word "control" as a moral failure if their blood glucose was not in the target range recommended by their physician. This caused much anguish among the study participants and prompted many not to be forthcoming to their caregivers with their self-management challenges.

People with diabetes also report being stigmatized solely because of their chronic condition. In a quantitative study, 5,422 responded to a survey soliciting their perceptions of diabetes stigma and its psychological effects. The most frequently cited experience with stigma (regardless of diabetes type) was the perception that the person was flawed with an inability to assume responsibility for their diabetes (81%), followed by a perception of burdening the health system (65%). Individuals with T1DM reported that they frequently encountered misinformation about diabetes, most notably that T1DM is contagious and that there are no differences in the types of diabetes. Parents of children with T1DM reported the highest rate of stigma (83%), and those with T2DM not requiring insulin reported experiencing the least (49%). Respondents reported feeling judged and shamed for causing their diabetes by being passive, lazy, overeating, and obese. While these behaviors are usually associated with T2DM, 83% of people with T1DM reported feelings of blame, shame, and being judged.

Strength-based language focuses on the positive attributes of an individual (Hie, 2013). Caregivers have been enculturated into a healthcare world that uses deficit-based language. When communicating with other caregivers, patients may be described by their inabilities, "patient is unable to walk, to eat, or toilet." Moreover, we often use judgment-laden labels to describe behaviors: "uncooperative," "unmotivated," "noncompliant." How caregivers communicate with patients can impact their health. Person-centered, strength-based language is a life-affirming intervention that offers hope, encouragement, and validation. A person, with DMT2, after visiting her doctor and reading the postencounter summary, commented, *"Why does my doctor always write on all my papers, 'uncontrolled diabetes'? This scares me, and I am already nervous all the time."* When the person was asked what it meant, she replied. *"I think it means I cannever get better"* (DeSmit & Andrews, 2018).

The American Medical Association adopted person-centered language in 2019, stating that its use reduces the stigma associated with certain conditions and fosters the caregiver/patient relationship. Nurses must collectively advocate using the language that patients prefer, as not all disability advocacy groups embrace the person-centered language. The National Federation of the Blind espouses the use of identity-first language because they believe that a disability such as blindness is "intertwined into their identity," and the word "blind" is not offensive when used as an adjective (Collier, 2012; Ferrigan, 2019; Jernigan, 2009).

Diabetes Self-Management Education and Support

The diabetes literature is replete with studies that indicate that people diagnosed with T2DM are not consistently referred to DSMES programs. Approximately 42% of people diagnosed with T2DM are not directed to a DSMES program, and only 5% of all Medicare recipients have received DSMES. It is posited that physicians do not provide referrals because there is a poor translation of evidence-based practice guidelines to clinical practice, so they are unaware of recommendations. Additionally, due to the brief office encounter, physicians do not have sufficient time to explore patient concerns regarding the daily worries, fears, and anxieties that patients with diabetes often confront (Powers et al., 2020). In a study examining the referral rate and participation of 105 patients with a new T2DM diagnosis, only 53% were referred to DSMES (Hassan et al., 2020).

It is recommended that people with diabetes participate in DSMES programs at four critical times during their lives: at the time of diagnosis, if not meeting mutually established goals, when complicating factors emerge, or during life or care transitions (Association of Diabetic Educators, 2020). The ADCES created a framework known as the ADCES7 Self-Care Behaviors® (Mulcahy et al., 2003). Each behavior is predicated on the successful adoption of the others. In 2020, ADCES examined the seven self-care behaviors, reviewed the literature, and assessed the impact of each behavior on outcomes of patients with T2DM. The working group determined that reordering the seven self-care behaviors was warranted, and healthy coping is now the first behavior to be addressed. Outcomes studies have revealed that healthy coping is integral to learning and performing the other six self-care behaviors.

The impact of DSMES on specific diabetes management outcomes—reduction in A1C, increase in physical activity, and healthy eating—are well documented in the literature (Creamer et al., 2016; Ueleman & Macleod, 2020). Innovative strategies, including peer educators and community health workers (CHWs), have been used to provide education, offer support, and assist in problem-solving. CHWs are individuals who reside in the patient's community and may also be referred to as "lay advocates." CHWs are effective peer teachers because they often share similar values, characteristics, and experiences with the individuals for whom they are providing care (Palmas et al., 2015). CHWs have also been integral in delivering culturally tailored mobile health (mHealth) DMSE programs. Fortmann et al. (2020) described the effective use of CHWs in introducing tablet technology and problem-solving tools to Hispanic individuals enrolled in asynchronous DSME programs resulting in improved A1C values and medication adherence.

A range of technologies provides diabetes education, monitoring, and support services. Telehealth can reach far more individuals than traditional in-person patient education programs. Vulnerable populations can now be connected to a diabetes healthcare professional, peer teacher, or CHW via mobile phone, smartphone app, websites, virtual visits, or virtual videos (CDC, n.d.-a; Modic & Knapp, 2015).

CASE STUDY 15.1: A 44-YEAR-OLD MAN WITH T2DM

Mr. George Jackson is a 44-year-old man admitted to the hospital after presenting to the emergency department (ED) with numbness in his feet. He has a history of asthma, hypertension, and T2DM. He was diagnosed with T2DM 4 years before his presentation at the ED. His blood glucose in the ED was 580 mg/dL. His insulin plan is insulin Glargine 75 units at bedtime and insulin Lispro 10 units with meals. His most recent A1C was 14.5 mg/dL (blood glucose 369 mg/dL).

Mr. Jackson lives alone and is unemployed due to a back injury he received while working construction 2 years ago. He receives Medicaid benefits. Both of his parents had T2DM. Mr. Jackson attributes his mother, who was incapacitated by a stroke, as the person who saved his life. She urged him to seek medical attention when he told her about his blurry vision. Upon presentation to the ED at the time of diagnosis, his blood glucose was 1,073 mg/dL.

Mr. Jackson admits to feeling lonely and isolated since the death of both parents and the end of a serious relationship. He says he knows what to do but "loves sweets, hates to poke his fingers" and does not exercise for "fear of getting killed" as his neighborhood has a high rate of crime. He "knows he is going to die from diabetes, it is just a matter of time." He feels better when his glucose "runs high" as he experiences symptoms of hypoglycemia at a blood glucose of 180 mg/dL.

He goes to the ED when his diabetes is out of control and admits to not being consistent with taking his insulin. He has not been back to the healthcare clinic for over a year. He felt ashamed by the provider, who admonished him for being "noncompliant" and told him he would eventually need dialysis if he did not take better care of himself.

Mr. Jackson is admitted to the hospital because of numbness in his feet and diabetic ketoacidosis (DKA). This is the first admission for DKA; he feels frightened and remorseful that his diabetes is out of control.

Discussion Questions:

1. What are the circumstances and characteristics of vulnerable populations that contribute to the development of diabetes?
2. What barriers are affecting Mr. Jackson's ability to self-manage his diabetes successfully?
3. Using the R.E.D.E. Model described in this chapter, what might be three empathic statements that could be used to promote a person-centered relationship?
4. What healthcare and support services would be beneficial to Mr. Jackson?

CASE STUDY 15.2: A 22-YEAR-OLD WOMAN WITH T1DM

Ms. Sarah Harris is 22-year-old woman who lives in the Diabetes Belt in southeastern Kentucky, also known as Appalachia. Sarah lives at home with her mother and four younger siblings. At 16, she dropped out of high school when her dad was diagnosed with pancreatic cancer to help her mother care for him. Her dad died six months after diagnosis. Sarah works at a local restaurant as a waitress and is the wage earner for the family.

Ms. Harris was diagnosed with T1DM when she was 15. She is on 70/30 insulin (a combination insulin of NPH and regular insulin) which she takes twice a day. She admits to rationing her insulin to save money. Her A1C from a year ago was 9.3% (blood glucose 220 mg/dL). She receives Medicaid benefits. She has been working overtime, picking up two to three extra shifts a week for several months. She has been experiencing several hypoglycemic events a week, two events that required assistance from a coworker. Sarah is exhausted, frightened, and embarrassed. She is distressed that a coworker had to come to her aid and give her orange juice to treat her hypoglycemia. While three of her coworkers know that she has T1DM, she is very private about having a diabetes diagnosis. Sarah is worried that her diabetes is out of control since she is not eating regularly or sleeping well.

Sarah's mother is frightened for her daughter and insists that she go to the doctor. Sarah seeks medical attention at a clinic an hour away. She takes a day off from work as she must travel by bus, and she anticipates the visit will take most of the day.

Discussion Questions:

1. What are the circumstances contributing to Sarah's hypoglycemic events?
2. What healthcare and support services would benefit Sara? What changes can be made to her diabetes plan?
3. Using the R.E.D.E. Model described in this chapter, what might be three empathic statements that could be used to validate Sarah's struggles?

Key Points

The activities listed in the following help promote successful self-management practices in people with diabetes.

◆ Create an accepting and welcoming atmosphere when engaging with patients, so they feel comfortable expressing concerns, asking questions, and admitting struggles.
◆ Assess for the SDH and their impact on an individual's ability to follow the prescribed plan of care.
◆ Use a myriad of teaching approaches to educating patients. There is not just one approach that yields success.
◆ Engage patients using relationship-centered communication techniques.
◆ Obtain referrals for DSMES and encourage participation.

CONCLUSION

Diabetes is a chronic, life-altering condition that disproportionately affects the poor and burdens individuals, the health system, and society. It is a condition that requires an individual to be educated, empowered, and self-reliant so that wise choices are made throughout the day, every day, 365 days of the year. There is no vacation from managing diabetes.

Individuals must be attentive to what they eat, incorporate physical activities into their daily routine, monitor their blood glucose, take medications several times a day, and adjust insulin dosages based upon glucose values obtained throughout the day. Diabetes management is time consuming, with up to 2 hours devoted to managing diabetes if insulin therapy is required.

Couple the daily diabetes activities with the worries that underserved people encounter daily—transportation, food insecurity, the potential for eviction, affording medications, an unsafe neighborhood polluted and filled with noise, or isolation due to living in a rural or dangerous environment. The demands are exhausting.

This chapter has emphasized the importance of diabetes education and support and described the techniques used to facilitate learning and offer ongoing assistance. It has also highlighted numerous barriers that vulnerable populations face in their daily lives and their impact on diabetes management. While the advent of innovative technologies and medications offer optimism and excitement in the specialty of diabetes care, there remain formidable obstacles for vulnerable populations. Significant changes to life inequities and racial disparities must happen for optimal diabetes care. A combination of fiscal policies, new laws, and regulations, along with urban and rural healthcare redesign, will make this happen.

REFERENCES

94th Congress. (1975). Education for all children act of 1975. (E.A.H.C.A.). https://www.govinfo
.gov/content/pkg/STATUTE-89/pdf/STATUTE-89-Pg773.pdf

Aaby, A., Friis, K. Christensen, B., Rowlands, G., & Maindal, H. T. (2017). Health literacy is associated with health behaviors and self-reported health: A large population-based strength in individuals with cardiovascular disease. *European Journal of Preventive Cardiology*, 24(17), 1880–1888. https://doi.org/10.1177/2047487317729538

Agarwal, S., Schlechter, C., Gonzalez, J., & Long, J. (2021). Racial-ethnic disparities in disparities in diabetes technology among young adults with type 1 diabetes. *Diabetes Technology and Therapeutics*, 23(4), 306–313. https://doi.org/10.1089/dia.2020.0338

American Diabetes Association. (2018a). Economic costs of diabetes in the U.S. in 2017. *Diabetes Care*, 41(5):917–928.

American Diabetes Association. (2018b). Statistics about diabetes. https://www.diabetes.org/resources/statistics/statistics-about-diabetes

American Diabetes Association. (2018c). Standards of care. http://diabetesed.net/wp-content/uploads/2017/12/2018-ADA-Standards-of-Care.pdf

American Diabetes Association. (2020). Management of type 2 diabetes. Author.

American Medical Association. (2019). Use of person-centered language. https://www.ama-assn.org/system/files/2019-05/a19-006.pdf

Andrae, S. J., Andrae, L. J., Cherrington, A., Richman, J., & Safford. M. (2020). Peer coach delivered storytelling program for diabetes medication adherence intervention development and process outcomes. *Contemporary Clinical Trials Communication*, 12(20), 1–8. https://doi.org/10.1016/j.conctc2020.100653

Association of Diabetic Educators. (2020). Consensus statement. https://www.diabeteseducator.org/practice/practice-tools/app-resources/a-consensus-report

Aunt Bertha. (2020). Aunt Bertha celebrates a decade of growth and service with major user milestone. https://www.prnewswire.com/news-releases/aunt-bertha-celebrates-a-decade-of-growth-and-service-with-major-user-milestone-301120773.html

Berkowitz, S. A., Karter, A. J., Corbie-Smith, G., Seligman, H. K., Ackroyd, S. A., Barnard, L. S., Atlas, S. J., & Wexler, D. J. (2018). Food insecurity, food "deserts," and glycemic control in patients with diabetes: A longitudinal analysis. *Diabetes Care*, 41(6), 1188–1195. https://doi.org/10.2337/dc17-1981

Boissy, A., Windover, A., Bokar, D., Karafa, M., Neuendorf, K., Frankel, R., Merlino, J., & Rothberg, M. (2016). Communication skills training improves patient satisfaction. *Journal of General Internal Medicine*, 31, 755–761. https://doi.org/10.1007/s11606-016-3597-2

Broom, D., & Whittaker A. (2004). Controlling diabetes, controlling diabetics: Moral language in the management of diabetes. *Social Science Medicine*, 58(11), 2371–2382. https://doi.org/10.1016/j.socscimed.2003.09.002

Butler, A. M. (2017). Social determinants of health and racial/ethnic disparities in type 2 diabetes in youth. *Current Diabetes Reports*, 17(8), 60. https://doi.org/10.1007/s11892-017-0885-0

Buttermore, E., Campanella, V., & Priefer, R. (2021). The increasing trend of type 2 diabetes in youth: An overview. *Diabetes & Metabolic Syndrome*, 15(5), 1022253. https://doi.org/10.1016/j.dsx.2021.102253

Carson, L. D., Henderson, J. N., King, K., Kleszynski, K., Thompson, D. M., & Mayer, P. (2015). American Indians diabetes beliefs and practices: Anxiety, fear, and dread in pregnant women. *Diabetes Spectrum*, 28(4), 258–263. https://doi.org/10.2337/diaspect.28.4.258

Cavanaugh, K. L. (2011). Health literacy in diabetes care; explanation, evidence and equipment. *Diabetes Management (London)*, 1(2), 191–199. https://doi.org/10.2217/dmt.11.5

Cavanaugh, K., Huizinga, M.,Walls ton, K. A., Gebrestsadik, T., Shintani, A, Davis, D., Gregory, R. P., Fuchs, I., Malone, R., Cherrington, A., Pignone, M., DeWalt, D. A., Elasy, T. A., & Rothman, R. L. (2008). Association of numeracy and diabetes control. *Annals of Internal Medicine*, 148(5), 737–746. https://doi.org/10.7326/0003-4819-148-10-20080-5200-0002

Centers for Control and Prevention. (n.d.-a). A guide for using telehealth technologies in diabetes delf-management education and support and the national diabetes prevention program lifestyles change program. https://www.cdc.gov/diabetes/pdfs/programs/E_Telehealth_translation_product_508.pdf

Centers for Control and Prevention. (n.d.-b). Stories to reach, teach and heal: A guide for diabetes health educators. https://www.cdc.gov/diabetes/ndwp/pdf/ebstoriestoreachteachandheal.pdf

Centers for Control and Prevention. (n.d.-c). Visual communication resources. https://www.cdc.gov/healthliteracy/developmaterials/visual-communication.html

Centers for Disease Control and Prevention. (2020a). National diabetes statistics report, 2020. Centers for Disease Control and Prevention, U.S. Department of Health and Human Services. https://www.cdc.gov/diabetes/library/features/diabetes-stat-report.html

Centers for Disease Control and Prevention. (2020b). Prediabetes: Your chance to prevent diabetes. https://www.cdc.gov/diabetes/basics/prediabetes.html

Collier, R. (2012). Person-first language: Noble but to what effect? *Canadian Medical Association Journal*, 184(12), 1977–1978. https://doi.org/10.1503/cmaj.109-4319

Cornell, S., Halstenson, C., & Miller, D. (Eds.) (2020). The art and science of diabetes care (5th ed.). Association of Diabetes Care and Education Specialists.

Creamer, J., Attridge, M., Ramsden, M., Cannings-John, R., & Hawthorne, K. (2016). Culturally appropriate health education for type 2 diabetes in ethnic minority groups: An updated cochrane review of randomized control trials. *Diabetic Medicine*, 33(2), 169–183. https://doi.org/10.111/dme.12865

Critser, G. (2003). *Fat land: How Americans became the fattest people in the world.* Houghton Mifflin.

Crocker, A. F., and Smith, S. (2019). Person-first language: Are we practicing what we preach? *Journal of Multidisciplinary Healthcare*, 12, 125–129. https://doi.org/10.2147.JMDH.5140067

Day, V. (2009). Health literacy through storytelling. *The Online Journal Issues in Nursing*, 16(3), 713–717. https://doi.org/3912/OJIN.Vol14No03Man06

Dendup, T., Feng, X., Clingan, S., & Ashell-Burt, T. (2018). Environmental risk factors for developing type 2 diabetes mellitus: A systematic review. *International Journal of Environmental Research and Public Health*, 15, 78. https://doi.org/10.3390/ijerph15010078

DeSmit, M., & Andrews, L (2018). What language are you speaking? Poster presentation, American association of diabetes educators annual meeting. https://healthyinteractions.com/what-language-are-you-speaking

Dickinson, J. K., Guzman, S. S., Maryniuk, M., O'Brien, C. A., Kadohiro, J. K., Jackson, R. A., D'Hondt, N., Montgomery, B., Close, K. L, & Funnell, M. M. (2017). The use of language in diabetes care and education. *Diabetes Care*, 40(12) 1790–1799. https://doi.org/10.2337/dci 17-0041

Donahue, J. A., Severson, T., & Martin, L. P. (2021). The food pharmacy: Theory, implementation, and opportunities. *American Journal of Preventive Cardiology*, 5(suppl 2), 10014.5. https://doi.org/10.1016/j.ajpc.2020.100145

DPP Research Group. (2002). Reduction in the incidence of type 2 diabetes with metformin or lifestyle intervention. *New England Journal of Medicine*, 346(6), 393–403. https://doi.org/10.1056?NEJM0912512

Fang, M., Wang, D., Coresh, J., & Selvin, E. (2021). Trends in diabetes treatment and control in U.S. adults, 1999–2018. *New England Journal of Medicine*, 384(23), 2219–2228. https://doi.org/10.1056/NEJMsa2032271

Ferrigan, P. (2019). Person first language versus identity first language. An examination and drawbacks of disability laws in society. https://jtds.commons.gc.cuny.edu/person-first-language-vs-identity-first-language-an-examination-of-the-gains-and-drawbacks-of-disability-language-in-society/

Fortmann, A. L., Walker, C., Barger, K., Robacker, M., Morrisey, R., Ortwine, K., Loupasi, I., Lee, I., Hogrefe, L., Strohmeyer, C., & Philis-Tsimikas. (2020). Care team integration in primary care improves one-year clinical and financial outcomes in diabetes: A case for value-based care. *Population Health Management*, 23(6), 467–475. https://doi.org/10.1089/pop.2019.0103

Geisinger Health. (2021). Fresh food farmacy. https://www.geisinger.org/freshfoodfarmacy/learn-more

Granello, D. H. & Gibbs, T. A. (2016). The power of language and labels: "The mentally ill" versus "people with mental illness." *Journal of Counseling and Development, 94*(1), 31–40. https://doi:org/10.1002/cad.12059

Gray, E. (2014). TED blog: Need help? Aunt Bertha helps people in need find social services in their area. https://blog.ted.com/need-help-ask-aunt-bertha-erine-gray-helps-people-in-need-find-social-services-in-their-area/

Gucciardi, E., Reynolds, E., Karam, G, Beanlands, H., Sidani, S., & Espin, S. (2019). Group-based storytelling in disease self-management. *Chronic Illness, 17*(3), 306–320. https://doi.org.10.1177/14742395319859395

Guidi, J., Lucente, M., Sonino, N., & Fava, G. A. (2021). Allostatic load and its impact on health: A systematic review. *Psychotherapy and psychosomatics, 90*(1), 11–27. https://doi.org.10.1159/000510696

Hassan, D. A., Curtis, A., Karver, J., & Vangsnes, E. (2020). Diabetes self-management education and support: Referral and attendance at a patient-centered medical home. *Journal of Primary Care and Community Health, 11*, 1–6. https://doi.org/10.1177/2150132720967232

Herrick, C. J., Yount, B. W., & Eyler, A. A. (2016). Implications of supermarket access, neighbourhood walkability and poverty rates for diabetes risk in an employee population. *Public Health Nutrition, 19*(11), 2040–2048. https://doi.org/10.1017/S1368980015003328

Hie, X. (2013). Strengths-based approach to mental health recovery. *Iranian Journal of Psychiatry and Behavioral Science, 7*(2), 5–10.

Hill-Briggs, F., Adler, N. E., Berkowitz, S. A., Chin, M. H., Gary-Webb, T. L. Navas-Acien, Thornton, P. L., & Haire- Joshu, D. (2021). Social determinants of health and diabetes: A scientific review. *Diabetes Care, 44*(1), 258–279. https://doi.org/10.2337/dci20-0053

Holt, R. E. I., & Speight, J. (2017). The language of diabetes: The good, the bad and the ugly. *Diabetic Medicine, 34*(11), 1495–1497. https://doi.org/10.111/dme.13520

Hsu, W. C., Araneta, M. R., Kanaya, A. M., Chiang, J. L., & Fujemoto, W. (2015). BMI cutpoints to identify at risk Asian Americans for type 2 diabetes. *Diabetes Care, 38*(1), 150–155. https://doi.org/10.2337/dc14-2391

Ideastream Public Media. (2017). Zip code as the hidden vital sign. https://www.ideastream.org/tags/zip-code-the-hidden-vital-sign

International Diabetes Federation. (2019). IDF diabetes atlas (9th ed.). International Diabetes Foundation. https://diabetesatlas.org/

International Diabetes Federation. (2021). IDF diabetes atlas (10th ed.). https://diabetesatlas.org/

Isaacs, D. (2019). New clinician resource and insulin cost saving guide. https://www.diabeteseducator.org/news/perspectives/aade-blog-details/adces-perspectives-on-diabetes-care/2019/03/28/new-clinician-resource-insulin-cost-savings-guide

Jagai, J., Krajewski, A. K., Shaikh, S., Lobdell, D. T., & Sargis, R. M. (2020). Association between environmental quality and diabetes in the US. *Journal of Diabetes Investigation, 11*(2), 315– 322. https://doi.org/10.111/jdi.13152

Jernigan, K. (2009). The pitfalls of political correctness: Euphemisms excoriated. *Braille Monitor, 52*(3). https://nfb.org//sites/default/files/images/nfb/publications/bm/bm09/bm0903/bm090308.htm

Kapitan, A. (2017). On person first language: It's time to put the person first. https://radicalcopyeditor.com/2017/07/03/person-centered-language

Kolb, H., & Martin, S. (2017). Environmental/lifestyle factors in the pathogenesis and prevention of type 2 diabetes. *BMC Medicine, 15*(1), 131. https://doi.org/10.1186/s12916-017-0901-x

Kriska, A. M., Rockette-Wagner, B., Edelstein, S. L., Bray, G. A., Delahanty, L. M., Hoskin, M. A., Horton, E. S., Venditti, E. M., & Knowles, W. C., DPP Research Group. (2021). The impact of physical activity on the prevention of type 2 diabetes: Evidence and lessons learned from the diabetes prevention program, a long-standing clinical trial incorporating subjective and objective measures. *Diabetes Care, 44*(1), 43–49. https://doi.org/10.2337/dc20-1129

Kruger, D. F., LaRue, S., & Estepa, P. (2015). Recognition of and steps to mitigate anxiety and fear of pain in injectable diabetes treatment. *Diabetes, Metabolic Syndrome and Obesity: Target and Therapy, 8*, 49–56. https://doi.org/10.2147/DMSO.571923

Laposky, A. D., Van Cauter, E., & Diez-Roux, A. V. (2016). Reducing health disparities: The role of sleep deficiency and sleep disorders. *Sleep Medicine, 18*, 3–6. https://doi.org/10.1016/j.sleep.2015.01.007

Lilly Pharmaceutical Company. (2021). How much should I expect to pay for non-branded insulin? https://www.lillypricinginfo.com/insulin-lispro

Lindenfield, J., & Jessup, M. (2017). Drugs don't work in patients who don't take them. *European Journal of Heart Failure, 19*(11), 1412–1413. https://doi.org/10.1002/ejhf.920

Lobo, J. M., Soyoun, K. M., Kang H., Ocker, G., McMurry, T. L., Balkrishnan, R., Anderson, R., Lobo, J. M., Soyoun, K. M., Ocker, G. M., Kang, H., McMurry, T. & Sohn, M. (2019). Effects of medicaid expansion on uninsured rates: Diabetes belt vs. non-belt counties. *Diabetes, 68*(supp 1). https://doi.org/10.2337/db19-1235-P

Lohr, L. (2017). Farmers markets: Teaching kids where food comes from. United States Department of Agriculture. https://www.usda.gov/media/blog/2013/08/08/farmers-markets-teaching-kids-where-food-comes

Martino, J., Pegg, J., & Frates, E. P. (2017). The connection prescription: Using the power of social interactions and the deep desire for connectedness to empower health and wellness. *American Journal of Lifestyle Medicine, 11*(6), 466–475. https://doi.org/10.1177/1559827615608788

Modic, M. B., & Knapp, S. (Eds.). (2015). Healthy you: A guide to diabetes self-care. Maximum Velocity Press.

Mulcahy, K., Maryniuk, M., Peeples, M., Peyrot, M., Tomky, D., Weaver, T., & Yarbrough, P. (2003). Position statement: Standards for outcome measurement of D.S.M.E. *Diabetes Educator, 29*(5), 804–818. https://doi.org/10.1177/014572170302900510

Myers, C. A., Slack, T., Broyles, S. T., Heymsfield, S. B., Church, T. S., & Martin, C. K. (2017). Diabetes prevalence is associated with different community factors in the diabetes belt versus the rest of the U.S. *Obesity, 25*(2), 452–459. https://doi.org/10.1002/oby.21725

Nandyala, A. S., Nelson, L. A., Lagotte, A., & Osborn, C. (2017). An analysis of whether health literacy and numeracy are associated with diabetes medication adherence. *Health Literacy Research and Practice, 2*(1), e15–e20. https://doi.org/10.3928/24748307-20171212-01

National Academies of Sciences, Engineering, and Medicine. (2019). Investing in interventions that address non-medical, health-related social needs: Proceedings of a workshop. Washington, DC: The National Academies Press. https://doi.org/10.17226/25544

National Academy of Medicine. (2021). The future of nursing 2020–2030. Charting a path to achieve equity. https://nam.edu/publications/the-future-of-nursing-2020-2030/

Nelson, A. (2013). They are what they eat? Ensuring our children get the right nutrients. *The Journal of Family Health Care, 23*(2), 14–16.

Office of Disease Prevention and Health Promotion. (2021). Healthy people 2030. https://health.gov/healthypeople/objectives-and-data/browse-objectives/sleep/increase-proportion-adults-who-get-enough-sleep-sh-03

Ogilvie, R. P., & Patel, S. R. (2018). The epidemiology of sleep and diabetes. *Current Diabetes Reports, 18*(10), 82. https://doi.org/10.1007/s11892-018-1055-8

Ohayon, M. M., & Milesi, C. (2016). Artificial outdoor nighttime lights associate with altered sleep behavior in the American general population. *Sleep, 39*(6), 1311–1320. https://doi.org/10.5665/sleep.5860

Osborn, C. Y., Cavanaugh, K., Wallston, K. A., White, R. O. & Rothman, R. L. (2009). Diabetes numeracy. *Diabetes Care, 32*(9), 1614–1619. https://doi.org/10.2337/dc09-0425

Palmas, W., March, D., Darakjy, S., Findley, S. E., Teresi, J., Carrasquillo, O., & Luchsinger, J. A. (2015). Community health worker interventions to improve glycemic control in people with diabetes: A systematic review and meta-analysis. *Journal of General Medicine, 30*(7), 1004–1012. https://doi.org/10.1007/s11606-015-3247-0

Paulis, G. (2020). Meal appeal: Patterns of expenditures on food away from home. US Bureau of Labor Statistics. https://www.bls.gov/spotlight/2020/food-away-from-home/home.htm

Popkin, B. M., Adair, S., & Ng, S. W. (2012). Now and then: The global nutrition transition: The pandemic of obesity in developing countries. *Nutrition Review, 71*(1), 3–21. https://doi.org/10.111/j.1753-4887.2071.00456.x

Powers, M. A., Bardsley, J. K., Cypress, M., Funnell, M. A., Harms, D., Hess-Fischl, A., Hooks, B., Isaacs, D. Mandel, E. D., Norton, A., Rinker, J., Siminerio, L. M., & Uelmen, S. (2020). Diabetes self-management education and support in adults with type 2 diabetes: A consensus report of the American Diabetes Association, the Association of Diabetes Care & Education Specialists, The Academy of Nutrition and Dietetics, the American Academy of Family Physicians, the American Academy of Physician Assistants, the American Association of Nurse Practitioners, and the American Pharmacists Association. *Diabetes Care, 43*(7), 1636–1649. https://doi.org/10.2337/dci20-0023

Rafferty, A. P., Winterbauer, N. L., Luo, H., Bell, R. A., & Gaskins-Little, N. R. (2021). Diabetes self-care and clinical care among adults with low health literacy. *Journal of Public Health Management and Practice, 27*(2), 144–153. https://doi.org/10.1097/PHH0000000000001352

Rajkumar, S. V. (2019). The high cost of insulin in the United States; an urgent call to action. *Mayo Clinic Proceedings, 95*(11), 22–28. https://doi.org/10.1001/j.mayocp.2019.11.013

Ratzan, S. C., & Parker, R. M. (2000). Introduction. In national library of medicine current bibliographies in medicine. National Institutes of Health, U.S. Department of Health and Human Services.

Rebolledo, J., & Arellano, R. (2016). Cultural differences and considerations when initiating insulin. *Diabetes Spectrum, 29*(3), 185–190. https://doi.org/10.2337/diaspect.29.3.185

Reusch, J. (2019). The diabetes story: A call to action. *Diabetes Care, 42*(5), 713–717.

Sandberg, J. C., Talton, J. W., Quandt, S., & Chen, H., Weir, M., Douman, W. R., Chatterjee, A., & Acury, T, (2014). Association between housing quality and individual health characteristics on sleep quality among Latino farmworkers. *Journal of Immigrant and Minority Health, 16*(2), 265–272, https://doi.org/10.10007/s`0903-0`2-9746-8

Satterfield, D., Debruyn, L., Francis, C. D., & Allen, A. A (2014). A stream is always giving life: Communities reclaim native science. *American Indian Culture and Research Journal, 38*(1), 157–190. https://doi.org/10.17953?aicr.38.1.hp318040258r

Spanakis, E. K., & Golden, S. H. (2013). Race/ethnic difference in diabetes and diabetic complications. *Current Diabetes Report, 13*(6), 814–823. https://doi.org/10.1007/s11892-013-0421-9

Statista.com. (2021). Countries with the highest number of diabetics worldwide in 2021. https://www.statista.com/statistics/281082/countries-with-highest-number-of-diabetics/

Trust for America's Health. (2021). https://www.tfah.org/report-details/publichealthfunding2020/

U.S. Department of Agriculture Economic Research Service. (2022). Definitions of food security. https://www.ers.usda.gov/topics/food-nutrition-assistance/food-security-in-the-u-s/definitions-of-food-security/

U.S. Preventive Services Task Force. (2021). Prediabetes and type 2 diabetes: Screening. https://www.uspreventiveservicestaskforce.org/uspstf/recommendation/screening-for-prediabetes-and-type-2-diabetes

Ueleman, S., & Macleod, J. (2020). Diabetes education reimagined: Educator- led, technology-enabled diabetes population health management services. *Diabetes Digital Health*, 25–36. https://doi.org/10.2026/8978-0-12-817485-2.00002x

Wahl, S., Englehardt, M., Schaupp, P., Lappe, C., & Ivanov, I. V. (2019). The inner clock-blue light sets the human rhythm. *Journal of Biophotonics, 12*(12). https://doi.org/10.1002/jbio.201900102

Walker, M. (2017). *Why we sleep: Unlocking the power of sleep and dreams*. Scribner.

Walker, R. J., Garacci, E., Campbell, J. A., Harris M., Mosley-Johnson, E., & Egede, L. (2020). Relationship between multiple measures of financial hardship and glycemic control in older adults with diabetes. *Journal of Applied Gerontology, 40*(2), 162–169. https://doi.org/10.1177/0733464820911545

Walker, R. J., Williams, J. S., & Egede, L. E. (2016). Influence of race, ethnicity and social determinants of health on diabetes outcomes. *American Journal of the Medical Sciences, 351*(4), 366–373. https://doi.org/10.1016/j.amjms.2016.01.008

Whinnery, J., Jackson, N., Rattanaumpawan, P., & Grander, M. A. (2014). Short and long sleep duration associated with race/ethnicity, sociodemographics, and socioeconomic position. *Sleep, 37*(3), 601–611. https://doi.org/10.5665/sleep.3508

White, R. O., Wolff, K., Cavanaugh, K., & Rothman, R. (2010). Addressing health literacy and numeracy to improve diabetes care. *Diabetes Spectrum, 23*(4), 238–243. https://doi.org/10.2337/diaspect.23.4.233

Wieland, M., Njeru, J., Hanza, M., Boehm, D., Sigh, D., …, Yawn, G. (2017). Pilot feasibility study of a digital storytelling intervention for immigrant and refuge adults with diabetes. *Diabetes Educator, 43*(4), 349–359. https://doi.org/10.1177?0145721717713317

Williams, D. R., Mohammed, S. A., Leavell, J., & Collins, C. (2010). Race, socioeconomic status, and health: Complexities, ongoing challenges, and research options. *Annals of the New York Academy of Science, 1186*, 24–36. https://doi.org/10.1111/j.1749-6632.2009.05339.x

Windover, A., Boissy, A., Rice, T., Gilligan, T., Velez, V. J., & Merlino, J. (2014). The REDE model of healthcare communication: Optimizing relationship as a therapeutic agent. *Journal of Patient Experience, 1*(1), 8–13. https://doi.org/10.1177/2374373431400100103

Yafi, M. (2015). Abstract 303: A toddler with type 2 diabetes. Presented at *European Association for the Society of Diabetes (EASD)*, Stockholm, Sweden. https://www.sciencedaily.com/releases/2015/09/150916215548.htm

Zaugg, S. D., Dogbey, G., Collins, K., Reynolds, S., Batista, C., Brannan, G., & Shubrook, J. H. (2014). Diabetes numeracy and blood glucose control: Association with type of diabetes and source of care. *Clinical Diabetes, 32*(4), 152–157. https://doi.org/10.2337/diaclin.37.4.152

CHAPTER 16

Intersections Among Sociocultural and Environmental Issues in Adulthood and Childhood Cardiovascular Health and Hypertension

Carolyn Harmon Still and Jackson T. Wright

LEARNING OBJECTIVES

- Describe the changing prevalence of cardiovascular disease among adults and children in the United States.

- Understand the racial and ethnic differences in cardiovascular disease among adults and children.

- Analyze the dynamic nature of risk factors, including social, economic, environment, health risk behaviors, and provider-level factors that influence racial/ethnic differences in cardiovascular health and outcomes.

- Describe the role of health inequities and how they emerge to influence cardiovascular health disparities.

- Discuss nonpharmacological and pharmacological options needed to reduce cardiovascular risk factors, promote lifestyle modifications, and improve the quality of healthcare in adults and children with cardiovascular disease and hypertension.

- Describe the influence of health professionals on improving health outcomes in adults and children with cardiovascular disease and hypertension.

INTRODUCTION

Cardiovascular disease (CVD), heart and blood vessel disorders, are the leading cause of death and disability globally and in the United States (Virani et al., 2020). CVD includes coronary artery disease, stroke, heart failure, peripheral arterial disease, and other vascular conditions, and it accounts for approximately 17.9 million deaths worldwide and one out of three deaths in the United States (Fullman et al., 2018; Virani et al., 2020). In this chapter, we highlight the complexity and scope of CVD and issues that contribute to the burden of health disparities in the United States. We also illuminate race and ethnicity at the interconnection of these outcomes with socioeconomic, environmental, cultural, and other determinants of health that directly and indirectly influence population-level differences in cardiovascular risk and health outcomes.

PREVALENCE AND RISK OF CARDIOVASCULAR DISEASE

In the United States, CVD affects nearly half (48%) of American adults. Of these, one in three adults have one or more types of CVD, and the prevalence increases with advancing age (i.e., 40% from 40–59 years to 86% in 80-plus years; Virani et al., 2020). Overall, CVD affects more men than women, with minorities, in particular non-Hispanic Black persons, disproportionately burdened. Major CVD diseases make up approximately 31% of the top 10 leading causes of death. In 2018, the majority of these deaths were attributed to coronary heart disease (665,381) and cerebrovascular disease (147,810), the first and third leading causes of death; combined, they represent one third of all deaths in the United States (Heron, 2019). Figure 16.1 presents the percentage of deaths by specific CVD condition. CVD is the most costly disease in terms of direct (healthcare services, medicines) and indirect (lost productivity/missed workdays, disabilities, death) costs. It is estimated to have cost $363.4 billion and accounted for 14% of total U.S. health expenditures in 2017 (Virani et al., 2020).

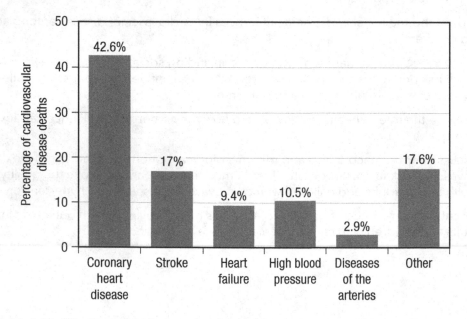

Figure 16.1 Distribution of cardiovascular disease deaths by type in the United States in 2017.
Source: Data from the American Heart Association, National Center for Health Statistics, and National Heart, Lung, and Blood Institute.

Prevalence of Cardiovascular Disease by Race/Ethnicity and Age

While there has been a decline in CVD mortality over the last decade across all populations, these trends differ by race and ethnicity, as well as by morbidity (the occurrence of specific health conditions) and mortality (incidence of death due to a specific health condition). Health statistics regarding mortality continue to show that non-Hispanic Black persons lag behind in the reduction of CVD when compared to other racial/ethnic groups (non-Hispanic Whites, Asian/Pacific Islanders, and Native Americans, including American Indians and Alaska Natives) and have a twofold higher incidence of CVD morbidity and mortality. It is important to mention that while Asian/Pacific Islanders and Native Americans are also considered minority populations, epidemiological statistics are inconsistent and sparse due to the lack of reporting of disease status or death rates. Among various racial and ethnic groups, non-Hispanic Black adults have the highest prevalence rate of CVD compared with other racial groups. In 2017, of non-Hispanic Black adults age 20 years and older, 60.1% of men and 58.8% of women had CVD. For non-Hispanic White adults, this number was lower: 50.6% of men and 43.4% of women had CVD. Hispanic and Asian men and women had the lowest prevalence of CVD rates. Figure 16.2 shows the age-adjusted death rates for CVD that vary by race/ethnicity. Among the data that are available, 4.4% of Asians Americans and Pacific Islanders age 18 years and older have CVD, with a 40% higher chance of death from CVD for men compared with women. There are even fewer data available on the health status of Native Americans. However, Native Americans have a similar or slightly higher disease burden of CVD compared to the general U.S. population (Virani et al., 2020).

In addition to disparities between racial and ethnic groups by sex, the relative excess mortality rates of CVD occur prematurely in people younger than 70 years and increase sharply with age. For example, the age-specific rates of CVD are higher in men than in women in most age group strata. At age 60 to 79 years, CVD prevalence doubles in women,

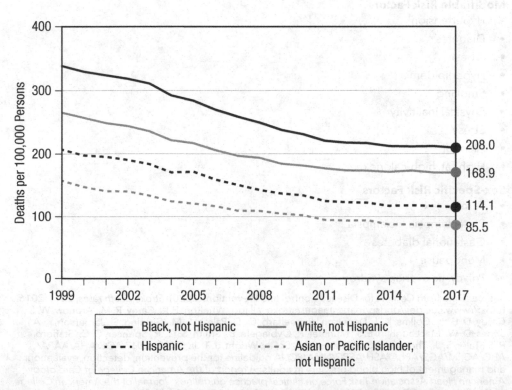

Figure 16.2 Age-adjusted death rates for heart disease by race and Hispanic origin, 1999 to 2017.
Source: Data from National Center for Health Statistics.

surpassing men. The higher incidence is associated with the increase of older adults living longer, especially women, who have a life expectancy 5 years longer than that of men. Data reveal that about two thirds of CVD deaths occur in people age 75 and older. With longevity gains, the aging population is projected to increase dramatically, and about one in five Americans (21.9% of the U.S. population) will be age 65 and older by 2040 (Ortman et al., 2014). The racial/ethnic differences in CVD morbidity and mortality cannot be completely explained by high incidents of CVD risk factors, but by the interactions of psychosocial and biological factors and the social determinants of health—conditions where people live, learn, work, and play—that have a profound effect on health risks and outcomes (Marmot, 2017). These factors are described later on in this chapter.

Cardiovascular Disease Risk Factors

The high prevalence of CVD is frequently associated with a myriad of complex risk factors, including both modifiable and nonmodifiable risk factors (Box 16.1). These risk factors play a key role in the burden of CVD and include conditions such as hypertension, diabetes, hyperlipidemia, and obesity (Ritchey et al., 2020; Whelton et al., 2018). Figure 16.3

BOX 16.1: Cardiovascular Disease Major Risk Factors

Nonmodifiable Risk Factors
- Sex
- Age
- Heredity or family history
- Race and ethnicity

Modifiable Risk Factors
- Hypertension
- Diabetes
- Obesity
- Hyperlipidemia
- Smoking
- Physical inactivity
- Stress
- Alcohol
- High-fat, high-calorie diet

Sex-Specific Risk Factors
- Female sex
- Pre-eclampsia, eclampsia
- Gestational diabetes
- Menopause
- Polycystic ovarian syndrome

Source: Data from Centers for Disease Control and Prevention. (2020). *Stroke death rates, 2014–2016.* https://www.cdc.gov/dhdsp/maps/images/stroke_all.jpg; Whelton, P. K., Carey, R. M., Aronow, W. S., Casey, D. E. Jr., Collins, K. J., Dennison Himmelfarb, C., DePalma, S. M., Gidding, S., Jamerson, K. A., Jones, D. W., MacLaughlin, E. J., Muntner, P., Ovbiagele, B., Smith, S. C. Jr., Spencer, C. C., Stafford, R. S., Taler, S. J., Thomas, R. J., Williams, K. A. Sr., ..., Wright, J. T. Jr. (2018). 2017 ACC/AHA/AAPA/ABC/ACPM/AGS/APhA/ASH/ASPC/NMA/PCNA guideline for the prevention, detection, evaluation, and management of high blood pressure in adults: *A report of the American College of Cardiology/American Heart Association Task Force on clinical practice guidelines. Journal of the American College of Cardiology,* 71(19), e127–e248. https://doi.org/10.1016/j.jacc.2017.11.006.

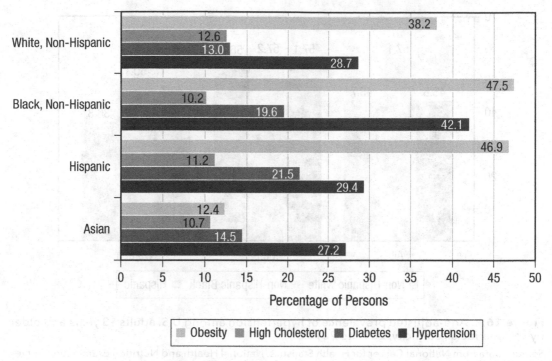

Figure 16.3 Prevalence of cardiovascular risk factors among U.S. adults in 2017.

Source: Data from National Center for Health Statistics.

shows selected CVD risk factors by race and ethnicity. This figure demonstrates that in 2017, non-Hispanic Black persons had the highest rates of most CVD risk factors compared with other groups, with the exception of high cholesterol. Among disadvantaged populations, women are more likely to be at greater risk of CVD related to sex-specific and unique pathophysiological changes as they age (Ahmad & Oparil, 2017). Substantial racial/ethnic differences are observed in CVD mortality in women, with African American women having the highest burden, followed by non-Hispanic White, Hispanic, Asian American/Pacific Islander, and Native American women. Misperceptions still exist that CVD does not affect women and that it is a man's disease. This is often because women are more likely to experience atypical symptoms (e.g., fatigue; shortness of breath; subtle discomfort in the throat, jaw, neck, arms, back, and stomach; muscle aches), are underdiagnosed, and are more likely to not be treated for CVD compared with men (see Figure 16.3).

Hypertension

Among CVD risk factors, hypertension is the leading contributor to CVD and related vascular diseases such as coronary heart disease (CHD), heart failure, stroke, chronic kidney disease (CKD), and dementia (Virani et al., 2020; Whelton et al., 2018). Hypertension, also called high blood pressure, occurs when the force (pressure) of the blood against the artery walls is high; if left untreated, the long-term consequences can result in adverse health conditions. In efforts to target earlier interventions and to account for adverse complications related to hypertension, stricter blood pressure guidelines were developed in 2017 by the American College of Cardiology and the American Heart Association (ACC/AHA). These criteria define hypertension as 130/80 millimeters of mercury (mmHg) and higher for all adults, compared with the previous definition of hypertension as 140/90 mmHg or greater. Further, this guideline changed the way in which high blood pressure is treated and managed. With the stricter blood pressure guidelines, the prevalence rates of hypertension in U.S. adults from 2014 to 2018 increased from 32% to 47.3%, respectively. According to 2018

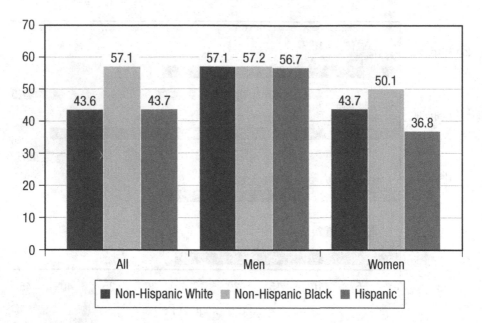

Figure 16.4 Age-adjusted prevalence of hypertension among U.S. adults 18 years and older by sex and racial/ethnicity, 2017 to 2018.

Source: Data from National Center for Health Statistics. National Health and Nutrition Examination Survey 2017-2018.

data, among American adults 20 years of age and older, 47% of men and 43% of women had hypertension, affecting approximately 108 million adults in the United States.

Figure 16.4 shows age-adjusted prevalence of hypertension, and non-Hispanic Black Americans continue to be disproportionately affected by the disease. Non-Hispanic Black Americans have higher rates of hypertension (54%) than non-Hispanic White (46%), non-Hispanic Asian (39%), and Hispanic Americans (36%). Non-Hispanic Black men currently account for the largest portion of U.S. adults diagnosed with hypertension when compared with non-Hispanic White and Hispanic populations (Centers for Disease Control and Prevention [CDC], 2020). For all people, the risk of hypertension increases markedly with age. Hypertension and related adverse conditions are associated with increased healthcare use, loss of years of healthy life and working, and premature death (CDC, 2021). These trends, in fact, may be attributed to a recent reversal in hypertension awareness and control. Data from the National Health and Nutrition Examination Survey (NHANES; a continuous program of assessment of health and nutritional status from a large, nationally representative sample) taken between 1999 and 2018 demonstrate that there has been a decline in the percentage of awareness of having hypertension from 85% in 2013 to 2014 to 77% in 2017 to 2018 (Muntner et al., 2020). Similar patterns of decline were observed in individuals in terms of blood pressure control (54%–44%) and being treated with antihypertensive medications (72%–65%). Non-Hispanic Black Americans continue to have lower proportions of controlled hypertension when compared with other subgroups. The high unawareness and uncontrolled hypertension rates can be explained by lack of health insurance or a primary care provider or by infrequent healthcare visits (Artiga et al., 2015; Fiscella & Sanders, 2016).

The magnitude of population differences in hypertension regarding early onset, severity, and subsequent clinical sequelae are due to biophysiological and pathophysiological mechanisms. Important factors influencing hypertension include familial and genetic dispositions, activation of neurohormonal systems such as the sympathetic nervous system (due to stress), the renin-angiotensin-aldosterone system controlling blood pressure, and salt intake sensitivity (Oparil et al., 2003). Considerable evidence suggests that hypertension has a strong familial and genetic component, and the heritability accounts for about 30% to 40% of hypertension risk and prevalence. In addition, the genetic epidemiology of hypertension has been linked to several candidate genes and accounts for a small percentage (approximately 6%) of the genetic contribution to blood pressure regulation and variance (Zilbermint et al., 2019). One example is the angiotensinogen (AGT) gene identified as a causative factor for hypertension susceptibility; its genetic variant, T235, is twice as likely to be found in Black people and is suggested to contribute to racial/ethnic differences observed in persons with hypertension (Bloem et al., 1997; Zilbermint et al., 2019). Environmental stimuli (sodium and potassium intake, stress) interact with gene variants, and the dynamic relationship (gene-environmental interaction) triggers biological processes to alter phenotypes, accounting for approximately 20% of the development of hypertension (Chobanian et al., 2003).

Diabetes

Another important CVD risk factor is diabetes. Diabetes is the seventh leading cause of death in the United States. In 2018, approximately, 4.2 million (34.2%) U.S. adults 18 years and older had diabetes. In contrast, one in five adults are unaware that they had the condition. Some racial/ethnic minorities are more likely to have diabetes and experience increased morbidity and mortality compared with non-Hispanic Whites. According to the 2018 National Health Interview Survey, higher age-adjusted percentages of diabetes are reported in American Indians or Alaska Natives (23.3%), Native Hawaiians or Other Pacific Islanders (19.8%), and Mexicans or Mexican Americans (14.9%). While only 13.1% of non-Hispanic Black people have diabetes, paradoxically, they are twice as likely to have secondary complications (limb amputation, end-stage renal disease) and concomitant CVD-related diseases (hypertension, stroke) from diabetes compared with non-Hispanic Whites. It is important to point out that the same factors (e.g., sociocultural and environmental factors, hypertension) that influence CVD also play a role in the incidence and prevalence rates of diabetes in U.S. adults.

Overall, the 2017 age-adjusted diabetes death rates in the United States for non-Hispanic Blacks were 38.8/100,000 compared with 18.8/100,000 non-Hispanic Whites (CDC, 2017). A recent report suggests that diabetes differs greatly by age and sex, with disproportionate numbers occurring in non-Hispanic Black men. For example, diabetes is the sixth leading cause of death for non-Hispanic Black men age 20 to 44 years, then ascends to the fourth leading cause of death for individuals age 45 to 84 years. Notably, evidence suggests that the higher rates observed in non-Hispanic Black men are also driven by individual CVD risk factors and health behaviors, as well as social, environmental, and biological determinants, which are discussed later in this chapter.

Hyperlipidemia

High blood cholesterol, also called hyperlipidemia, has been well-documented as a risk factor for CVD. Approximately 12% of U.S. adults age 20 years and older have high cholesterol, with higher rates in non-Hispanic White woman (14.9%) and Hispanic men (13.9%), while lower rates are observed in non-Hispanic Black men (10.6%) and Hispanic women (9.0%). Racial and ethnic differences observed in cholesterol incidence and treatment are partly explained by the lower screening rates among minority populations, suggesting that there is an underestimation of prevalence rates for high cholesterol (Kenik et al., 2014). For this reason, minority populations have lower rates of awareness, treatment, and control of their cholesterol compared with non-Hispanic Whites (Kim et al., 2018). Epidemiological data suggest that conditions such as high levels of cholesterol and high blood pressure increase the risk for coronary heart disease and mortality (Virani et al., 2020).

Obesity

There has been an unprecedented increase in obesity prevalence in the United States, with 42.4% of adults regarded as clinically obese (Hales et al., 2017, 2020). The degree and incidence

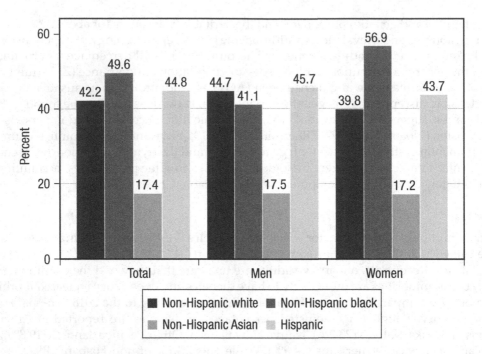

Figure 16.5 Age-adjusted prevalence of obesity among U.S. adults 20 years and older by sex and racial/ethnicity, 2017 to 2018.

Source: Data from National Health and Nutrition Examination Survey, 2017–2018.

of obesity remains high in minority populations, regardless of age. Nearly half of non-Hispanic Black adults (49.6%) had the highest age-adjusted prevalence of obesity, followed by Native Americans (48.1%), Hispanic adults (44.8%), and non-Hispanic White adults (42.2%), while non-Hispanic Asian adults (17.0%) have the lowest rates. Data also reveal that minority women, especially non-Hispanic Black women and Hispanic women, are more likely to be overweight or obese (Figure 16.5). Further, obesity plays a major role in mortality and is recognized as a risk factor for several health conditions, including CHD, hypertension, dyslipidemia, diabetes, stroke, and cancer. Among many other factors, adverse economic and social conditions (poverty, unemployment, underemployment), individual behaviors (unhealthy dietary patterns, physical inactivity), and community and environmental factors (food insecurity, exposure to the marketing of unhealthy products) contribute to the high rates of obesity, especially in minority populations (LaVeist, 2005; Marmot & Wilkinson, 2006).

Behavioral Risk Factors

CVD is frequently associated with a myriad of risk factors, including behavioral health risk factors—behaviors that can potentially have negative effects on health (see Box 16.1). For example, smoking (tobacco use), physical inactivity, alcohol consumption, and unhealthy diet, while modifiable, contribute to a large proportion of CVD disease burden (Virani et al., 2020). Smoking remains the leading modifiable risk factor that contributes to a large portion of premature CVD and mortality, followed by both physical inactivity and poor dietary patterns. The burden of these three risk factors accounts for one third of all CVD deaths and partly explains the observed differences in CVD health outcomes between minority populations and non-Hispanic Whites (Virani et al., 2020). For example, physical activity has been shown to significantly reduce all-cause mortality by 33%, yet less than half of U.S. adults (46%) engage in the recommended level of physical activity (American Heart Association, 2018). Carnethon et al. (2017) found that disparities in physical inactivity prevalence are generally highest for Hispanic Americans (31.7%), followed by non-Hispanic Black Americans (30.3%), relative to non-Hispanic White Americans (23.4%). Overall, the pronounced differences in health risk behaviors are also related to economic status and sociocultural environmental factors, such as affordability of and access to healthy foods, unsafe and disadvantaged neighborhoods, and cultural and family influences (Gary-Webb et al., 2021; Hawes et al., 2019).

Cardiovascular Disease in Children and Adolescents

CVD risk factors often present during early childhood and persist through adulthood. In children, the principal causes of CVD are similar to those of adults, with many factors having a direct relationship to the probability of cardiac disease later in life. These novel risk factors include obesity, physical inactivity, sedentary lifestyle, smoking, high blood pressure, and high cholesterol. Intrinsic to the direct relationship between subclinical disease state and CVD are the constellation of cardiometabolic risk factors (hyperglycemia, increased central adiposity, elevated triglycerides, decreased high-density lipoprotein cholesterol, and elevated blood pressure), all conditions noted to be increasingly high in minority children as well as in adults. Recent trends demonstrate an increase in prevalence of obesity rates in children, with approximately 13.7 million (18.5%) children and adolescents age 2 to 19 years being overweight or obese. By way of comparison, in descending order, 25.6% of Hispanic children, 24.2% of non-Hispanic Black children, 16.1% of non-Hispanic White children, 11.0% Native American children, and 8.7% Asian American children are obese or overweight. In terms of cholesterol, 7% of U.S. children age 6 to 19 years were diagnosed with high total cholesterol in 2018 (Virani et al., 2020). Evidence suggests that striking disparities persist in patterns of CVD risk factors and health, especially for children of color and those who are from low-income families (Jackson et al., 2018). Equally important, children who reside in rural and southern geographical U.S. locations (Kentucky, Mississippi, South Carolina, Tennessee, and Arkansas) tend to have the highest obesity rates, well above the national average; that is, greater than or equal to 20% (Dwyer-Lindgren et al., 2017). Further, the CVD health of children and adolescents is inextricably linked to their parents' physical, emotional, and social health, as well as their social and environmental circumstances: living in poverty, food insecurity, limited health literacy, and access to care (Expert Panel on Integrated Guidelines for Cardiovascular Health and Risk Reduction in Children and Adolescents, 2011). A more in-depth discussion of the intersectionality of CVD and determinants of health occurs later in this chapter.

Hypertension in Children

Historically, hypertension or elevated blood pressure has been associated with adults. However, over the last decade there has been a steady increase in younger populations diagnosed and treated for high blood pressure. The diagnosis of hypertension in children is complex and is defined as a systolic and/or diastolic blood pressure greater than or equal to the 95th percentile by sex, age, and height (Sun et al., 2017). According to the 2017 American Academy of Pediatrics Clinical Practice Hypertension Guideline, one in 25 people age 12 to 19 has hypertension, and one in 10 has elevated blood pressure (Flynn et al., 2017). When considering age and sex, epidemiological data suggest racial/ethnic groups do not differ in prevalence of hypertension until adolescence (Hansen et al., 2007; Song et al., 2019). In general, boys tend to have slightly higher blood pressure compared with girls during the first decade of life, and then differences are more pronounced by the age of puberty (Perng et al., 2019). Relative to the adult population, non-Hispanic Black and Hispanic children have a greater prevalence of high blood pressure and hypertension than non-Hispanic White children, largely due to the surge in obesity (Al Kibria et al., 2019).

Similar to adults, lifestyle and health risk behaviors of children contribute to the development of hypertension from childhood into adulthood. Obesity, low physical activity, and dietary intake of high sodium foods and saturated fats are leading risk factors and are the precursors to lifelong CVD adverse health conditions and morbidity and mortality. Of particular importance, numerous interrelated risk components and perinatal health conditions such as pre-eclampsia/eclampsia, gestational diabetes, and maternal obesity predispose children to early onset of high blood pressure (Davis et al., 2015; Geelhoed et al., 2010). While the data are not robust for children, there is a strong association between sleep disorders (e.g., obstructive sleep apnea, sleep deprivation, insomnia) and high blood pressure, known factors that increase CVD risk (Matthews & Pantesco, 2016; Paciência et al., 2013). In addition, sleep characteristics (duration, continuity, quality) coupled with stress and diet influence increase rates of hypertension in children across all racial and ethnic groups (Matthews et al., 2014).

THE INTERSECTIONALITY OF CARDIOVASCULAR DISEASE AND DETERMINANTS OF HEALTH

Disparities in CVD health and outcomes have been well-documented. In fact, these trends—CVD prevalence, morbidity, and mortality—are rooted in sociocultural environmental issues at the individual, provider, and system levels. Many theories have conceptually explained and linked empirically broad patterns of health and outcomes to distinct mechanisms and pathways driven by social, environmental, and biological factors (Glass & McAtee, 2006; Marmot & Wilkinson, 2006; Thorpe et al., 2008). Collectively, these models focus on how causal influences flow metaphorically upstream (macrosocial factors that limit personal resources) and downstream (individual factors that affect health outcomes over time). Thus, increased risk for CVD in turn rests on social structure and limited personal resources. Income level, educational attainment, employment status, access to care, health literacy, and neighborhood conditions (e.g., community violence, food deserts) exert a strong influence on health and may partly explain racial/ethnic gaps in CVD morbidity (obesity, heart disease, hypertension).

Low socioeconomic status has been associated with the development of CVD (Havranek et al., 2015). Broadly speaking, minority groups disproportionately live in poverty and are more likely to live in disadvantaged neighborhoods that lack stores to purchase healthy foods and places to exercise, with exposure to deteriorating housing, and high crime and related safety issues. In 2019, 12.3% of U.S. adults lived in poverty, with highest rates among Native Americans (25.4%), non-Hispanic Black Americans (21.2%), and Hispanic Americans (17.2%) compared with non-Hispanic White Americans (9.0%). Similar trends are observed in children's populations. Poverty dramatically inhibits one's ability to afford a wide range of material goods or basic necessities such as decent housing, healthy foods, medications, adequate education, and medical care essential to health and well-being. Research has also suggested that conditions (high-poverty neighborhoods, urban and high-violence areas) and place of residence—living in the southern region of the United States (Mississippi, Louisiana, Kentucky, Arkansas, West Virginia, Alabama, Oklahoma, Tennessee, South Carolina, and Puerto Rico)—play an important contributing role in racial/ethnic disparities in CVD risk and outcomes such as hypertension and stroke (Elkind et al., 2020; Kaiser et al., 2016; Ko et al., 2016).

One study, the REasons for Geographic And Racial Differences in Stroke (REGARDS) study, found evidence that Black people were twice to four times as likely to die from stroke when compared with White people (Howard et al., 2007). This excessive stroke mortality persists 20 years later, largely in part due to lower socioeconomic status and higher incidence of CVD-related risk factors such as obesity, hypertension, and diabetes, which contribute to the observed differences in stroke by geographical region. Specifically, a collection of southeastern states with increased stroke risk and related mortality, known as the "Stroke Belt," includes 11 states: Alabama, Arkansas, Georgia, Kentucky, Louisiana, Mississippi, Missouri, North Carolina, South Carolina, Texas, and Tennessee (Howard & Howard, 2020). Furthermore, non-Hispanic Black people, as well as other disadvantaged groups, have the highest burden of CVD mortality due to one or more risk factors (Virani et al., 2020).

The literature further suggests that social inequalities and a range of health risk exposures perpetuate downstream factors—the psychosocial and biophysiological mechanisms

BOX 16.2: Social, Environmental, and Biological Determinants Affecting Cardiovascular Health

Social
- Social economic status
- Education attainment
- Employment status
- Cultural beliefs/attitudes
- Health behaviors
- Health literacy

Environment
- Residential environment and geographic location
- Community violence and safety
- Food insecurity
- Levels of overt or explicit racism, discrimination
- Healthcare access and inequalities

Biological
- Genetics (family history)
- Gene-environmental interaction
- Sex

Source: Data from LaVeist, T. (2005). *Minority population and health: Introduction to health disparities in the United States.* Jossey-Bass; Marmot, M., & Wilkinson, R. (2006). *Social determinants of health* (2nd ed.). Oxford University Press.

that lead to health outcomes (Box 16.2). Stress has been shown to affect health, especially the development of hypertension that is brought on by work-related and life stressors, inadequate social support, and adverse experiences such as racism, discrimination, and social unrest (Adhikari et al., 2020; Schoenthaler & Rosenthal, 2018). Several studies have demonstrated an association between psychological and physiological states on health. The impact of such interaction subsequently disrupts the body's homeostasis, activating the hypothalamic-pituitary-adrenal (HPA) axis and the sympathetic nervous system. Over time, chronic stressors elicit stress-induced cardiovascular reactivity responses (i.e., excessive cortisol and catecholamine release, elevated heart rate and blood pressure) and exacerbate the stress/ hypertension relationship (Gehlert et al., 2008; Spruill, 2010). The potential synergistic effects of psychosocial factors and health risk behaviors (e.g., physical inactivity, smoking, unhealthy eating, alcohol and substance use) help to create the backdrop for ill health and predicts poor CVD outcomes.

The circumstances in which children are born, live, learn, and grow, as well as their parents' unmet psychosocial needs, have adverse consequences on their health outcomes. Much of the research that has explored the influence of determinants of health on children's morbidity and mortality suggest it coincides with the parents' socioenvironmental circumstances, and diseases in children originate during intrauterine development (Barker, 2007; Marmot & Wilkinson, 2006). For example, children's adverse early life exposure (undernutrition in utero, low birth weight, failure to thrive) coupled with socioeconomic environmental disadvantages (poor housing, food insecurity), and the accumulation of multigenerational cycles of poverty shape their health over the life course. Contributions of early life, chronic stressors, and unhealthy lifestyles add to the rising unfavorable health outcomes (CVD, diabetes, hypertension) in children that demonstrate similar patterns of poor health observed in adults. It is these childhood circumstances that may explain the early onset of unfavorable health and premature death related to CVD (Barker, 2007).

Other Underlying Causes of Disparities in Cardiovascular Disease

Despite advances in the prevention and treatment of CVD, there is increasing awareness that the benefits (reduction in CVD-related health conditions and an increase in longevity) are not equal across racial/ethnic groups in the United States. With the recognition that lifestyle behavioral factors do not fully explain CVD risk, explanatory models have shifted to focus on healthcare disparities (Marmot, 2017). Growing evidence suggests that a complex and interrelated set of individual, provider, and health system level factors fuel persistent healthcare disparities. Racial/ethnic differences in healthcare are closely linked with access, use, and quality of care (Fiscella & Sanders, 2016). For example, a large proportion of health disparities is associated with suboptimal insurance coverage and poor access to healthcare, which has several dimensions, such as the lack of transportation, limited health literacy, inadequate cultural acumen among providers, and language barriers. According to the U.S. Census Bureau, 29.6 million Americans did not have health insurance coverage in 2019, with Hispanic American and Black American populations having the highest uninsured rates, 16.7% and 9.6%, respectively, compared with 5.2% of White Americans. Although after the Affordable Care Act (ACA) coverage expansion (including Medicaid) vulnerable populations' insurance coverage status somewhat improved, the data show that minorities still tend to delay or forego care (e.g., preventive care) due to perceived health status, a sense of susceptibility about disease conditions, or healthcare cost (Artiga et al., 2015; Fiscella & Sanders, 2016).

Other explanations for healthcare disparities go beyond lack of insurance and include predisposing and enabling factors such as individuals' cultural beliefs, health literacy, lack of a healthcare provider, and availability and access to primary care. A combination of these factors ultimately affects healthcare service utilization. For those individuals who seek care, health inequalities arise at the provider level. In various reports, linguistic and cultural competency, perceived discrimination, provider's attitude, and poor patient/provider communication have been suggested to have major influence on the underuse of healthcare services (Carnethon et al., 2017; Schoenthaler et al., 2012). The degree of difference in racial/ethnic disparities may also be explained by the confluence of the providers' decision-making and clinical inertia (failure to intensify therapy to achieve treatment goals), which greatly affects the quality of care (Smedley et al., 2003). For example, recent research such as the Systolic Blood Pressure Intervention Trial (SPRINT), found that aggressive treatment for hypertension can reduce all-cause mortality by 27%, regardless of race/ethnicity or age. Treatment would require, on average, two antihypertensive medications for most adults, and at least three antihypertensive medications on average for non-Hispanic Black persons (Still et al., 2017; Wright et al., 2015). However, minorities are less likely to be prescribed appropriate drugs that are known to be more efficacious at lowering blood pressure, such as diuretics and calcium channel blockers (Whelton et al., 2018; Wright et al., 2005), for many reasons mentioned previously. Other factors, such as lack of provider awareness, cultural sensitivity, or patients' unintentional noncompliance to prescribed medications (because of inability to afford medication or possible side effects) influence high rates of hypertension.

PREVENTION AND TREATMENT OF CARDIOVASCULAR DISEASE

Overall, trends in CVD health have shown steady improvements for most Americans. The key factor in reducing morbidity and mortality from CVD and related conditions is prevention, especially the incorporation of nonpharmacological treatment (e.g., physical activity, healthy diet, stress reduction). Research has clearly demonstrated the benefits of lifestyle modifications in the prevention and reduction of CVD (Mensah et al., 2017). Calls to improve prevention of CVD have led to national efforts and guidelines to modify health behaviors, such as "Life's Simple 7," developed by the American Heart Association (Georgiadis, 2013), and the Million Hearts initiative to improve primary and secondary prevention of CVD and related risk factors (Lloyd-Jones et al., 2010). Such programs target health behaviors and metrics to improve health with regard to smoking status, physical activity, weight, diet, blood glucose, cholesterol, and blood pressure. National efforts have also extended to reach children, as seen with the former First Lady Michelle Obama's "Let's Move!" campaign to address childhood obesity and food insecurity to improve overall health of the nation's children (Georgiadis, 2013). However, strategic goals aimed at reducing CVD deaths by 20% in 2022 might not be met (Lloyd-Jones et al., 2010; Wright et al., 2018). While there have been modest declines in cardiovascular mortality over time by race and sex, data continue to demonstrate poorer compliance in terms of lifestyle modifications among minorities, especially for non-Hispanic Black women (Muntner et al., 2020; Pool et al., 2017). Given that hypertension is associated with many CVD-related health conditions, a recent health priority and strategic goal put forth by Healthy People 2030 is to target controlling blood pressure in 60% of adults age 18 years and older with hypertension to less than 130/80 mmHg (Office of Disease Prevention and Health Promotion [ODPHP], 2020).

Because of increased longevity, most adults in the United States have one out of three key CVD risk factors, with hypertension as the leading risk factor. Evidence suggests that the relationship between blood pressure and risk of CVD is linear. Thus, lifestyle modifications alone will not markedly lower CVD risk. In conjunction with lifestyle modifications, pharmacological approaches play an important role in the treatment of risk factors and the achievement and maintenance of cardiovascular health. Research has demonstrated that antihypertensive therapy is associated with a 30% to 50% reduction in CVD complications such as stroke, myocardial infarction, and heart failure (Virani et al., 2020). Yet these benefits are not seen in all populations. For example, evidence suggests that determinants of hypertension treatment in non-Hispanic Black persons extend to beliefs about blood pressure, such as perception of hypertension severity and symptoms (e.g., headache, vision changes, dizziness), and prior experience, communication, and satisfaction with provider/patient interaction regarding hypertension management (Flynn et al., 2013; Ogedegbe, 2008). Similar beliefs are deeply rooted in other groups, such as Hispanic Americans, Native Americans, and Asian Americans/Pacific Islanders (LaVeist, 2005). Notably, across all populations, beliefs and attitudes can affect adherence to a prescribed treatment regimen and the adoption of lifestyle modifications (Ferdinand et al., 2017; LaVeist, 2005; Whelton et al., 2016). Another important factor is the consideration of drug selection for the treatment of CVD and related conditions. This may include assessing circumstances in which individuals live and work and the consideration of dose timing and drug agents known to be more effective in certain populations (National Academies of Sciences, Engineering, and Medicine, 2019), as well as medication side effects. Furthermore, nurses and all other health professionals are in a unique position to consider culturally appropriate interventions to prevent and treat CVD while taking into account determinants of health in order to improve cardiovascular health of populations.

SUMMARY

In this chapter, we examined the sociocultural environmental factors that influence CVD health in adults and children living in the United States. Racial/ethnic disparities in CVD and hypertension are pervasive and remain a public health challenge. Despite declines in cardiovascular mortality over the last four decades, minorities, especially non-Hispanic Black people, continue to have higher mortality rates related to CVD and hypertension. We discussed the contributions of health risk factors and lifestyle behaviors, and how these factors have the propensity to accelerate the incidence of CVD morbidity and mortality rates. This chapter also highlighted the underlying causes of racial/ethnic differences in CVD as they relate to access, use, and quality of healthcare.

CASE STUDY 16.1: AN ENCOUNTER WITH A PATIENT WITH UNCONTROLLED HYPERTENSION

Alex Crossing (not his real name) is a 45-year-old African American man who lives in South Carolina with his wife and three children. He completed his associate's degree and has been self-employed as a truck driver for 10 years.

Mr. Crossing visited a healthcare provider, who asked Mr. Crossing, "So, you're here for a headache?" and then continued to talk, barely letting Mr. Crossing get in a word. Mr. Crossing complained of intermittent headaches for about 4 months. The nature and attributions of Mr. Crossing's symptoms were missed due to the closed-ended questions asked by the provider, which elicited "yes" or "no" responses. Mr. Crossing's chart revealed that he had a history of being overweight and of smoking since age 18 years, but he had not been to the doctor in almost 7 years. Mr. Crossing's blood pressure was 145/90 mmHg. Given that the focus of Mr. Crossing's visit was complaints of headaches, the provider rushed him through the visit, then prescribed ibuprofen and recommended that Mr. Crossing return to the clinic if the headaches persisted.

Mr. Crossing returned to the office 4 weeks later and was seen by another healthcare provider. This time he complained of frequent headaches and urination, and weight loss of 15 lb, although there had been no change in his diet. Mr. Crossing revealed that he ate mostly fast food due to being on the road as a truck driver. During this visit, he also disclosed that he had a positive family history of hypertension (both parents and his two sisters). In addition, his father suffered a stroke at age 45 years. Upon assessment, Mr. Crossing's blood pressure was 160/91 mmHg, and his hemoglobin A1C was 7.4%. Mr. Crossing was diagnosed with type 2 diabetes and hypertension. Mr. Crossing's initial treatment regimen consisted of metformin 500 mg daily for diabetes and lisinopril 10 mg daily for hypertension. Additional blood tests indicated high cholesterol.

Discussion

An important observation is that Mr. Crossing would have benefited from a more patient-centered, culturally sensitive approach to care. Vital statistics indicate that minority populations, especially African Americans, have higher incidence of most chronic diseases, often due to a number of reasons including access to care, distrust of healthcare systems/ providers, and inadequate clinical encounters, including providers failing to elicit a comprehensive and accurate history. An in-depth history from Mr. Crossing would have been beneficial to elucidate the information deficit regarding his health, as well as to allow him an opportunity to voice his health concerns in detail.

During the clinical encounter, it is important to create a welcoming environment, establish provider/patient communication, and consider the patient as an equal partner in managing their care. Such efforts have been shown to improve the patient/provider relationship and health outcomes (Pérez-Stable & El-Toukhy, 2018). A thorough and comprehensive approach to eliciting medical information (patient-centered medical interviewing) should be used to collect pertinent background information, such as an individual's present and past medical history, social determinants of health, and current health practices and cultural beliefs, all factors that can influence health outcomes. If the provider is unable to collect a complete history during the initial encounter, every effort should be made to collect data at each subsequent visit. The lack of assessment limits a provider's conscious effort to view the patient in terms of their individual characteristics and symptoms and may provoke medical inaction or clinical inertia. Importantly, research has suggested that provision for the continuity of care helps establish rapport, builds trust, allows the provider to accumulate knowledge, improves patient satisfaction, and influences quality of care and outcomes over time. In terms of Mr. Crossing, another important consideration is that after a diagnosis is given,

(continued)

CASE STUDY 16.1: AN ENCOUNTER WITH A PATIENT WITH UNCONTROLLED HYPERTENSION (*CONTINUED*)

there is an opportunity to explore the patient's understanding of the diagnosed condition and offer shared decision-making of how to manage the disease.

Discussion Questions

1. What additional data would you want to collect related to possible CVD risk factors?
2. Prior to managing Mr. Crossing's concomitant conditions, what are some sociocultural considerations the primary provider should take into considerations?
3. What should be goal of treatment and care for this patient with diabetes and hypertension?

ADDITIONAL RESOURCES

Several resources and guidelines offer best practices to prevent, manage, and treat CVD risk factors. The guidelines listed are intended to be used by health professionals to improve quality of care of patients at risk for or diagnosed with CVD:

National Hypertension Guideline

2017 American College of Cardiology and American Heart Association Guideline for the Prevention, Detection, Evaluation, and Management of High Blood Pressure in Adults.

www.acc.org/-/media/Non-Clinical/Files-PDFs-Excel-MS-Word-etc/Guidelines/2017/Guidelines_ Made_Simple_2017_HBP.pdf

Primary Prevention of Cardiovascular Disease

2019 ACC/AHA Guideline on the Primary Prevention of Cardiovascular Disease: A Report of the American College of Cardiology/American Heart Association Task Force on Clinical Practice Guidelines. www.ahajournals.org/doi/pdf/10.1161/CIR.0000000000000678

Cardiovascular Risk Assessment

Heart risk calculation is a great resource to calculate an individual's risk for 10-year atherosclerotic CVD (ASCVD) and estimate the potential impact of different interventions on patient risk. https://tools.acc.org/ASCVD-Risk-Estimator-Plus/#!/calculate/estimate

REFERENCES

Adhikari, S., Pantaleo, N. P., Feldman, J. M., Ogedegbe, O., Thorpe, L., & Troxel, A. B. (2020). Assessment of community-level disparities in Coronavirus disease 2019 (COVID-19) infections and deaths in large US metropolitan areas. *JAMA Network Open*, 3(7), e2016938–e2016938. https:// doi.org/10.1001/jamanetworkopen.2020.16938

American Heart Association. (2018). American heart association recommendations for physical activity in adults and kids. https://www.heart.org/en/healthy-living/fitness/fitness-basics/ aha-recs-for-physical-activity-in-adults

Ahmad, A., & Oparil, S. (2017). Hypertension in women: Recent advances and lingering questions. *Hypertension*, 70(1), 19–26. https://doi.org/10.1161/hypertensionaha.117.08317

Al Kibria, G. M., Swasey, K., Sharmeen, A., & Day, B. (2019). Estimated change in prevalence and trends of childhood blood pressure levels in the United States after application of the 2017 AAP Guideline. *Preventing Chronic Disease*, 16, E12. https://doi.org/10.5888/pcd16.180528

Artiga, S., Young, K., Garfield, R., & Majerol, M. (2015). Racial and ethnic disparities in access to and utilization of care among insured adults. The Kaiser Commission on Medicaid and the Uninsured (Issue Brief). https://www.kff.org/report-section/racial-and-ethnic-disparities-in-access-to-and -utilization-of-care-among-insured-adults-issue-brief/

Barker, D. J. (2007). The origins of the developmental origins theory. *Journal of Internal Medicine*, 261(5), 412–417. https://doi.org/10.1111/j.1365-2796.2007.01809.x

Bloem, L. J., Foroud, T. M., Ambrosius, W. T., Hanna, M. P., Tewksbury, D. A., & Pratt, J. H. (1997). Association of the angiotensinogen gene to serum angiotensinogen in blacks and whites. *Hypertension (Dallas, Tex.: 1979), 29*(5), 1078–1082. https://doi.org/10.1161/01.hyp.29.5.1078

Carnethon, M. R., Pu, J., Howard, G., Albert, M. A., Anderson, C. A. M., Bertoni, A. G., Mujahid, M. S., Palaniappan, L., Taylor, H. A. Jr., Willis, M., & Yancy, C. W., & American Heart Association Council on Epidemiology and Prevention; Council on Cardiovascular Disease in the Young; Council on Cardiovascular and Stroke Nursing; Council on Clinical Cardiology; Council on Functional Genomics and Translational Biology; and Stroke Council. (2017). Cardiovascular health in African Americans: A scientific statement from the American Heart Association. *Circulation, 136*(21), e393–e423. https://doi.org/10.1161/cir.0000000000000534

Centers for Disease Control and Prevention. (2017). National diabetes statistics report, 2017. Centers for Disease Control and Prevention, U.S. Dept of Health and Human Services. https://dev .diabetes.org/sites/default/files/2019-06/cdc-statistics-report-2017.pdf

Centers for Disease Control and Prevention. (2021, March 1). Hypertension. National Center for Health Statistics. https://www.cdc.gov/nchs/fastats/hypertension.htm

Centers for Disease Control and Prevention. (2020). Stroke death rates, 2014–2016. https://www.cdc .gov/dhdsp/maps/images/stroke_all.jpg

Chobanian, A. V., Bakris, G. L., Black, H. R., Cushman, W. C., Green, L. A., Izzo, J. L. Jr., Jones, D. W., Materson, B. J., Oparil, S., Wright, J. T. Jr., Roccella, E. J., National Heart, Lung, Blood Institute Joint National Committee on Prevention, Dectection, and Evaluation and Treatment of High Blood, Pressure, & National High Blood Pressure Education Program Coordinating Center. (2003). The seventh report of the joint national committee on prevention, detection, evaluation, and treatment of high blood pressure: The JNC 7 report. *JAMA, 289*(19), 2560–2572. https://doi.org/10.1001/jama.289.19.2560

Davis, E. F., Lewandowski, A. J., Aye, C., Williamson, W., Boardman, H., Huang, R. C., Mori, T. A., Newnham, J., Beilin, L. J., & Leeson, P. (2015). Clinical cardiovascular risk during young adulthood in offspring of hypertensive pregnancies: Insights from a 20-year prospective follow-up birth cohort. *BMJ Open, 5*(6), e008136. https://doi.org/10.1136/bmjopen-2015-008136

Dwyer-Lindgren, L., Bertozzi-Villa, A., Stubbs, R. W., Morozoff, C., Mackenbach, J. P., van Lenthe, F. J., Mokdad, A. H., & Murray, C. (2017). Inequalities in life expectancy among US counties, 1980 to 2014: Temporal trends and key drivers. *JAMA Internal Medicine, 177*(7), 1003–1011. https://doi .org/10.1001/jamainternmed.2017.0918

Elkind, M. S. V., Lisabeth, L., Howard, V. J., Kleindorfer, D., & Howard, G. (2020). Approaches to studying determinants of racial-ethnic disparities in stroke and its sequelae. *Stroke, 51*(11), 3406–3416. https://doi.org/10.1161/strokeaha.120.030424

Expert Panel on Integrated Guidelines for Cardiovascular Health and Risk Reduciton in Chidren and Adolescents, & National Heart, Lung Blood, Institute. (2011). Expert panel on integrated guidelines for cardiovascular health and risk reduction in children and adolescents: Summary report. *Pediatrics, 128*(suppl 5), S213–S256. https://doi.org/10.1542/peds.2009-2107C

Ferdinand, K. C., Yadav, K., Nasser, S. A., Clayton-Jeter, H. D., Lewin, J., Cryer, D. R., & Senatore, F. F. (2017). Disparities in hypertension and cardiovascular disease in blacks: The critical role of medication adherence. *Journal of Clinical Hypertension (Greenwich), 19*(10), 1015–1024. https://doi .org/10.1111/jch.13089

Fiscella, K., & Sanders, M. R. (2016). Racial and ethnic disparities in the quality of health care. *Annual Review of Public Health, 37*(1), 375–394. https://doi.org/10.1146/annurev-publhealth-032315-021439

Flynn, J. T., Kaelber, D. C., Baker-Smith, C. M., Blowey, D., Carroll, A. E., Daniels, S. R., de Ferranti, S. D., Dionne, J. M., Falkner, B., Flinn, S. K., Gidding, S. S., Goodwin, C., Leu, M. G., Powers, M. E., Rea, C., Samuels, J., Simasek, M., Thaker, V. V., & Urbina, E. M. (2017). Clinical practice guideline for screening and management of high blood pressure in children and adolescents. *Pediatrics, 140*(3). https://doi.org/10.1542/peds.2017-1904

Flynn, S. J., Ameling, J. M., Hill-Briggs, F., Wolff, J. L., Bone, L. R., Levine, D. M., Roter, D. L., Lewis-Boyer, L., Fisher, A. R., Purnell, L., Ephraim, P. L., Barbers, J., Fitzpatrick, S. L., Albert, M. C., Cooper, L. A., Fagan, P. J., Martin, D., Ramamurthi, H. C., & Boulware, L. E. (2013). Facilitators and barriers to hypertension self-management in urban African Americans: Perspectives of patients and family members. *Patient Preference Adherence, 7*, 741–749. https://doi.org/10.2147/ppa.s46517

Fullman, N., Yearwood, J., Abay, S. M., Abbafati, C., Abd-Allah, F., Abdela, J., Abdelalim, A., Abebe, Z., Abebo, T. A., & Aboyans, V. (2018). Measuring performance on the healthcare access and quality index for 195 countries and territories and selected subnational locations: A systematic analysis from the Global Burden of Disease Study 2016. *The Lancet, 391*(10136), 2236–2271. https:// doi.org/10.1016/S0140-6736(18)30994-2

Gary-Webb, T. L., Baumann, S. E., Rodriquez, E. J., Isaac, L. A., & LaVeist, T. A. (2021). In I. Dankwa-Mullan, E. J. Pérez-Stable, K. L. Gardner, X. Zhang, & A. M. Rosario (Eds.), *Racial/ethnic, socioeconomic, and other social determinants: The Science of Health Disparities Research* (pp. 39–57). John Wiley & Sons, Inc. https://doi.org/https://doi.org/10.1002/9781119374855.ch3

Geelhoed, J. J., Fraser, A., Tilling, K., Benfield, L., Davey Smith, G., Sattar, N., Nelson, S. M., & Lawlor, D. A. (2010). Preeclampsia and gestational hypertension are associated with childhood blood pressure independently of family adiposity measures: The avon longitudinal study of parents and children. *Circulation*, 122(12), 1192–1199. https://doi.org/10.1161/circulationaha.110.936674

Gehlert, S., Sohmer, D., Sacks, T., Mininger, C., McClintock, M., & Olopade, O. (2008). Targeting health disparities: A model linking upstream determinants to downstream interventions. *Health Affairs (Millwood)*, 27(2), 339–349. https://doi.org/10.1377/hlthaff.27.2.339

Georgiadis, M. (2013). Motivating behavior change: A content analysis of public service announcements from the Let's move! campaign. *Elon Journal of Undergraduate Research in Communications*, 4(1). http://www.inquiriesjournal.com/a?id=791

Glass, T. A., & McAtee, M. J. (2006). Behavioral science at the crossroads in public health: Extending horizons, envisioning the future. *Social Science & Medicine*, 62(7), 1650–1671. https://doi.org/10.1016/j.socscimed.2005.08.044

Hales, C. M., Carroll, M. D., Fryar, C. D., & Ogden, C. L. (2017). Prevalence of obesity among adults and youth: United States, 2015–2016. *NCHS Data Brief*, (288), 1–8.

Hales, C. M., Carroll, M. D., Fryar, C. D., & Ogden, C. L. (2020). Prevalence of obesity and severe obesity among adults: United States, 2017–2018. *NCHS Data Brief*, (360), 1–8.

Hansen, M. L., Gunn, P. W., & Kaelber, D. C. (2007). Underdiagnosis of hypertension in children and adolescents. *JAMA*, 298(8), 874–879. https://doi.org/10.1001/jama.298.8.874

Havranek, E. P., Mujahid, M. S., Barr, D. A., Blair, I. V., Cohen, M. S., Cruz-Flores, S., Davey-Smith, G., Dennison-Himmelfarb, C. R., Lauer, M. S., Lockwood, D. W., Rosal, M., & Yancy, C. W. (2015). Social determinants of risk and outcomes for cardiovascular disease. *Circulation*, 132(9), 873–898. https://doi.org/10.1161/CIR.0000000000000228

Hawes, A. M., Smith, G. S., McGinty, E., Bell, C., Bower, K., LaVeist, T. A., Gaskin, D. J., & Thorpe, R. J. (2019). Disentangling race, poverty, and place in disparities in physical activity. *International Journal of Environment Research and Public Health*, 16(7), 1193. https://www.mdpi.com/1660-4601/16/7/1193

Heron, M. (2019). Deaths: Leading causes for 2017. National vital statistics reports: From the Centers for Disease Control and Prevention, National Center for Health Statistics, *National Vital Statistics System*, 68(6), 1–77. https://stacks.cdc.gov/view/cdc/79488

Howard, G., & Howard, V. J. (2020). Twenty years of progress toward understanding the stroke belt. *Stroke*, 51(3), 742–750. https://doi.org/10.1161/STROKEAHA.119.024155

Howard, G., Labarthe, D. R., Hu, J., Yoon, S., & Howard, V. J. (2007). Regional differences in African Americans' high risk for stroke: The remarkable burden of stroke for Southern African Americans. *Annals of Epidemiology*, 17(9), 689–696. https://doi.org/10.1161/STROKEAHA.119.024155

Jackson, S. L., Yang, E. C., & Zhang, Z. (2018). Income disparities and cardiovascular risk factors among adolescents. *Pediatrics*, 142(5), e20181089. https://doi.org/10.1542/peds.2018-1089

Kaiser, P., Diez Roux, A. V., Mujahid, M., Carnethon, M., Bertoni, A., Adar, S. D., Shea, S., McClelland, R., & Lisabeth, L. (2016). Neighborhood environments and incident hypertension in the multi-ethnic study of atherosclerosis. *American Journal Epidemiology*, 183(11), 988–997. https://doi.org/10.1093/aje/kwv296

Kenik, J., Jean-Jacques, M., & Feinglass, J. (2014). Explaining racial and ethnic disparities in cholesterol screening. *Preventive Medicine*, 65, 65–69. https://doi.org/10.1016/j.ypmed.2014.04.026

Kim, E. J., Kim, T., Conigliaro, J., Liebschutz, J. M., Paasche-Orlow, M. K., & Hanchate, A. D. (2018). Racial and ethnic disparities in diagnosis of chronic medical conditions in the USA. *Journal of General Internal Medicine*, 33(7), 1116–1123. https://doi.org/10.1007/s11606-018-4471-1

Ko, Y. A., Mukherjee, B., Smith, J. A., Kardia, S. L., Allison, M., & Diez Roux, A. V. (2016). Classification and clustering methods for multiple environmental factors in gene-environment interaction: Application to the multi-ethnic study of atherosclerosis. *Epidemiology*, 27(6), 870–878. https://doi.org/10.1097/ede.0000000000000548

LaVeist, T. (2005). *Minority population and health: Introduction to health disparities in the United States*. Jossey-Bass.

Lloyd-Jones, D. M., Hong, Y., Labarthe, D., Mozaffarian, D., Appel, L. J., Van Horn, L., Greenlund, K., Daniels, S., Nichol, G., Tomaselli, G. F., Arnett, D. K., Fonarow, G. C., Ho, P. M., Lauer, M. S., Masoudi, F. A., Robertson, R. M., Roger, V., Schwamm, L. H., Sorlie, P., …, Rosamond, W. D. (2010). Defining and setting national goals for cardiovascular health promotion and disease reduction: The American Heart Association's strategic impact goal through 2020 and beyond. *Circulation*, 121(4), 586–613. https://doi.org/10.1161/circulationaha.109.192703

Marmot, M. (2017). The health gap: The challenge of an unequal world: The argument. *International Journal of Epidemiology*, 46(4), 1312–1318. https://doi.org/10.1093/ije/dyx163

Marmot, M., & Wilkinson, R. (2006). *Social determinants of health* (2nd ed.). Oxford University Press.

Matthews, K. A., Hall, M., & Dahl, R. E. (2014). Sleep in healthy black and white adolescents. *Pediatrics*, 133(5), e1189–e1196. https://doi.org/10.1542/peds.2013-2399

Matthews, K. A., & Pantesco, E. J. (2016). Sleep characteristics and cardiovascular risk in children and adolescents: An enumerative review. *Sleep Medicine, 18*, 36–49. https://doi.org/10.1016/j.sleep.2015.06.004

Mensah, G. A., Wei, G. S., Sorlie, P. D., Fine, L. J., Rosenberg, Y., Kaufmann, P. G., Mussolino, M. E., Hsu, L. L., Addou, E., Engelgau, M. M., & Gordon, D. (2017). Decline in cardiovascular mortality: Possible causes and implications. *Circulation Research, 120*(2), 366–380. https://doi.org/10.1161/circresaha.116.309115

Muntner, P., Hardy, S. T., Fine, L. J., Jaeger, B. C., Wozniak, G., Levitan, E. B., & Colantonio, L. D. (2020). Trends in blood pressure control among US Adults with hypertension, 1999–2000 to 2017–2018. *JAMA, 324*(12), 1190–1200. https://doi.org/10.1001/jama.2020.14545

National Academies of Sciences, Engineering, and Medicine. (2019). Integrating social care into the delivery of health care: Moving upstream to improve the nation's health. The National Academies Press. https://doi.org/10.17226/25467

Office of Disease Prevention and Health Promotion. (2020). Increase control of high blood pressure in adults. Healthy people 2030. U.S. Department of Health and Human Services. https://health.gov/healthypeople/objectives-and-data/browse-objectives/heart-disease-and-stroke/increase-control-high-blood-pressure-adults-hds-05

Ogedegbe, G. (2008). Barriers to optimal hypertension control. *Journal of Clinical Hypertension (Greenwich), 10*(8), 644–646. https://doi.org/10.1111/j.1751-7176.2008.08329.x

Oparil, S., Zaman, M. A., & Calhoun, D. A. (2003). Pathogenesis of hypertension. *Annals of Internal Medicine, 139*(9), 761–776. https://doi.org/10.7326/0003-4819-139-9-200311040-00011 %m 14597461

Ortman, J. M., Velkoff, V. A., Hogan, H. (2014). An aging nation: The older population in the United States, Current Population Reports (pp 25–1140). Washington, DC: U.S. Census Bureau.

Paciência, I., Barros, H., Araújo, J., & Ramos, E. (2013). Association between sleep duration and blood pressure in adolescents. *Hypertension Research: Official Journal of the Japanese Society of Hypertension, 36*(8), 747–752. https://doi.org/10.1038/hr.2013.36

Pérez-Stable, E. J., & El-Toukhy, S. (2018). Communicating with diverse patients: How patient and clinician factors affect disparities. *Patient Education and Counseling, 101*(12), 2186–2194. https://doi.org/10.1016/j.pec.2018.08.021

Perng, W., Rifas-Shiman, S. L., Hivert, M. F., Chavarro, J. E., Sordillo, J., & Oken, E. (2019). Metabolic trajectories across early adolescence: Differences by sex, weight, pubertal status and race/ethnicity. *Annual of Human Biology, 46*(3), 205–214. https://doi.org/10.1080/03014460.2019.1638967

Pool, L. R., Ning, H., Lloyd-Jones, D. M., & Allen, N. B. (2017). Trends in racial/ethnic disparities in cardiovascular health among US adults from 1999–2012. *Journal of the American Heart Association, 6*(9), e006027. https://doi.org/10.1161/JAHA.117.006027

Ritchey, M. D., Wall, H. K., George, M. G., & Wright, J. S. (2020). US trends in premature heart disease mortality over the past 50 years: Where do we go from here? *Trends Cardiovascular Medicine, 30*(6), 364–374. https://doi.org/10.1016/j.tcm.2019.09.005

Schoenthaler, A., Allegrante, J. P., Chaplin, W., & Ogedegbe, G. (2012). The effect of patient-provider communication on medication adherence in hypertensive black patients: Does race concordance matter? *Annuals of Behavioral Medicine, 43*(3), 372–382. https://doi.org/10.1007/s12160-011-9342-5

Schoenthaler, A. M., & Rosenthal, D. M. (2018). Stress and hypertension. In A. E. Berbari & G. Mancia (Eds.), Disorders of blood pressure regulation: Phenotypes, mechanisms, therapeutic options (pp. 289–305). Springer International Publishing. https://doi.org/10.1007/978-3-319-59918-2_19

Smedley, B. D., Stith, A. Y., & Nelson, A. R. (2003). *Unequal treatment: Confronting racial and ethnic disparities in health care.* Washington, D.C: The National Academies Press.

Song, P., Zhang, Y., Yu, J., Zha, M., Zhu, Y., Rahimi, K., & Rudan, I. (2019). Global prevalence of hypertension in children: A systematic review and meta-analysis. *JAMA Pediatric, 173*(12), 1154–1163. https://doi.org/10.1001/jamapediatrics.2019.3310

Spruill, T. M. (2010). Chronic psychosocial stress and hypertension. *Current Hypertension Reports, 12*(1), 10–16. https://doi.org/10.1007/s11906-009-0084-8

Still, C. H., Rodriguez, C. J., Wright, J. T. Jr., Craven, T. E., Bress, A. P., Chertow, G. M., Whelton, P. K., Whittle, J. C., Freedman, B. I., Johnson, K. C., Foy, C. G., He, J., Kostis, J. B., Lash, J. P., Pedley, C. F., Pisoni, R., Powell, J. R., & Wall, B. M. (2017). Clinical outcomes by race and ethnicity in the systolic blood pressure intervention trial (SPRINT): A randomized clinical trial. American Journal of Hypertension. https://doi.org/10.1093/ajh/hpx138

Sun, J., Steffen, L. M., Ma, C., Liang, Y., & Xi, B. (2017). Definition of pediatric hypertension: Are blood pressure measurements on three separate occasions necessary? *Hypertension Research, 40*(5), 496–503. https://doi.org/10.1038/hr.2016.179

Thorpe, R. J. Jr., Brandon, D. T., & LaVeist, T. A. (2008). Social context as an explanation for race disparities in hypertension: Findings from the exploring health disparities in integrated communities (EHDIC) study. *Sococial Science Medicine, 67*(10), 1604–1611. https://doi.org/10.1016/j.socscimed.2008.07.002

Virani, S. S., Alonso, A., Benjamin, E. J., Bittencourt, M. S., Callaway, C. W., Carson, A. P., Chamberlain, A. M., Chang, A. R., Cheng, S., Delling, F. N., Djousse, L., Elkind, M. S. V., Ferguson, J. F., Fornage, M., Khan, S. S., Kissela, B. M., Knutson, K. L., Kwan, T. W., Lackland, D. T., …, Tsao, C. W. (2020). Heart disease and stroke statistics-2020 update: A report from the American Heart Association. *Circulation, 141*(9), e139–e596. https://doi.org/10.1161/cir.0000000000000757

Whelton, P. K., Carey, R. M., Aronow, W. S., Casey, D. E. Jr., Collins, K. J., Dennison Himmelfarb, C., DePalma, S. M., Gidding, S., Jamerson, K. A., Jones, D. W., MacLaughlin, E. J., Muntner, P., Ovbiagele, B., Smith, S. C. Jr., Spencer, C. C., Stafford, R. S., Taler, S. J., Thomas, R. J., Williams, K. A. Sr., …, Wright, J. T. Jr. (2018). 2017 ACC/AHA/AAPA/ABC/ACPM/AGS/APhA/ASH/ASPC/NMA/PCNA guideline for the prevention, detection, evaluation, and management of high blood pressure in adults: A report of the American College of Cardiology/American Heart Association Task Force on Clinical Practice Guidelines. *Journal of the American College of Cardiology, 71*(19), e127–e248. https://doi.org/10.1016/j.jacc.2017.11.006

Whelton, P. K., Einhorn, P. T., Muntner, P., Appel, L. J., Cushman, W. C., Diez Roux, A. V., Ferdinand, K. C., Rahman, M., Taylor, H. A., Ard, J., Arnett, D. K., Carter, B. L., Davis, B. R., Freedman, B. I., Cooper, L. A., Cooper, R., Desvigne-Nickens, P., Gavini, N., Go, A. S., …, National Heart, Lung, and Blood Institute Working Group on Research Needs to Improve Hypertension Treatment and Control in African Americans. (2016). Research needs to improve hypertension treatment and control in African Americans. *Hypertension (Dallas, TX: 1979), 68*(5), 1066–1072. https://doi.org/10.1161/HYPERTENSIONAHA.116.07905

Wright, J. S., Wall, H. K., & Ritchey, M. D. (2018). Million hearts 2022: Small steps are needed for cardiovascular disease prevention. *JAMA, 320*(18), 1857–1858. https://doi.org/10.1001/jama.2018.13326

Wright, J. T. Jr., Dunn, J. K., Cutler, J. A., Davis, B. R., Cushman, W. C., Ford, C. E., Haywood, L. J., Leenen, F. H., Margolis, K. L., Papademetriou, V., Probstfield, J. L., Whelton, P. K., Habib, G. B., & Group, A. C. R. (2005). Outcomes in hypertensive black and nonblack patients treated with chlorthalidone, amlodipine, and lisinopril. *JAMA, 293*(13), 1595–1608. https://doi.org/10.1001/jama.293.13.1595

Wright, J. T. Jr., Williamson, J. D., Whelton, P. K., Snyder, J. K., Sink, K. M., Rocco, M. V., Reboussin, D. M., Rahman, M., Oparil, S., Lewis, C. E., Kimmel, P. L., Johnson, K. C., Goff, D. C. Jr., Fine, L. J., Cutler, J. A., Cushman, W. C., Cheung, A. K., & Ambrosius, W. T. (2015). A randomized trial of intensive versus standard blood-pressure control. *New England Journal of Medicine, 373*(22), 2103–2116. https://doi.org/10.1056/NEJMoa1511939

Zilbermint, M., Hannah-Shmouni, F., & Stratakis, C. A. (2019). Genetics of hypertension in African Americans and others of African descent. *International Journal of Molecular Science, 20*(5), 1081. https://doi.org/10.3390/ijms20051081

CHAPTER 17

Population Health in Rural and Urban Communities

June G. Hopps, Ruby M. Gourdine,* Christopher Strickland, Latrice Rollins, and
Kevin Linder

LEARNING OBJECTIVES

◉ Discuss the demographics of rural and urban populations relative to each cohort's
needs and access to quality healthcare among children and adults.

◉ Explain factors related to deaths from despair and suicidal behaviors among rural
and urban populations and barriers to access to care.

◉ Examine common and unique health problems in rural and urban populations.

◉ Highlight best practices for engaging communities in plans for health promotion,
disease prevention, and treatment to enhance well-being.

INTRODUCTION

Rural and urban populations have numerous points of intersectionality, including race,
socioeconomic status, location, age, sex, and access to education and healthcare. Throughout
this chapter, reference is made to these constructs as related to both populations. The base
of society in America is rural communities, but future projections indicate that urban communities will eventually be dominant. This chapter also focuses on rural and urban health
issues, primarily in the United States. It provides a historical and contemporary perspective and highlights variations in health outcomes among individuals in both settings.
Characteristics of rural and urban communities are explained, and emphasis is placed on
the future of communities created in urban environments. Barriers to healthcare for both
populations are discussed, and exemplary programs that focus on improving health outcomes conclude the chapter.

RURAL AND URBAN PERSPECTIVES

In the United States, about 46 million people live in rural communities, accounting for
15% of the nation's population (Centers for Disease Control and Prevention [CDC],

---

*Dr. Gourdine passed away before the publication of this book.

2019). Rural communities can have varied definitions. The Census Bureau utilized statistical data for its definition of rural, which consists of population density and size. In 2012, according to the 2010 decennial census data, rural was defined as open country or settlements where less than 2,500 residents reside (USDA Economic Research Service, 2019). Rural and rural development is also a space where culture, economy, and geographical locations overlap and create a gestalt of health-related disparities (Murdock et al., 2012).

In the United States, an urban population typically encompasses groups ranging from 2,000 to 10,000 and beyond (Guest, 2012). Economic advancement and urbanization are closely linked in the United States and the world community (Guest, 2012). In the United States, urban development has historically been associated with growing income, educational achievement, mass media and communications, availability of health systems, and large numbers of people living in a designated area. Additionally, urban centers have tended to provide physical access to a variety of goods and services. Across the world, urbanization has also been pervasive. According to the United Nations, in 2019, about one half of the global population—4.2 billion people—lived in urban areas. It is estimated that by 2041, more than 6 billion people will reside in urban settings (Kuddus et al., 2020). Some writers such as Guest (2012) suggest that it is getting more challenging to determine where urban communities end and rural communities begin.

Some discerning characteristics help to pinpoint health issues in both rural and urban communities. According to the CDC, in rural America (a) higher rates of unhealthy behaviors are manifest, (b) there are problems with reduced access to healthcare, (c) fewer resources for purchasing healthy foods are available, and (d) demographic data suggest that people in rural areas tend to be older, poorer, and less educated. Collectively, these considerations contribute to higher rates of illnesses and untimely deaths. The five leading causes of death among rural populations are heart disease, cancer, unintentional injuries, chronic lower respiratory disease, and stroke (CDC, 2019; Garcia et al., 2017). In rural America, these five causes are associated with more people not participating in physical activities, partly because of chronic health problems, compared with urban populations (Meit et al., 2014). In addition, health-related behaviors and social circumstances can negatively influence morbidity and mortality among rural people (Li et al., 2020).

Common sources of mortality and morbidity associated with social determinants of health in both rural and urban areas include motor vehicle crashes, opioid and other drug use, unemployment, and lack of access to quality healthcare (Kuddus et al., 2020). To improve health outcomes in both settings, health professionals should promote motor vehicle safety by encouraging adults to wear seat belts and instruct parents about the added protection of age-appropriate car seats and booster chairs. Additionally, health professionals can promote the safer use of opioid medications for pain control. Nonpharmacologic therapies are options, along with education and patient teaching about the benefits and risks of opioids (MacKinney et al., 2021). Finally, health professionals should more robustly address the social determinants of health, including underemployment and unemployment, lack of access to healthcare, and safer environments.

In rural and urban communities across the world, noncommunicable diseases are responsible for about 71% of deaths—41 million people annually. As in the United States, the annual leading causes of death worldwide include cardiovascular diseases (17.9 million), cancer (9.3 million), respiratory diseases (4.1 million), and diabetes (1.5 million). These four conditions are responsible for 80% of noncommunicable disease deaths, which are often preventable. Consequently, the development and proliferation of chronic diseases present demanding challenges to the world and local communities. To address this burden, most communities will require greater attention to early detection and prompt treatment (World Health Organization [WHO], 2021).

In rural and urban communities throughout the United States and across the world, some lifestyle factors—including tobacco use, lack of physical exercise, inadequate diets, and alcohol misuse—produce poor health outcomes, disability, morbidity, and mortality. These factors are also associated with obesity, a significant health problem in both rural and urban American communities and an antecedent to numerous other illnesses (Bauer et al., 2014; Parekh & Goodman, 2013; WHO, 2021). In many instances, individuals with health insurance and more sustained incomes access preventive and routine healthcare that includes health-promoting and disease-preventing services. On the other hand, marginalized populations using "safety net" emergency department care services do not have continuity of care and are less likely to benefit from health promotion and disease prevention programs (Burns, 2017). Healthcare for more immediate problems can also be elusive and difficult to address because of their urgency and the limited resources.

History suggests that healthcare systems in the United States are filled with disparities, complications, and challenges. The scenario is evident in rural and urban settings and impacts all population cohorts throughout the life span, affecting more than 300 million people. Moreover, since the shaping of the nation, healthcare systems have been filled with inequities, access issues, cost constraints, and varied notions about who is worthy and who is not worthy of care (Germain & Knight, 2021).

CONTEMPORARY ISSUES

Disparities in healthcare delivery persist today and are tied to the structure of healthcare delivery systems across the nation. A critical issue in the absence of universal healthcare is the number of uninsured people in the United States, approximately 26.1 million in 2019; that number is expected to increase significantly in 2020 due to the COVID-19 pandemic and resulting surges in national unemployment rates. One population of particular concern is essential workers, or those who perform a range of services that are necessary for infrastructure operations in healthcare, agriculture, transportation, defense and energy (www. cisa.gov/identifying-critical-infrastructure-during-covid-19). These workers are notable because they are often low-wage service employees who are uninsured.

In the United States, the uninsured population has an increased cardiac death rate relative to their insured counterparts. In 2019, patients hospitalized because of heart attacks but with no insurance had a 25% higher death rate than insured patients with comparable illnesses. The uninsured population cohort, whether rural or urban, participates in several healthcare scenarios characterized by a lack of regular or routine medical care and consequential increases in the use of hospitalization and emergency department visits (Karger & Stoesz, 2018). In such scenarios, health problems that are preventable, avoidable, and acute, such as uncontrolled diabetes and pneumonia, are treated in emergency departments. Misuse and overuse of hospital emergency departments increase other health and social problems, including medical expenses and debt (costs can range from $150 to $3,000 or more per visit, depending on the diagnoses and interventions).

Another challenge for the uninsured is postponement in receiving care when needed or in securing prescribed medications, often owing to the lack of ability to pay and transportation matters. Ambulance services, for example, represent additional costs and are used for transportation in both rural and urban communities. Most insurance will cover the cost of ambulance service, but the individual is responsible for the copay, which is, on average, about $150. Location, type of transfer (emergency or scheduled transportation), the number of miles the patient must travel to an emergency department, and the extent to which basic or advanced life support is used are some variables that determine the charges for the health service. Fees for the service, on average, range from less than $400 to $1,200 and more per mile (Costhelper Health, n.d.) in some communities. When complex equipment is used and further distances are connected with greater costs of transportation, the burden on uninsured people and/or lower income residents of rural populations may increase. In particular, rural residents are limited in their health seeking by a lack of transportation or resources to access available services, including telehealth (Harrington et al., 2020). Ambulance services are often unavailable, and hospitals and clinics can sometimes be many miles away from residents with rugged terrain to maneuver before a vehicle arrives. In some communities, the ambulance drivers are volunteers, and vehicles might not always be available. Paid personnel is not yet a reality in many rural communities. A lack of coordination among local, regional, and federal agencies complicates the development and maintenance of reasonable plans for ambulance transportation in rural America (Costhelper Health, n.d.; MacKinney et al., 2021).

Other factors that affect survival and create divides across the insured and uninsured include the traumatic nature of injury and household wealth. Uninsured individuals with traumatic injuries are twice as likely to lose their lives (even when controlled for the seriousness of injury across cohorts). In 2019, the average medical expenses for a significant illness in an uninsured household was slightly over $42,000 but, by contrast, less than $27,000 for the insured home—a sizeable difference. Diagnoses of health conditions such as cancer, heart attack, diabetes, stroke, and lung disease were associated with a 20% reduction in household wealth among the uninsured, in contrast to 2% for the insured (Karger & Stoesz, 2018).

Uninsured children require special consideration. Children younger than 18 years who live in poverty are most often uninsured, representing some 15.4% of the population compared with 9.8% of adults. Those who recently reached young adult status (i.e., the 19- to 25-year-old age group) were more likely than other age cohorts to be uninsured (Karger & Stoesz, 2018). Lack of insurance in the child population is associated with poorer health outcomes across the life course; children who lack healthcare insurance experience developmental delays in more significant numbers than those who have healthcare insurance. They are also more likely to have unattended chronic illness such as asthma, diabetes, cardiovascular disease, or other debilitating conditions (Pate et al., 2020).

To address these challenges, the Affordable Care Act (ACA) provides additional coverage for young adults (coverage until age 26 years under a parent's plan). Moreover, the ACA covers free preventive services, such as immunizations; screening for certain conditions, including depression and obesity; services for pregnant patients, such as vitamin and iron supplements; expanded benefits covering ambulatory and emergency department care, maternity services, and mental healthcare; and medical, dental, and vision coverage (Johns Hopkins Medicine, n.d.). Over the past several decades, Medicaid and the Children's Health Insurance Program (CHIP) have also expanded their range of preventive services and treatment offered to children (Kaiser Family Foundation State Health Facts, CDC, 2021). Consequently, the uninsured rate for children is currently at historically low levels. However, 60% of their uninsured parents live in states that have not expanded Medicaid. See Box 17.1 for a listing of states that have not expanded Medicaid through the ACA.

There are numerous benefits to the expansion of Medicaid for people in all settings, including (a) *access to care*, including preventive healthcare and management of chronic health conditions; (b) *improved health outcomes*, such as reduction of premature deaths among older adults and improved health status for individuals with diabetes, hypertension, and mental illnesses; (c) *short-term financial security* through fewer payments toward medical debt from personal income and fewer evictions among renters; (d) *long-term economic stability and improved financial status* as evidenced by better credit scores and lower interest rates for home mortgages and car loans; and (e) *significant reductions* in uncompensated healthcare for hospitals and improved budgets for health systems, especially for rural hospitals

BOX 17.1: Status of Lack of Medicaid Expansion by State in 2021

Alabama	South Carolina
Florida	South Dakota
Georgia	Tennessee
Kansas	Texas
Mississippi	Wisconsin
North Carolina	Wyoming

Source: Data from Kaiser Family Foundation. (2021). www.kff.org/medicaid/issue-brief/status-of-state-medicaid-expansion-decisions-interactive-map.

and clinics (Cross-Call, 2020); Wang et al., 2015). For in-depth information, see Kaiser Family Foundation State Health Facts, CDC (2021).

The following brief perspective on rural and urban health is one straightforward approach to examining contributing social factors that affect health outcomes, which intersects with the social determinants of health as promulgated by the National Institute of Minority Health and Health Disparities (see Chapters 5, 7, 10, and 20). This section uses three variables to explicate universal and particular factors associated with rural and urban health: social environment, physical environment, and access to quality healthcare and social services (Global Health University, n.d.).

RURAL AND URBAN HEALTH: A BRIEF PERSPECTIVE

Rural Health

Social Environment

Across the nation, rural older adults have poorer health than their urban counterparts. They are more likely to have a history of tobacco use, participate in less exercise, consume less-healthy diets, and be more obese than suburban residents. These health behaviors and outcomes are likely to be addressed through interventions targeting social determinants of health, including efforts to promote health, prevent disease, and improve healthy lifestyles (Bauer et al., 2014; Hartley, 2004; James, 2017). However, numerous health benefits are associated with rural living, including extensive social networks of extended duration, a "self-help" attitude, and task sharing among family and neighbors. These attributes could be used to structure novel health-related programs to strengthen the health, public health structures and programs, and economic and educational needs of people in rural America (Lichter & Ziliak, 2017; Weiss-Laxer et al., 2020).

Physical Environment

Despite benefits like open spaces, better air quality, lower crime levels, and less noise from vehicles, people in rural areas are less likely to benefit from built physical environments, including household and community resources and structures. In rural areas, barriers such as limited access to health systems, pharmacies, and recreation facilities could compromise health-seeking behaviors. Generally, nutrition and exercise habits are not supported by built environmental assets (e.g., structures, natural resources) that facilitate healthier habits (Barnett et al., 2017; Stankov et al., 2017).

Access to Quality Healthcare and Social Services

Individuals residing in rural communities have limited access to health and social services. Many factors overlap to interrupt access to care. For example, there are fewer primary care physicians, nurse practitioners, social workers, and other health professionals practicing in rural areas, which places rural individuals in these areas at a disadvantage for accessing and securing needed services. Additionally, transportation needs, health insurance, and health literacy issues need to be considered with a sense of urgency (Brown et al., 2019; Vohra et al., 2020).

Urban Health

Social Environment

Urban communities face many challenges, including crime and violence among residents, the presence of marginalized and poorer groups, health risk behaviors (e.g., sex trafficking, drugs, gangs, firearms), and increased stressors associated with activities of daily living. As urbanization continues to increase, people live closer to each other in sometimes substandard housing—many in unhygienic and unsafe environments where the potential for transmission of infectious disease is higher and more frequent than in rural areas. Rapid growth in urban areas has also produced poorer working conditions, creating environments in which contagious diseases and chronic illnesses such as asthma associated with mold and lead in older buildings are more prevalent. Because residents of urban populations are generally living longer, chronic illnesses associated with aging are also prevalent among people in these communities (Case & Deaton, 2017; U.S. Conference of Mayors, 2019). Despite denser populations, social isolation can still occur in urban areas.

Physical Environment

Urbanization also brings environmental pollution and climate change (Adams et al., 2017; Global Health University, n.d.; Kuddus et al., 2020). In many urban areas, increased pollution leads to poor air quality, which is associated with premature mortality and adverse health outcomes such as pulmonary disease and asthma, especially among children. Hispanic American, Asian American, and Black American populations tend to have higher morbidity and mortality rates related to air particle pollution than their White counterparts (Di et al., 2017). In urban areas, housing often consists of high-rise buildings, and people of various socioeconomic levels are usually found in different sections of the city. Consequences of overcrowding include more frequent use of public transportation, greater pollution from industry and noxious odors, and limited home ownership, all of which are linked to higher mortality and morbidity and overall poorer well-being (American Lung Association, 2020; Miranda et al., 2011).

Access to Healthcare and Social Services

Individuals with limited incomes in underresourced communities are more likely to live in urban areas and be uninsured; many do not consistently access healthcare. These factors are barriers to better health outcomes and contribute to higher morbidity and mortality rates among many people, including American Indian, Alaska Native, Asian American, Black American, and Hispanic American populations. Much of the housing stock in urban America is old and is therefore more likely to be associated with lead and mold problems. These are the places and spaces where people in minority groups and people living in poverty are likely to reside. Redlining, segregated education, discrimination, and other race-driven policies and practices are responsible for many factors that are associated with variations and disparities in access to healthcare and social services (American Lung Association, 2020; Ludwig et al., 2012). (See Chapter 22 for a discussion of redlining.)

RURAL AND URBAN HEALTH SCENARIOS

The following discussion presents a more detailed review of health-related scenarios for rural and urban populations in the United States, including demographic information, health needs and priorities, racial and ethnic disparities, and the impact of COVID-19. The country has seen rapid demographic changes, fluctuating between rural and urban areas according to longitudinal statistical estimates. In 1950, for example, approximately 54 million people resided in rural areas, while more than 68 million people identified as urban residents. By 2020, the rural population had seen a slight increase to more than 57.2 million, while urban areas witnessed a dramatic increase to 272.9 million people (CDC, 2017a; Johnson & Lichter, 2019; MacKinney et al., 2021).

From a historical perspective, more than 90% of the U.S. population resided in rural areas in 1790. By 1920, that number had plummeted to 50%. Currently, rural counties represent 14% of the country's total population (Johnson & Lichter, 2019). Several factors influenced rapid urban growth, including the perception of enhanced economic and social opportunity in the industrialized North and the urban South (Center for American Progress, 2015; Johnson & Lichter, 2019; Runde, 2015). Additionally, cities are sometimes referred to as "incubators of talent" because they facilitate access to goods and services, embody diversity, are culturally vibrant, advocate for innovation and futuristic planning, and are home to clusters of organizations, businesses, universities, and other vital establishments. However, not all people in cities benefit from these substantial assets. More innovation is needed to enhance the lives of city residents who live in poor, unsafe, and nonproductive environments (U.S. Conference of Mayors, 2020).

Rural Populations

Rural generally describes areas with low or geographically diffuse populations. Rural can also be characterized as a space with no urban center (Harrington et al., 2020). Using this description, about 14% of the U.S. population and nearly three quarters of U.S. land is considered rural (Harrington et al., 2020; Health Resources and Services Administration, 2021). The total U.S. population living in rural counties ranges from 46.2 million to 59 million people (Coughlin et al., 2019). Additionally, rural areas tend to have a lower population growth rate (3%) than urban (13%) and suburban (16%) regions (Harrington et al., 2020). Approximately two thirds of rural counties in the United States have experienced a population drop during the past decade (Cushing, 2021; Figure 17.1).

There are countless assets in rural communities, as they contain many natural resources and manufacturing industries. These communities are economically diverse, ranging from deeply impoverished to wealthier communities (Mueller et al., 2021). While urban areas are more racially and ethnically diverse than rural areas, rural America is also home to various populations. White individuals comprise almost 80% of the population, compared with 68% of suburban and 44% of urban populations. However, there are also long-established indigenous communities in Oklahoma, the Great Plains, the American Southwest, and Alaska, and predominantly Black communities in the South. Hispanic American communities have also grown in the Southwest and in parts of California (Harrington et al., 2020).

Rural Health Issues

Rural community residents tend to be older and sicker and have less income than their urban counterparts. In 2017, 19% of the rural population was older than 65 years, compared with 15% in urban areas (Harrington et al., 2020). Poverty rates in rural counties also averaged 18%, compared with 17% in urban regions and 14% in suburban communities (Harrington et al., 2020). Compared to urban areas, rural communities also have lower educational attainment, lack adequate transportation, and have less accessible healthcare

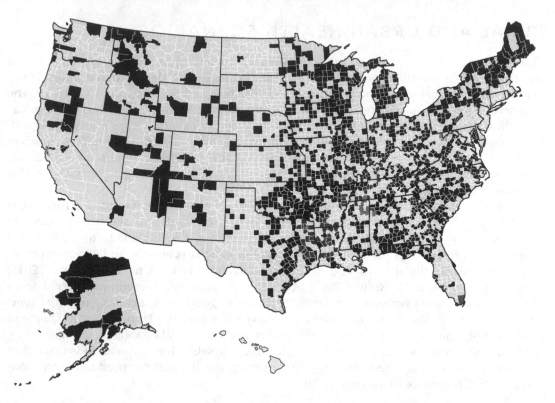

Figure 17.1 Map of mostly rural counties in the United States.

Source: U.S. Census Bureau. (2016). www.census.gov/newsroom/blogs/random-samplings/2016/12/life
_off_the_highway.html.

(Coughlin et al., 2019). Additionally, the uninsured rate for rural community residents younger than age 65 years is 12%, compared with 10% for urban community residents (Cheeseman Day, 2019). Rural community residents are more likely to have jobs that do not offer employer-sponsored insurance (Foutz et al., 2017; Medicaid and CHIP Payment and Access Commission [MACPAC], 2021). Many rural states also have not expanded Medicaid. Notably, between 2013 and 2015, the uninsured rate in rural areas within Medicaid expansion states fell by nearly half, from 16% to 9%, primarily because of increased Medicaid coverage in these states (Foutz et al., 2017; MACPAC, 2021).

Chronic diseases are health priorities in rural communities (Harrington et al., 2020). In the Rural Healthy People 2020 initiative, chronic diseases like diabetes and high blood pressure were top priority (Bolin et al., 2015). Older adults in rural communities have a higher prevalence of comorbid chronic diseases, such as diabetes and heart disease, than urban older adults (Coughlin et al., 2019). This population is more likely to show a higher prevalence of obesity, with the percentage being 29% in rural counties compared to 24% in urban counties (Coughlin et al., 2019).

Mental health service access in rural areas is a significant issue. The Rural Healthy People 2020 initiative ranked mental health and mental disorders as another vital priority (Bolin et al., 2015). The Healthy People 2030 initiative also lists suicide as a leading health indicator. Suicide is one of the foremost causes of death nationwide, particularly among young people (U.S. Department of Health and Human Services [DHHS], n.d.). Rural youth suicide rates are nearly double urban rates for both males and females, and longitudinal analyses suggest that the disparity will continue to rise (Coughlin et al., 2019). Increased rates among rural youth have been attributed to the significant impact of interpersonal factors such as social isolation, loneliness, lack of belonging, and perceived burdensomeness that have been identified in these communities (Monteith et al., 2020a, b). Furthermore, interpersonal violence (e.g., childhood abuse, intimate partner violence) is severe and chronic in many kinds of communities; however, such conditions are associated with worse health and psychosocial outcomes in rural areas compared with urban areas (Monteith et al., 2020a, b).

Telehealth is a powerful tool that expands availability of health and social services. Therefore, the use of this modality should be encouraged to reduce disparities, make services more available and convenient, and remove barriers associated with transportation, travel time, additional costs, and workforce shortages (Catalyst, 2018). In a 2019 study, researchers reported that about 24% of rural adults stated that they had used telehealth sometime during the past year, and 14% of them indicated that they had received either a diagnosis or treatment information from a healthcare provider through this technology. Furthermore, among the 24% of adults who had used telehealth during the past year, about 69% of them indicated that the modality was convenient; another 30% used the service because an in-person healthcare professional visit was not otherwise possible at that time. About 26% of adults posited that they used telehealth because it was difficult to travel to a health professional or a hospital for healthcare (Harvard T.H. Chen School of Public Health, 2019). Further studies are needed to methodologically evaluate the impact and efficacy of telehealth among people in rural communities (Butzner & Cuffee, 2021). It is important to remember that many rural communities are not connected to internet services, and residents might not have adequate technology or skills, including older adults and individuals with disabilities. All of the aforementioned factors are barriers to healthcare services (Behrman et al., 2021).

Rural Mortality Rates

For nearly 30 years, there have been widening mortality disparities in rural areas compared with urban communities, with moderately sized rural populations being the most negatively affected (Gong et al., 2019; James & Cossman, 2017). A possible explanation for this trend is that some rural counties are not keeping pace with the health improvements of their urban counterparts. In 2016, the health improvement rate for rural low-income areas was approximately 2 decades behind the levels observed in urban areas (Cosby et al., 2019). Various interconnected societal, geographic, behavioral, and structural factors may contribute to higher mortality rates in rural districts, including differences in health-related behaviors, access to healthcare services, and environmental exposures (Harrington et al., 2020; Long et al., 2018). Notably, the mortality rates for the five leading causes of death in the United States (heart disease, cancer, unintentional injury, chronic lower respiratory disease, and stroke) are generally higher in rural areas than in urban areas (Coughlin et al., 2019; Garcia et al., 2017; Ma et al., 2022).

Racial and Ethnic Health Disparities in Rural America

Racial and ethnic disparities in health and healthcare quality are well documented and persistent (Baciu et al., 2017; James et al., 2017). Racial and ethnic minorities, which account for 20% of the U.S. rural population, are often geographically isolated and face significant health challenges (Cheng et al., 2020; Henning-Smith et al., 2019). Across many health indicators, including access to care and healthcare quality, racial and ethnic minorities fare worse than their White counterparts. However, certain populations in rural communities face specific health challenges, such as heart disease and stroke among Black Americans, tuberculosis among Asian Americans, opioid overdose among White Americans, suicide among American Indians/Alaska Natives, and access issues among Hispanic Americans, such as not having a primary healthcare provider (Case & Deaton, 2017; James et al., 2017). Therefore, while health outcomes, quality of care, and access to healthcare have improved over time for all populations, disparities remain constant among racial and ethnic communities (James et al., 2017).

URBAN HEALTHCARE

NARRATIVE 17.1: THINKING OUT LOUD: A DAY IN THE LIFE OF A HEALTH PROFESSIONAL IN URBAN AMERICA

Providing healthcare to individuals and families who live in urban communities can be both daunting and rewarding. Many older adults live alone, are on fixed incomes, and reside in older houses that may need repair or are in "senior living" high-rise buildings, which are often moldy, poorly maintained, inadequately lighted, and situated in noisy communities. Too often, older adults struggle to access quality food because of their limited income, being located in food deserts, lacking reliable transportation, and having access to only inadequate supports. Common comorbidities among older adults are hypertension, heart disease, cancer, diabetes, and arthritis, all of which tend to restrict mobility, reduce opportunities for physical activity, and increase chances of further deterioration of overall health status. Falls can be a substantial problem. Poor eyesight and lack of dental care contribute to other health conditions, such as deficient nutrition. Noise levels are a significant concern, as police and emergency vehicle sirens are often heard throughout the day and night. "There never seems to be any peace in my house," reported an older adult patient during my home visit. Moreover, pollution contaminates the thick air, which can be smoke-filled and tainted with annoying odors. As a result, windows are often closed, which can be a safety issue when older adults may become overheated and dehydrated. Management of medications and other home-based procedures such as wound dressing (related to diabetes) often require the attention of professionals who can help older adults administer treatments safely and efficiently.

Concerns proliferate when individuals "stretch their medications" to create more dosages, or reduce their recommended number of daily doses per day to save money. Older adults might also cut pills in half, dilute insulin, reuse contaminated needles, and miscalculate measurements—all of which can have harmful consequences. Social workers are needed to assist with securing support for older adults to help with activities of daily living, including house cleaning, financial management of funds, socialization activities, and other life events. Knowledge about community resources is an essential component of care of older adults. The older adult population is an invisible but vulnerable group. Many do not have access to computers and internet services or the skills to use the technology. Some are afraid that personal details of their lives might "get out" and negatively expose them in their communities. Even when living in urban neighborhoods, proximity to resources may not always mean that the services are accessible. Also, costs are a constant concern, as is the possibility that the "doctor or nurse will find something else wrong." A comment about costs from one older person: "These doctors and nurses are 'come-back people.' They say, 'You got this disease—come back ... . Then, the next time you see them, they say, 'you got that disease—come back!' They can worry you to death—they can make you sick!" Often, decisions are made to delay healthcare visits, which might increase older adult morbidity and mortality. They deserve better!

Discussion Questions

1. How would you, as a health professional, plan policy change in your community to address the realities of millions of older adults living in urban communities?
2. What are the significant points of concern that would need immediate and long-range interventions? Be specific; document your findings, including the outcomes.
3. Using the National Institute on Minority Health and Health Disparities Research Framework as discussed in Chapters 5 and 10, or a theoretical framework of your choice, develop a research program that could address selected variables extracted from the healthcare provider's narrative.

Urban Populations

According to the *Urban Areas for the 2020 Census: Proposed Criteria,* "urban communities represent densely developed territory and encompass residential, commercial, and other non-residential land uses" (Bureau of the Census, Department of Commerce, 2021). Boundaries used to determine urban zones have been mainly defined by measures based on population counts, residential population density, and standards centered on nonresidential urban land use criteria, such as commercial, industrial, transportation, and open space. All of these are included as part of the urban landscape, first defined in the 1950 census (Bureau of the Census, Department of Commerce, 2021).

Recent estimates purport that more than 80% of the U.S. population resides in urban environments; it is projected that by the year 2050, almost 90% of the total U.S. population will live in metropolitan cities (Center for Sustainable Systems, 2021). In the United States, urban economies have accounted for more than 90% of the nation's gross domestic product (GDP), almost 92% of total generated wage income, and approximately 88% of jobs in the country (U.S. Conference of Mayors, 2020). The median household income in urban centers is approximately $66,164, which is over $10,000 more than localities outside these municipalities (U.S. Census Bureau, 2019). Since 2000, poverty has dramatically increased in suburban communities when compared with rural regions. However, the overall poverty rate is higher in rural and urban areas relative to suburban regions (Parker et al., 2018). According to Horowitz, people in rural America without a college degree are "not optimistic about their future financial well-being" (Parker et al., 2018).

According to recent Pew Research Center data, U.S. urban counties have no significant racial or ethnic majority. However, White citizens made up approximately 44% of urban regions from 2012 to 2016, followed by Hispanic American citizens (almost 27% of urban populations). Black Americans made up 17% of people in urban neighborhoods, while metropolitan areas have the highest rates of foreign-born inhabitants (22% from 2012–2016). Regarding educational attainment, 35% of urban residents have a bachelor's degree or higher, compared with 21% of rural residents (Parker et al., 2018; USDA Economic Research Service, 2019). A map of urban counties in the United States is displayed in Figure 17.2.

Urban Health Issues

In recent years, urban health researchers have employed a prevailing social-ecological framework to identify the pressing health priorities of metropolitan environments. The social-ecological model considers the effects of interplay among individual, relationship, community, and societal factors on health outcomes in different populations (CDC, 2021). The linkages of the functionality of urban spaces to human health have been enumerated pervasively, but the mechanisms that undergird this relationship are opaque, at best (Bentley, 2014). According to the CDC, the past 10 years have ushered in various health priorities for urban localities. The CDC suggests five priorities for these environments: strengthen essential public health services, enrich capacity to respond to urgent threats to health, develop a nationwide prevention network and program, promote women's health, and invest in our nation's youth (Speers & Lancaster, 1998). These priorities are reflected in the bulk of public health literature on health issues specific to densely populated metropolitan areas, as perceived through social-ecological lenses and as have been examined over the past two decades. For example, a global systematic literature review conducted by Vilar-Compte et al. (2021) uncovered 68 papers from international perspectives that identified four overarching concerns: urban poverty, food insecurity, urban risk factors of nutritional status, and coping strategies for food scarcity. The researchers posited that urban poverty is related to poorer health outcomes, which raises questions about the "urban advantage"—perhaps an advantage for some, but not all, people.

Although not reflected explicitly in the health priorities of the U.S.'s predominant public health institutions, researchers have found that urban environments experience significant

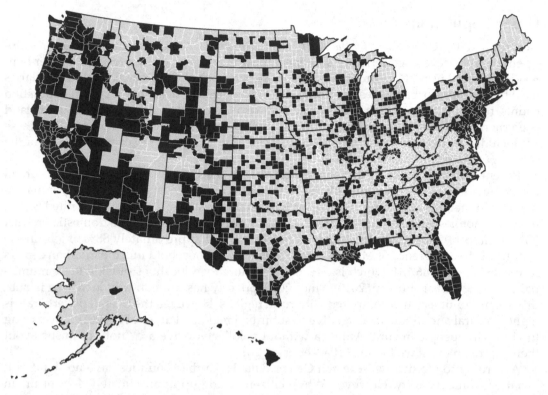

Figure 17.2 Map of mostly urban counties in the United States.

Source: U.S. Census Bureau. (2016). www.census.gov/newsroom/blogs/random-samplings/2016/12/life _off_the_highway.html.

obstacles in the conjoined realms of clean water accessibility and homelessness. From 2013 to 2017, approximately 1.2 million people in the United States lacked consistent access to clean water, about half of whom were located in urban places and spaces. Within a sample of U.S. cities from 2017 to 2019 that controlled for persons experiencing homelessness and poor housing, at least 930,000 people lacked consistent access to basic sanitation, and 610,000 also lacked access to clean water (Capone et al., 2020; Meehan et al., 2020).

Relevant urban public health research embeds the elevation of urban well-being through social cohesion as an essential intervention in the new era. For example, Leviton et al. (2000) suggested over 2 decades ago that the future well-being of U.S. urban centers rests in the enrichment of positive connections throughout metropolitan regions via coalition building; however, little has changed to this day, and disparities have persisted. A more recent systematic review exploring the effectiveness of community-based health promotion interventions in urban areas posited exciting findings when individuals are involved in decision-making. However, although community-based interventions are promising for health promotion and disease prevention, they have been far from fully actualized (Nickel & von dem Knesebeck, 2020). Barten et al. (2011) acknowledge that the physical environment, social conditions, and dynamics of climate change often contribute to health inequities in urban contexts. Successful urban governance consists of understanding and managing the intersectionality of these factors, which can be a difficult charge. Urban health interventions must focus on systemic poverty, food scarcity, and nutrition with a conceptualized understanding of community connectedness and resource availability (Bentley, 2014; Evans et al., 2020; Rice & Hancock, 2016).

Interventions from the CDC are significant. Since the creation of the CDC's 1998 priorities, substantial progress has been made in attaining their objectives. For example, the

CDC's *Racial and Ethnic Approaches to Community Health (REACH)* initiative commenced the year after publication of the urban priorities. Its purpose was to increase the capacity of locally based, sustainable solutions designed to address health status gaps among culturally diverse communities in urban, rural, and tribal areas in the United States (CDC, 2020a). According to evaluation data compiled from 2014 to 2018, approximately 3 million people have experienced better access to healthy foods and beverages, and 322,000 people have benefitted from smoke- and tobacco-free interventions. Almost 1.4 million people have more access to consistent opportunities to be physically active. A million additional participants have access to local health promotion, chronic disease prevention, and treatment programs (CDC, 2020a).

Similarly, the *State Public Health Actions to Prevent and Control Diabetes, Heart Disease, Obesity, and Associated Risk Factors and Promote School Health* initiative was launched in 2013. The initiative is a multidimensional program designed to improve the health of American communities through synchronized chronic disease prevention programs, including childhood and adult obesity, diabetes, heart disease, and stroke prevention projects (Park, 2017) and is currently implemented in all 50 states. The CDC has worked with state agencies to implement environmental approaches to support healthy behaviors among participants to accomplish its metrics. The program's focus has also been on enriching health systems interventions, efficient care delivery, and improved community-to-health linkages to support local urban environments, including built communities. As a result, although national adult and adolescent obesity rates have increased by more than 2%, the CDC reports a significant decrease in adolescent and adult overweight classification since the beginning of the program (CDC, 2019). Additional reports show that minor improvements related to clean water access have occurred in urban cities (Capone et al., 2020), but more efforts are needed.

Urban Mortality Rates

As discussed previously, the urban environment has lower mortality rates and elevated rates of well-being across a spectrum of health indicators. In several studies using a retrospective analysis of age-adjusted death rates for all-cause mortality and deaths by cardiovascular disease, cancer, unintentional injuries, chronic lower respiratory disease, and stroke, urban populations experience lower mortality rates across all variables (Probst et al., 2020; Shah et al., 2020). When exploring education, race, and rurality as predictors of mortality, research indicates that rural counties with high-level poverty encompass populations with higher mortality rates—yet, rural/urban mortality and ongoing disparities continue. Compared to residents of urban centers, people of rural counties were significantly less likely to have consistent access to care. They traveled longer distances to their healthcare providers than did urbanites (Gong et al., 2019). Furthermore, the prevalence of disabilities of any kind, even controlling for age, sex, race, education, and federal poverty level, is significantly lower in large metropolitan centers than in rural communities (Zhao et al., 2019). Overall, urban areas have experienced very high indicators of health and well-being over the past few decades (Salgado et al., 2020).

Notably, as urbanization increases, infant mortality rates in many places have decreased incrementally, including neonatal and postneonatal mortality rates (Ely et al., 2017). One explanation is related to the more significant socioeconomic disadvantage that rural groups experience, rather than limited healthcare access or increased individual health indicators among childbearing women (Ehrenthal et al. (2020). The Kozhimannil studies (2019, 2020) also found that mortality rates of infants of non-Hispanic White and non-Hispanic Black mothers were lowest in large urban counties. Ultimately, maternal morbidity and mortality were lower in urban than in rural populations (Kozhimannil et al., 2019, 2020), but concerns about existing rates in both communities still persist, particularly in underresourced areas and in populations such as American Indians and Alaska Natives.

Racial and Ethnic Disparities in Urban America

In general, national and statewide population studies show significant racial and ethnic disparities in urban environments related to socioeconomic status, maternal and child health, and a wide variety of mortality indicators over the past 5 years. Generally speaking, a lack of education and training and unemployment are related to lower economic status and poorer health status (Allard & Brundage, 2019; van Zon et al., 2017). Native Americans and Alaska Natives experience a 200% higher poverty rate than the general population in select urban counties. Moreover, in a study investigating the effects of residential segregation on urban youth and children, researchers found that Black children and adolescents experienced worse outcomes across all health indicators as segregation increased. A study conducted in metropolitan Atlanta found that non-Hispanic Black women, regardless of socioeconomic status, died at twice the rate of their White counterparts (Collin et al., 2019). Although influenza and pneumonia were concurrently the eighth leading causes of death in the United States for all Americans, non-Hispanic Black populations experienced the highest mortality rates associated with these maladies (Lippert et al., 2022). Children from underresourced communities continue to be subjected to disproportionate health disparities. For example, asthma is the primary reason children seek treatment in emergency departments (DeLaroche et al., 2021). The root cause of asthma among minority children is associated with unhealthy housing and air pollution and is considered one of the most impactful health disparities in the nation (Bryant-Stephens et al., 2021).

At all levels of society, disproportionate socioeconomic barriers persist in historically marginalized communities, including Black, Latino/Hispanic, Native American and Alaskan Native, and Native Hawaiian and Pacific Islander populations. After controlling for household, neighborhood, and metropolitan nuances, Hess et al. (2020) found that, from 1980 to 2017, Black American families experienced a higher housing cost burden than their White counterparts. These findings may partly explain why 104 out of every 10,000 Black people in major cities in the United States are homeless (Moses, n.d.).

COVID-19 IN RURAL AND URBAN AMERICA

In 2019, the coronavirus disease became a global pandemic and a significant public health crisis in the United States, severely affecting many Americans' health and socioeconomic well-being (Peters, 2020). By 2021, COVID-19 made a worldwide impact, with deaths linked to the novel coronavirus at more than 2.5 million people, and socioeconomic and political effects unsurpassed by any other health issue in modern times. People age 65 years and older account for 50% of hospital and intensive care unit admissions and 80% of deaths (Peters, 2020). However, regardless of age, of those hospitalized with COVID-19, 75% have some underlying medical condition, typically diabetes or chronic lung or cardiovascular disease (Peters, 2020). Due to the more significant number of cases and deaths, urban areas in the United States have garnered more attention about the impact of COVID-19 on their communities (Peters, 2020).

Rural areas have also been negatively impacted by the COVID-19 pandemic. The number of COVID-19 cases is low in most rural areas compared with urban communities, likely due to remoteness, open space, and low population density that initially limited the spread in these locations (Ameh et al., 2020). However, a third of rural counties are in the White House Coronavirus Task Force "red zone," and rural areas may experience higher COVID-19 case fatality rates when outbreaks occur (Cheng et al., 2020). The red zone designation is given to a community when more than 100 new cases per 100,000 population is reported within the week. Even before COVID-19, death rates were high in rural areas. Data indicate that the gap between death rates among rural and urban populations has increased during the last 2 decades, with urban residents experiencing significant improvement in health outcomes while drugs and disease spread throughout rural areas. Life expectancy fell particularly among less-educated White men, primarily because of "deaths of despair" due to substance use-related casualties or suicide (Case & Deaton, 2020; CDC, 2021b).

Notably, the pandemic occurred in a world that is vastly connected and codependent. The closing of many workplaces, schools, universities, religious institutions, and other organizations was made possible by modern technology that expanded remote service delivery capacities in pivotal enterprises. New and critical pharmaceutical and medical research resulted in the rapid development of effective vaccines that have reduced the spread of the COVID-19 virus where effective vaccination programs have been implemented. The economic impact of the COVID-19 pandemic, which began in 2020, has been the most significant economic contraction since World War II. World output in 2020 was 8% lower than what it would have been if the pandemic had not occurred. Economic growth was forecast to be about 3%; instead, the decline was approximately 5%. In comparison, the world economy declined by 0.1% during the Great Recession of 2009 (*The Economist*, 2020).

Deaths of Despair and Suicidal Behaviors and the COVID-19 Pandemic

In 2019 across the United States, one person died every 11 minutes from suicide, 12 million people gave serious thought to suicide, 3 million individuals planned to commit suicide, and 1.4 million people attempted suicide. Suicide is the second leading cause of death among individuals age 10 to 34, the fourth leading cause of death among individuals age 34 to 54, and the fifth leading cause among 45- to 54-year-olds (CDC, 2020b). Suicidal behaviors consist of attempts at self-injury with the intent to die or self-injury itself that produces death; this outcome is preventable, involves all ages, happens in rural and urban communities, and can occur across the life course. In rural communities, factors associated with suicide include access to firearms and substance use at the individual level, as well as economic tensions and lack of mental health services at the community level. More research is needed to help unravel and quantify how risk factors influence suicidal behaviors in these areas (Mohatt et al., 2021). Stigma associated with suicide and help-seeking behaviors, especially among veterans in rural communities, remains a barrier to prevention and efficient treatment that health professionals will need to address to more robustly reduce deaths by suicide (Monteith et al., 2020a).

By contrast, data from urban communities suggest that adults who live in cities, live in poverty, and have limited family contact and support have higher odds of committing suicide than their adult counterparts who live in more resourced urban areas. Other factors, such as marital status, employment, family size, and health status, including mental health conditions, further influence outcomes in this population (Denney et al., 2015).

The COVID-19 pandemic has exacerbated the health and mental health issues of rural and urban communities. For example, depressive disorders increased by four times in one quarter in 2019 (24.4% compared to 6.5%). There was also a rise in substance use, and suicidal thoughts increased with about twice as many people reporting suicidal behaviors than in 2018. Some populations, such as young adults, Hispanic Americans, Black Americans, essential workers, caregivers who were unpaid, and people with pre-existing mental health conditions, were unduly impacted by this malady.

The Ecological Model (see Chapter 10) provides a framework for conceptualizing suicide because it is associated with multiple risk factors, such as those included here:

◆ *Individual Level:* Many factors, such as a history of mental health conditions, chronic health illnesses, previous self-harm attempts, and biological determinants, are evident.

◆ *Relationship Level:* Excessive conflict, tensions, or violent relationships; a sense of loneliness and sporadic social support; and a family history of suicide, economic stress, and work strain are essential factors.

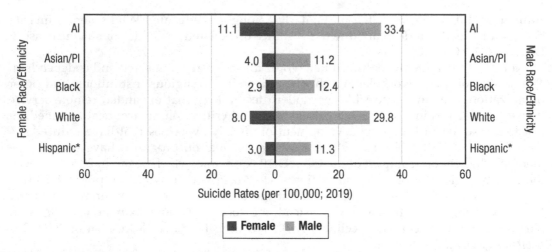

Figure 17.3 Overview of suicidal rates among race/ethnic groups.

*Persons of Hispanic origin may be of any race; all other racial/ethnic groups are non-Hispanic

AI, American Indian; PI, Pacific Islander

Source: Centers for Disease Control and Prevention. www.nimh.nih.gov/health/statistics/suicide; WISQARS Fatal Injury Data Visualization Tool.

◆ *Community Level:* Limited connections and interactions with community people and organizations, health and social services barriers, and inadequate community resources such as housing.

◆ *Societal Level:* Access to lethal means of self-harm, the stigma of health-seeking for mental health and substance abuse/use, unsafe use of the portrayal of suicidal ideation and behaviors, distance from social service and health systems.

Figure 17.3 provides an overview of suicidal rates among race/ethnic groups, suggesting that the highest rates occur among Native American and Alaska Native people, followed by non-Hispanic White people. People who live in rural areas have high rates of suicide as well. Males in all categories are more likely to commit suicide than females. Again, treatment is often delayed or not forthcoming because the early warning signs of suicide are missed by families, friends, and others, along with its accompanying stigma and feelings of shame among youth and adults (Simes et al., 2021).

Rural Hospitals and Challenges for Health Services During COVID-19

Rural regions often lack hospital access to the interstate system, making transportation of patients, health providers, and supplies difficult (Peters, 2020). These regions have also had lower COVID-19 testing rates than urban areas and lack the healthcare infrastructure to deal with a high number of severe cases (Cheng et al., 2020). Since 2010, 126 rural hospitals have closed (Cheng et al., 2020). Even when hospitals are available, most do not have the capacity to address surges in cases, and only 1% of the nation's intensive care unit beds are in rural areas (Cheng et al., 2020). While the death toll of COVID-19 in rural areas has not been as high as that in more densely populated urban settings, inequities of healthcare access could ultimately make the virus's impact more harmful in rural communities (Mueller et al., 2021). The case study that follows highlights some of the concerns that rural families confront when trying to meet their needs and respond to a plethora of crises that the virus and other external forces have created.

CASE STUDY 17.1: CHALLENGES WITH ACCESS TO HEALTH SERVICES IN RURAL AMERICA

Ray is a 28-year-old married man. He and his wife, Tonya, moved from an urban center to a rural town in southern Georgia because the corporate staff of the restaurant that Ray manages promoted him. He was asked to open a new restaurant in a smaller community, about 100 miles east of the city, without access to comprehensive healthcare facilities. Tonya is pregnant and now travels 50 miles to the nearest obstetrician for prenatal care visits. Her pregnancy is considered high-risk due to a history of high blood pressure controlled by a special diet, exercise, medications, and a sleep plan. Ray is very supportive of her prescribed routine, and Tonya is following the health plan. Unfortunately, just 3 months after their move, the COVID-19 pandemic forced all restaurants in the area to close, leaving Ray unemployed. With tight finances and numerous obligations, the couple worries about keeping their health insurance, purchasing medications and the food items needed for Tonya's diet, and paying for gas and car repairs required for travel to healthcare facilities for prenatal care. They must also pay for the new home that they purchased in their recently acquired community. Ray is overwhelmed with worry and has begun to complain about feelings of anxiety, difficulty sleeping, and brief bouts of depression. He says that his highest priority is the overall health of his wife and unborn child. In just a few days, their life, once stable and relatively well planned, became a "nightmare" for both of them. Ray goes on to say that because they're a new family in the community, finding assistance will be complex, and they will have to "start from scratch" when it comes to seeking aid for healthcare, housing, and social support. Ray has begun to search for employment, which has not yet produced any positive outcomes. He admits that frightening thoughts enter his head, but will not comment further.

Discussion Questions

1. When you've constructed a plan of care for this family and identified priorities based on a family-centered approach, what steps would you take to ensure that Ray and Tanya agree with the program and work with a social worker and other health professionals to address their needs?
2. Are there immediate issues that need attention? What are the long-term problems that should be discussed at this time?
3. Is there a need to discuss with them the COVID-19 virus and its implications for Tonya's and Ray's safety as determined by the CDC guidelines?
4. Identify Ray's and Tonya's physical, mental/emotional, and social/interpersonal needs and delineate their priorities with documented, evidence-based practices.
5. Would the needs of Tonya's and Ray's unborn infant be a component of the comprehensive plan (including its birth delivery at a nearby health facility)? If yes, describe that component. If not, provide a rationale for not including the infant's health concerns in the plan.
6. Could telehealth be used to support this couple? Could you determine whether there are barriers to the use of telehealth for them? What concerns might emerge?
7. How will the family pay for health services? What about services for the unborn infant?
8. What are your next steps? What community resources and supports would you suggest for this couple? How long do you think they will need assistance before their level of overall stability is restored to its original, precrisis state?

THE CULTURE OF HEALTH

In recent years, a focus on developing a culture of health for all people in the United States has emerged. This approach suggests that every person should have a chance to live to their healthiest potential (National Academy of Medicine, 2021). Health equity is the cornerstone to the creation of this culture of health. The National Academy of Medicine (2021) has proposed a model that is effective in helping communities achieve a culture of health through the reduction and elimination of health disparities at the community level. Seven steps are proposed for the development of a community-driven health equity plan that has value for both rural and urban communities. The steps include questions and examples. The questions follow; a more complete document is available on National Academy of Medicine's website. The questions are (a) vision and goals (what is to be achieved); (b) community context (identify the unique challenges and opportunities that exist); (c) research grounding (use best practices and evidence-based data and approaches); (d) strategies and tactics (develop cultural approach strategies for goal achievement); (e) stakeholders (who is needed for planning, implementing, evaluating, and sustaining the plan); (f) timeline (develop a timeline with milestones for all aspects of the plan); and (g) sustainability (at the beginning of the plan, develop communication approaches, additional resources, and how evaluation data could be used to sustain and enhance all aspects of the action plan (Chandra et al., 2017; National Academy of Medicine, 2021; Plough, 2015). Examples of community health plans in four regions of the nation can be viewed at nam.edu/healthequityactionplans.

CONCLUSION

This chapter emphasizes issues related to rural and urban health population, as well as numerous disparities from the past to the present (Brown et al., 2019). Although significant, individual-based disparities persist, there have been improvements over time. For example, U.S. healthcare coverage for older adults and those living in poverty—Medicare and Medicaid—have been significant resources for individuals and families for more than 50 years. Still, gaps in service and health outcomes continue. In more recent times, the Patient Protection and Affordable Care Act, which expanded government-based funding and healthcare regulations, has helped narrow gaps in access to healthcare. Private insurance continues to be available to individuals through their employment or direct, market-driven purchases. These efforts have been significant and have improved healthcare for many, but not all. A plethora of evidence about continuing disparities between and among rural and urban health outcomes are supported by research, including that individuals with low education and socioeconomic status are more likely to have poorer health outcomes regardless of residence in rural or urban settings. There is no clear path forward for further significant public healthcare legislation; vulnerable populations, poverty, and lack of access to quality healthcare need to be addressed with a sense of urgency.

ADDITIONAL RESOURCES

Rural America at a Glance. www.ers.usda.gov/webdocs/publications/80894/eib-162.pdf?v=42684

Rural Health Promotion and Disease Prevention Toolkit.

Preventing Suicide: A Technical Package of Policy, Programs, and Practice www.cdc
   .gov/suicide/pdf/suicideTechnicalPackage.pdf
Stone, D. M., Holland, K. M., Bartholow, B. N., Crosby, A. E., Davis, S. P., & Wilkins, N. (2017).
   Preventing suicide: A technical package of policies, programs, and practice.

To learn more about preventing suicide, call 1-800-CDC-INFO or visit CDC's violence prevention pages at www.cdc.gov/violenceprevention. AK2017 TM National Center for Injury Prevention and Control Division of Violence Prevention www.cdc.gov/suicide/pdf/suicideTechnicalPackage.pdf

Kaiser Family Foundation State Health Facts, The Centers for Disease Control and Prevention. (2021). *Medicaid & chip*. https://www.kff.org/state-category/medicaid-chip/

The Economist. (2020). The peril and the promise: The world economy. https://www.economist.com/search?q=The+Peril+and+the+Promise+

REFERENCES

Adams, J. D., Greenwood, D. A., Thomashow, M., & Russ, A. (2017). Chapter 7: Sense of Place. In *Urban environmental education review* (pp. 68–75). Cornell University Press.

Allard, M. D., & Brundage, Jr. V. (2019). American Indians and Alaska natives in the US labor force. *Monthly Labor Review*, 142, 1.

Ameh, G. G., Njoku, A., Inungu, J., & Younis, M. (2020). Rural America and coronavirus epidemic: Challenges and solutions. *European Journal of Environment and Public Health*, 4(2), em0040.

American Lung Association. (2020). Disparities in the impact of air pollution. https://www.lung.org/clean-air/outdoors/who-is-at-risk/disparities

Baciu, A., Negussie, Y., Geller, A., Weinstein, J. N., & National Academies of Sciences, Engineering, and Medicine. (2017). *The state of health disparities in the United States. In Communities in action: Pathways to health equity*. National Academies Press (US).

Barnett, D. W., Barnett, A., Nathan, A., Van Cauwenberg, J., & Cerin, E. (2017). Built environmental correlates of older adults' total physical activity and walking: A systematic review and meta-analysis. *International Journal of Behavioral Nutrition and Physical Activity*, 14(1), 1–24.

Barten, F., Akerman, M., Becker, D., Friel, S., Hancock, T., Mwatsama, M., Rice, M., Sheuya, S., & Stern, R. (2011). Rights, knowledge, and governance for improved health equity in urban settings. *Journal of Urban Health: Bulletin of the New York Academy of Medicine*, 88(5), 896–905. https://doi.org/10.1007/s11524-011-9608-z

Bauer, U. E., Briss, P. A., Goodman, R. A., & Bowman, B. A. (2014). Prevention of chronic disease in the 21st century: Elimination of the leading preventable causes of premature death and disability in the USA. *The Lancet*, 384(9937), 45–52.

Behrman, P., Fitzgibbon, M. L., Dulin, A., Wang, M. L., & Baskin, M. (2021). Society of behavioral medicine statement on COVID-19 and rural health. *Translational Behavioral Medicine*, 11(2), 625–630.

Bentley, M. (2014). An ecological public health approach to understanding the relationships between sustainable urban environments, public health and social equity. *Health Promotion International*, 29(3), 528–537. https://doi.org/10.1093/heapro/dat028

Bolin, J. N., Bellamy, G. R., Ferdinand, A. O., Vuong, A. M., Kash, B. A., Schulze, A., & Helduser, J. W. (2015). Rural healthy people 2020: New decade, same challenges. *The Journal of Rural Health*, 31(3), 326–333.

Brown, A. F., Ma, G. X., Miranda, J., Eng, E., Castille, D., Brockie, T., & Trinh-Shevrin, C. (2019). Structural interventions to reduce and eliminate health disparities. *American Journal of Public Health*, 109(S1), S72–S78. https://doi.org/10.2105/AJPH.2018.304844

Bryant-Stephens, T. C., Strane, D., Bhambhani, S., & Kenyon, C. C. (2021). Housing and asthma disparities. *Journal of Allergy and Clinical Immunology*.

Bureau of the Census, Department of Commerce. (2021). Urban areas for the 2020 census-proposed criteria. https://www.federalregister.gov/documents/2021/02/19/2021-03412/urban-areas-for-the-2020-census-proposed-criteria

Burns, T. R. (2017). Contributing factors of frequent use of the emergency department: A synthesis. *International Emergency Nursing*, 35, 51–55.

Butzner, M., & Cuffee, Y. (2021). Telehealth interventions and outcomes across rural communities in the United States: Narrative review. *Journal of Medical Internet Research*, 23(8), e29575.

Capone, D., Cumming, O., Nichols, D., & Brown, J. (2020). Water and sanitation in urban America, 2017–2019. *American Journal of Public Health*, 110(10), 1567–1572.

Case, A., & Deaton, A. (2017). Mortality and morbidity in the 21st century. *Brookings Papers on Economic Activity*, 2017, 397.

Case, A., & Deaton, A. (2020). Deaths of despair and the future of capitalism. Princeton University Press.

Catalyst, N. E. J. M. (2018). What is telehealth? *NEJM Catalyst*, 4(1).

Centers for Disease Control and Prevention. (2019). Rural health: Preventing chronic diseases and promoting health in rural communities. https://www.cdc.gov/chronicdisease/resources/publications/factsheets/rural-health.htm

Centers for Disease Control and Prevention. (2020a). REACH program impact. Centers for Disease Control and Prevention. https://www.cdc.gov/nccdphp/dnpao/state-local-programs/reach/program_impact/index.htm

Centers for Disease Control and Prevention. (2020b). Racial and ethnic approaches to community health. Centers for Disease Control and Prevention. https://www.cdc.gov/nccdphp/dnpao/state -local-programs/reach/index.htm

Centers for Disease Control and Prevention. (2021). The social-ecological model. Centers for Disease Control and Prevention. https://www.cdc.gov/violenceprevention/about/social- ecologicalmodel.html

Center for American Progress. (2015). Expanding opportunities in America's urban areas. https://www .americanprogress.org/issues/poverty/reports/2015/03/23/109460/expanding-opportunities -in-americas-urban-areas/

Center for Sustainable Systems. (2021). U.S. cities factsheet. https://css.umich.edu/publications/ factsheets/built-environment/us-cities-factsheet

Chandra, A., Acosta, J., Carman, K. G., Dubowitz, T., Leviton, L., Martin, L. T., Miller, C., Nelson, C., Orleans, T., Tait, M., Trujillo, M., Towe, V., Yeung, D., & Plough, A. L. (2017). Building a national culture of health: Background, action framework, measures, and next steps. *Rand Health Quarterly*, 6(2), 3.

Cheeseman Day, J. (2019). Rates of uninsured fall in rural counties, remain higher than urban counties. Washington, DC: US Census Bureau. https://www.census.gov/library/ stories/2019/04/health-insurance-rural-america.html

Cheng, K. J. G., Sun, Y., & Monnat, S. M. (2020). COVID-19 death rates are higher in rural counties with larger shares of Blacks and Hispanics. *The Journal of Rural Health*, 36(4), 602–608.

Collin, L. J., Jiang, R., Ward, K. C., Gogineni, K., Subhedar, P. D., Sherman, M. E., Gaudet, M. M., Breitkopf, C. R., D'Angelo, O., Gabram-Mendola, S., Aneja, R., Gaglioti, A. H., & McCullough, L. E. (2019). Racial disparities in breast cancer outcomes in the metropolitan Atlanta area: New insights and approaches for health equity. *JNCI Cancer Spectrum*, 3(3). https://doi.org/10.1093/jncics/ pkz053

Cosby, A. G., McDoom-Echebiri, M. M., James, W., Khandekar, H., Brown, W., & Hanna, H. L. (2019). Growth and persistence of place-based mortality in the United States: The rural mortality penalty. *American Journal of Public Health*, 109(1), 155–162.

Costhelper Health. (n.d). Ambulance cost. https://health.costhelper.com/ambulance.html

Coughlin, S. S., Clary, C., Johnson, J. A., Berman, A., Heboyan, V., Benevides, T., Moore, J., & George, V. (2019). Continuing challenges in rural health in the United States. *Journal of Environment and Health Sciences*, 5(2), 90.

Cross-Call, J. (2020). Medicaid expansion has helped narrow racial disparities in health coverage and access to care. *Center on Budget and Policy Priorities*. https://www.cbpp.org/research/health/ medicaid-expansion-has-helped-narrow-racial-disparities-in-health-coverage-and

Cushing, R. (2021, April 27). Regional population loss 'Metastasizes' in the last decade. The Daily Yonder. https://dailyyonder.com/regional-population-loss-metastasizes-in-the-last-decade/2021/ 04/27/

DeLaroche, A. M., Mowbray, F. I., Bohsaghcheghazel, M., Zalewski, K., & Obudzinski, K. (2021). Early versus delayed administration of intravenous magnesium sulfate for pediatric asthma. *The American Journal of Emergency Medicine*, 50, 36–40.

Denney, J. T., Wadsworth, T., Rogers, R. G., & Pampel, F. C. (2015). Suicide in the city: Do characteristics of place really influence risk? *Social Science Quarterly*, 96(2), 313–329.

Di, Q., Wang, Y., Zanobetti, A., Wang, Y., Koutrakis, P., Choirat, C., Dominici, F., & Schwartz, J. D. (2017). Air pollution and mortality in the medicare population. *New England Journal of Medicine*, 376(26), 2513–2522. https://doi.org/10.1056/NEJMoa1702747

Ehrenthal, D. B., Kuo, H. H. D., & Kirby, R. S. (2020). Infant mortality in rural and nonrural counties in the United States. *Pediatrics*, 146(5), e20200464. https://doi.org/10.1542/peds.2020-0464

Ely, D. M., Driscoll, A., & Matthews, T. J. (2017). Infant mortality rates in rural and urban areas in the United States, 2014. *NCHS Data Brief*, 285, 8.

Evans, B. E., Huizink, A. C., Greaves-Lord, K., Tulen, J. H. M., Roelofs, K., & van der Ende, J. (2020). Urbanicity, biological stress system functioning and mental health in adolescents. *PLoS ONE*, 15(3). https://doi.org/10.1371/journal.pone.0228659

Foutz, J., Artiga, S., & Garfield, R. (2017). The role of Medicaid in rural America. Washington, DC: Kaiser Family Foundation. https://www.kff.org/medicaid/issue-brief/ the-role-of-medicaid-in-rural-america/

Garcia, M. C., Faul, M., Massetti, G., Thomas, C. C., Hong, Y., Bauer, U. E., & Iademarco, M. F. (2017). Reducing potentially excess deaths from the five leading causes of death in the rural United States. *MMWR Surveillance Summaries*, 66(2), 1.

Germain, C., & Knight, C. (2021). Chapter 1: Social work practice and its historical traditions. In *The life model of social work practice* (pp. 1–53). Columbia University Press.

Global Health University. (n.d). Urban health online course. https://www.uniteforsight.org/ global-health-university/urban-health-certificate

Gong, G., Phillips, S. G., Hudson, C., Curti, D., & Philips, B. U. (2019). Higher US rural mortality rates linked to socioeconomic status, physician shortages, and lack of health insurance. *Health Affairs*, 38(12), 2003–2010.

Guest A. M. (2012) World urbanization: Destiny and reconceptualization. In L. Kulcsár, & K. Curtis (Eds.), *International Handbook of Rural Demography. International Handbooks of Population*, vol. 3. Springer. https://doi.org/10.1007/978-94-007-1842-5_5

Harrington, R. A., Califf, R. M., Balamurugan, A., Brown, N., Benjamin, R. M., Braund, W. E., Hipp, J., Konig, M., Sanchez, E., & Joynt Maddox, K. E. (2020). Call to action: Rural health: A presidential advisory from the American Heart Association and American Stroke Association. *Circulation, 141*(10), e615–e644.

Hartley, D. A. (2004). Rural health disparities, population health, and rural culture. *American Journal of Public Health, 94,* 1675–1678.

Harvard T.H. Chen School of Public Health. (2019). Life in rural America: Part II. National public radio. Robert Wood Johnson Foundation. https://www.rwjf.org/content/dam/farm/reports/surveys_and_polls/2019/rwjf454285

Health Resources and Services Administration. (2021). Defining rural population. https://www.hrsa.gov/rural-health/about-us/definition/index.html

Henning-Smith, C. E., Hernandez, A. M., Hardeman, R. R., Ramirez, M. R., & Kozhimannil, K. B. (2019). Rural counties with majority Black or Indigenous populations suffer the highest rates of premature death in the US. *Health Affairs, 38*(12), 2019–2026.

Hess, C., Colburn, G., Crowder, K., & Allen, R. (2020). Racial disparity in exposure to housing cost burden in the United States: 1980–2017. *Housing Studies, 0*(0), 1–21. https://doi.org/10.1080/02673037.2020.1807473

James, C. V., Moonesinghe, R., Wilson-Frederick, S. M., Hall, J. E., Penman-Aguilar, A., & Bouye, K. (2017). Racial/ethnic health disparities among rural adults—United States, 2012–2015. *MMWR Surveillance Summaries, 66*(23), 1.

James, L. (2017). Books: The health gap: The challenge of an unequal world: Unjust sense. *The British Journal of General Practice, 67*(662), 415.

James, W., & Cossman, J. S. (2017). Long-term trends in Black and White mortality in the rural United States: Evidence of a race-specific rural mortality penalty. *The Journal of Rural Health, 33*(1), 21–31.

Johns Hopkins Medicine. (n.d.). How can the affordable care act help kids? https://www.hopkinsallchildrens.org/Patients-Families/Health-Library/HealthDocNew/How-Can-The-Affordable-Care-Act-Help-Kids

Johnson, K. M., & Lichter, D. T. (2019). Rural depopulation: Growth and decline processes over the past century. *Rural Sociology, 84*(1), 3–27.

Kaiser Family Foundation. (2021). Status of state medicaid expansion decisions: Interactive map. https://www.kff.org/medicaid/issue-brief/status-of-state-medicaid-expansion-decisions-interactive-map/

Karger, H., & Stoesz, D. (2018). American social welfare policy: A pluralist approach. Pearson.

Kozhimannil, K., Interrante, J., Henning-Smith, C., & Admon, L. (2019). Rural-urban differences in severe maternal morbidity and mortality in the US, 2007–15 | Health Affairs. https://www.healthaffairs.org/doi/10.1377/hlthaff.2019.00805

Kozhimannil, K. B., Interrante, J. D., Tofte, A. N., & Admon, L. K. (2020). Severe maternal morbidity and mortality among indigenous women in the United States. *Obstetrics & Gynecology, 135*(2), 294–300. https://doi.org/10.1097/AOG.0000000000003647

Kuddus, M. A., Tynan, E., & McBryde, E. (2020). Urbanization: A problem for the rich and the poor? *Public Health Reviews, 41*(1), 1–4.

Leviton, L. C., Snell, E., & McGinnis, M. (2000). Urban issues in health promotion strategies. *American Journal of Public Health, 90*(6), 863–866. https://doi.org/10.2105/ajph.90.6.863

Li, J., Auchincloss, A. H., Rodriguez, D. A., Moore, K. A., Roux, A. V. D., & Sánchez, B. N. (2020). Determinants of residential preferences related to built and social environments and concordance between neighborhood characteristics and preferences. *Journal of Urban Health, 97*(1), 62–77.

Lichter, D. T., & Ziliak, J. P. (2017). The rural-urban interface: New patterns of spatial interdependence and inequality in America. *The ANNALS of the American Academy of Political and Social Science, 672*(1), 6–25.

Lippert, J. F., Buscemi, J., Saiyed, N., Silva, A., & Benjamins, M. R. (2022). Influenza and pneumonia mortality across the 30 biggest U.S. cities: Assessment of overall trends and racial inequities. *Journal of Racial and Ethnic Health Disparities, 9*(4), 1152–1160. https://doi.org/10.1007/s40615-021-01056-x

Long, A. S., Hanlon, A. L., & Pellegrin, K. L. (2018). Socioeconomic variables explain rural disparities in US mortality rates: Implications for rural health research and policy. *SSM-Population Health, 6,* 72–74.

Ludwig, J., Duncan, G. J., Gennetian, L. A., Katz, L. F., Kessler, R. C., Kling, J. R., & Sanbonmatsu, L. (2012). Neighborhood effects on the long-term well-being of low-income adults. *Science, 337*(6101), 1505–1510. https://doi.org/10.1126/science.1224648

Ma, J., Yabroff, K. R., Siegel, R. L., Cance, W. G., Koh, H. K., & Jemal, A. (2022). Progress in reducing disparities in premature mortality in the USA: A descriptive study. *Journal of General Internal Medicine, 37,* 2923–2930. https://doi.org/10.1007/s11606-021-07268-5

MacKinney, A. C. Mueller, K. J., Coburn, A. F., Knudson, A., Lundblad, J. P., & McBride, T. D. (2021). Characteristics and challenges for rural ambulance agencies—a brief review and policy consideration. https://rupri.org/wp-content/uploads/Characteristics-and-Challenges-of-Rural-Ambulance-Agencies-January-2021.pdf

Medicaid and CHIP Payment and Access Commission (MACPAC). (2021). Medicaid and rural health. https://www.macpac.gov/wp-content/uploads/2021/04/Medicaid-and-Rural-Health.pdf

Meehan, K., Jurjevich, J. R., Chun, N. M. J. W., & Sherrill, J. (2020). Geographies of insecure water access and the housing-water nexus in US cities. *Proceedings of the National Academy of Sciences of the United States of America*, 117(46), 28700–28707. https://doi.org/10.1073/pnas.2007361117

Meit, M., Knudson, A., Gilbert, T., Yu, A. T.-C., Tanenbaum, E., Ormson, E., & Popat, S. (2014). *The 2014 update of the rural-urban chartbook*. Rural Health Reform Policy Research Center.

Mohatt, N. V., Kreisel, C. J., Hoffberg, A. S., & Beehler, S. J. (2021). A systematic review of factors impacting suicide risk among rural adults in the United States. *The Journal of Rural Health*, 37(3), 565–575.

Monteith, L. L., Holliday, R., Brown, T. L., Brenner, L. A., & Mohatt, N. V. (2020a). Preventing suicide in rural communities during the COVID-19 pandemic. *The Journal of Rural Health*. https://doi.org/10.1111/jrh.12448

Monteith, L. L., Smith, N. B., Holliday, R., Dorsey Holliman, B. A., LoFaro, C. T., & Mohatt, N. V. (2020b). "We're afraid to say suicide": Stigma as a barrier to implementing a community-based suicide prevention program for rural veterans. *Journal of Nervous and Mental Disease*, 208(5), 371–376. https://doi.org/10.1097/nmd.0000000000001139

Moses, J. (n.d.). Part IV: The Role of Geography (Demographic Data Project, p. 5). Homelessness Research Institute.

Mueller, J. T., McConnell, K., Burow, P. B., Pofahl, K., Merdjanoff, A. A., & Farrell, J. (2021). Impacts of the COVID-19 pandemic on rural America. *Proceedings of the National Academy of Sciences*, 118(1).

Murdock, S. H., Cline, M., & Zey, M. (2012). Challenges in the analysis of rural populations in the United States. In *International handbook of rural demography* (pp. 7–15). Springer.

National Academy of Medicine. (2021). Culture of health: Community-driven health equity action plan. https://nam.edu/programs/culture-of-health/community-driven-health-equity-action-plans/

Nickel, S., & von dem Knesebeck, O. (2020). Effectiveness of community-based health promotion interventions in urban areas: A systematic review. *Journal of Community Health*, 45(2), 419–434. https://doi.org/10.1007/s10900-019-00733-7

Parekh, A. K., & Goodman, R. A. (2013). The HHS strategic framework on multiple chronic conditions: Genesis and focus on research. *Journal of Comorbidity*, 3(2), 22–29. https://doi.org/10.15256/joc.2013.3.20

Park, B. Z. (2017). State public health actions to prevent and control diabetes, heart disease, obesity and associated risk factors, and promote school health. *Preventing Chronic Disease*, 14. https://doi.org/10.5888/pcd14.160437

Parker, A., Horowitz, J., Brown, A., Fry, R., Cohn, D., Igielnik, R. (2018). *What unites and divides urban, suburban, and urban communities*. https://www.pewresearch.org/social-trends/2018/05/22/demographic-and-economic-trends-in-urban-suburban-and-rural-communities/

Pate, C. A., Qin, X., Bailey, C. M., & Zahran, H. S. (2020). Cost barriers to asthma care by health insurance type among children with asthma. *Journal of Asthma*, 57(10), 1103–1109. https://doi.org/10.1080/02770903.2019.1640730

Peters, D. J. (2020). Community susceptibility and resiliency to COVID-19 across the rural-urban continuum in the United States. *The Journal of Rural Health*, 36(3), 446–456.

Plough, A. L. (2015). Building a culture of health: A critical role for public health services and systems research.

Probst, J. C., Zahnd, W. E., Hung, P., Eberth, J. M., Crouch, E. L., & Merrell, M. A. (2020). Rural-urban mortality disparities: Variations across causes of death and race/ethnicity, 2013–2017. *American Journal of Public Health*, 110(9), 1325–1327. https://doi.org/10.2105/AJPH.2020.305703

Runde, D. (2015). Urbanization, opportunity, and development. Urbanization, Opportunity, and Development. Center for Strategic & International Studies.

Salgado, M., Madureira, J., Mendes, A. S., Torres, A., Teixeira, J. P., & Oliveira, M. D. (2020). Environmental determinants of population health in urban settings. A systematic review. *BMC Public Health*, 20, 1–11.

Shah Nilay, S., Carnethon, M., Lloyd-Jones, D. M., & Khan Sadiya, S. (2020). Widening rural-urban cardiometabolic mortality gap in the United States, 1999 to 2017. *Journal of the American College of Cardiology*, 75(25), 3187–3188. https://doi.org/10.1016/j.jacc.2020.03.080

Simes, D., Shochet, I., Murray, K., & Sands, I. G. (2021). A systematic review of qualitative research of the experiences of young people and their caregivers affected by suicidality and self-harm: Implications for family-based treatment. *Adolescent Research Review*, 1–23.

Speers, M. A., & Lancaster, B. (1998). Disease prevention and health promotion in urban areas: CDC's perspective. *Health Education & Behavior: the Official Publication of the Society for Public Health Education, 25*(2), 226–233. https://doi.org/10.1177/109019819802500209

Stankov, I., Howard, N. J., Daniel, M., & Cargo, M. (2017). Policy, research and residents' perspectives on built environments implicated in heart disease: A concept mapping approach. *International Journal of Environmental Research and Public Health, 14*(2), 170.

U.S. Conference of Mayors. (2020). The United States conference of Mayors: Supporting, protecting, and advocating for America's cities and their residents. https://www.usmayors.org/2020-vision/

U.S. Conference of Mayors. (2019). Mayor's vision for America: A 2020 call to action.

U.S. Census Bureau. (2019). Mostly urban counties: American community survey, 2011–2015 five-year estimates. https://www.census.gov/programs-surveys/acs/technical-documentation/table-and-geography-changes/2015/5-year.html

U.S. Department of Health and Human Services. (n.d.). Healthy People 2030. https://health.gov/healthypeople

USDA Economic Research Service. (2019). What is rural? https://www.ers.usda.gov/topics/rural-economy-population/rural-classifications/what-is-rural.aspx

van Zon, S., Reijneveld, S. A., Mendes de Leon, C. F., & Bültmann, U. (2017). The impact of low education and poor health on unemployment varies by work life stage. *International Journal of Public Health, 62*(9), 997–1006. https://doi.org/10.1007/s00038-017-0972-7

Vilar-Compte, M., Burrola-Méndez, S., Lozano-Marrufo, A. et al. (2021). Urban poverty and nutrition challenges associated with accessibility to a healthy diet: A global systematic literature review. *International Journal for Equity in Health, 20*(40). https://doi.org/10.1186/s12939-020-01330-0

Vohra, S., Pointer, C., Fogleman, A., Albers, T., Patel, A., & Weeks, E. (2020). Designing policy solutions to build a healthier rural America. *Journal of Law, Medicine & Ethics, 48*(3), 491–505.

Wang, Y. C., Pamplin, J., Long, M. W., Ward, Z. J., Gortmaker, S. L., & Andreyeva, T. (2015). Severe obesity in adults cost state medicaid programs nearly $8 billion in 2013. *Health Affairs, 34*(11), 1923–1931.

Weiss-Laxer, N. S., Crandall, A., Hughes, M. E., & Riley, A. W. (2020). Families as a cornerstone in 21st century public health: Recommendations for research, education, policy, and practice. *Frontiers in Public Health, 8.*

World Health Organization. (2021, April 13, 2021). Noncommunicable diseases. https://www.who.int/news-room/fact-sheets/detail/noncommunicable-diseases

Zhao, G. X., Okoro, C. A., Hsia, J., Garvin, W. S., & Town, M. (2019). Prevalence of disability and disability types by urban-rural county classification—US, 2016. *American Journal of Preventive Medicine, 57*(6), 749–756.

CHAPTER 18

Historical Trauma and Indigenous Health

Gary L. Lawrence and Faye A. Gary

LEARNING OBJECTIVES

- Define the term *historical trauma* and discuss the influence it has had on the health and well-being of American Indians (AI) and Alaskan Natives (AN).

- Discuss the meaning of cultural identity and connectedness.

- Describe the concept of soul wound and how it relates to intergenerational trauma.

- Discuss the concept of cultural buffers and how it relates to AI and AN health and well-being.

- Define the roles that the Indian Health Service plays and the responsibilities that it has in the provision of healthcare services to AI and AN.

- Explain the key elements of the Indigenist Stress-Coping Model and how they contribute to the promotion and maintenance of desired health outcomes.

THE HONORABLE CHIEF GARY BATTON OF THE CHOCTAW NATION SPEAKS

Healthcare is a necessity for all people, and it should be provided within the context of a community where people will be treated with respect and dignity. The Choctaw Nation continues to make bold steps in offering care for its people. We have survived hardships and atrocities across the ages and have overcome them. The historical traumas that have been imposed on us across the centuries are addressed through our health, education, and social service systems and through other community-based programs such as organized biking, jogging, and other physical fitness programs. Attention to nutrition and diet habits is also essential, as are academic, social, and emotional learning for the youth of our communities. We continue to believe in spiritual connections, the holistic approach to wellness, and the harmonious relationship between traditional and Western medicine. The Choctaw Nation is a self-respecting group of Native Americans, who live, work, play, and pray in peace among themselves, with other Native communities, and with others across this vast land. We are proud of our heritage, our capacity to endure, and our vision of a dynamic future, and we have an abiding hope for people and for the prosperity of all humankind.

As Chief of this great sovereign nation, I hope you will learn more about Native Americans and other Native communities, all of whom have faced universal yet particular tragedies but have overcome and now thrive. We are extraordinarily proud of our heritage, our language, our indigenous cultures, and other traditional customs embedded in our ways of life. We all are connected to the earth and each other. Peace and good health. Chahta Sia Hoke (I am Choctaw)!

—*Gary Batton, Chief*
Choctaw Nation of Oklahoma
August 11, 2021

INTRODUCTION

Divided into two sections, this chapter acknowledges the universal challenges of all American Indians (AI) and Alaskan Natives (AN) and the attributes and efforts used by selected tribes to overcome adversity. The first section provides information about AI and AN groups and highlights health challenges that confront both groups. The second section focuses on the five "civilized tribes," which should help to point out particulars about some of the tribes.

The purpose of this chapter is to introduce the relationship between historical trauma and indigenous health including the perspective of indigenous peoples and historical traumas as experienced by AI and AN. It also addresses the history of the Indian Health Service (IHS), the prevalence of disease, cultural coping mechanisms, and the cultural buffers used as protective measures to promote health and prevent disease that threatens the mind, spirit, and body. Emphasis is placed on the intersectionality between historical traumas and the physical and psychological health of the AI and AN people.

Throughout the nation, about 200 AI groups are home to tens of thousands of people but are not federally recognized and therefore do not qualify for support, including healthcare that is available to other tribes that are federally recognized. There are seven required criteria that must be favorably considered before a tribe can have federal status in the United States. For example, several federal criteria require that political influence or authority rest within the tribal leadership and that the leaders have sufficient influence over their groups. The tribal group must be an autonomous body, and records must show that the tribe has existed since 1900. The tribal leadership is responsible for producing legitimate copies of its governing documents, along with membership criteria and names on rolls.

Preparing all necessary documents for review by the U.S. Department of Interior Committee, which is composed of anthropologists, historians, genealogists, and administrators, can be a daunting task. Numerous tribes have not yet satisfied the federal government's approval threshold. See "Additional Resources" for more details.

Across the nation, about 5.2 million persons self-identify as AI and AN as one group or in combination with other groups and ethnicities. About 45,000 AI and AN report being age 65 years or older, and they qualify for Medicare. They account for about 1% of the nation's total population. About 22% live on reservations or trusted land, and more than 60% reside in urban communities. Many AI and AN people are affiliated with federally recognized tribes, others belong to state-recognized tribes, and still others are not enrolled in any tribe. Individuals who are enrolled in federally recognized tribes have access to more benefits and goods and services than their counterparts (Kaiser Family Foundation [KFF], 2019; Schmidt, 2011; Smedley, 2007). Currently, 2,907,272 individuals identify as AI or AN, belonging to one or more of the 574 federally recognized tribes in the United States. Some individuals identify with more than one tribe. Approximately one half of these individuals live in specific urban areas where access to health and social services is limited (U.S. Departement of Health and Human Services [DHHS], 2022). Throughout the chapter, the terms *AI* and *AN* are used to describe this group collectively and do not refer to a specific group unless otherwise identified. Although not a homogeneous group, AI and AN are grouped together statistically regardless of tribal affiliation and other distinct attributes (Srinivasan, 2018). Although the grouping together of all tribes is a common practice in research, scholarly writings, and policy, it does not provide a robust approach for discussing the universal and particular characteristics of the collective groups. Hence, many unique practices and cultures of each group are somewhat compromised, a caveat that remains a concern.

The AN tribes are a smaller population than the AI tribes, which, again, comprise 574 federally recognized communities. AI tribes are located throughout the United States, with concentrations in specific areas of the nation. It is important to remember that there are unique identities within each tribe, a presence in all geographical regions, singular challenges, and a variety of health disparities. With the annexation of Alaska as a state on January 3, 1959, Alaska Natives became citizens of the United States. They experienced some of the same adverse events that are detailed about AN populations, which occurred centuries earlier when Europeans entered the United States. (Precious few lessons have been learned from the traumatic past.) The AN population is estimated at 138,000 with more than 20 language groups and five major tribes: the Inuit, Tlingit, Haida, Alaskan Athabaskan, and Aleut. AN people make up approximately 15% of the total Alaskan population. (See https://minority-rights.org/minorities/alaska-natives.)

While this chapter delineates numerous characteristics and historical truths of most AI tribes, their healthcare, and their health outcomes, it highlights the five so-called "civilized tribes" (the Choctaw, Cherokee, Chickasaw, Creek, and Seminole Indians of Oklahoma)—a degrading designation coined by the U.S. government. These five tribes were deemed "civilized" because they were initially more amenable to negotiations with the federal government and had begun to develop economic and social activities with White people, including the practice of Christianity and the enslavement of Black people (Doran, 1978).

HISTORICAL PERSPECTIVE

Indigenous historians agree that the first contact with European invaders initiated the decline in AI health and well-being. AI people helped the Europeans to survive the bitter cold, assisted with securing and preparing food, and befriended the new arrivals. Despite the acceptance and support offered by AI people, the wave of Europeans brought with them religion, which eventually resulted in AI's loss of culturally protective beliefs and practices; unfamiliar foods; alcohol; and disease, to which Native Americans had no resistance. Their hospitality was initially appreciated but soon discounted by the Europeans, and the colonization of native peoples began to occur when the Europeans began to seize the land and use it as their own without regard for the indigenous tribes (Bird, 2003; Brave Heart & Debruyn, 1998; Duran, 2006; Jacobs, 2004; Lomawaima, 1994; Mitchell & Kaufman, 2002; Skewes & Blume, 2019; Weaver & Yellow Horse-Brave Heart, 1999; Whitbeck et al., 2004).

The colonization of North America continued in various forms. The U.S. government and numerous private religious institutions bear a heavy responsibility for the systematic destruction of the AN and AI culture and identity. Government actions such as poisoning AI people's blankets, seizing their land, and other atrocities linked with the demise of the AI were devastating, with their own deleterious impacts. Across the tribes, each of these actions was devastating, forcing tribes to relocate on reservations and prohibiting them from hunting and gathering off the reservation by making it illegal to leave the reservation or own weapons. Equally dangerous were providing unhealthy and nontraditional food choices and "legally" taking children from their families and placing them in boarding schools that were established and operated throughout the United States (Skewes & Blume, 2019).

Boarding school policies were especially cruel and devastating to children, families, and community sustainability. The devastation intensified when Andrew Jackson became president of the United States in 1829, and the forcible removal of AI from their ancestral lands was initiated and culminated in the Indian Removal Act of 1830. Under the guise of this treaty, the uprooting of the Choctaw, Chickasaw, Cherokee, Creek, and Seminole tribes from their homes to land west of the Mississippi was carried out. The land is now known as the state of Oklahoma. The Choctaws were the first to take this forced march, which was poorly planned and occurred in deplorable weather conditions, and it resulted in the loss of nearly 2,500 lives along the way (Debo, 1940). This ill-conceived and life-threatening journey became known as the "Trail of Tears and Death" (Choctaw Nation, 2011). All five "civilized tribes" eventually endured their own trails of tears, being forcibly displaced from their native lands and relocated. These relocations led to massive loss of human life (see www.history.com/topics/native-american-history/trail-of-tears; www.nationalgeographic.org/thisday/may28/indian-removal-act). To help reinforce the oppression imposed on Native Americans from the earliest appearance of Western civilization and then exacerbated by the U.S. government, treaties were signed between the government and AI. The treaties were considered by the tribes to be promises by the federal government, which used phrases such as "as long as the waters run" in the treaties, an expression that the tribes interpreted to mean *forever*. However, the government repeatedly broke these promises, which the tribes considered betrayals and which led to a mistrust of the government (Debo, 1934; Skewes & Blume, 2019). For example, the Indian Territory that is now Oklahoma and parts of Arkansas was originally ceded to the tribes in exchange for their native lands. But Europeans, eager to develop the lands, sought to acquire them, and so they schemed to accomplish this goal by colluding with corrupt politicians. Knowing little of land ownership, the AI people held their properties in common to be shared by all and worked together. They viewed themselves as stewards of the land and sought to protect it. Thoughts of owning a piece of land individually were not a consideration for them (Debo, 1940). Chief Seattle's speech exemplified the AI perspective of their relationship with the land (see https://passionistfamily.org.nz/resources/downloads/Chief%20Seattle.pdf).

The Dawes Severalty Act of 1887 was one of the schemes designed to separate the AI and AN from their lands. The first step of this act was to create a roll of all the members of each tribe to determine land allotments. These allotments consisted of 180 acres for heads of families, 80 acres for unmarried adults, and 40 acres for children (Debo, 1940). The rest of the lands were bought back from the tribes by the government and opened to homesteading by settlers. The allocation was done by a series of "land runs," in which individuals started at a specific time and location and raced others to stake their claim on a section of the property. Between 1886 and 1906 there were five land runs in Oklahoma, followed by a land lottery and land auction (see https://nationalcowboymuseum.org/explore/rushes-statehood-oklahoma-land-runs). In this way, the AI land was seized by White Americans and used at their discretion. Other manipulative and rapacious policies and practices were implemented as well.

Blood Quantum and Its Meaning

Many "full-blooded" Native Americans, distrustful of the government because they had lived through all the broken promises and forcible removals, refused to sign the Dawes Rolls and thereby forfeited their right to land. These decisions had far-reaching consequences.

The Dawes Roll, also known as the "Final Roll," was used to determine the degree to which a person was deemed to be a member of a Native American tribe. It was an essential component of the documentation that provided "proof" of being Native American. Certificates of Degree of Indian Blood (CDIB) were issued to individuals and families and were important government documents that served as a gateway to goods and services for the population (see www.archives.gov/research/native-americans/dawes/tutorial/final-rolls.html).

The five "civilized tribes" continue to use the Dawes Roll to document the degree of one's Indian blood and to establish whether one qualifies for the Certificate of Membership in one of the tribes. Concerns about the accuracy and reliability of the Dawes Roll remain, and therefore some individuals and groups refuse to participate. (See www.archives.gov/research/native-americans/dawes/tutorial/intro.html for a detailed discussion about the Dawes Roll and its past and current use.)

The Dawes Roll requires demographic data such as name, age, birth date, degree of Indian blood (which was not scientifically established), and a roll and a census card number for everyone. The complexities associated with ascertaining who is an authentic Native American continue to be elusive. One approach, however, has been to use the blood quantum documentation, which is considered by many to be a metaphorical construction—or a fanciful creation—for tracking and documenting individual, family, and group ancestry (Schmidt, 2011), although it has been used for almost a century. For example, Dawes Roll membership was intent on documenting a person's appearance and level of cultural involvement. The lack of a systematic method and little scientific evidence is associated with the generation and maintenance of the Dawes Roll and the dissemination of the CDIB. These two documents are used to demonstrate one's "Indianness," but neither requires authentic documentation.

Over the years, many tribes have become more autonomous, and their nation status is more likely to be recognized by the federal government. One outcome of this recognition is that each tribe can control its own criteria for enrollment into its particular tribal group. Some tribes have elected to create variability in their blood quantum. Other tribes, such as the Navajo, insist on a minimum of 25% or a one fourth degree of "Indian blood"; some others have no minimum requirement to be eligible for membership and the related benefits. Still other tribes demand documentation of a blood relationship with a relative who was an original enrollee on the Dawes Roll (National Public Radio [NPR], 2018; Schmidt, 2011).

Given this backdrop, a common school of thought among some government officials has concluded that the mechanisms that were developed were designed with the hope that over time the AI people would literally breed themselves out of existence. Because of the variability in requirements and the disappearance of a unique "physical appearance," there is a possibility that communities might lose their identities and remaining close relationships and thus forfeit the specific federal and state benefits allocated to those who have acquired or maintained the identity of being AI. Throughout the history of America, representative physical characteristics have been important. Consider, for example, the history of the "one-drop rule" that was applied to Black people. If a person had one drop of "Black blood" in their veins, they were classified as Black, without regard for other physical and mental characteristics or any other criteria. The one-drop rule was a hard-and-fast way to enforce harsh rules of discrimination and oppression. The principle of determining racial identity through specified physical characteristics helped to reinforce the blood quantum concept among AI. Some were shocked and others were energized by the practice. The action might have also helped to ensure their survival, reinforce their identity, and maintain their linkage to the federal treaties during that period of history (Byrd & Clayton, 2000; NPR, 2018; Schmidt, 2011).

Another dynamic was operative as well. The Dawes Roll with its associated CBID was used to separate indigenous people from their lands. The question of how indigenous people were maneuvered (or manipulated) into participating in the loss of their land through this process emerges. One response is to examine the requirement of numerous documents that had to be approved by the federal government. Without government validation, no land ownership or other privileges would be forthcoming. At the same time, other dynamics were also occurring, including marriages among AI and White people and the adoption of AI children. With the closure of AI boarding schools in the 1950s and 1960s, the federal government enacted the Indian Adoption Project, with the intent of establishing a mechanism through which White people could adopt AI children. The law provided a pathway for the adoption of "one little, two little, three little Indians" by White families who had "taken the Indian waifs as their own" (see www.vox.com/identities/2020/2/20/21131387/indian-child-welfare-act-court-case-foster-care). Both realities, intermarriage and adoption, helped to create additional opportunities that facilitated the loss of ownership of indigenous land. As a protective measure, the tribal leaders would examine the European man's (White man's) moral character and would pronounce approval of the person before the marriage would be allowed and the couple could become members of the group. Specific traits for "approval" were scant. Regarding AI children who were adopted by White people, history suggests that most of them were enrolled in AI boarding schools and might not have received their land allotments (Debo, 1940). Currently, more than half of AI who decide to marry choose not to marry other Native people. Linkage and ownership through blood levels and other criteria conduce to bring about complex issues regarding land usage, tribal identities, and the preservation of cultural practices and values. Marriages to non-Indian people raise questions about who can qualify over time as being AI. The Native American identity will begin to expire at each non-Indian marriage in the next generation, and by the third generation, more identity issues are likely to arise. Issues abound about AI benefits and protections through treaties and other rights including free healthcare, educational assistance, and land ownership. These concerns come about because of questions about authentic identity and methods of documentation that are satisfactory to the tribes and the federal government.

If, for example, an AI woman marries a White man and has children with him, the offspring will be one-half AI, assuming the woman is "full-blooded." If the children marry White people, the next generation's offspring will be one-fourth AI, which is the minimum blood quantum required for tribal membership in most populations.

In the next generation, if the children marry a non-Indian, their grandchildren will not be, by definition, AI; this uncertain and ongoing refashioning of identity is a problematic tendency that is increasing (Schmidt, 2011). Recall that the concept of race was developed as a de facto method for differentiating human groups, and the data could be used in federal, state, and local jurisdictions to determine the allocation of goods and services. The concept negates the unique sociopolitical and cultural histories, geographical characteristics, and differences among the tribes. These race-driven approaches have been used in medicine, nursing, and all health systems over the centuries (Gampa et al., 2020). (See Chapter 15 for an in-depth discussion of race; see also www.npr.org/2011/03/31/134421470/native-american-intermarriage-puts-benefits-at-risk.)

Other factors, such as acculturation and assimilation through the development and use of boarding schools across the United States and Canada, are briefly highlighted in the following. Most of the schools are closed, but their lingering impact is evident in the minds and hearts of AI people.

Acculturation, Assimilation, and Boarding Schools

Acculturation is described as a cultural change occurring when two or more cultures are in constant contact and both cultures change gradually because of that interaction. Acculturation involves a cultural exchange between groups and can occur with or without the acceptance of the broader society. Acculturation can take place voluntarily or by force, as was the case with AI and AN, which was done to establish and maintain control of a people. It can lead to three possible outcomes: acceptance, adaption, or reaction. Acculturation is a group-level activity and affects systems or communities, not individuals. *Assimilation* can involve forced acculturation, in which one culture changes significantly more than the other culture and could end up losing most of its distinctive heritage and identity. Over time, the less dominant cultural group is more likely to resemble the dominant culture. For assimilation to occur, the dominant culture must be willing to accept the assimilating group. The process depends on the nature of the "reward" as related to being able to function in the dominant culture. Assimilation can refer to both group and individual processes (Garcia & Ahler, 1992).

The establishment of Indian boarding schools exemplified forced acculturation. The phrase "Kill the Indian and save the man" was attributed to Richard Pratt, the founder of the Carlisle Indian School in Pennsylvania (Brunhouse, 1939; Skewes & Blume, 2019; White, 2018) (see www.nps.gov/articles/the-carlisle-indian-industrial-school-assimilation-with-education-after-the-in-dian-wars-teaching-with-historic-places.htm).

Agents of the government forcibly removed children from their homes, cut their hair, and dressed them in European clothing, which sometimes consisted of discarded military uniforms. The children were forbidden under penalty of harsh punishment to speak their native languages (Skewes & Blume, 2019; Walls & Whitbeck, 2012). They were usually removed from their homes by age 4 to 5 years for a minimum of 8 years spent away from their families and Native communities. Often by violent methods, these schools compelled the children to absorb and integrate into European culture (Deloria, 1988; Herring, 1989; Skewes & Blume, 2019; Sue & Sue, 1990). Being separated from their families and forbidden to practice their cultural beliefs or to speak their Native language, except at designated times, resulted in a devastating loss of cultural identity and healing practices—two essential inherited means that are historically responsible for AI and AN health, which consists of physical, mental, and spiritual realms, or body, mind, and spirit. These factors, considered buffers that could offset harmful incidents and effects, were mostly eradicated with the boarding school experience and other sources of cultural loss (Lomawaima, 1994; Mitchell & Kaufman, 2002; Skewes & Blume, 2019; Weaver & Yellow Horse Brave Heart, 1999; Whitbeck et al., 2004).

Cultural identity has been identified as an essential protective quality that fosters a sense of belonging and connectedness but is lost through the process of assimilation. It is developed and passed on to others through the sharing of traditions, customs, heritage, and language (Bassett et al., 2012; Chen, 2014). The damage—physical, mental, and spiritual—caused by the extirpation of cultural identity is illustrated in a story about the Chilocco Indian School by K. Tsianina Lomawaima. The author describes the experiences of Native children in the government school by encouraging them to speak for themselves in the form of recollections and storytelling. What the students recall is a sense of loneliness, forced labor, and the feeling of being an outsider when returning home. Their lives were regimented and filled with military-type discipline. Their days were devoted to prayer and studies, which included agriculture for the boys and cooking and sewing for the girls. The school adhered to the Pratt theory of civilization, which advocated "immersing the Indians in our civilization and when we get them under, holding them there until they are thoroughly soaked" (see https://upstanderproject.org/firstlight/pratt). From a traditional American perspective herein lies implicit imagery of violence. The immersion in water suggests baptism and purification, and yet the vicious metaphor of holding the AI people under the water exposes the ruthless and destructive intentions concealed beneath the civilizing efforts. The implicit symbolism of baptism conveys the message that without the cleansing power of Western civilization, the Indians are morally stained and spiritually cursed.

Following the traditional line of thinking at the time, this approach decreed that the only way to "civilize" the AI people was to kill the "red man" inside. Realized in the repressive and callous education administered in the boarding schools, this philosophy led to the inability of the children to function independently. Much as when a prisoner is let out of jail, the children were left estranged both from their indigenous community and culture and from the Western community—a culture that they were expected to appreciate and join as its members. During the 1960s and 1970s, social conditions provoked changes in policy that resulted in the closing of many of these schools, and by the end of the 20th century, only a handful remained. Currently, four such schools are still in operation, scattered about the United States and controlled by the Bureau of Indian Affairs (BIA). Fortunately, they no longer follow the horrendous educational practices and standards of the past. Even today the tragic history of the boarding schools persists in the haunting of its victims. The school's damaging effects on the mental health of the attendees can be measured by their stories and the trauma they continue to experience (Charbonneau-Dahlen et al., 2016; Gampa et al., 2020; Gregg, 2018; Lomawaima, 1994; Lomawaima & Cantley, 2018; Schmidt, 2011; Skewes & Blume, 2019; Williams, 2020). The voices of boarding school survivors can be heard at www .spokesman.com/stories/2021/jul/08/all-these-children-matter-discovery-of-indian-boar.

HISTORICAL TRAUMA

This discussion begins by introducing the Four Arrows concept, which emphasizes the connections among all living creatures and plants and the material presence of all elements that compose one Earth family. The Four Arrows concept (Jacobs, 2006) is used to describe the systematic destruction of the indigenous people of North America as coming in four distinct waves. Jacobs (2006) states that the first wave began with the arrival of European invaders, soldiers, and settlers, an arrival that brought violence and disease to the land of the indigenous people. The greed of these new occupiers led to the genocide of the Native people, the denial of any claims made by them to their ancestral lands, and the erasure of any signs that indicated that they were the original inhabitants. The second wave came in the form of government, military, and corporate attempts to control every aspect of Native life, including culture, natural resources, land, and sovereignty.

The third wave is considered by some scholars to be extremely devastating and one of the most important waves. At the hands of academics, researchers, policymakers, and thought workers, the AI and AN cultures and peoples were decimated. Widely accepted but thoroughly erroneous "scholarly" publications and presentations misrepresent the traditions and histories of the Native people and attack the philosophies and world views by which they have lived for centuries (Fleming, 2006; Jacobs, 2006; White, 2018). These misrepresentations are created through generalizations and stereotypes that suggest that Native tribes are homogeneous, are not yet "worthy," and do not fit a Eurocentric perspective. Hence, boarding schools and other mechanisms were developed to "socialize, educate, and orientate" them to a more "civilized" way of living, which was primarily based on Christianity. Europeans often described an individual by characteristics attributed to the group (Fleming, 2006; White, 2018), such as considerable variations in linguistic patterns; physical features, including hair color and texture and skin tone; and varied attitudes about accepting Christianity (Huddleston, 2015; see www.infoplease.com/encyclopedia/history/north-america/indigenous). Grouping the members of the tribes negated cultural differences such as customs, languages, and traditions, along with rights and privileges that were naturally granted their White counterparts. There are more than 574 recognized tribes and about 200 nonfederally recognized tribes; they all have distinct languages, religious practices, customs and folkways, and guidelines for daily living (Gampa et al., 2020; Gregg, 2018; Schmidt, 2011). In fact, in some cases, the distinctive ways of communicating developed by Native Americans were called on to benefit the entire country, especially in times of crisis. Native American people have been active citizens in our nation. Choctaw Code Talkers in World War I (Archambeault, 2008) and Navajo Code Talkers in World War II, for example, played crucial military roles because of their traditional languages that were unique ways of communicating and thus never broken when used as codes (see www.ushistory.org/us/1a.asp).

The fourth wave extends and reinforces the first three waves, serving to continue the climate of "anti-Indian" sentiment through misinformation and negative portrayals of Native people in films, classrooms, media, public opinion, and legislation, thus resulting in a cultural genocide (Gregg, 2018; Jacobs, 2006; White, 2018).

Again, the third wave is often considered to be one of the most detrimental of the four waves because it relates to the education of the public and the dissemination of information through social media and scientific and scholarly publications and presentations. From a different perspective, the authors believe that the wave is dangerous also because it has the potential to continue its devastating damage to the AI and AN nations by presenting Native culture and its people in a negative light, through stereotypes, and by denying opportunities for quality education and access to healthcare. Certainly, the first two waves (arrival of the Europeans and systematic massacre of Native people, and government policies and practices) were more destructive because they "struck at the heart" of the Native people, and in some instances, occasioned genocide. But through the dissemination of misinformation disguised as scholarly work, the mistrust and misunderstanding of Native culture continue (Jacobs, 2006; Schmidt, 2011; Walters et al., 2020). In this same context, the systematic and persistent defacement of Native American people is unlike any other historical ill usage that has occurred in this nation: Europeans invaded and wreaked havoc on the AI people and their lands.

Some positive actions have emerged that are designed to help address a multitude of the nation's maladies that have been systematically thrust upon AI and AN people. Self-protection laws and policies regarding research with the population are one example (Him et al., 2019). In recent times, tribal institutional review boards, such as the one operated by the Choctaw Nation of Oklahoma, require that researchers obtain approval for their study protocol prior to research. All researchers are further required to submit to the tribal chiefs for review of all results of studies conducted with Native populations for additional approval prior to publication to ensure that tribes are depicted in a respectful manner.

Moreover, the National Institutes of Health (NIH) recently published a guidebook authored by Native researchers and titled *American Indian and Alaskan Native Research in the Health Sciences Critical Considerations for Review of Research Applications* at https://dpcpsi .nih.gov/sites/default/files/Critical_Considerations_for_Reviewing_AIAN _Research_508.pdf. It is intended to provide a framework to make certain that research is conducted in an ethical and meaningful way that has value to AI and AN people while protecting this vulnerable population (Walters et al., 2020). Research-related projects are often associated with the health and well-being of children and families and the environment in Native communities. One of the frequent topics of interest is adverse childhood experiences and how they are manifested through the life course. The concept of historical trauma, a phenomenon that is cited in the literature, follows in a brief discussion.

Historical trauma is a term that refers to the cumulative and collective emotional and psychological trauma suffered by a society over time because of genocide and dispossession (Weaver & Yellow Horse Brave Heart, 1990). The historical trauma suffered by AI and AN can be linked to every realm of the current circumstances being experienced by them, including, for example, disparities related to physical and psychological health, substance use, and loss of spiritual and cultural practices. The past agonies endured by indigenous people have contributed to the troubles that continue to afflict them: physical health diseases, mental health/behavioral health disorders, poverty, unemployment, and other hardships, including lack of access to healthcare and quality education (Hartmann et al., 2019). Historical trauma has been described by Native scholars such as Eduardo Duran as a "soul wound" that, if not healed in one generation, will have to be dealt with in the next. Because it is passed on from one generation to the next, it has spurred the emergence of interest in intergenerational trauma by Native researchers (Duran, 2006; Skewes & Blume, 2019; Walters et al., 2002).

One of the key components of historical trauma concerns the concept of dispossession. Defined as a loss of culture, dispossession is viewed by tribal leaders and Native scholars as the root of the health disparities and social, physical, and mental disorders experienced by AI and AN populations today (Akee, 2020; Bird, 2003; Jones, 2006). From the time that AI people were removed from their ancestral lands and deprived of their Native culture, the impact of dispossession has been felt through physical disease, mental illness, and economic poverty. Contact with European Americans began the pestilence and destitution that are still evident across the population. Having had no previous exposure to communicable diseases, the indigenous people had little or no immunities, which resulted in highly contagious afflictions like smallpox killing entire tribes. Often such contagions were induced intentionally through tainted food and infected blankets. Along with this significant loss of life, culture was also wiped out through the death of tribal elders and spiritual leaders. AI and AN are storytellers, and the primary way that knowledge and instruction are shared or passed down is through the oral tradition of storytelling. With the death of tribal leaders, familiarity with cultural and traditional ways of life was eradicated, and this led to the destruction of the Native American society (Duffy, 1997, Jones, 2004; Schmidt, 2011). As we have seen, further destruction of Native culture was ensured by the government-established "Indian" boarding schools (Mitchell & Kaufman, 2002; Schmidt, 2011; Skewes & Blume, 2019; Weaver & Yellow Horse Brave Heart, 1999; Whitbeck et al., 2004).

The historical trauma experienced by the AI and AN is historical only in the sense that it began long ago, not that it remains in the past. The trauma did not end with military defeat and the subsequent removal of indigenous people from their native homes. These past acts of oppression and expulsion were only preludes to one of the most successful ethnic cleansing programs of all time. The ethnic cleansing of the American Indians was sanctioned by the government in the name of progress and civilization. The historic loss felt by the elders persists in a sense of hopelessness and mistrust. The sense of hopelessness stems from the loss of lands, the buffalo, indigenous languages, cultural practices, and traditional family values and customs. It also arises from and reflects the loss of community and caring for one another. The hopelessness is further engrained due to the widespread use of drugs and alcohol in Indian country and the shame that is associated with such abuse and addiction (Jacobs, 2006; Novins et al., 2016; Whitbeck et al., 2004).

Although the children and grandchildren are several generations removed from the original sources of trauma, they still experience the detrimental effects today in the form of discrimination, poverty, and health disparities, including mental illness, substance use, generational poverty, and domestic violence related to historical loss (Gampa et al., 2020; Garcia et al., 2017; Gregg, 2018; Jacobs, 2006; Schmidt, 2011; Whitbeck et al., 2004).

NARRATIVE 18.1: A NATIVE AMERICAN GIRL AT RISK FOR CULTURAL IDENTITY LOSS

An Indian agent arrives at the home of a Native couple who have a 6-year-old female Native child named Velma. According to law, Velma must attend an "Indian" boarding school, which is 25 miles from their home. Velma is forcibly removed from her home and family, flailing and crying for her parents, who are both visibly upset. She is transported to a government "Indian" boarding school. Upon her arrival, Velma is told to remove her clothing. She is "deloused" and clothed in an ill-fitting dress and hard leather lace-up shoes. Velma is then taken to have her hair cropped short and is then brought to a dormitory with many other girls of various ages and tribes. Velma is told that if she needs anything, she must ask for it in English, which is a language she doesn't speak or understand.

The mornings are spent with housekeeping duties and the afternoons with classwork and learning homemaking skills. The nights are filled with sadness, and the sounds of Velma's sadness mix with those of others in her dormitory. One night Velma flees the school and makes her way home. The next afternoon the Indian agent arrives with law enforcement, and Velma is returned to the "Indian" boarding school. This process is repeated several times until Velma finally accepts her fate. With the exception of a visit during the holidays, she doesn't see her parents or home for the next 8 years.

When Velma finally "graduates" from the boarding school, she is a stranger in her own home and community, fitting in neither with her Native family nor with the White community.

(continued)

NARRATIVE 18.1: A NATIVE AMERICAN GIRL AT RISK FOR CULTURAL IDENTITY LOSS (*CONTINUED*)

Discussion Questions

1. Using what has been described about acculturation or assimilation, identify three factors that make it difficult for Velma to "fit in at her home."
2. Describe two risk factors that acculturation and assimilation contribute to the health status of Native American people.
3. Discuss historical trauma from the perspective of providing care for AI children in foster care.

Health Disparities Related to Historical Trauma

Reducing health disparities is identified as one of four overarching goals of Healthy People 2030, together with achieving health equity and improving the health of all groups (U.S. Department of Health and Human Services [DHHS], 2011 para 4; DHHS, 2020). A significant decrease in disparities is also one of the four foundational health measures for achieving the goals, with a disparity defined as occurring "if a health outcome is seen to a greater or lesser extent between populations" (DHHS, 2011 para 4; DHHS, 2020). AI and AN populations have been plagued by many disparities, including inadequate mental health care, economic and educational disadvantage, family and community disruption, violence, suicide, and substance use. These can be attributed to the governmental policies and treaties that have affected AI and AN people and shaped the future of this population for generations. The health disparities arise largely from a lack of availability of and access to culturally appropriate care. It is estimated that only one in five AI and AN people has access to care provided by the IHS, the government agency responsible for delivering care to AI and AN people (National Indian Health Board [NIHB], 2020). The IHS is underfunded, operating on approximately one third of the funds necessary to meet the needs of the Native people. And of this inadequate funding, only a small portion is used for the treatment of mental health disorders and substance use (NIHB, 2020).

A similar deficiency in funding results in economic and educational disparities among Native people, which diminish substantially and persistently the income levels necessary for the acquisition of knowledge and skillsets from which their White counterparts benefit. Approximately 90% of Native Americans complete high school or higher education, which is looked upon as an indicator of employment success. Although this percentage is higher than in past generations, it is still below the national average of 95% and is significantly lower than the percentage of students who graduate from the nation's more affluent schools. By comparison, pupils in the Bureau of Indian Education (BIE) schools on Indian reservation lands experience about a 53% graduation rate (Camera, 2015). AI and AN people continue to face higher levels of unemployment and low-paying jobs than the general population, especially in reservation communities, with 28.3% living below the poverty level (National Center for Education Statistics [NCES], 2018; Partnership With Native Americans, 2022). Native people also continue to suffer higher rates of morbidity and mortality than their White counterparts; this trend has persisted since the arrival of Europeans. Improved access to quality healthcare and high-performing schools are the keystones for healthier AI and AN people.

Family disruption, violence, suicide, and substance use can also be viewed as interrelated and mutually reinforcing. The presence of any one of these dysfunctions can lead to another due to the despondency and misery associated with devaluing and marginalizing people who lack the necessary resources to bolster resilience, autonomy, and economic sufficiency. Approximately 50% of AI and AN children live in single-parent homes, with as high as 30% being removed from the family home because of violence and substance use and being forced to live in governmental group homes or foster care (Cross et al., 2000; Foster Care Facts, 2021; Kids Count Data Center, 2019). These social determinants of health indicators work against creating viable families and communities, which are the bedrock of any society. Single-parent homes, often female-headed, along with the widespread removal of children from their homes because of various forms of child maltreatment, give rise to conditions that militate against thriving families and communities. These factors help lay the foundation for a multitude of health disparities such as school failure, unemployment, and higher morbidity and mortality rates across the life course. The challenges associated with these identified maladies—family dysfunction, violence, and so forth—lead directly to the need to develop culturally congruent programs that are designed to "target" each of these factors over time and work toward the reduction and elimination of them. Specific laws, health policies, attention to improved educational opportunities, and economic stability are the bedrocks for improved sustainability (Brayboy & Lomawaima, 2018; Marmot, 2015). The goals of Healthy People 2020 and 2030 are yet to be met.

The high rates of alcohol and substance use, violence, and suicide are well documented in Native populations and have been major contributors to the morbidity and mortality of AI and AN people. Substance use is also a malady that negatively impacts the AI and AN nations. In recent years, with regard to people age 12 years and older, substance dependence or misuse among AI and AN people might be the highest it has ever been in the nation at 14.9%. By comparison, the lowest rate is at 4.6% among Asian Americans. Regarding violence, 39% of AI and AN women report exposure to intimate partner violence, which is also the highest in the United States. Associated with these other disparities is suicide. The rate of suicide for AI and AN is 1.7 times higher than the rate for the rest of the nation and can be related to the social despair caused by the other factors (IHS, 2015; Manson, 2004; Skewes & Blume, 2019). Inadequate housing, poor nutrition, low health literacy, enduring poverty, limited access to behavioral and mental health services, and lower income are some of the factors that converge to create these health disparities. For years, AN and AI people have endured a lower health status than others in the United States. Again, these quality of life issues and higher morbidity and mortality rates are deeply rooted in systems that fail to address adequate education and healthcare. Their failures are evidenced in deficient socioeconomic resources, fewer career opportunities, more stress and daily burdens, and a shorter life span than other American groups experience (Brayboy & Lomawaima, 2018; Hartmann et al., 2019; Marmot, 2015).

Heart disease, other cardiovascular conditions, and diabetes are troublesome chronic health conditions and the leading causes of mortality among the population (2009–2011). The life expectancy among this population is about 5.5 years below that of all other groups in the country, at 73.0 years to 78.5 years, respectively (see www.ihs.gov/newsroom/fact-sheets/disparities; www.samhsa.gov/sites/default/files/topics/tribal_affairs/ai-an-data-handout.pdf).

The severe and endemic health problems found among Native Americans can be explained by the prevalence of other social, physical, and psychological dysfunctions, including a prevailing sense of despair, limited income, isolation, and inadequate access to quality healthcare and educational opportunities. Some interventions, however, are having a positive impact on some illness conditions. The prevalence of diabetes, for example, has actually declined from 15.4% in 2013 to 14.6% in 2017, an impact that can be attributed largely to the Special Diabetes Program for Indians (SDPI), which is administered by the IHS and tribal and urban programs, which are federal programs. Yet even with the decline in the rate of diabetes, it is still twice that of the White non-Hispanic population, and diabetes-related mortality, though once as high as 54%, remains high at 34% as of 2017 (Dong et al., 2016; IHS, 2020a). Depression is more common among people with diabetes than among the general population, and past research has suggested that a relationship may exist between depression and hyperglycemia. The exact nature of that relationship remains unclear; it may be as simple as a decreased ability to practice self-care or as biopsychological as depression-induced changes in endocrine and neurotransmitter function (Engrum et al., 2005, Williams et al., 2004). Studies have suggested that people with diabetes experience depression at rates twice those of their nondiabetic cohort (Harper-Jaques, 2004; Lin et al., 2004). Diabetes has also been shown to be a contributing factor in the development of depression. Studies have revealed that patients with a diagnosis of diabetes are forced to undergo increased self-care rigors and lifestyle changes and to deal with healthcare directives. They may be subject to a sense of helplessness and loss of control, which may result in discouragement and a feeling of being overwhelmed. Access to healthcare, or the lack thereof, may also serve as a contributing factor. AI and AN people have one of the highest rates of being uninsured, and one in three lives below the poverty level (Redbird, 2020). Food insecurity is also a major concern. One in four experience problems caused by lack of access to healthy foods as compared with one in nine in the general population (Move for Hunger, 2022). Without adequate support systems, the unavailability of nutritious food may place additional burdens on an already stressed psyche (Harper-Jaques, 2004; Polonsky et al., 2005). AI and AN individuals with depression also have a high incidence of alcohol misuse, and similarly, those with alcoholism tend to have a higher rate of depression. At least 20% to 30% of those with diagnosed alcoholism concurrently suffer from depression (Gray & Nye, 2001). This comorbidity makes for difficulty in the diagnosis and treatment of either and, because of low adherence to treatment, creates an increased burden of symptoms, which may lead to suicide (Goldstein et al., 2006). AI and AN endure 49.1 alcohol-related deaths per 1 million each year (Spillane et al., 2020). One of the explanations for the high incidence of comorbidity is that alcohol is used for the self-medication of depressive symptoms. Another is the theory that there may be an inherited genetic predisposition for depression and alcohol or other substance use (Westermeyer, 2001). Those with comorbidities are at risk for medical morbidities related to increased stress and poor self-care, which reduce the rate of recovery significantly (Gregg, 2018; Schmidt, 2011).

The residual effects of historical trauma have been associated with the diagnosis of posttraumatic stress disorder (PTSD) by recognized Native scholars who seek to bring to light the collective effects of that trauma. The benefit of acknowledging this association is that it offers researchers a recognizable framework of PTSD with which to link the current mental health, domestic violence, and substance use problems present in the AI and AN culture and thus obtain valuable exposure and funding for projects. The problem with acknowledging this association is that, although it tends to make sense of the effects of historical trauma on the mental health of AI and AN people, it does not address the issue of intergenerational trauma and the continued trauma being perpetuated by the majority culture and the resulting self-perpetuation by the AI and AN people themselves (Evans-Campbell, 2008; Van Styvendale, 2008).

PTSD is a diagnosis made on the basis of a group of symptoms linked with and arising from a single past traumatic event. The historical trauma experienced by the AI and AN people, however, cannot be reduced to a single event; in fact, viewed through the conceptual lens of intergenerational trauma, it is a recurring, self-perpetuating problem, a reality that complicates both the PTSD diagnosis and the potential solutions to the problem (Manson et al., 2005). The problem is diagnosed as a psychic dislocation or relocation of the individual's essential sense of identity as an AI or AN person and the culture associated with that identity (Van Styvendale, 2008). It is that historical loss or dislocation that can be established as the source of the current mental health disorders, substance use, and domestic violence plaguing the AI and AN populations and resulting in health disparities and high mortality rates (Van Styvendale, 2008; Whitbeck et al., 2004).

Other cultural barriers are also responsible for the mental health and behavioral health disparities affecting AI and AN people. The stigma placed on mental illness and behavioral health and the associated complications experienced by AI and AN people with the maladies contribute to a reduction in health-seeking behaviors and also play a role in the effectiveness of treatment modalities. For example, the seeking of help is often delayed or might not occur, and recommended interventions, including psychotropic involvement with supportive and psychodynamic therapies, are often curtailed after a few sessions (Barnett et al., 2018). Cultural differences between the patient and the provider figure prominently in the effectiveness or ineffectiveness of mental health programs. These cultural differences can also undermine the productiveness of carefully planned mental health initiatives. AI and AN people believe that to live in health is to follow core cultural values in order to maintain balance and stability and give meaning to life's events. They believe that illness results from the disruption of the harmony between the individual and the surrounding physical and spiritual world. This harmony can be restored only through ritual and ceremony, traditional sacred elements that are glaringly absent in most mental healthcare programs intended for AI and AN but that are essential to any successful program involving this population group (Avery, 1991; Walters et al., 2020). An example of a successful program is the Inter-tribal Talking Circle, in which the customary talking circle is used in a group setting as a safe space to openly discuss experiences with mental health issues and substance use. Another type of approach that involves the potential participants in all phases of the research continues to gain credibility: Community-Based Participatory Research (CBPR). The conceptualization of ideas, research questions, design, interpretation of data, and so forth of planned interventions and other types of programs can fruitfully include the use of CBPR. The methodology should be crafted to reflect the tribal culture in which the intervention is being conducted. The healthcare program should involve tribal elders, healthcare providers, and community members, who work jointly to shape the instrument and interventions in accord with the needs, practices, and traditions of the specific tribe. The intervention then reflects culturally relevant material that has meaning for the participants (Pacheco et al., 2013; Sahota, 2010; Satcher, 2005; Wiley et al., 2007).

Indian Health Service

Health services for AI and AN began in the early 1800s during outbreaks of diseases when U.S. Army physicians provided care to AI and AN people residing in the vicinity of military posts. Later, healthcare services were exchanged for rights and property ceded to the government via treaty. In 1849, the Bureau of Indian Affairs, which had responsibility for the provision of Native healthcare, was transferred from the War Department (now known as the Department of Defense) to the Department of the Interior, and the first Indian hospital was built in Oklahoma (Kuschell-Hayworth, 1999). The Snyder Act of 1921 authorized the permanent provision of healthcare to Native American tribes (CRS Report, 2016; Kuschell-Hayworth, 1999). In 1955, the Public Health Service (PHS) assumed responsibility for the provision of Native healthcare from the Department of the Interior by establishing the IHS. This decision was in response to the Indian Health Facilities Act (Transfer Act) of 1954. During this period, it was decided that services were inadequate to meet the needs of AI and AN people and that the PHS was better suited to the task. In 1975, the Indian Self-Determination and Education Assistance Act was initiated, which created opportunities for tribes to contract with the federal government for programs that address the needs of the tribes. Hence, tribes assumed more autonomy and responsibility for their own communities through collaboration with the Bureau of Indian Affairs and the federal government. The Assistance Act of 1975 supplied provisions for the tribes to take control of their own healthcare services and directly receive the funds that were allocated for that program, which resulted in the expansion of services for many of those tribes calling for the change (CRS Report, 2016). The five "civilized tribes" in Oklahoma have made use of this Act and have seen their access to health services and the quality of services increase over time.

Established in 1955, the IHS is the federal agency tasked with providing healthcare services for AI and AN people (Box 18.1). It is made up of a system of hospitals, outpatient clinics, and primary care units that function under the aegis of the IHS, tribes, or tribal groups. These facilities are located across the United States in urban, rural, and reservation

BOX 18.1: Indian Health Service (IHS)

- Created in 1955
- Services approximately 3 million people
- Services 574 federally recognized tribes
- Operates 670 IHS and tribal healthcare facilities in 36 states in rural areas
- Operates 31 hospitals, 52 health centers, two school health centers, and 31 health stations
- Operates 41 grant-funded urban health centers under contract
- Approximately 50% of the IHS system is operated by tribal entities
    - Tribes operate 15 hospitals, 256 health centers, nine school centers, and 288 health stations, including 166 Alaska Native village clinics

Source: Data from National Indian Health Board.

locations. As a rule, services provided by the IHS are limited to individuals who are members of federally recognized tribes that live on reservations, while urban health services provide care to AI and AN individuals who cannot access the services that are available on reservations or tribally operated facilities that are not located on tribal lands. The programs are also designed for those who do not qualify for services or are located outside of a designated service area. There is no cost for the use of these health resources; an individual can receive care that should help to limit the number of days of disability and loss of life, and the individual is not charged for the care that is rendered (Honeycutt et al., 2019;Trimbie et al., 2018). The IHS provides services to approximately 2.56 million AI and AN people who are enrolled in one of the 574 federally recognized tribes that are spread across the nation and in 22 states. The IHS also consists of 12 area offices and 170 tribally managed service units (IHS, 2020b). The obligation to offer these health-based resources is derived from various federal statutes, treaties, court decisions, and the U.S. Constitution. The Constitution assigns the specific responsibility to Congress, which has a legal obligation to provide healthcare to the tribes (CRS Report, 2016). The 2020 IHS budget was $6 billion, which equates to approximately $4,078 per patient annually. The allocation does not compare with the $9,726 spent per nontribal person annually on the national level (IHS, 2020b). Although the IHS fulfills its legal duty to meet the healthcare needs of the tribes, it does so only minimally, as evidenced by this disparity.

Prior to the 1950s, the majority of AI and AN people lived on reservations in rural areas or within tribal jurisdictions like Oklahoma. In the 1950s and 1960s, however, legislation terminated legal responsibilities to the tribes, with the intent of encouraging Native American Indians to relocate to urban areas (IHS, 2020b). Things did change. Today, approximately 60% of tribal members reside in areas other than reservations and are served by tribal or urban healthcare centers. The Urban Indian Health Program (UIHP) consists of 41 centers funded through health consortium grants, contracts, and fees for services. The health facilities are owned or leased by urban organizations (IHS, 2021).

MODELS FOR RESEARCH, EDUCATION, PRACTICE, AND POLICY: ENVISIONING A HEALTHIER FUTURE

In recent years, the National Institute of Minority Health and Health Disparities has developed a theoretical and practical framework that has utility for conducting research, for planning and evaluating clinical services, and for promulgating policy, all of which are intended to reduce or eliminate health disparities. The framework in Exhibit 18.1 appears in

EXHIBIT 18.1: National Institute for Minority Health and Health Disparities Research Framework for American Indian and Alaska Native Nations

	NIH National Institute on Minority Health and Health Disparities	**NIMHD Minority Health and Health Disparities Research Framework** Adapted to reflect historic and socio-cultural influences for American Indian and Alaska Native Nations *Spero M. Manson, Ph.D., University of Colorado Denver's Anschutz Medical Center*		
Domains of Influence	**Levels of Influence**			
	Individual	**Interpersonal**	**Community**	**Societal**
Biological	Biological Vulnerability and Mechanisms *Metabolic Syndrome*	Caregiver-Child Interaction *Out-of-Indian Home Adoption* *Grandparent / Child-Rearing* Family Microbiome	Community Illness Exposure *Exxon Valdez Oil Spill* *Gold King Mine Waste Water Spill* Herd Immunity	Sanitation Immunization Pathogen Exposure *Uranium and Coal Mining*
Behavioral	Health Behaviors *External Locus of Control* *Drug Preferences* Coping Strategies *Resilience* *Spirituality* *Community-Mindedness*	Family Functioning *Extended Family* School / Work Functioning	Community Functioning *Collective Resilience* *Cultural Forms of Social Control* *Language Revitalization*	Policies and Laws *Termination and Relocation 1953* *Indian Self-Determination &* *Education Assistance Act 1975* *American Indian Religious* *Freedom Act 1978*
Physical / Built Environment	Personal Environment *Subsistence Activities*	Household Environment *HUD Housing Clusters* School / Work Environment *Boarding School Education*	Community Environment *Natural Resources* Community Resources *Gaming* *Tribal Commercial Enterprise*	Societal Structure *Matrilineal, Patrilineal, &* *Bilateral Systems of Descent* *and Jural Authority*
Sociocultural Environment	Sociodemographics *Per Capita Payments* Limited English Cultural Identify Response to Discrimination *Historical Trauma*	Social Networks Family / Peer Norms *Traditional Men's / Women's* *Societies* Interpersonal Discrimination *Stereotyped Threat* *Racial Prejudice*	Community Norms *Progressives and Traditionalists* *Alcohol Prohibition* Local Structural Discrimination *Border Town Economics*	Societal Norms *Hollywood Indian* *Firewater Myth* Societal Structural Discrimination *Sports Mascots*
Health Care System	Insurance Coverage Health Literacy Treatment Preferences	Patient-Clinician Relationship *Implicit Bias* Medical Decision-Making *Cultural Construction of Health*	Availability of Health Services *Direct, Contracted, and* *Compacted Services* Safety Net Services	Quality of Care Healthcare Policies *Reimbursement of Tribal Healing* *Ceremonies* *Indian Health Care* *Reauthorization Act*
Health Outcomes	**Individual Health**	**Family/Organizational Health**	**Community Health**	**Population Health**

Lifecourse (vertical label on left axis)

Health Disparity Populations: Race/Ethnicity, Low SES, Rural, Sexual/Gender Minority
Other Fundamental Characteristics: Sex/Gender, Disability, Geographic Region

Source: National Institute on Minority Health and Health Disparities. (n.d.). www.nimhd.nih.gov/about/overview/research-framework/adaptation-framework.html.

its generic form in Chapter 5 and is specifically adapted here for the AI and AN populations. Other groups will also find the framework useful when variables that are pertinent to their own purposes and populations are carefully pinpointed.

The Indigenist Stress-Coping Model

The Indigenist Stress-Coping Model (Walters et al., 2002) is unique in incorporating historical trauma and other adverse events in a model that helps to illuminate the sources of stress that Native Americans and Alaska Natives have endured. The model also explicates the cultural buffers that serve as moderators or retardants that can help balance and reduce stress and that facilitate culturally appropriate coping mechanisms that help to positively influence health outcomes (Fernandez et al., 2020). The majority of the literature on stress coping is largely irrelevant to the indigenous world because it is based on the use of Eurocentric values and theories (Walters et al., 2002). The Eurocentric view focuses on negative factors such as disease and pathology, or, if the factor is positive, it emphasizes the individual or individual behavior instead of communal or cultural behaviors and folkways. The Eurocentric stress-coping paradigm does not recognize the relationship between culture and trauma and how they can serve as predictors of substance use/misuse and mental health disorders (Fernandez et al., 2020; Walters et al., 2002,

2011). In the Indigenist Stress-Coping Model, sources of stress such as historical trauma, violent crimes/assault, traumatic life events, child abuse/neglect, discrimination, and unresolved grief and mourning are moderated by coping mechanisms described as cultural buffers (Walters et al., 2002). These cultural buffers include family/community support, spiritual coping, traditional health practices, identity attitudes, and enculturation, all of which help to create and sustain a sense of belonging and community. In the model, enculturation is described as the process by which individuals learn about and identify with their minority culture of original practices, and the process is the foundation for sustaining one's identity and self-worth (Bird, 2003; Brave Heart & DeBruyn, 1998; Duran, 2006; Jacobs, 2006; Jones, 2004; Lomawaima, 1994; Mitchell & Kaufman, 2002; Weaver & Yellow Horse Brave Heart, 1999; Whitbeck et al., 2004). These cultural buffers are incorporated into the Indigenist Stress-Coping Model, which emphasizes the strengths of the Native culture rather than its weaknesses, and their presence or absence serve as a predictor of health outcomes such as depression and alcohol misuse (Fernandez et al., 2020; Walters et al., 2002, 2011).

CASE STUDY 18.1: RHONDA, A PATIENT WITH COMORBID OR DUAL DIAGNOSES

Patient's chief complaints: "My blood sugars are always high, and they say I need to exercise, but I just don't seem to have any energy. I always feel tired, and I just sit around the house, watch television, and eat. I am not really hungry, but I can't think of anything else to do, so I eat. I have gained almost 50 pounds in the last year, and my BMI is over 50. I am only 40 years old, but I act like an old woman, I never get out of the house anymore, and I don't have any friends. I don't know what is wrong with me. I do not have a job, but I think that would help me. I am afraid of this COVID-19 virus. It is killing people."

Patient's history of present illness: Since the pandemic began, Rhonda has been isolated from her family because of COVID-19 restrictions, and she has lost two family members to the virus. She was not able to see them before they died because of the visitor restrictions at the nearby IHS hospital. There were restrictions determining the number of people who could attend the funeral services and determining the number of people who could come together and celebrate the joy of the family members' lives and pray to the ancestors about their spirits that will enter another realm. Rhonda recognizes that she has withdrawn from people and is not interested in much of anything. Despite her insights about her overall health status, she has continued to gain weight, and her BMI has increased to more than 50. Rhonda's hemoglobin A1C is 13.5, and she states that her anxiety and fears get in the way of her following the dietician's or nurse's recommendations. Rhonda also mentions that she has started to exhibit signs of vision changes and peripheral neuropathy, which frighten her.

Discussion Questions

1. Based on the chief complaints and clinical findings, which two comorbid conditions would you suggest are the primary concerns?
2. Identify possible causes for Rhonda's withdrawal and lack of energy or ambition.
3. Based on her history and your knowledge, design a plan of care that is culturally relevant for Rhonda and that might help to improve her mood and activity level.
4. What planned actions could be developed with Rhonda that might mitigate the effects of her disease burden?
5. Using the Indigenous Stress-Coping Model, develop a comprehensive plan of care that would potentially improve Rhonda's overall health status and quality of life. Provide a rationale for your care plan.

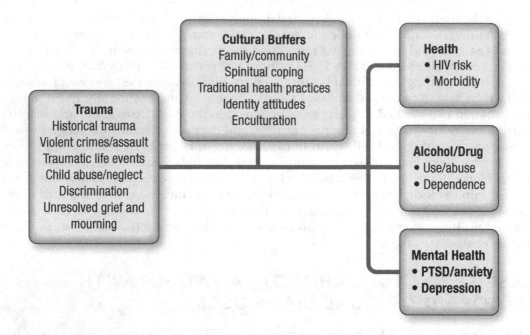

Figure 18.1 Relationship among sources of stress, cultural buffers, and negative outcomes.

The Indigenous Stress-Coping Model highlights stress and coping from a "fourth world" or indigenous perspective (Walters et al., 2002). The "fourth world" is defined as a world in which an Indigenous population resides within its own nation-state, and the nation-state maintains power and control over its people and the environment. Although acknowledging the powerlessness and colonized position that has been devastating, an indigenous perspective actively advocates for empowerment and sovereign rights. The model creates a framework through which AI and AN people can continue to cope with traumatic events and life stressors while planning for a healthier and more productive future (WFieland et al., 2007; Walters et al., 2002).

The model is built on the earlier work of Dinges and Joos (1988) that expanded a stress and coping model to include traumatic life events. They proposed that certain internal and external factors pre-exist and may serve as buffers between traumatic events and health outcomes. There is a linkage between historical and present trauma such as discrimination and unresolved grief related to historical loss, and negative health outcomes such as alcohol use/misuse and depression (Walters et al., 2002). Such an approach also helps to define the importance of moderators or retardants, such as traditional health practices, enculturation practices, and ceremonies, which conduce to strengthen attitudes and behaviors related to the cultures of origin and to apply them as buffers and protective factors between trauma and health outcomes (Fieland et al., 2007; Walters et al., 2002). The Indigenist Stress-Coping Model provides a culturally appropriate framework that serves as a lens through which Native researchers and others can examine these relationships and avoid the pitfalls associated with Eurocentric models that do not address the lived experiences and historical realities of Native people. Figure 18.1 shows the relationship among sources of stress, cultural buffers, and negative outcomes.

Community-Based Practice

Talking Circles

The use of talking circles in Native American populations has a long and rich tradition. In fact, this is a cultural practice that is innate to the Native culture. Traditionally, talking circles are described as individuals coming together to share stories in a respectful and nonjudgmental manner in order to learn from one another and provide support and acceptance for those experiencing difficult circumstances (Lowe, 2006; Luna et al., 2020). They have a sacred function of healing or cleansing while also serving to bring people together (Ywahoo, 1987). Talking circles allow the participants to experience the feelings of the other members and to develop and maintain a trusting relationship that lends itself to active listening and mutual respect among members (Hodge et al., 1999; Winters, & America, 2014).

Talking circles can be used for a variety of purposes and afflictions. From type 2 diabetes to HIV and substance use, talking circles have proven to be an effective method to provide comfort and healing. The approach can also be used as an educational tool to share information about disease processes and to promote understanding and resolve conflicting ideas about diseases such as diabetes and heart disease. Talking circles can be used, too, as an intervention to find the root causes of problems or as a means of data collection about a particular phenomenon.

Many tribes avail themselves of talking circles in their diabetic education programs, and Struthers et al. (2003) described the experiences of talking circle facilitators offering diabetic wellness education to Native Americans from the Pine Ridge Reservation in South Dakota and the Winnebago Reservation in Nebraska. Of the many functions associated with talking circles, a major function is as a forum for the processing of personal emotions surrounding diabetes.

Among the experiences described by the participants are isolation, depression, or a strong sense of punishment for some wrongdoing. A common complaint of many people with diabetes is that there is no place for the care of the emotional reactions that are evident when the diagnosis is made and that intensifies during the long and taxing treatment process (Sittner et al., 2018; Struthers et al., 2003). Through the sharing of feelings and information, additional strategies that are culturally appropriate, continued support from among the group, new insights, and creative decisions emerge.

Sweat Lodges

The sweat lodge ceremony is a traditional healing practice that is used by tribes from coast to coast in North America. There is evidence that it was practiced by indigenous peoples as early as 400 BCE. It is used as a means of healing the body, mind, emotion, and spirit. Although there is little scientific evidence of its efficacy, it is widely accepted as a means of Indigenous healing. The sweat lodge serves the sacred purpose of cleansing the body, mind, and spirit while bringing people together to share their life experiences (Marsh et al., 2018). The "sweat" is usually guided by a medicine man or elder and consists of the participants being exposed to intense heat created by heated stones. The ceremony involves "rounds," and periodically the tent flap is opened to allow the heat to escape and to add more stones before another round begins. The goal is to create an altered state of consciousness in which participants can let their pain go. The sweating is thought to help physically rid the body of impurities.

During the rounds, the participants take turns sharing, and after each sharing, they thank the creator for the healing (Garrett et al., 2011; Marsh et al., 2018; Sabucedo, 2017).

CONCLUSION

AI and AN people have a long history of being traumatized and marginalized in American culture. This chapter has highlighted links among the invasion of the Europeans, federal treaties, boarding schools, and the lack of adequate healthcare and educational opportunities, which has been glaring and detrimental for centuries. These factors lead to numerous health disparities that continue to exist. The forced assimilation and acculturation that have occurred over time have resulted in the devaluation and dismissal of cultural and spiritual practices and folkways that traditionally served as protective barriers for Native people's physical and psychological health. The perceived loss of culture has bred a sense of hopelessness that is exacerbated by the demise of the traditional family and the lack of quality healthcare and educational opportunities, which are linked to economic success. The widespread rates of violence, suicide, underemployment, and substance use remain major health disparities that need urgent attention. These conditions will be self-perpetuating unless culturally congruent and sustained interventions are implemented.

The health disparities experienced by AI and AN people can be corrected when the cycle of intergenerational trauma is broken. Researchers need to focus on developing culturally relevant interventions aimed at restoring the cultural beliefs and practices of the past as part of any health and social services plan of care. In order to return Native people to harmony with the spiritual and physical worlds, the soul wounds of the past and present must heal. This chapter has provided topics that all healthcare professionals should consider when interacting with AI and AN people for the purpose of improving their health and overall well-being.

ADDITIONAL RESOURCES

www.kff.org/medicaid/issue-brief/medicaid-and-american-indians-and-alaska-natives/
https://minorityrights.org/minorities/alaska-natives
https://theredroad.org/
https://nationalcowboymuseum.org/explore/rushes-statehood-oklahoma-land-runs/
www.npr.org/2021/04/17/988123599/unrecognized-tribes-struggle-without-federal-aide-during-pan demic
https://minorityrights.org/minorities/alaska-natives/
www.nationalgeographic.org/thisday/may28/indian-removal-act/
www.history.com/topics/native-american-history/trail-of-tears
www.ihs.gov/newsroom/factsheets/disparities/
www.samhsa.gov/sites/default/files/topics/tribal_affairs/ai-an-data-handout.pdf
https://passionistfamily.org.nz/resources/downloads/Chief%20Seattle.pdf
https://nationalcowboymuseum.org/explore/rushes-statehood-oklahoma-land-runs/
www.archives.gov/research/native-americans/dawes/tutorial/final-rolls.html
www.npr.org/sections/codeswitch/2018/02/09/583987261/so-what-exactly-is-blood-quantum
www.npr.org/2011/03/31/134421470/native-american-intermarriage-puts-benefits-at-risk
www.differencebetween.net/miscellaneous/culture-miscellaneous/
    difference-between-acculturation-and-assimilation/
www.nps.gov/articles/the-carlisle-indian-industrial-school-assimilation-with-education-after-the-in dian-wars-teaching-with-historic-places.htm
www.culturalsurvival.org/publications/cultural-survival-quarterly/
    they-called-it-prairie-light-story-chilocco-indian-school
https://upstanderproject.org/firstlight/pratt
www.spokesman.com/stories/2021/jul/08/all-these-children-matter-discovery-of-indian-boar/
www.ushistory.org/us/1a.asp
www.dpcpsi.nih.gov/sites/default/files/Critical_Considerations_for_Reviewing_AIAN_Research_5 08.pdf
www.nimhd.nih.gov/about/overview/research-framework/adaptation-framework.html
www.nimhd.nih.gov/about/overview/research-framework/adaptation-framework.html
www.powwows.com/main/native-american-pow-wow/
www.nanticokeindians.org/page/what-powwow
www.differencebetween.net/miscellaneous/culture-miscellaneous/
    difference-between-acculturation-and-assimilation/
www.nps.gov/articles/the-carlisle-indian-industrial-school-assimilation-with-education-after-the-inhttps://www.bia.gov/sites/bia.gov/files/assets/as-ia/ofa/admindocs/25CFRPart83_2015_abbrev.pdf
www.npr.org/2021/04/17/988123599/unrecognized-tribes-struggle-without-federal-aide-during-pan demicdian-wars-teaching-with-historic-places.htm

Muhammad, D., Tec, R., & Ramirez, K. (2019). Racial Wealth Snapshot: American Indians/
Native Americans. National Community. Reinvestment Coalition. https://ncrc.org/
racial-wealth-snapshot-American-Indians-Native-Americans/
ushistory.org. Diversity of Native American groups. U.S. history online textbook. www.ushistory
.org/us/1a.asp

REFERENCES

Akee, R. (2020). Land titles and dispossession: Allotment on American Indian Reservations. *Journal of Race, Economics and Policy*, 3, 123–143.

Archambeault, M. (2008). World War I choctaw code talkers: 36th division of the national guard. *Whispering Wind*, 37(5).

Avery, C. (1991). Native American medicine: Traditional healing. *Journal of the American Medical Association*, 265(17), 2271–2273.

Barnett, M., Gonzalez, A., Miranda, J., Chavira, D., & Lau, A. (2018). Mobilizing community health workers to address mental health disparities for underserved populations: A systematic review. *Administration and Policy in Mental Health and Mental Health Services Research*, 45(2), 195–211.

Bassett, D., Tsosie, U., & Nannauck, S. (2012). "Our culture is medicine": Perspectives of native healers on post-trauma recovery among American Indian and Alaska native patients. *The Permanente Journal*, 16(1), 19–27.

Bird, M. (2003, October 17). Statement of Michael E. Bird, MSW, MPH, Executive Director, National Native American AIDS Prevention Center to the United States Commission on Civil Rights.

Brave Heart, M., & DeBruyn, L. (1998). The American Indian holocaust: Healing unresolved historical grief. *The Journal of the National Center American Indian and Alaska Native Programs*, 60(8) 2, 60–82.

Brayboy, B., & Lomawaima, K. (2018). Why don't more Indians do better in school? The battle between US schooling & American Indian/Alaska native education. *Daedalus*, 147(2), 82–94.

Brunhouse, R. L. (1939). The Founding of the Carlisle Indian school. *Pennsylvania History: A Journal of Mid-Atlantic Studies*, 6(2), 72–85.

Byrd, W., & Clayton, L. (2000). An American health dilemma: Race, medicine and health care in the United States. Routledge.

Camera, L. (2015). Native American students left behind. US News and World Report. https://www.usnews.com/news/articles/2015/11/06/native-american-students-left-behind

Charbonneau-Dahlen, B., Lowe, J., & Morris, S. (2016) Giving voice to historical trauma through storytelling: The impact of boarding school experience on American Indians. *Journal of Aggression, Maltreatment & Trauma*, 25(6), 598–617.

Chen, V. (2014). Cultural identity: Key concepts in intercultural dialogue (22). http://centerforinterculturaldialogue.org

Choctaw Nation. (2011). Choctaw Nation of Oklahoma Website: History. http://www.choctawnation.com/

Cross, T., Earle, K., & Simmons, D. (2000). Child abuse and neglect in Indian country: Policy issues. *Families in Society*, 81, 49–58.

CRS Report. (2016). The Indian Health Service (IHS): An overview. https://www.everycrsreport.com/reports

Debo, A. (1934). The rise and fall of the Choctaw republic. University of Oklahoma Press.

Debo, A. (1940). "And still the waters run". University of Oklahoma Press.

Deloria, V. (1988). Custer died for your sins: An Indian Manifesto. University of Oklahoma Press.

Dinges, N., & Joos, S. (1988). Stress coping and health: Models for interaction for Indian and Native Populations. *American Indian and Alaska Native Mental Health Research*, 1, 8–64.

Dong, Y., Collado, M., & Branscum, P. (2016). Native American diabetes prevention intervention programs: A systematic review. *California Journal of Health Promotion*, Vol. 10(3), 26–36.

Doran, M. F. (1978). Negro slaves of the five civilized tribes. *Annals of the Association of American Geographers*, 68(3), 335–350.

Duffy, J., (1997). Smallpox and the Indians in American colonies. *Biological Consequences of European Expansion, 1450–1880* (pp. 233–250). Ashgate.

Duran, E. (2006) Healing the soul wound: Counseling with American Indians and other Native peoples. Teachers College Press.

Engrum, A., Holen, A., Myletun, A., Dahl, A. A., & Midthjell, K., (2005). Depression and diabetes. *Diabetes Care*, 28(8), 1904–1909.

Evans-Cambell, T. (2008). Historical trauma in American Indian/Native Alaska communities: A multilevel framework for exploring impacts on individuals, families, and communities. *Journal of Interpersonal Violence, 23*, 316.

Fernandez, A., Evans-Campbell, T., Johnson-Jennings, M., Beltran, R., Schultz, K., Stroud, S., & Walters, K. (2020). "Being on the walk put it somewhere in my body": The meaning of place in health for Indigenous women. *Journal of Ethnic & Cultural Diversity in Social Work.* https://doi.org/10.1080/15313204.2020.1770652

Fieland, K. C., Walters, K. L., & Simoni, J. M. (2007). Determinants of health among two-spirit American Indians and Alaska Natives. *The Health of Sexual Minorities: Public Health Perspectives on Lesbian, Gay, Bisexual, and Transgender Populations,* 268–300.

Fleming, W. (2006). Myths and stereotypes about native Americans, *Phi Delta Kappan, 88*(3), 213–217.

Foster Care Facts. (2021). Disproportionate representation of Native Americans in foster care across the United States. http://www.potawatomi.org/

Gampa, V., Bernard, K., & Oldani, M. J. (2020). Racialization as a barrier to achieving health equity for native Americans. *AMA Journal of Ethics, 22*(10), 874–881.

Garcia, M. C., Faul, M., Massetti, G., Thomas, C. C., Hong, Y., Bauer, U. E., & Iademarco, M. F. (2017). Reducing potentially excess deaths from the five leading causes of death in the rural United States. *MMWR Surveillance Summaries, 66*(2), 1.

Garcia, R., & Ahler, J. (1992). Indian education: Assumptions, ideologies, strategies. In J. Reyhner (Ed.), *Teaching American Indian students* (pp. 13–32). University of Oklahoma Press.

Garrett, M., Torres-Rivera, E., Brubaker, M., Portman, T., Brotherton, D., West-Olatunji, C., Conwill, W., & Grayshield, L. et al. (2011). Crying for a vision: The Native American sweat lodge ceremony as a therapeutic intervention. *Journal of Counseling & Development, 89*(3), 318–325.

Goldstein, B., Diamantouros, A., Sahffer, A., & Naranjo, C. (2006). Pharmacotherapy of alcoholism in patients with co-morbid psychiatric disorders. *Drugs, 66*(9), 1229–1237.

Gray, N., & Nye, P. (2001). American Indian and Alaska native substance abuse: Co-morbidity and cultural issues. *The Journal of the National Center American Indian and Alaska Native Programs, 10*(2), 67–84.

Gregg, M. (2018). Long-term effects of American Indian boarding schools. *Journal of Development Economics, 130*, 17–32.

Harper-Jaques, S. (2004). Diabetes and depression: Addressing the depression can improve glycemic control. *American Journal of Nursing, 104*(9), 56–59.

Hartmann, W., Wendt, D., Burrage, R., Pomerville, A., & Gone, J. (2019). American Indian historical trauma: Anti-colonial prescriptions for healing, resilience, and survivance. *American Psychology, 74*(1), 6–19.

Herring, R. D. (1989). The American native family: Dissolution by coercion. *Journal of Multicultural Counseling and Development, 17*, 4–13. https://doi.org/10.1002/j.2161-1912.1989.tb00411.x

Him, D., Aguilar, T., Frederick, A., Larsen, H., Seiber, M., & Angal, J. (2019). Tribal IRBs: A framework for understanding research oversight in American Indian and Alaska Native communities. *American Indian Alaskan Native Mental Health Resources, 26*(2), 71–95.

Hodge, F., Stubbs, H., & Fredericks, L. (1999). Talking circles: Increasing cancer knowledge among American Indian women. *Cancer Research and Therapy, 8*(1–2), 103–111.

Honeycutt, A., Khavjou, O., Neuwahl, S., King, G., Anderson, M., Lorden, A., & Reed. (2019). Incidence, deaths, and lifetime costs of injury among American Indians and Alaskan natives. *Injury Epidemiology, 6*(1), 1–12.

Huddleston, L. E. (2015). Origins of the American Indians: European Concepts, 1492–1729 (Vol. 11). University of Texas Press.

Indian Health Services. (2015). History of HIS. https://www.ihs.gov/urban/history/

Indian Health Services. (2020a). *Changing the course of diabetes: Charting remarkable progress.* https://www.ihs.gov/sites/newsroom/themes/responsive2017/display_objects/documents/SDPI2020Report_to_Congress.pdf.

Indian Health Services. (2020b). IHS profile. https://www.ihs.gov

Jacobs, D. (Ed.). (2006). *Unlearning the language of conquest: Scholars expose anti-Indianism in America.* University of Texas Press.

Jones, D. (2004). Rationalizing epidemics: Meanings and uses of American Indian mortality since 1600. Harvard University Press.

Jones, D. S. (2006). The persistence of American Indian health disparities. *American Journal of Public Health, 96*(12), 2122–2134. https://doi.org/10.2105/AJPH.2004.054262

Kaiser Family Foundation. (2019). Health and health care for American Indians and Alaska Natives (AIANs) in the United States. https://www.kff.org/wp-content/uploads/2019/05/health-and-health-care-for-american-indians-and-alaska-natives-AIANs-in-the-united-states-may-2019.png

Kids Count Data Center. (2019). Children in single-parent families by race in the United States. https://www.datacenter.kidscount.org

Lin, E., Katon, W., Von Korff, M., Rutter, C., Simon, G., Oliver, M., Ciechanowski, P., Ludman, E. J., Bush, T., & Young, B. et al. (2004). Relationship of depression and diabetes self-care, medication adherence, and preventative care. *Diabetes Care, 27*(9), 2154–2160.

Lomawaima, K. T. (1994). The story of Chilocco Indian School: They called it prairie light. University of Nebraska Press.

Lomawaima, K., & Cantley, J. (2018). Remembering our Indian school days: The boarding school Experience: A landmark exhibit at the Heard Museum. *Journal of American Indian Education, 57*(1), 22–29.

Lowe, J. (2006). Teen intervention project—cherokee (TIP-C). *Pediatric Nursing, 32*(5), 495–500.

Luna, W., Malvezzi, C., Teixeira, K., Almeida, D., & Bezerra, V. (2020). Identity, care and rights: The experience of talking circles about the health of Indigenous people. *Revista Brasileira de Educação Médica, 44.*

Manson, S. (2004). Meeting the mental health needs of American Indians and Alaska natives. Report for the National Technical Assistance Center (NTAC) for State Mental Health Planning.

Manson, S., Beals, J., Klein, S., & Croy, C. et al. (2005). Social epidemiology of trauma among 2 American Indian reservation populations. *American Journal of Public Health, 2005*(95), 851–859.

Marmot, M. (2015). The health gap: The challenge of an unequal world. *The Lancet, 386*(10011), 2442–2444.

Marsh, T., Marsh, D., Ozawagosh, J., & Ozawagosh, F. et al. (2018). The sweat lodge ceremony: A healing intervention for intergenerational trauma and substance use. *The International Indigenous Policy Journal, 9*(2).

Mitchell, C., & Kaufman, C. (2002). Structure of HIV knowledge, attitudes, and behaviors among American Indian young adults. *AIDS Education Prevention, 14*(5), 401–418.

Move for Hunger. (2022). How hunger affects Native American communities. https://moveforhunger.org/one-in-4-native-americans-is-food-insecure

National Indian Health Board. (2020). Indian health care 101. www.nihb.org; National Center for Educational Statistics (NCES). Fast facts https://nces.ed.gov/fastfacts/display.asp?id=16

National Public Radio. (2018). *So what exactly is "blood quantum"?* https://www.npr.org/sections/codeswitch/2018/02/09/583987261/so-what-exactly-is-blood-quantum

Novins, D. K., Croy, C. D., Moore, L. A., & Rieckmann, T. (2016). Use of evidence-based treatments in substance abuse treatment programs serving American Indian and Alaska native communities. *Drug and Alcohol Dependence, 161,* 214–221.

Pacheco, C., Daley, S., Brown, T., Filippi, M., Greiner, K., & Daley, C. M. (2013). Moving forward: Breaking the cycle of mistrust between American Indians and researchers. *American Journal of Public Health, 103*(12), 2152–2159.

Partnership With Native Americans. (2022). Living conditions. http://www.nativepartnership.org/site/PageServer?pagename=naa_livingconditions

Polonsky, W. H., Fisher, L., Earles, J., Dudl, R. J., Lees, J., Mullan, J., & Jackson, R. A. et al. (2005). Assessing psychosocial distress in diabetes. *Diabetes Care, 28*(3), 626–631.

Redbird, B. (2020). What drives native poverty? https//www.ipr.northwestern.edu/news/2020/redbird-what-drives-native-american-poverty.html

Sabucedo, P. (2017). The psychological flexibility model from a cultural prospective: An interpretive analysis of two native American healing rituals. *International Journal of Culture and Mental Health, 10*(4), 367–375.

Sahota, P. (2010). Community-based participatory research in American Indian and Alaska Native communities. Washington, DC: NCAI Policy Research Center.

Schmidt, R. (2011). American Indian identity and blood quantum in the 21st century: A critical review. *Journal of Anthropology, 2011,* 9.

Sittner, K. J., Greenfield, B. L., & Walls, M. L. (2018). Microaggressions, diabetes distress, and self-care behaviors in a sample of American Indian adults with type 2 diabetes. *Journal of Behavioral Medicine, 41*(1), 122–129.

Skewes, M., & Blume, A. (2019). Understanding the link between racial trauma and substance use among American Indians. *American Psychologist, 74*(1), 88–100.

Smedley, A. (2007). Race in North America: Origin and evolution of a worldview (3rd ed.). Westview Press.

Spillane, S., Shiels, M. S., Best, A. F., Haozous, E. A., Withrow, D. R., Chen, Y., Berrington de González, A., & Freedman, N. D. (2020). Trends in alcohol-induced deaths in the United States, 2000–2016. *JAMA Network Open, 3*(2), e1921451. https://doi.org/10.1001/jamanetworkopen.2019.21451

Srinivasan, S. (2018). Cancer Control in American Indian and Alaska Native Populations. https://www.cancer.gov/news-events/cancer-currents-blog/2018/american-indian-alaskanative-cancer-control

Struthers, R., Kaas, M., Hill, D., Hidge, F., DeCora, L., & Geeishirt-Cantrell, B. et al. (2003). Providing culturally appropriate education on type 2 diabetes to rural American Indians: Emotions and racial consciousness. *Journal of Rural Community Psychology, E6*(1).

Sue, D., & Sue, D. (1990). Counseling the culturally different: Theory and Practice (2nd ed.). Wiley.

Trimbie, J., Mahmud, A., Buttorff, C., & Meza, E. (2018). Implementation of patient-centered medical homes in small and rural practices: The experience of Indian Health Service clinics. In 2018 Annual Research Meeting, Academy Health.

U.S. Department of Health and Human Services. (2011). Nation prevention strategy: Elimination of health disparities. http://www.healthcare.gov/prevention/nphpphc/strategy/health-disparities .pdf

U.S. Department of Health and Human Services. (2020). About Healthy People 2030. https://health .gov/healthypeople/about

U.S. Department of Health and Human Services. (2022). Profile: American Indian/Alaska Native. https://minorityhealth.hhs.gov/omh/browse.aspx?lvl=3&lvlid=62

Van Styvendale, N. (2008). The trans/historicity of trauma in Jeanette Armstrong's slash and Sherman Alexie's Indian killer. *Studies in the Novel*, 40(1&2), 203–223.

Walls, M., & Whitbeck, L. (2012). Advantages of stress process approaches for measuring historical trauma. *The American Journal of Drug and Alcohol Abuse*, 38(5), 416–420.

Walters, K., Mohammed, S., Evans-Campbell, T., Beltran, R., Chae, D., & Duran, B. (2011). Bodies don't just tell stories, they tell histories. *Du Bois Review: Social Science Research on Race*, 8(1).

Walters, K., Walls, M., Dillard, D., & Kaur, J. (2020). American Indian and Alaskan native research in the health sciences: Critical considerations for the review of research applications. https://dpcpsi .nih.gov/sites/default/files/Critical_Considerations_for_Reviewing_AIAN_Research_508.pdf

Weaver, N., & Yellow Horse Brave Heart, M. (1999). Examining two facets of American Indian identity: Exposure to other cultures and the influence of historical trauma. *Journal of Human Behavior in the Social Environment*, 2(1/2), 19–33.

Westermeyer, J. (2001). Alcoholism and comorbid psychiatric disorders among American Indians. *The Journal of the National Center American Indian and Alaska Native Programs*, 10(2), 27–51.

Whitbeck, L., Adams, G., Hoyt, D., & Chen, X. (2004). Conceptualizing and measuring historical trauma among American Indian people. *American Journal of Community Psychology*, 33(3/4), 119–130.

White, L. (2018). Who gets to tell the stories? Carlisle Indian school: Imagining a place of memory through descendant voices. *Journal of American Indian Education*, 57(1), 122–144.

Wiley, J., Sons Noe, T., Manson, S., Croy, C., McGough, H., Henderson, J., & Buchwald, D. (2007). The influence of community-based participatory research principles on the likelihood of participation in health research in American Indian communities. *Ethnicity & Disease*, 17(1 suppl 1), S6–S14.

Williams, J., Katon, W., Lin, E., Noel, P., Worchel, J., Cornell, J., Harpole, L., Fultz, B, Hunkeler, E., Mika, V., & Unutzer, J. et al. (2004). The effectiveness of depression care management on diabetes-related outcomes in older patients. *Annals of Internal Medicine*, 140(12), 1015–1025.

Williams, S. (2020). Native American boarding schools: Some basic facts and statistics. https://www .samanthawilliams.com/blog/native-american-boarding-schools-some-basic-fact s-and-statistics

Winters, A., & America, N. (2014). Using talking circles in the classroom. Heartland Community College.

Ywahoo, D. (1987). Voices of our ancestors: Cherokee teachings from the wisdom fire. Shambhala.

CHAPTER 19

Environmental Health: Neighborhoods and Communities

Irene C. Felsman, Schenita Randolph, AnnMarie L. Walton, Amie Koch, Donna Biederman, and Rosa M. Gonzalez-Guarda

LEARNING OBJECTIVES

- Examine historical, physical, and social contributors to environmental health.
- Examine theoretical frameworks describing environmental health from a health equity lens.
- Describe how environmental injustice contributes to health disparities.
- Analyze how structural racism continues to impact health outcomes related to the environment.
- Evaluate differences among rural, urban, and suburban factors influencing environmental health and wellness.
- Appraise the role of the nurse in addressing environmental health disparities and promoting community resilience through an environmental justice lens.

INTRODUCTION

This chapter aims to (a) discuss the impact of environmental issues on the health of individuals, families, neighborhoods, and communities with an emphasis on social, environmental, and climate justice, and (b) highlight the importance of the role of the nurse in response to these issues. Concerns related to environmental hazards globally have never been as urgent as they are in the 21st century. Health concerns related to water contamination, climate change, deforestation, fossil fuel pollution, and animal and human waste disposal are topics that dominate news coverage. Extreme changes in the environment have exacerbated geographic and socioeconomic health disparities. In response, global environmental targets have been intentionally integrated into each of the 17 United Nations Sustainable Development Goals (United Nations Department of Economic and Social Affairs, 2022), which aim to increase health for all people (Menton et al., 2020).

Environmental health, defined as freedom from injury due to toxic agents and hazardous environmental conditions (American Public Health Association, n.d.), is affected by numerous physical, chemical, biological, and psychosocial determinants. Assessment of individual, family, and community health must include consideration of:

◆ Physical, legal, and social factors influencing the living environment, such as zoning laws governing housing, green spaces, and recreational sites; neighborhood placement and affordability; transportation; accessibility of nutritious food and health care; commerce; industrial waste; and toxic farming practices;
◆ Psychosocial consequences of environmental deficits or hazards, including structural violence, toxic stress, social isolation, and racism embedded in the history and structure of a society; and
◆ Physical and mental health effects of natural and manmade environmental disasters such as floods, tornadoes, earthquakes, and fires, which may increase anxiety and stress or result in suicide, particularly for those with chronic mental health conditions (Liu et al., 2020) and members of other vulnerable populations (e.g., people who are visually impaired, developmentally delayed, or experiencing homelessness).

Historically, people who live in poverty and are disenfranchised, such as Black people, Indigenous people (in Australia, New Zealand, and the Americas, including Native Hawaiians and Pacific Islanders), and other people of color—collectively referred to as BIPOC (Black, Indigenous, and people of color)—and new immigrants, often live in geographic areas, both urban and rural, characterized by unsafe housing, increased environmental hazards, and limited access to healthcare (*The Lancet Planetary Health*, 2018; Shavers, 2007). Schools and healthcare institutions in these areas are often underequipped, and safety standards found in more prosperous settings are lacking, disproportionately exposing residents to health hazards. People living in poverty are more likely to be in substandard housing with mold, lead paint contamination, and insect debris, or in settings affected by flooding and fires caused by climate change–related high temperatures (Dodson et al., 2017). Policies that govern environmental hazards are frequently lagging and subject to lobbying on the part of significant corporate interests that ignore environmental risks. Thus, there is a great need for policy development on a global scale (Vardoulakis et al., 2016). Given that environmental, social, and health issues are closely linked, only a holistic, multisectoral approach to addressing these issues can significantly change populations health.

THEORETICAL FRAMEWORK

As a concept in the overarching framework, or metaparadigm, of the profession of nursing (Fawcett, 1984), the environment has been central to nursing care since Florence Nightingale's early work recognized the importance of environmental factors (e.g., sanitization, warfare, social exploitation) in health. Indeed, evaluation of the theoretical tenets used by Nightingale has highlighted essential strategies such as mobilizing people, resources, and power and generating evidence to prompt social justice (Hegge, 2013). Recognition of the importance of environmental health underlies the perspective of the social determinants of health approach, focusing increased attention on how people live, work, and play (World Health Organizaiton [WHO] Commission on Social Determinants of Health, 2008).

Myriad theories and frameworks proposed across various disciplines have focused on neighborhood- and community-level influences to guide a comprehensive approach to healthcare, including nursing care of individuals, families, and communities. These theories delineate the roles of built and social environments on health and well-being. The built environment refers to the physical environment created by people (e.g., objects, buildings, spaces) or modified by people (e.g., sidewalk and green space creation, building maintenance; Gilbert & Stephens, 2018; Sallis, 2009). Its influence on health has been incorporated into several models for change in the United States and at WHO (see Chapters 5 and 21) and is related to the types of frameworks used in urban planning. Urban planning frameworks that are intentionally developed to foster health and well-being focus on three major domains: physical activity, social interaction, and access to healthy food (Kent & Thompson, 2012). For example, as most of the global population increasingly resides in urban settings, WHO has developed policy frameworks and guidance on interventions to increase green spaces to meet sustainable development goals for 2030 (WHO, 2017). However, unless a life course perspective (e.g., playground vs. a running trail) and equity lens (e.g., distance to green space) are employed in their design, the benefits of these green spaces may not reach all portions of the population (Douglas et al., 2017; Lachowycz & Jones, 2014). This well-documented trend is discussed later in the chapter.

In addition to addressing the built environment, social aspects of communities and neighborhoods, such as their deficits (e.g., neighborhood disorder) and strengths (e.g., community resilience), can be leveraged to guide healthcare and nursing care and enhance health and well-being. For example, the "broken window theory," based on criminology research and literature, purports that the deterioration of buildings and public incivilities such as breaking windows of stores and homes leads to increased crime. In addition to predicting overall health outcomes, this theory has shown value in predicting outcomes of mental health treatment and substance misuse prevention and management (O'Brien et al., 2019). Similarly, theories that focus on community cohesion, organization, and resilience can drive strengths-based interventions. Health professionals, including nurses, have become increasingly focused on fostering resilience. The Society-to-Cell Resilience Model (Szanton & Gill, 2010) is one example of a nursing model that delineates multilevel influences on resilience. In addition to the built environment, this model incorporates important community-level factors, including institutions, social capital, social support, and diversity that influence biological outcomes such as cellular and physiological resilience among individuals.

Interestingly, the biology of the environment, including the human microbiome within a community, also appears to influence the health of community members (Dowd & Renson, 2018). The microbiome is defined as the collective genomes of the microbes that live inside and on the human body (National Human Genome Research Institute, n.d.). Given the increased attention to precision health, which focuses on an individual's genetic, behavioral, and environmental determinants of health (Gambhir et al., 2018), there have been recent calls to consider and leverage the integration of the microbiome of neighborhood and community spaces to promote environmental and human health (Horve et al., 2020).

ENVIRONMENTAL JUSTICE VERSUS ENVIRONMENTAL INJUSTICE

The U.S. Environmental Protection Agency (EPA) Office of Environmental Justice defines *environmental justice* as "the fair treatment and meaningful involvement of all people regardless of race, color, national origin, or income concerning the development, implementation, and enforcement of environmental laws, regulations, and policies" (EPA, n.d.). For environmental justice to be achieved, all people must benefit from the same protections and be included in decisions regarding healthy living, working, and learning environments. "Environmental injustice," in contrast, is the disproportionate exposure of people, often those who are BIPOC or living in low-income communities, to adverse environmental conditions and substances. Conditions such as lead paint, air pollution, hazardous waste sites, improper disposal of solid waste, substandard housing, dangerous jobs, and polluting industries are of primary concern (Environmental Justice Organizations, Liabilities and Trade, n.d.; Landrigan et al., 2010). Environmental injustice across all populations contributes significantly to well-documented disparities in health. It is linked to increased risks for many diseases (Liddell & Kington, 2021) and the prevalence of adverse health conditions, such as asthma, mental health disorders, developmental delays, lung cancer, malnutrition, obesity, and lead poisoning. Pregnant people, fetuses, children, adolescents, and seniors are particularly susceptible to the impact of environmental injustice on health (Tilburg, 2017).

Environmental injustice is highly correlated with many factors that link poverty to poor health. Inadequate access to quality education and healthcare, lack of safe play spaces for children, lack of access to nutritious foods and clean water, absence of work opportunities that pay a living wage, and high exposure to crime and violence (Rosner, 2016) are primary concerns. The economy of the United States is based on capitalist systems, policies, and laws that are inherently designed to emphasize profit over environmental protection and thus benefit wealthier communities to the detriment of lower-income communities (Bell, 2015). Lower-income communities, by definition, are communities in which at least 20% of residents have a median family income of 80% or lower than the area against which they are benchmarked in the U.S. Census (Benzow et al., 2020). Lower-income communities often have limited political or economic power; therefore, companies that produce higher pollution rates may operate without the level of regulatory attention they would receive in higher-income communities (Collins et al., 2016). This same phenomenon applies to low- and low-middle income countries as well.

Children's Health and the Environment

The rate of childhood obesity is increasing each year in the United States, with significant disparities related to race, ethnicity, income, and geographic location. Children in historically marginalized populations, specifically those who are BIPOC, have a higher prevalence of obesity than do non-Hispanic White populations (Lane et al., 2021). A lack of access to nutritious foods, sufficient grocery stores, financial resources, adequately stocked food banks, neighborhoods promoting physical activity, and nutritional and educational support has contributed to the current rate of childhood obesity.

Children are at risk of increased absorption of toxins from the environment; they drink more water per body weight than adults and often play on the floor or in soil and runoff water. In addition, children cannot excrete toxic compounds that accumulate in the bloodstream. Examples of environmental injustice can be found in marginalized, low-income BIPOC communities, Native American reservations, migrant farmworker camps, and older cities with water systems that have not been upgraded (McOliver et al., 2015; Ruckart et al., 2019; Sattler, 2019; see Chapters 5 and 24).

An example of environmental justice to improve children's health outcomes is regulating well water to ensure decreased exposure to arsenic, thereby reducing the rates of skin and liver cancer in children (Flanagan et al., 2016). Other environmental regulations and practices that have reduced disease and improved health include the delivery of safe drinking water in some cities, access to fresh fruits and vegetables at farmers markets, mobile delivery of food to neighborhoods, safer sewage systems, the control of insect vectors, and the construction of safer housing (Miller et al., 2021).

Today, children are at risk for exposure to more than 80,000 synthetic chemicals, most of which have been introduced since the 1970s. These synthetic chemicals are plastics, pesticides, motor fuels, building materials, antibiotics, chemotherapeutic agents, flame retardants, and synthetic hormones. Information about the toxicity of chemicals in communities is not widely available to the public. Some environmental toxins lead to neurodevelopmental impairment, shortened attention span, and disruption in behavior. Parental pesticide exposure may cause preterm birth, low birth weight, smaller head circumference, and developmental delays in children (Qu et al., 2017). For example, bisphenol, a chemical used to make plastics, and phthalates, used to soften plastics, disrupt the endocrine system; these chemicals have been found in high levels in children with diabetes and obesity in the United States (Kahn et al., 2020).

Research shows that the most socioeconomically disadvantaged areas face the highest burdens of disease associated with poor air quality (Mitchell et al., 2015), including automotive exhaust and ambient air pollution. Historically, in New York City, virtually all diesel bus depots, or places where buses may idle for hours emitting pollutants, are located in low-income, disadvantaged neighborhoods (Kheirbek et al., 2016). Well-described environmental risk factors for asthma include ambient air pollution from industrial and vehicular sources, indoor air pollution, secondhand cigarette smoke, mold, mildew, and cockroach droppings (Lavigne et al., 2021). Air pollution is a significant environmental hazard to human health and a leading cause of asthma-related morbidity and mortality (Zheng et al., 2021). Asthma, one of the most common childhood conditions, has increased due to air pollution and secondhand smoke; the risk for sudden infant death syndrome has also increased due to air pollution (Chen et al., 2020). Policy changes, including instituting low pollutant-emitting or electric buses, are ways to improve environments.

CLIMATE CHANGE

Climate change is a primary threat to public health in the 21st century (Centers for Disease Control and Prevention [CDC], n.d.; Wu et al., 2016). Injustices are associated with climate change, energy use, natural disasters, urban greenspaces, and public policies adversely and disproportionately affecting people who are BIPOC, minority low-income communities, and socially disadvantaged groups (Chakraborty, 2017).

Although coastal flooding and hurricanes impact all communities, they have a far more significant effect on economically disadvantaged communities due to residents' insecure and often unsafe living conditions and lack of insurance. For example, during the recent flooding on the U.S. east coast during Hurricane Ida, dozens of people perished; most of the 13 people who died in New York City were immigrants trapped in subdivided, illegal basement apartments (*New York Times*, 2021). Another example is renters and low-income households in Puerto Rico that were more vulnerable to storm damage than higher-income households during Hurricane Maria (Ma & Smith, 2020). Forest fires can cause the displacement of families, and the strain of rebuilding ravaged homes may cause long-term displacement and housing insecurity. Smoke from forest fires contributes to poor air quality, leading to increased rates of chronic respiratory illness. Nurses and other healthcare professionals must learn about the harm caused by natural disasters, which are increasing in number and severity due to climate change. The integration of climate change content into nursing education and training is becoming more and more critical (Wu et al., 2016). Learning how to assess climate change's current or previous harm to individuals and communities can help health professionals, including nurses, evaluate the risk for future damage and plan public health interventions.

RACISM AND ENVIRONMENTAL INJUSTICE

Too often, individuals who are BIPOC and people who live in lower socioeconomic communities work, play, or attend school near sources of harmful environmental conditions. A disproportionate share of the most dangerous pollution comes from a few sources that exploit a legacy of racism and powerlessness to inflict devastating harm on vulnerable communities (Collins et al., 2016). BIPOC communities are impacted to a substantially greater degree by the most harmful 10% of pollutants, including arsenic, benzene, cadmium, and other dangerous toxins from industrial production (Collins et al., 2016). Sacrifice zones, a term used to identify areas where super polluters operate below the radar, impose enormous health burdens on the environment and on majority/minority, low-income neighborhoods and communities with little power to offer resistance (Oyarzo-Miranda et al., 2020). For example, in Chicago's South Side, Black and Latino residents are more likely to live close to industrial pollution, with 50 documented landfills, hundreds of hazardous waste sites, and leaking underground storage tanks contributing to higher rates of chronic health conditions such as asthma, and the highest rates of cancer in the United States (Natural Resources Defense Council [NRDC], 2020). Local, state, and national governments determine where super polluters, landfills, and hazardous waste sites can be located. Therefore, these decisions are made intentionally and reflect the disproportionate value placed on some lives over others by elected officials and policymakers at all levels of government. All health professionals can communicate with local, state, and national elected officials to influence how and where the hazardous waste will be disposed of and how existing sites will be safely managed. Writing policy letters and editorials, attending civic meetings, voting, and participating in elected boards are a few activities that could be impactful. Healthcare professionals and community advocates should be encouraged to join organizations that influence and guide health policy and practice.

Structural Racism

Structural racism refers to "the totality of ways in which societies foster racial discrimination through mutually reinforcing systems of housing, education, employment, earnings, benefits, credit, media, health care, and criminal justice; these patterns and practices, in turn, reinforce discriminatory beliefs, values, and distribution of resources" (Bailey et al., 2017, p. 1455). Structural racism accounts for many inequities experienced by individuals who are BIPOC, particularly regarding housing, education, healthcare, and community development in the United States. The communities in which people of color are born, live, work, and age are often segregated and receive inequitable resources and attention compared with predominantly White neighborhoods, resulting in inequities in environmental health outcomes. One example of structural racism is the ongoing residential segregation of Black Americans in the United States. Residential segregation separates communities by social groups and class, significantly affecting the availability of resources that ensure positive health outcomes. Racial segregation is associated with adverse birth outcomes, increased exposure to air pollutants, heightened risk for chronic diseases (e.g., cardiovascular disease), decreased access to healthcare, and raised rates of crime and homicide (Bailey et al., 2017). Redlining is one of the historical dynamics that has helped create underresourced neighborhoods. (See Chapter 22 for further information about redlining and the role of the federal government.)

Current statistics reflect the severe effects of social determinants of health (SDH) on people of color and their health status. Although all people, especially children, who are exposed to high pollution rates can experience asthma, people who are Black are twice as likely to have asthma and three times more likely to die from asthma-related conditions than people who are White (Blessett & Littleton, 2017). Other chronic conditions, such as diabetes and heart disease, exhibit similar rates of racial disparity (Blessett & Littleton, 2017). For example, non-Hispanic Black Americans are twice as likely as non-Hispanic White Americans to die from diabetes. Similarly, cardiovascular disease is a common illness and cause of death in all U.S. communities; however, people who are BIPOC experience the disease in a more brutal way and at younger ages. The trend in health outcomes is clear: Individuals who are BIPOC are more likely than individuals who are White to be struck by illness and much more likely to die from ill health, often at an earlier age. This ongoing trend results from intergenerational racial inequities within social institutions that policymakers and politicians have consistently ignored. In their 2017 study, Bailey et al. conducted a Web of Science search on race and health. They found that "racism" and "racial discrimination" are terms that are silenced in the literature and in reports on health and health disparities. To address racial discrimination as a social contributor to poor health, healthcare professionals must first acknowledge and expose it. Failure to do so will allow health inequities to become increasingly entrenched and harmful.

Historic methods used in urban planning to segregate communities of color from White communities bear a heavy responsibility for health inequities. Redlining is a term used to describe racial segregation and discrimination against minority populations. Redlining was first implemented in the 20th century when banks and insurers used this phenomenon to concentrate Black residents and other people of color within specific neighborhoods (Cusick, 2020). Additionally, the Home Owners Loan Corporation used redlining to categorize neighborhoods during the Great Depression era (*The Lancet*, 2020); banks withheld loans to people in redlined communities, a policy supported by federal government policies. Redlining was used to warn non-Black people away from neighborhoods primarily inhabited by Black residents. Inner-city areas with predominantly Black and immigrant residents were considered to be redlined. Low-income Black people in these communities suffered from "diminished educational attainment, disparaging health outcomes, limited employment opportunities, stifled political participation" and other inequities (Blessett & Littleton, 2017). Black people living in redlined communities are at very high risks for illness and failure due to harmful community conditions, lack of community development and resources, and inadequate education and healthcare (Blessett & Littleton, 2017). (See Chapter 20 for further discussion of redlining in the United States.)

Although the Fair Housing Act of 1968 was created to ban redlining, the practice continues to negatively affect people of color because banks and other organizations maintain it. Because the Fair Housing Act has failed to ameliorate segregation issues, economic setbacks, and inequitable access to community services, residents of redlined communities lack access to the resources necessary to live healthy lives (Cusick, 2020). Residents in these areas are more likely to experience poor health outcomes, limited economic opportunities, and inadequate public school education.

Racial inequities have persisted over the past few decades. As climate change increasingly influences human conditions, the gap between the health outcomes of people who are White and people who are BIPOC in the United States has widened. As referenced previously, climate change affects residents of redlined communities because these communities are exposed to increased air pollution and extreme heat (Cusick, 2020). Studies show that, on average, redlined areas are 5 degrees warmer than nonredlined districts (Cusick, 2020), placing residents in these communities at a higher risk of experiencing health issues without being able to seek treatment. Given the lack of proper ventilation and air conditioning in redlined neighborhoods, residents are more likely to suffer from heatstroke. In recent years, the gap in homeownership for families who are BIPOC versus those who are White has increased to rates higher than in the pre-1960s era of redlining, and substandard rental housing carries higher environmental risks than owned homes (Bhutta et al., 2020; Urban Institute, n.d.). Unstable housing, employment disparities, and the high cost of homeowner or rental insurance disproportionately affect BIPOC communities (Urban Institute, n.d.). Redlined neighborhoods lack the financial resources needed to maintain a safe and healthy life. Yet the effects of heightened climate change make the availability of healthcare resources an ever-growing priority. Laws and policies are not protective mechanisms for these communities; instead, they support deleterious practices.

Research has demonstrated that communities with a history of redlining are less likely to contain grassy areas and parks (Nardone et al., 2021). Their proximity to industrial plants, landfills, and urban highways causes these communities to suffer from additional air and water pollution (Cusick, 2020). It might explain the increased temperature in these neighborhoods and the lack of improvement in their air quality despite an overall decline in national air pollution over several years (Thompson, 2019). These conditions present profound health implications for future generations; recent research has linked living in historically redlined communities with preterm birth (Krieger et al., 2020). It is important to note that the creation of the interstate highway system and other roadways in the United States was instrumental in the destruction of historically minority neighborhoods and the consequent disruption of these communities' economic and environmental structure (Evans, 2021). The grave results of disparities suffered by people who are BIPOC due to environmental issues are increasingly apparent, yet continue to be largely ignored by policymakers (Bailey et al., 2021).

Structural racism in the United States exists across all institutions. Structures work together, simultaneously, to support inequities that have substantial implications for the health outcomes of historically marginalized people of color. Policymakers must address inequities through increased support to communities of color by implementing urban planning, housing opportunities, education, access to healthcare, community development, and resource efforts to undo the perpetuation of poor environmental health (Nardi et al., 2020). Additionally, given that structural racism has intergenerational effects on people of color, it can be extrapolated that health issues faced due to poor environmental health will negatively impact future generations. There is a need for additional research in this area, particularly regarding the health effects of exposure to pollution and increased temperature on children and adults of reproductive age and interventions to improve these outcomes (Williams et al., 2019; Williams & Cooper, 2019).

Rural, Urban, and Suburban Priorities

Before engaging in discussions of rural, urban, and suburban environmental health concerns, healthcare providers should recognize that residents may prioritize environmental health concerns differently than ecological health professionals do. Collaboration between community members and environmental health professionals is critical to successfully prioritize needs and design effective interventions to improve environmental health in communities. It is also suggested that community involvement in environmental health decision-making may foster community awareness of environmental health services (Wu et al., 2017).

Recent evidence shows that rural areas in the United States have superior air quality to some urban areas, including lower population mean nitrous oxide concentrations in parts per billion (ppb) of 4.4 versus 14.2 (Clark et al., 2014). The number of days with delicate particulate matter ($PM_{2.5}$) levels greater than EPA National Ambient Air Quality Standards (NAAQS) is lower. Also, the mean ambient concentrations of $PM_{2.5}$ in micrograms per cubic meter (mean $PM_{2.5}$) are lower, and the total number of days with maximum 8-hour average ozone concentrations greater than NAAQS is lower (Strosnider et al., 2017). In conclusion, lower nitrous oxide concentrations and fewer days with fine particulate matter levels higher than desired contribute to superior air quality in rural areas.

However, rural counties do experience greater exposure to agriculture-related pollution than do urban counties. Although people commonly associate exposure to pesticides with agricultural areas, exposure to other physical toxicants, including organic and inorganic fertilizers, dust, grains, animals, diesel exhaust, and solvents, must be considered (Cushing et al., 2015; Guidry et al., 2018; Merchant et al., 2006). Unlike workers in many other industries, people in agriculture generally live where they work and may carry occupational contaminants into their home setting. Furthermore, agricultural contributions to water pollution are often more significant than contributions made by cities or industries (Food and Agriculture Organization of the United Nations, 2018). Many who work in agriculture in the United States are non-English speakers with low levels of formal education and limited or no healthcare. Thus, education and training about these hazards may be insufficient for their needs. These workers are often unprotected by labor laws and protection standards enacted through federal and state governments because agricultural employers are exempt, placing their workers at greater risk (MHP Salud, 2014). Several toxicants unique to Concentrated Animal Feeding Operations (CAFOs) emerge in rural areas. CAFOs produce an immense amount of manure that can contaminate groundwater (veterinary antibiotics, pathogens, and nitrates). Manure management problems also impact surface water by (a) increasing ammonia to levels that can kill aquatic life, (b) releasing hormones that affect fish, and (c) introducing bacteria that disrupt the ecological balance of lakes and rivers. The air around CAFOs contains ammonia, hydrogen sulfide, methane, and particulate matter, which are associated with human health risks. CAFOs emit greenhouse gases that contribute to climate change and odors far worse than smaller livestock farms due to anaerobic reactions when large amounts of manure are stored in pits or lagoons over long periods. There are more than 150 pathogens in manure that can affect human health and a host of insects (such as flies) that breed in manure and bedding (Hribar, 2010). The effects of CAFOs on environmental health cannot be overstated, and they are disproportionately experienced by people who are BIPOC (Wing & Johnston, 2014). According to the Clean Water Act, the federal government regulates discharge from CAFOs through the EPA. Local governments can use zoning ordinances, detailed permitting schemes, and odor controls to defend local communities from the effects of CAFOs (Kottwitz & Jarchow, n.d.). Local boards of health can monitor and investigate health problems, engage in research, create health-related policies and regulations, mobilize community partnerships, and engage in education about the health dangers of CAFOs (Hribar, 2010). Furthermore, individuals can take action by gathering information, conducting water sampling, organizing with others, and reporting illegal behavior (Sierra Club, 2021).

Urban areas generally have superior drinking water to rural areas because of infrastructure resources; however, in urban areas with substandard housing, the water may be contaminated by inadequate sanitation, poor solid waste disposal services, air pollution, inadequate trash collection systems, and congested traffic. Other urban area health risks include crowded living conditions, noise pollution, traffic accidents, and contaminated food. Significant health inequities often exist within cities, such as differences in life expectancy for people living in poor versus affluent conditions (Owens-Young, 2018). These health inequities can be traced to differences in social and living conditions among urban dwellers and variable environmental qualities in cities (Clark et al., 2014). Trees, green roofs, and vegetation can help reduce urban heat island effects by shading buildings, deflecting radiation from the sun, and releasing moisture into the atmosphere (EPA, 2020). Efficient public transportation can also minimize emissions, noise pollution, air pollution, and traffic accidents.

Suburban areas have a combination of environmental health issues. Suburban areas have an increased dependence on automobiles for goods and services than urban areas, increasing greenhouse gas emissions and depleting fossil fuels. Suburban regions, on average, emit more greenhouse gases per person than urban or rural areas (Pahl, 2020). Suburban areas cause water pollution due to sprinklers and irrigation systems that carry fertilizers, pesticides, and other potentially harmful substances into adjacent bodies of water (Pahl, 2020). Furthermore, viable agricultural land is being destroyed to create more suburban development. As this land cannot easily be restored to agricultural land, the trend is concerning while the population continues to expand (Pahl, 2020). Solutions include more use of renewable energy and electric vehicles, efficient public transportation systems for cities and suburbs, bans on harmful chemicals and pesticides, and stricter land development regulations (Pahl, 2020).

ROLE OF HEALTHCARE PROFESSIONALS

Healthcare professionals' roles in environmental health and climate change issues are broad and include policy development; advocacy for healthy communities, workplaces, families, and individuals; ecological assessment of homes and communities; and research. Most healthcare professionals affirm the urgency of environmental and climate change issues and believe that their representative organizations must address them (Kotcher et al., 2021; Terry et al., 2019). There are many such organizations. Some of the more prominent cross-professional coalitions include The Medical Society Consortium on Climate and Health, Health Professionals for a Healthy Climate, Health Care Without Harm, and Practice Greenhealth (see References section for website access). An important interprofessional initiative is the Robert Wood Johnson Foundation's *Culture of Health Action Framework* (Robert Wood Johnson Foundation, n.d.), which sets a national plan for scalable solutions to improve health, equity, and well-being for all communities in the United States and includes foundational principles for safe environments.

The American Nurses Association (ANA) standards of practice clearly define the commitment of nursing to protect the health of populations, communities, and individuals through engaging with coalitions and partnerships (ANA, n.d.). One of its significant roles is to inform policy and support nurse-led development of healthcare practice innovations. The guidelines enumerated in the ANA Principles of Environmental Health for Nursing Practice (2007) address the nurse's role in environmental health and justice. The principles present guidance for environmentally safe nursing care, methods to address issues and consequences of global climate change and the chemical burden of disease, and implementation strategies for nursing practice.

The International Council of Nurses (ICN, 2018), an organization representing the global voice of nurses, issued a position statement in 2018 outlining areas of importance for policy change and intervention by nurses. These include building climate-resilient health systems, developing models of care to reduce unnecessary travel, developing climate-informed health programs for emerging infectious and contagious diseases, and engaging in sustainable practices in the health sector. Other initiatives include building the health workforce's response capacity, engaging in health and climate research, and participating in intersectoral policy and governance responses (ICN, 2018). The effects of climate change on health are broad and increasingly important for healthcare professionals to address (Angelini, 2017). The Alliance of Nurses for Healthy Environments (AHNE, n.d.) supports nurses in the specialty practice of occupational and environmental health nursing through policy development and advocacy. AHNE focuses on health and safety programs and services that prevent work-related and environmental hazards for worker populations and community groups (AHNE, n.d.). The Nurses Climate Challenge is a global partnership between the AHNE and Health Care Without Harm (Health Care Without Harm, n.d.) that aims to mobilize nurses to educate health professionals worldwide about the effects of climate change on health.

The physical environment is an essential determinant of health (Castner et al., 2019), making assessment and identification (diagnosis) of environmental risks in homes, communities, and workplaces a key priority for nursing and healthcare professionals (Agency for Toxic Substances Disease Registry, n.d.). The IPREPARE environmental assessment (Paranzino et al., 2005) is one example of a tool used to guide environmental assessment, and this tool is used in both public health and clinical settings.

Another important role for nurses and other healthcare professionals is the development of educational resources and the planning and delivery of programs about environmental health and risk factors for individuals, communities, and the broader population (Williamson et al., 2020). Resource identification and referral for community members and organizations are essential to achieving risk reduction and addressing environmental health concerns (immediate crises or long-term issues). Nurses are well placed to promote health literacy and build community resilience through an environmental justice lens to support the most vulnerable populations. Environmental health literacy (EHL) is a specialty area that uses principles and practices from the fields of risk communication, health literacy, environmental health sciences, communications research, and safety culture (Finn & O'Fallon, 2017) to promote prevention and improve health. EHL is a distinct form of health literacy to prevent environmentally induced diseases. Its approach includes increasing knowledge among community partners, investigators, health professionals, educators, and decision-makers about root environmental causes of illness and disabilities and mitigating environmental hazards. In contrast, other forms of health literacy focus on improving the understanding of diagnosed individuals and families about their medical conditions.

Nursing and public/population health research is key in defining the best evidence-based practices for promoting a safe and healthy environment. Community-Based Participatory Research, often referred to as CBPR, is an effective way to engage community stakeholders in the process of creating healthy environments. CBPR principles emphasize equitable group dynamics, including shared leadership and power, participatory decision-making, and two-way open communication and health equity in the research process (Ward et al., 2018).

One example of CBPR is found in a study of air quality and information dissemination in a California community (Madrigal et al., 2020). A collaboration of community members, researchers, and scientists developed a community air-monitoring network. High school students were engaged in a program to learn about air quality science, respiratory health, community air monitoring, and policies intended to improve air quality and communicate this information to community members. The effort was impactful for the students and the community. Another example of CBPR is a study that focused on the effectiveness of communicating the dangers of phthalate exposure in a community setting, which showed an improvement in participants' knowledge of environmental health and a reduction in their risk behaviors (Claudio et al., 2018).

In summary, advocacy is an influential role for all healthcare professionals, including nurses, and involves working alongside community members, government and policy agencies, and special issue organizations focused on environmental concerns. Important advocacy activities include promoting policy change and development related to environmental issues such as climate change, safer chemicals, food sustainability, energy and health (e.g., mining), and safe work environments. As one of the most trusted professions worldwide, nurses are ideal advocates for increased climate action in the healthcare sector. Nurses and other healthcare professionals possess strong values of social justice, generational fairness, and a will to alleviate suffering, coupled with the skills to create system change and solutions to mitigate the harm of environmental hazards (National Resource Defense Council, 2019). Nurses are often leaders in building coalitions and partnerships across public and private sectors and promoting collaboration to advocate for and create healthy environments (Dressel et al., 2020; Sefcik et al., 2019), but more action is needed. All healthcare professionals must step forward with an equity lens to mitigate harmful environmental health effects using the ADPIE nursing process (assessment, diagnosis, planning, intervention, and evaluation) to build and support programs and interventions that ensure health for all.

CASE STUDY 19.1: INCREASED CARBON MONOXIDE LEVELS IN A PUBLIC HOUSING COMMUNITY

Situation

McDougald Terrance is one of 14 public housing properties owned and maintained by the Durham Housing Authority (DHA) in Durham, North Carolina. Built in 1954, McDougald Terrace was heralded as the city's first "Black project." In 2019, McDougald Terrace had 360 units occupied primarily by African American, female-headed families (DHA, 2021).

In 2018 and 2019, McDougald Terrace did not pass U.S. Department of Housing and Urban Development (HUD) health and safety inspections due to numerous noted deficiencies (Bridges, 2020). In late December 2019, Emergency Management Services (EMS) discovered an unusual cluster of carbon monoxide (CO) calls and developed a task force (Bridges, 2020). DHA launched an immediate response in an effort to protect their residents and ordered a full inspection of the property. Over 3 days, 296 apartments were inspected, and occupants' CO levels were assessed (Bridges, 2020). Several adults and

(continued)

CASE STUDY 19.1: INCREASED CARBON MONOXIDE LEVELS IN A PUBLIC HOUSING COMMUNITY (*CONTINUED*)

children had elevated CO levels, and some apartments had stoves and water heaters emitting higher than expected CO levels. After the inspections were completed, another call for unusual levels of CO prompted a voluntary evacuation of the property. Within the ensuing weeks, 270 families relocated to local hotels to allow property repairs (Bridges, 2020). Ultimately, an inspection of 346 units revealed 211 stoves, 38 furnaces, and 35 hot water heaters emitting high CO levels (Bridges, 2020). Appliances emitting high CO levels were repaired or replaced, and the original ventilation system was replaced to properly vent the gas appliances.

Background

The U.S. Housing Act of 1937 established government-funded permanent public housing under the U.S. Department of Housing and Urban Development (HUD, n.d.). The intent was to provide affordable and safe rental housing to eligible low-income families, older adults, and persons with disabilities. African Americans make up less than 15% of the population of the United States (U.S. Census Bureau, 2019) but account for 44% of people living in public housing (HUD, n.d.) in the United States. Public housing residents pay income-based rent, which is generally 30% of all adults' combined earnings or $25 to $50 per month for households where no adults earn wages (HUD, n.d.).

Over the years, a manifestation of structural racism and disinvestment in public housing has resulted in a $26 billion backlog of deferred maintenance to housing units across the nation (HUD, n.d.). The rental assistance demonstration (RAD) program is a policy solution that allows for private investment in public housing. RAD is being implemented in cities across the United States. Through RAD, private monies will help to offset critical public housing capital needs, which are estimated at over $70 billion nationwide (Schwartz & McClure, 2021).

Findings

The CO emergent situation at the McDougald Terrace apartments and the displacement of families into hotels, in some cases for up to 4 months, caused significant life disruptions. Regular routes for transportation and communication changed abruptly. A special bus route was established to provide transportation to school but resulted in children being ostracized and bullied. Many hotels had no cooking facilities, and families had to eat take-out, prepared, and processed foods for all meals. Residents feared for their families' health and safety and the security of their personal belongings, which remained in their apartments during renovation. The situation created an increased distrust of DHA and local government among some public housing residents. The McDougald Terrace property renovations, hotel room rentals, and necessities for the 270 displaced families cost millions. These monies were from the DHA budget intended to provide maintenance and upkeep to all their public and affordable housing properties.

Conclusions

Structural racism has resulted in disinvestment in public housing nationwide, jeopardizing the health and well-being of low-income families, older adults, and disabled persons. In Durham, substandard public housing caused the displacement of 270 families and more

(continued)

CASE STUDY 19.1: INCREASED CARBON MONOXIDE LEVELS IN A PUBLIC HOUSING COMMUNITY (*CONTINUED*)

than 1,000 individuals and resulted in major life disruptions and stress. Public housing properties across the United States are undergoing RAD conversion and are receiving renovations, resulting in improved health outcomes.

Discussion Questions

1. What implications for practice, research, and advocacy work stand out in this case study? Consider the following:
   a. Zoning laws governing housing,
   b. Green spaces and recreational sites,
   c. Neighborhood placement and affordability,
   d. Transportation,
   e. Access to nutritious food, and
   f. Access to healthcare.
2. In what ways does this case study illustrate inequity? Discuss the following:
   a. Systemic racism/redlining, and
   b. Social determinants/drivers of health.
3. Discuss the components of environmental risk assessments that you would focus on when assessing individuals living in public housing.
4. How does housing insecurity affect the health and well-being of individuals, families, and communities?
5. Discuss the psychosocial consequences of environmental hazards, including:
   a. structural violence,
   b. toxic stress, and
   c. social isolation.

ADDITIONAL RESOURCES

Food and Agricultural Organization of the United Nations. (2018). Pollutants from agriculture a serious threat to world's water. https://www.fao.org/news/story/en/item/1141534/icode/
Health Care Without Harm. (n.d.). https://noharm-global.org/documentresource
Hribar, C. (2010). National association of local boards of health: Understanding concentrated animal feeding operations and their impact on communities. https://www.cdc.gov/nceh/ehs/docs/understanding_cafos_nalboh.pdf

REFERENCES

Agency for Toxic Substances Disease Registry. (n.d.). https://www.atsdr.cdc.gov/csem/exposure-history/Components-of-an-Exposure-History.html
Alliance of Nurses for Healthy Environments. (n.d.). https://envirn.org/
American Nurses Association. (n.d.). https://www.nursingworld.org/practice-policy/
American Public Health Association. (n.d.). Building an understanding of environmental health. https://apha.org/topics-and-issues/environmental-health/understanding-environmental-health
ANA Principles of Environmental Health for Nursing Practice. (2007). https://www.nursingworld.org/practice-policy/work-environment/health-safety/environmental-health/
Angelini, K. (2017). Climate change, health, and the role of nurses. *Nursing for Women's Health*, 21(2), 79–83. https://doi.org/10.1016/j.nwh.2017.02.003

Bailey, Z. D., Feldman, J. M., & Bassett, M. T. (2021). How structural racism works – racist policies as a root cause of U.S. racial health inequities. *The New England Journal of Medicine, 384*(8), 768–773. https://doi.org/10.1056/NEJMms2025396

Bailey, Z. D., Krieger, N., Agénor, M., Graves, J., Linos, N., & Bassett, M. T. (2017). Structural racism and health inequities in the USA: Evidence and interventions. *Lancet (London, England), 389*(10077), 1453–1463. https://doi.org/10.1016/S0140-6736(17)30569-X

Bell, K. (2015). Can the capitalist economic system deliver environmental justice? *Environmental Research Letters, 10,* 125017.

Benzow, A., Fikri, K., & Newman, D. (2020). Meet the low-income communities eligible for powerful new small business relief in the Rubio-Collins Phase IV proposal. https://eig.org/news/meet-the-low-income-communities-eligible-for-powerful-new-small-business-relief-in-the-rubio-collins-phase-iv-proposal

Bhutta, N., Chang, A. C., Dettling, L. J., & Hsu, J. W. (2020). Disparities in wealth by race and ethnicity in the 2019 survey of consumer finances. *Board of Governors of the Federal Reserve System.* https://doi.org/10.17016/2380-7172.2797

Blessett, B., & Littleton, V. (2017). Examining the impact of institutional racism in black residentially segregated communities. *Ralph Bunche Journal of Public Affairs, 6*(1).

Bridges, V. (2020 February 17). McDougald Terrace inspection, carbon monoxide crisis timeline. https://www.newsobserver.com/article239315688.html

Castner, J., Amiri, A., Rodriguez, J., Huntington-Moskos, L., Thompson, L. M., Zhao, S., & Polivka, B. (2019). Advancing the symptom science model with environmental health. *Public Health Nursing (Boston, Mass), 36*(5), 716–725. https://doi.org/10.1111/phn.12641

Centers for Disease Control and Prevention. (n.d.). Climate effects on health. https://www.cdc.gov/climateandhealth/effects/default.htm

Chakraborty, J. (2017). Focus on environmental justice: New directions in international research. *Environmental Research Letters, 12*(3), 030201. https://doi.org/10.1088/1748-9326/aa63ff

Chen, Y. T., Liu, C. L., Chen, C. J., Chen, M. H., Chen, C. Y., Tsao, P. N., Chou, H. C., & Chen, P. C. (2020). Association between short-term exposure to air pollution and sudden infant death syndrome. *Chemosphere, 271,* 129515. https://doi.org/10.1016/j.chemosphere.2020.129515

Clark, L. P., Millet, D. B., Marshall, J. D. (2014). National patterns in environmental injustice and inequality: Outdoor NO2 air pollution in the United States. *PLoS One, 9*(4), e94431. https://doi.org/10.1371/journal.pone.0094431

Claudio, L., Gilmore, J., Roy, M., & Brenner, B. (2018). Communicating environmental exposure results and health information in a community-based participatory research study. *BMC Public Health, 18*(1), 784. https://doi.org/10.1186/s12889-018-5721-1

Collins, M. B., Munoz, I., & JaJa, J. (2016). Linking 'toxic outliers' to environmental justice communities. *Environmental Research Letters, 11*(1), 015004. https://doi.org/10.1088/1748-9326/11/1/015004

Cushing, L., Faust, J., August, L. M., Cendak, R., Wieland, W., & Alexeeff, G. (2015). Racial/ethnic disparities in cumulative environmental health impacts in california: Evidence from a statewide environmental justice screening tool (CalEnviroScreen 1.1). *American Journal of Public Health, 105*(11), 2341–2348. https://doi.org/10.2105/AJPH.2015.302643

Cusick, D. (2020, January 21). Past racist "redlining" practices increased climate burden on minority neighborhoods. https://www.scientificamerican.com/article/past-racist-redlining-practices-increased-climate-burden-on-minority-neighborhoods/

Dodson, R. E., Udesky, J. O., Colton, M. D., McCauley, M., Camann, D. E., Yau, A. Y., Adamkiewicz, G., & Rudel, R. A. (2017). Chemical exposures in recently renovated low-income housing: Influence of building materials and occupant activities. *Environment International, 109,* 114–127. https://doi.org/10.1016/j.envint.2017.07.007

Douglas, O., Lennon, M., & Scott, M. (2017). Green space benefits for health and wellbeing: A life-course approach for urban planning, design and management. *Cities, 66,* 53–62.

Dowd, J. B., & Renson, A. (2018). "Under the skin" and into the gut: Social epidemiology of the microbiome. *Current Epidemiology Reports, 5*(4), 432–441. https://doi.org/10.1007/s40471-018-0167-7

Dressel, A., Bell-Calvin, J., Lee, E., Hermanns, L., Anderko, L., Swaney, V., Steinberg, J., Hawkins, M., & Yeldell, S. (2020). Sustaining a nurse-led community partnership to promote environmental justice. *Public Health Nursing (Boston, Mass).* https://doi.org/10.1111/phn.12820

Durham Housing Authority. (2021). http://www.durhamhousingauthority.org/

Environmental Justice Organizations, Liabilities and Trade. (n.d.). http://www.ejolt.org/2013/02/environmental-injustice/

Evans, F. (2021). *How interstate highways gutted communities—and reinforced segregation.* History. https://www.history.com/news/interstate-highway-system-infrastructure-construction-segregation

Fawcett, J. (1984). The metaparadigm of nursing: Present status and future refinements. *Image: The Journal of Nursing Scholarship, 16*(3), 84–87.

Finn, S., & O'Fallon, L. (2017). The emergence of environmental health literacy-from its roots to its future potential. *Environmental Health Perspectives*, 125(4), 495–501. https://doi.org/10.1289/ehp.1409337

Flanagan, S. V., Spayd, S. E., Procopio, N. A., Marvinney, R. G., Smith, A. E., Chillrud, S. N., Braman, S., & Zheng, Y. (2016). Arsenic in private well water part 3 of 3: Socioeconomic vulnerability to exposure in Maine and New Jersey. *The Science of the Total Environment*, 562, 1019–1030. https://doi.org/10.1016/j.scitotenv.2016.03.217

Gambhir, S. S., Ge, T. J., Vermesh, O., & Spitler, R. (2018). Toward achieving precision health. *Science Translational Medicine*, 10(430), eaao3612. https://doi.org/10.1126/scitranslmed.aao3612

Gilbert, J. A., & Stephens, B. (2018). Microbiology of the built environment. *Nature Reviews. Microbiology*, 16(11), 661–670. https://doi.org/10.1038/s41579-018-0065-5

Guidry, V. T., Rhodes, S. M., Woods, C. G., Hall, D. J., & Rinsky, J. L. (2018). Connecting environmental justice and community health: Effects of hog production in North Carolina. *North Carolina Medical Journal*, 79(5), 324–328. https://doi.org/10.18043/ncm.79.5.324

Hegge, M. (2013). Nightingale's environmental theory. *Nursing Science Quarterly*, 26(3), 211–219.

Horve, P. F., Lloyd, S., Mhuireach, G. A., Dietz, L., Fretz, M., MacCrone, G., …, Ishaq, S. L. (2020). Building upon current knowledge and techniques of indoor microbiology to construct the next era of theory into microorganisms, health, and the built environment. *Journal of Exposure Science & Environmental Epidemiology*, 30(2), 219–235.

ICN Position Statement: Nurses, Climate Change and Health. (2018). https://www.icn.ch/sites/default/files/inline-files/PS_E_Nurses_climate%20change_health_0.pdf

Kahn, L. G., Philippat, C., Nakayama, S. F., Slama, R., & Trasande, L. (2020). Endocrine-disrupting chemicals: Implications for human health. *The Lancet: Diabetes & Endocrinology*, 8(8), 703–718. https://doi.org/10.1016/S2213-8587(20)30129-7

Kent, J., & Thompson, S. (2012). Health and the built environment: Exploring foundations for a new interdisciplinary profession. *Journal of Environmental and Public Health*, 2012, 958175. https://doi.org/10.1155/2012/958175

Kheirbek, I., Haney, J., Douglas, S., Ito, K., & Matte, T. (2016). The contribution of motor vehicle emissions to ambient fine particulate matter public health impacts in New York City: A health burden assessment. *Environmental Health: a Global Access Science Source*, 15(1), 89. https://doi.org/10.1186/s12940-016-0172-6

Kotcher, J., Maibach, E., Miller, J., Campbell, E., Alqodmani, L., Maiero, M., & Wyns, A. (2021). Views of health professionals on climate change and health: A multinational survey study. *The Lancet: Planetary Health*, 5(5), e316–e323. https://doi.org/10.1016/S2542-5196(21)00053-X

Kottwitz, J., & Jarchow, T. (n.d.). Concentrated animal feeding operation regulations.

Krieger, N., Wye, G. V., Huynh, M., Waterman, P. D., Maduro, G., Li, W., Bassett, M. T. (2020). Structural racism, historical redlining, and risk of preterm birth in New York City, 2013–2017. *American Journal of Public Health*, 110(7), 1046–1053. https://doi.org/10.2105/ajph.2020.305656

Lachowycz, K., & Jones, A. P. (2014). Does walking explain associations between access to greenspace and lower mortality? *Social Science & Medicine*, 107(100), 9–17. https://doi.org/10.1016/j.socscimed.2014.02.023

Landrigan, P. J., Rauh, V. A., & Galvez, M. P. (2010). Environmental justice and the health of children. *The Mount Sinai Journal of Medicine*, 77(2), 178–187. https://doi.org/10.1002/msj.20173

Lane, T. S., Sonderegger, D. L., Holeva-Eklund, W. M., Brazendale, K., Behrens, T. K., Howdeshell, H., Walka, S., Cook, J. R., & de Heer, H. D. (2021). Seasonal variability in weight gain among American Indian, Black, White, and Hispanic children: A 3.5-year study. *American Journal of Preventive Medicine*. https://doi.org/10.1016/j.amepre.2020.12.010

Lavigne, É., Talarico, R., van Donkelaar, A., Martin, R. V., Stieb, D. M., Crighton, E., Weichenthal, S., Smith-Doiron, M., Burnett, R. T., & Chen, H. (2021). Fine particulate matter concentration and composition and the incidence of childhood asthma. *Environment International*, 152, 106486. https://doi.org/10.1016/j.envint.2021.106486

Liddell, J. L., & Kingdon, S. G. (2021). "Something was attacking them and their reproductive organs": Environmental reproductive justice in an indigenous tribe in the United States Gulf coast. *International Journal of Environmental Research and Public Health*, 18(2), 666. https://doi.org/10.3390/ijerph18020666

Liu, J., Potter, T., & Zahner, S. (2020). Policy brief on climate change and mental health/wellbeing. *Nursing Outlook*, 68(4), 517–522. https://doi.org/10.1016/j.outlook.2020.06.003

Ma, C., & Smith, T. (2020). Vulnerability of renters and low-income households to storm damage: Evidence from Hurricane Maria in Puerto Rico. *American Journal of Public Health*, 110(2), 196–202. https://doi.org/10.2105/AJPH.2019.305438

Madrigal, D., Claustro, M., Wong, M., Bejarano, E., Olmedo, L., & English, P. (2020). Developing youth environmental health literacy and civic leadership through community air monitoring in

Imperial County, California. *International Journal of Environmental Research and Public Health, 17*(5), 1537. https://doi.org/10.3390/ijerph17051537

McOliver, C. A., Camper, A. K., Doyle, J. T., Eggers, M. J., Ford, T. E., Lila, M. A., Berner, J., Campbell, L., & Donatuto, J. (2015). Community-based research as a mechanism to reduce environmental health disparities in American Indian and Alaska native communities. *International Journal of Environmental Research and Public Health, 12*(4), 4076–4100. https://doi.org/10.3390/ijerph120404076

Menton, M., Larrea, C., Latorre, S. et al. (2020). Environmental justice and the SDGs: From synergies to gaps and contradictions. *Sustainable Science, 15*, 1621–1636. https://doi.org/10.1007/s11625

Merchant, J., Coussens, C., Gilbert, D. (Eds.) (2006). Rebuilding the unity of health and the environment in rural America: Workshop summary. National Academies Press. https://www.nap.edu/catalog/11596/rebuilding-the-unity-of-health-and-the-environment-in-ruraamerica

MHP Salud. (2014). Farmworkers in the United States. https://mhpsalud.org/who-we-serve/farmworkers-in-the-united-states/

Miller, J. D., Workman, C. L., Panchang, S. V., Sneegas, G., Adams, E. A., Young, S. L., & Thompson, A. L. (2021). Water security and nutrition: Current knowledge and research opportunities. *Advances in Nutrition (Bethesda, Md.), 12*(6), 2525–2539. https://doi.org/10.1093/advances/nmab075

Mitchell, G., Norman, P., & Mullin, K. (2015). Who benefits from environmental policy? An Environmental Justice Analysis of air Quality Change in Britain, 2001–2011. *Environmental Research Letters, 10*, 105009.

National Resource Defense Council. (2019). Transforming local policies to achieve environmental justice. Author. https://www.nrdc.org/sites/default/files/transforming-local-policies-achieve-environmental-justice-fs.pdf

Nardi, D., Waite, R., Nowak, M., Hatcher, B., Hines-Martin, V., & Stacciarini, J. R. (2020). Achieving health equity through eradicating structural racism in the United States: A call to action for nursing leadership. *Journal of Nursing Scholarship, 52*(6), 696–704. https://doi.org/10.1111/jnu.12602

Nardone, A., Rudolph, K. E., Morello-Frosch, R., & Casey, J. A. (2021). Redlines and greenspace: The relationship between historical redlining and 2010 greenspace across the United States. *Environmental Health Perspectives, 129*(1), 17006.

National Human Genome Research Institute. (n.d.). https://www.genome.gov/27549400/the-human-microbiome-project-extending-the-definition-of-what-constitutes-a-human

New York Times. (2021). As Ida deaths rise, N.Y. leaders look toward future storms. https://www.nytimes.com/live/2021/09/03/nyregion/nyc-flooding-ida

NRDC. (2020). https://www.nrdc.org/stories/environmental-justice-chicago-its-been-one-battle-after-another

O'Brien, D. T., Farrell, C., & Welsh, B. C. (2019). Broken (windows) theory: A meta-analysis of the evidence for the pathways from neighborhood disorder to resident health outcomes and behaviors. *Social Science & Medicine, 228*, 272–292. https://doi.org/10.1016/j.socscimed.2018.11.015

Owens-Young, J. (2018). Being born in the wrong ZIP code can shorten your life. The Conversation. https://theconversation.com/being-born-in-the-wrong-zip-code-can-shorten-your-life-104037

Oyarzo-Miranda, C., Latorre, N., Meynard, A., Rivas, J., Bulboa, C., & Contreras-Porcia, L. (2020). Coastal pollution from the industrial park Quintero Bay of central Chile: Effects on abundance, morphology, and development of the kelp Lessonia spicata (Phaeophyceae). *PLoS One, 15*(10), e0240581. https://doi.org/10.1371/journal.pone.0240581

Pahl, J. (2020, October 26). The detrimental impact of suburban sprawl on the environment. The Organization for World Peace. https://theowp.org/reports/the-detrimental-impact-of-suburban-sprawl-on-the-environment/

Paranzino, G. K., Butterfield, P., Nastoff, T., & Ranger, C. (2005). I prepare: Development and clinical utility of an environmental exposure history mnemonic. *AAOHN Journal, 53*(1), 37–42.

Practice Greenhealth. https://practicegreenhealth.org/

Qu, Y. M., Chen, S., Li, J. J., Jin, R. R., Pan, H., & Jiang, Y. (2017). *Zhonghua liu xing bing xue za zhi = Zhonghua liuxingbingxue zazhi. Relationship Between Pesticide Exposure and Adverse Pregnancy Outcomes among Reproductive Couples in Rural Areas of China, 38*(6), 732–736. https://doi.org/10.3760/cma.j.issn.0254-6450.2017.06.008

Robert Wood Johnson Foundation. (n.d.). Culture of health action framework. https://www.rwjf.org/en/cultureofhealth/taking-action.html

Rosner, D. (2016). Injurious inequalities. *The Milbank Quarterly, 94*(1), 47–50. https://doi.org/10.1111/1468-0009.12179

Ruckart, P. Z., Ettinger, A. S., Hanna-Attisha, M., Jones, N., Davis, S. I., & Breysse, P. N. (2019). The flint water crisis: A coordinated public health emergency response and recovery initiative. *Journal of Public Health Management and Practice, 25*(suppl 1), S84–S90. https://doi.org/10.1097/PHH.0000000000000871

Sallis, J. F. (2009). Measuring physical activity environments: A brief history. *American Journal of Preventive Medicine*, 36(4), S86–S92.

Sattler B. (2019). Farmworkers: Environmental health and social determinants. *Annual Review of Nursing Research*, 38(1), 203–222. https://doi.org/10.1891/0739-6686.38.203

Schwartz, A., & McClure, K. (2021). The rental assistance demonstration program and its current and projected consumption of low-income housing tax credits. *Cityscape*, 23(2), 9–26. https://www.huduser.gov/portal/periodicals/cityscpe/vol23num2/ch1.pdf

Sefcik, J. S., Kondo, M. C., Klusaritz, H., Sarantschin, E., Solomon, S., Roepke, A., South, E. C., & Jacoby, S. F. (2019). Perceptions of nature and access to green space in four urban neighborhoods. *International Journal of Environmental Research and Public Health*, 16(13), 2313. https://doi.org/10.3390%2Fijerph16132313

Shavers, V. L. (2007). Measurement of socioeconomic status in health disparities research. *Journal of the National Medical Association*, 99(9), 1013–1023.

Sierra Club. (2021). Michigan chapter: Stopping existing CAFOS. https://www.sierraclub.org/michigan/stopping-existing-cafos

Strosnider, H., Kennedy, C., Monti, M., Yip, F. (2017). Rural and urban differences in air quality, 2008–2012, and community drinking water quality, 2010–2015—United States. *MMWR Surveillance Summary*, 66(SS-13), 1–10. http://doi.org/10.15585/mmwr.ss6613a1

Szanton, S. L., & Gill, J. M. (2010). Facilitating resilience using a society-to-cells framework: A theory of nursing essentials applied to research and practice. *Advances in Nursing Science*, 33(4), 329–343.

Terry, L., Bowman, K., & West, R. (2019). Becoming and being an environmentally 'woke' nurse: A phenomenological study. *Nursing Outlook*, 67(6), 725–733. https://doi.org/10.1016/j.outlook.2019.04.011

The Lancet Planetary Health. (2018). Environmental racism: Time to tackle social injustice. *The Lancet: Planetary Health*, 2(11), e462. https://doi.org/10.1016/S2542-5196(18)30219-5

The Lancet. (2020, January 27). The lancet planetary health: Discriminatory redlining practices in the 1930s associated with present-day rates of emergency department visits due to asthma. https://www.eurekalert.org/pub_releases/2020-01/tl-pss012720.php

The Medical Society Consortium on Climate and Health. https://medsocietiesforclimatehealth.org/

Thompson, A. (2019, June 1). Minorities breathe more than their share of polluted air. https://www.scientificamerican.com/article/minorities-breathe-more-than-their-share-of-polluted-air/

Tilburg W. C. (2017). Policy approaches to improving housing and health. *The Journal of Law, Medicine & Ethics*, 45(suppl 1), 90–93. https://doi.org/10.1177/1073110517703334

U.S. Census Bureau. (2019). Quick facts: United States. https://www.census.gov/quickfacts/fact/table/US/IPE120219

U.S. Department of Housing and Urban Development. (n.d.). https://www.hud.gov/

United Nations Department of Economic and Social Affairs. (2022). Sustainable development goals 2022. https://unstats.un.org/sdgs/report/2022/

U.S. Environmental Protection Agency. (n.d.). Office of environmental justice. https://www.epa.gov/environmentaljustice

U.S. Environmental Protection Agency. (2020). Reduce urban heat island effect. https://www.epa.gov/green-infrastructure/reduce-urban-heat-island-effect

Urban Institute. (n.d.). Reducing the racial homeownership gap. https://www.urban.org/policy-centers/housing-finance-policy-center/projects/reducing-racial-homeownership-gap

Vardoulakis, S., Dear, K., & Wilkinson, P. (2016). Challenges and opportunities for urban environmental health and sustainability: The HEALTHY-POLIS initiative. *Environmental Health*, 15(suppl 1), 30. https://doi.org/10.1186/s12940-016-0096-1

Ward, M., Schulz, A. J., Israel, B. A., Rice, K., Martenies, S. E., & Markarian, E. (2018). A conceptual framework for evaluating health equity promotion within community-based participatory research partnerships. *Evaluation and Program Planning*, 70, 25–34. https://doi.org/10.1016/j.evalprogplan.2018.04.014

Williams, D. R., & Cooper, L. A. (2019). Reducing racial inequities in health: Using what we already know to take action. *International Journal of Environmental Research and Public Health*, 16(4), 606. https://doi.org/10.3390/ijerph16040606

Williams, D. R., Lawrence, J. A., & Davis, B. A. (2019). Racism and health: Evidence and needed research. *Annual Review of Public Health*, 40, 105–125. https://doi.org/10.1146/annurev-publhealth-040218-043750

Williamson, D., Yu, E. X., Hunter, C. M., Kaufman, J. A., Komro, K., Jelks, N. O., Johnson, D. A., Gribble, M. O., & Kegler, M. C. (2020). A scoping review of capacity-building efforts to address environmental justice concerns. *International Journal of Environmental Research and Public Health*, 17(11), 3765. https://doi.org/10.3390/ijerph17113765

Wing, S., & Johnston, J. (2014). Industrial hog operations in North Carolina disproportionately impact African-Americans, hispanics, and American Indians. The University of North Carolina at Chapel Hill. https://www.ncpolicywatch.com/wp-content/uploads/2014/09/UNC-Report.pdf

World Health Organization. (2017). Urban green space interventions and health: Review of impacts and effectiveness. https://www.euro.who.int/__data/assets/pdf_file/0010/337690/FULL -REPORT-for-LLP.pdf

World Health Organization Commission on Social Determinants of Health, & World Health Organization. (2008). Closing the gap in a generation: Health equity through action on the social determinants of health: Commission on Social Determinants of Health final report. World Health Organization.

Wu, C. Y. H., Evans, M. B., Wolff, P. E., & Gohlke, J. M. (2017). Environmental health priorities of residents and environmental health professionals: Implications for improving environmental health services in rural versus urban communities. *Journal of Environmental Health*, *80*(5), 28–36.

Wu, X., Lu, Y., Zhou, S., Chen, L., & Xu, B. (2016). Impact of climate change on human infectious diseases: Empirical evidence and human adaptation. *Environment International*, *86*, 14–23. https://doi.org/10.1016/j.envint.2015.09.007

Zheng, X. Y., Orellano, P., Lin, H. L., Jiang, M., & Guan, W. J. (2021). Short-term exposure to ozone, nitrogen dioxide, and sulphur dioxide and emergency department visits and hospital admissions due to asthma: A systematic review and meta-analysis. *Environment International*, *150*, 106435. https://doi.org/10.1016/j.envint.2021.106435

CHAPTER 20

Adverse Childhood Experiences: What Is an Ounce of Prevention Worth?

Mona Hassan and Faye A. Gary

LEARNING OBJECTIVES

- Examine recent patterns of health behaviors among adolescents in the United States in relation to risky behaviors, diet, health habits, sexual activities, and suicidal behaviors.

- Explain the impact of adverse childhood experiences (ACEs) across the life course.

- Analyze the features of ACEs concerning strategies that can be used in the prevention and cure of this societal tragedy.

- Discuss the origins and outcomes of mandatory reporting and the role of healthcare workers in this endeavor.

- Examine the difficulties and challenges encountered in dealing with child abuse victims, particularly child sexual abuse victims.

- Evaluate the profound effects of living in poverty and relate this dilemma to redlining policies and practices.

- Elucidate the far-reaching impact of education on well-being outcomes.

INTRODUCTION

Having access to healthcare is an essential component in the overall health status of all population groups. Many nations have developed and provided public health systems based on the premise that good health is a basic human right. In contrast to other economically and technologically advanced nations, the United States has a system that confers responsibility upon the individual to acquire access to fee-based private and government-funded health systems (e.g., healthcare benefits that are available to select employees; Medicare and Medicaid benefits provided to persons with disabilities and to older adults; Kiprop, 2018; Shvili, 2020).

The United States is the only country in the developed world that does not provide universal healthcare (Kiprop, 2018; Shvili, 2020). Differences in resources, laws, practices, and cultures at the state and local levels dictate who gets the goods and services and at what cost, thus influencing health outcomes (Miller et al., 2014; Shultz et al., 2021). The health of adolescents is linked to our nation's political system and the type of health structures that it provides. The mental health of children and adolescents is a key public health concern that encompasses prevention of illness and treatment of mental health conditions (Youth.gov, 2021).

Mental health promotion involves interventions designed to enhance the overall quality of life. The goal of prevention is to strengthen the overall mental health status of a group or population. The desired outcome is the reduction of future mental health problems at all levels (Miles et al., 2010). Prevention of mental health problems employs prompt and efficient interventions that target the determining factors of mental health issues before they become problems among individuals, families, communities, and populations (Miles et al., 2010; Patton et al., 2018; Satcher, 2020; Shultz et al., 2021). The purpose of this chapter is to illuminate the devasting impact of adverse childhoon experiences (ACEs). We will examine the domino effects of laws and policies that promote redlining (defining neighborhood borders according to social class), perpetuate poverty, and deprive individuals and families of education, employment, and health. These factors, combined with family dysfunction, disease, and unsafe surroundings, can have devastating effects on the lives of youth that are often manifested across the life course.

ADOLESCENT HEALTH

Adolescence and early adulthood (ages 16–24 years) represent the period of growth and development embedded with more potential changes and impactful decision-making than any other period in the life course. Physical and neurological developments accelerate, and brain function expands along with the extension of cognitive capacities. Extreme stress in children's and adolescents' lives can bring about physical changes in the brain structure through the expression of genes embedded in the individual's DNA, including impaired cognitive and neurological outcomes (Romeo, 2017). In addition, prenatal stress may alter fetal development and increase the risk of childhood respiratory disorders (Rosa et al., 2018). The intersectionality between early childhood hardships and future growth and development should be a core element in the overall approach to the protection of children and adolescents (Felitti et al., 2019; Ghebreyesus, 2020; Patton et al., 2018; Sciaraffa et al., 2018; Shultz et al., 2021).

Peers have dominating influences over the daily activities of adolescents. New relationships created during late adolescence and early adulthood often result in decreased connection to the family of origin. Adolescents are expected to pursue secondary and postsecondary education or vocational/technical training, acquire alternate living arrangements/negotiate remaining at home, woo and win partners for permanent relationships, and perhaps establish their own families. They are responsible for their social and emotional learning and their behaviors within the context of legal, political, and social norms (Patton et al., 2018; Shultz et al., 2021; Tang et al., 2019; Weiss-Laxer et al., 2020).

Across the global community and at every level in American society, unprecedented changes influence the future of youth. The timing of and quality of parenting and access to essentials such as education and healthcare are notable investments in this group. Adolescents are the largest cohort in history. From every perspective, they will profoundly impact the outcome of future generations (Patton et al., 2018).

ADVERSE CHILDHOOD EXPERIENCES

What follows is a focus on the ACEs study, which examined the impact of childhood abuse and neglect and other challenges on the health and well-being of individuals throughout the life course. Household dysfunction and experiences of abuse during childhood have been correlated with detrimental health outcomes in adulthood. Research studies have disclosed that early exposure to negative experiences can create antecedents that facilitate the development of undesirable long-term physical and psychological outcomes (Commission on Social Determinants of Health, 2008; Deighton et al., 2018; Felitti et al., 2019; Kalmakis & Chandler, 2015; Patton et al., 2018; Sciaraffa et al., 2018; Shultz et al., 2021; Weiss-Laxer et al., 2020). Such outcomes might include drug abuse, alcohol abuse, depression, suicide, bullying, interpersonal violence, and other maladaptive and risk-taking behaviors. Heart disease, respiratory problems, cancer, lung disease, skeletal fractures, liver disease, diabetes, obesity, and other maladies are also anticipated consequences (Figure 20.1).

Over the past few decades, research and practice data have posited that ACEs-related early life experiences among children have a lasting and harmful impact on their lives that is evident across the life course until death. The ACEs study is one of the largest research projects that has ever occurred in the United States investigating childhood abuse and neglect and household challenges that influence health outcomes and overall well-being in later life (Murphy et al., 2014). The effort was a collaboration between the Centers for Disease Control and Prevention (CDC) and the Kaiser Permanente Health Clinical Clinic, San Diego. Eighty-one percent of the participants were age 25 years or older. The three categories of childhood abuse included were psychological abuse, physical abuse, and contact sexual assault. The research survey included four categories related to overall household dysfunction during the early years of life: exposure to substance abuse; presence of someone in the home with mental illness; violent treatment of mother or stepmother; and one question about criminal

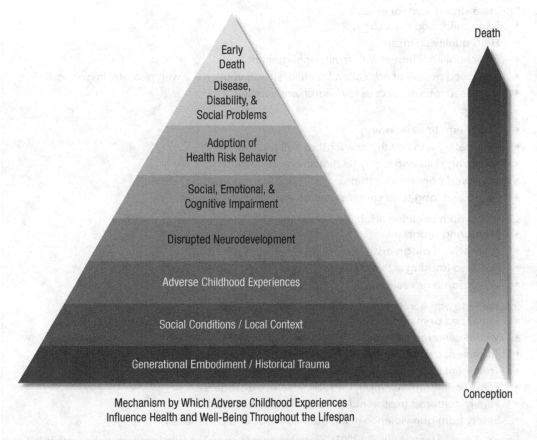

Figure 20.1 The Adverse Childhood Experiences (ACEs) pyramid.

Source: Centers for Disease Control and Prevention. (2020). *About the CDC-Kaiser ACEs study: The ACEs pyramid.* http://www.cdc.gov/violenceprevention/aces/about.html.

behavior (Felitti, 2019; Felitti et al., 2019; Shultz et al., 2021; Zarse et al., 2019). This and other research studies have documented the deleterious impact that ACEs have on children that are manifested throughout the entire span of life. Personal health behaviors, such as smoking, risky sexual behaviors, interpersonal violence, separation, and divorce, are among a plethora of health conditions that have been linked to ACEs (Assari et al., 2019; Case & Deaton, 2021a, 2021b; Deighton et al., 2018; Felitti et al., 2019; Fiocco et al., 2007; Horowitz, 2018; Murphy et al., 2014; O'Keefe et al., 2018; Park et al., 2019; Saito et al., 2018; Sciaraffa et al., 2018; Shultz et al., 2021; Skalamera & Hummer, 2016; Zajacova & Lawrence, 2018; Zarse et al., 2019). See Box 20.1 for a list of steps to help prevent ACEs.

BOX 20.1: An Ounce of Prevention for Adverse Childhood Experiences

Strengthen economic support to children and families.
- Strengthen household financial security.
- Improve family-friendly work policies.

Promote social norms that protect against violence and adversity.
- Public education campaigns.
- Legislative approaches to reduce corporal punishment.
- Bystander approaches.
- Men and boys as allies in prevention.
- Building safety and resource equity among neighborhoods.

Ensure a strong start for children.
- Early childhood education.
- High-quality childcare.
- Preschool enrichment with family engagement.
- Improved quality of education for children and youth K-12 with parental involvement.
- Increased internet access to children and families.

Teach skills.
- Social-emotional learning.
- Safe dating and healthy relationship skill programs.
- Parenting skills and family relationship approaches.
- Improved peer relationships.
- Short- and long-term career-planning approaches.

Connect youth to caring adults and activities.
- Mentoring programs.
- After-school programs.
- Focused tutoring activities.
- Wholesome recreation.

Intervene to ameliorate immediate and long-term harms.
- Enhanced primary care.
- Victim-centered services.
- Treatment to mitigate the harms of ACEs.
- Treatment to prevent problem behavior and future involvement in violence.
- Family-centered treatment for substance use disorders.
- Family-centered treatment for mental health disorders.
- Safety from gun violence in the home, school, and community.

Source: Adapted from Hursh, D. (2007). Exacerbating inequality: The failed promise of the no child left behind act. *Race, Ethnicity and Education*, 10, 295–308. https://doi.org/10.1080/13613320701503264.

NARRATIVE 20.1: A PSYCHIATRIC-MENTAL HEALTH NURSE PRACTITIONER'S ACCOUNT OF TEEN PATIENT

Brianna was a 16-year-old female patient admitted to an inpatient psychiatric unit for depression and suicidal behaviors. During my initial interview with Brianna, she revealed that the possible root of her depression stemmed from a history of sexual abuse. The death of her grandfather, who had been her abuser—and her caregiver/babysitter—triggered this depressive episode with suicidal behaviors and a variety of intermittent somatic symptoms. During the clinical interview, Brianna shared that her grandfather had sexually assaulted her from the time she was 8 years old until she turned 15. The experience made her feel as if there were something wrong with her. After all, even though she hated the abuse, she also loved her grandfather. After his death, she missed him, and psychiatric symptoms began to emerge.

Brianna could not understand how she could care for someone who had sexually abused her for so many years. She also blamed herself because, believing that she was "special" like her grandfather told her, she recalled enjoying the extra attention he gave her and the little gifts he shared with her. He had also admonished Brianna that their relationship was a secret and that she should never tell anyone. Brianna wanted to tell someone, but she had made a promise to her grandfather, and he was good to her. Although she was the child victim, she verbalized that she believed that she was the perpetrator because she allowed the abuse to happen year after year. Brianna also became suspicious of her grandfather's interest in a younger cousin whom he would "babysit" from time to time. She began to wonder if there would be another victim in her family. She also feared that he was losing interest in her. These were dangerous thoughts, and Brianna could not allow herself to think about these possibilities.

This clinical encounter left me, her nurse, with a myriad of emotions, including anger, disgust, revulsion, and sadness. I began to think about the family dynamics that maintained this relationship for more than 7 years. Initially, I couldn't fathom how this young girl could feel responsible for being a victim and blaming herself for her grandfather's devastating sexually abusive behavior. Brianna's story is like that of many others who experience sexual abuse, although most never share their story. Hard as it may be, sharing is the first step to recovery. Brianna has committed to working on her problems. I will be there to assist with her healing.

Mandatory Reporting Requirements for Child Maltreatment

One of the most significant public-generated policy initiatives occurred in 1962, when Kempe et al. (1962, 1985) advocated for mandatory reporting of child maltreatment. They asserted that child maltreatment was continuing to negatively impact the lives of children who were under the care of parents who were disturbed and unable to care for their children. They successfully advocated for mandatory reporting of egregious acts by all health professionals. Three years later, all states had instituted mechanisms for reporting child maltreatment (Melton, 2005; Murray & Gesiriech, 2004). Over the years, laws and protocols have been enacted, and best practices continue to evolve. Some issues that have emerged include lack of resources to adequately detect and monitor child maltreatment cases, concerns that some groups might conceal egregious acts due to fear of losing control over their child, and inadequacy of intervention strategies to address the concerns in the here and now and long term (Drake & Jonson-Reid, 2015; Lindenmeyer, 1997; Melton, 2005; Murray & Gesiriech, 2004). Child maltreatment remains a significant problem, and additional action is needed (Felitti, 2019; Felitti et al., 2019; Patton et al., 2018).

Precursor of Mandated Reporting

Competing narratives exist about how, in 1874, the state of New York used animal cruelty laws to remove a young girl, Mary Ellen Wilson, from her stepmother's home, where she had been beaten and abused daily. Perhaps the misinformation is related to the quagmire of agencies and agents that reported on their various roles as her tragedy unfolded. The most credible version affirms that the extrication of Mary Ellen from the home where she was subjected to daily abuse required collaboration from a valiant cohort that was made up of concerned neighbors; a missionary; a case worker; the head of the American Society for the Prevention of Cruelty to Animals (ASPCA), an individual who later became the attorney for the ASPCA; and a sympathetic judge in the New York Supreme Court. It took several attempts by concerned parties to find the correct authorities who would be willing to tackle Mary Ellen's case because jurisdiction over incidents of child abuse had not yet been clearly designated, nor were there explicit protocols for action. In part, this perilous course of events occurred because child welfare advocates in New York City had been reluctant to intervene, believing that parents and guardians had the unequivocal basic right to discipline their children. That Mary Ellen's guardian was eventually sentenced to 1 year in a penitentiary was a historic event itself because children, as property of their father, were expected to provide labor to offset the burdensome inconvenience of their existence (Jalongo, 2006; Murray & Gesiriech, 2004; Schuman, 2017; Watkins, 1990). Mary Ellen Wilson's case marked a turning point in history; it spawned such outrage among the citizens of New York that finally, in 1874, the New York Society for the Prevention of Cruelty to Children was founded (New York Society for the Prevention of Cruelty to Children, n.d.).

In 1962, another essential milestone occurred when an influential article was published in the *Journal of the American Medical Association* by Kempe et al. (1962, 1985) insisting that "battered child syndrome" be recognized as a medical diagnosis. This syndrome is described as a compilation of injuries that are the result of continued maltreatment or beatings (e.g., bone fractures, failure to thrive, bruises and other soft tissue injuries, even death—particularly when the child dies without a history of previous illness). Kempe (1975) emphasized that the dangers of battered child syndrome could persist over time; internalizing and externalizing behaviors are likely to follow, setting off a chain reaction of long-term negative outcomes. During the later developmental years, drug use, depression, anxiety, and suicidal thoughts may emerge; in addition, engagement in illegal, violent, and/or risky behaviors is a likely repercussion of the battered child syndrome (Greengard, 1964; Kempe, 1975; Kempe et al., 1962/1985; Levesque, 2011).

Over the next 10 years, most states refined laws against child abuse and neglect and mandated reporting. Professionals, including nurses, physicians, and teachers, are currently required to report any suspected child abuse or neglect to law enforcement agencies. These professionals are protected from retaliation by the accused when conforming to the mandatory reporting law (Texas Department of Family and Protective Services, 2020).

Another important concept, the "world of abnormal rearing (W.A.R.)," was coined in 1968 by Helfer (Helfer, 1987; Helfer et al., 1999). W.A.R. pertains to adults who have not acquired sufficient basic skills to interact with others in a normal, mature manner. It manifests as a reduplicating cycle, with attitudes and behaviors being perpetuated from one generation to the next, and to the next. Basically, W.A.R. children, from the moment of their conception, are expected to fulfill unmet needs of the parent. The emerging role of the W.A.R. child is to parent their own parent. The W.A.R. child who fails in this regard ends up being resented and is denied a nurturing environment. Child maltreatment is a condition that must be nipped in the bud, and devastating consequences must be eliminated (Greengard, 1964; Hayes, 1988; Helfer, 1987, Helfer et al., 1999). The parents of W.A.R. children may sometimes benefit from counseling or strategies learned in groups like Parents Anonymous (Helfer, 1987, Helfer et al., 1999). Attention must be given to children and adolescents who are caught in this behavioral maelstrom; healthy coping behaviors, age-appropriate communications, and plans for a productive future should be the prevailing blueprint.

In 1974, federal law directed states to provide shelter and protective services for abused children and families. Unfortunately, these services only come into play *after* the abuse, if then. Child maltreatment remains a major public health problem (CDC, 2019; World Health Organization [WHO], 2021). On many occasions, perpetrators of child sexual abuse are acquaintances known to the child victims. This is a troubling reality that delays the disclosure of maltreatment and complicates prosecution, as superficial genital injuries in children heal rapidly—usually within 3 to 4 days—leaving limited residual physical evidence (Alaggia et al., 2019; Hassan et al., 2020).

It has been established that victims are best served by a multidisciplinary collaboration of healthcare professionals, including physicians, nurses, and social workers, who have been trained to investigate abuse (Annapragada et al., 2021). Well-trained professional nurses who have advanced educational and mentoring experience in child sexual assault play an essential role in detection and intervention and in the appropriate use of community health services. For sexual abuse, forensic nurse examiners and sexual assault nurse examiners (SANEs) are specially trained experts who provide 24/7 services to children and their families. The primary responsibilities of SANEs include first-response crisis intervention and forensic medical examinations for children, adolescents, and adult male and female victims (Chandramani et al., 2020).

Sexual abuse disclosure is an unpredictable event influenced by many variables, including age, gender, and psychological and social factors. Children may delay disclosure of sexual abuse for many reasons: fear of not being believed, perpetrator threats (including threats to the child and their loved ones), or other forms of psychological abuse from adults in their environments (Hassan et al., 2015a; Morrison et al., 2018). The perpetrator's relationship to the child and the perpetrator's psychological and sociodemographic profile often prevail upon the experience of the sexually abused victim. A child's gender and age may also color sexual abuse experiences. Younger child victims present less frequently with vaginal injuries and more frequently with anal injuries than older child victims (Hassan et al., 2020). Male child victims are more likely to experience anal penis and finger penetration, whereas female child victims experience more mouth contact to their genitalia and body kisses (Hassan et al., 2015b). It is essential to identify the effects of everyday perpetrator activities and profiles to help sexually abused victims and their families cope with the physical and psychological aftereffects of abuse (Felitti et al., 2019; van Delft et al., 2015).

According to the National Children's Alliance, about 700,000 children in the United States are abused each year. The general perception among the experts is that child maltreatment is underreported. In 2017, child welfare and protection agencies conducted more than 3.5 million investigations and interventions; nearly 2 million children were provided protective services. Child sexual abuse is the most common type of maltreatment (National Children's Alliance, 2021). The primary goal, however, is to prevent sexual abuse from ever occurring. More data about the social and behavioral determinants of child sexual abuse could help nurses and other healthcare professionals identify vulnerable children and their families and provide appropriate interventions (Hassan et al., 2015a; Sciaraffa et al., 2018).

CASE STUDY 20.1: STORIES OF TWO SEXUALLY ABUSED CHILDREN

Kathy's Story

Kathy (not her real name) is a 9-year-old girl. She was admitted to the emergency department because of alleged sexual abuse. When the SANE asked her how the perpetrator started his acts, the child responded, "When he was mad at Mommy, he would tell me that he would take me away to another country and marry me." The SANE asked, "What country?" Kathy responded, "I don't know, but what country is going to let a kid get married? He told us if we have sex with him, we won't get AIDS. He tried to put his penis in my butt, but there were a lot of people running around making noise and it scared him. He said this was our

(continued)

CASE STUDY 20.1: STORIES OF TWO SEXUALLY ABUSED CHILDREN (*CONTINUED*)

secret. He said sex was an experience. He said he wanted to have sex with me when I was older. He makes us hold his penis when he goes to pee in the toilet" (Hassan et al., 2015a).

Lauren's Story

Lauren (not her real name) is an 8-year-old girl. During the interview, the SANE asked the child if she knew why she was in the emergency department. The child victim said, "For a checkup, because my brother touched me." The SANE asked, "How did he touch you?" Lauren responded, "He put his privates in mine." The SANE then asked, "Can you show me with your hand where?" Lauren took her index finger and placed it in her crotch. This victim was very fidgety, and was having trouble giving a proper history of the abuse, so the SANE engaged the child in a conversation on a different topic. The child victim said she cried when she found out that her brother was going to jail. She said she had tried to push him off her really hard (Hassan et al., 2015a).

Discussion

Kathy's responses to the SANE's concerns were informative. She was aware that the interaction was inappropriate and commented about the perpetrator's remark about marriage in another county one day. Kathy had also identified the family dynamics under which the sexual acts were likely to occur, such as the perpetrator's anger toward his partner, Kathy's mother.

From the perpetrator's perspective, keeping secrets is important, but families can also have a stake in helping to keep the secret a secret. Secret keeping in families can be examined through an intersectionality approach. Briefly, the survivor is in a position that creates feelings called the "pressure cooker effect," which produces the dilemma of wanting to tell the story, but this need becomes overshadowed by not feeling safe enough to set off a bombshell (McElvaney et al., 2012). The struggle is exacerbated by the need to avoid blame, to find someone who would understand the experience, and to trust that comfort will come from having revealed the secret. This can be a daunting endeavor for anyone, especially a young child or adolescent. Some of the dynamics that influence revealing or keeping the secret include:

◆ Identifying the right person—a trusted confidant—with whom the secret can be shared.
◆ Assessing family and community characteristics to determine the stability or capacity of the family/community to accept the information and respond in a facilitating manner. Potential reactions to disclosure can range from being helpful and engaging to shaming, blaming, and other negative attitudes and behaviors.
◆ Being constrained by religious dogma, practices, and taboos.
◆ Fear of legal consequences.
◆ Fear of retaliation from the perpetrator or anyone whose allegiance lies with the perpetrator.

Delaying disclosure is associated with avoiding physical and emotional harm and with the lack of a trusted confidant with whom to communicate the devastating event. Some individuals might not ever disclose the secret, while others may share bits and pieces of the experience over time. Some victims may not share the experience until years or even decades later when situations threaten the once-buried secret, which surfaces during child, family, and marriage therapy sessions initiated to address other antecedent events (Tener, 2018).

(*continued*)

CASE STUDY 20.1: STORIES OF TWO SEXUALLY ABUSED CHILDREN (*CONTINUED*)

Lauren's conversation with the SANE occurred in a private and safe place. She was frightened and did not know what to expect during the clinical encounter; embedded in the reporting of sexual abuse and other types of child maltreatment are concerns about shaming and blaming. The shaming comes with the sense that others might not believe them, thus placing responsibility for the act upon the victim. Lauren expressed feelings of shame. She did not have the vocabulary to fully explain the incident, but she tried. Her feelings of remorse related to her brother's pending incarceration heightened the burden of blame she carried for the abuse, even though she had attempted to foil his attempt by pushing him away.

In addition to a physical examination and documentation of clinical findings is the need for a culturally informed, age-specific psychological assessment; this could be facilitated within the context of the Minority Health and Health Disparities Research Framework (Alvidrez et al., 2019; see Chapter 5, Figure 5.4). Despite such devastating experiences, there are opportunities for healing. Quality healthcare creates a probability that education centered on the prevention and early detection of critical health issues in specific communities would be therapeutic. A focused approach highlighting children, youth, and their families could evolve into a community-based program. Importantly, healthcare providers are needed who present themselves as empathetic, caring, and knowledgeable; who have proactive attitudes and behaviors; who are natural advocates; and who are willing to serve as informed confidants for children and their families. School-based intervention programs guided by social workers, counselors, psychologists, and physicians are proven options. Nurse-centered health clinics addressing a holistic approach to health and illness are also ideal options.

Case Study Questions

1. Regarding safe home environments and adequate supervision, how would you begin to unravel the perpetrator's access to the child in the home? What additional information would be helpful to know when interviewing Kathy's mother?
2. What are some essential considerations that should be addressed when interacting with children and youth who report to a health facility or a school clinic with complaints about the occurrence of "issues" that are potentially harmful to them?
3. How could social media be used to expand new methods for disseminating health information, providing interventions for improving health behaviors, and reducing violence and risks that are harmful to the self and others?
4. Do you think Lauren should receive additional counseling regarding her feelings of shame and blame related to her brother's impending incarceration?

POVERTY

One of the most devastating influences on the lives of children and adolescents—and families—is poverty. It affects most of the lived experiences that ensue and is likely to impact the person's well-being for a lifetime (see Figure 20.1). Adverse components of poverty are multifaceted and include risks for biological and neurocognitive development, inadequate nutrition, multiple stressors related to familial and physical environmental challenges, and exposure to pathogens. Parenting practices are seldom optimal, with poverty becoming physically, biologically, and psychologically transmitted from one generation to the next. Among low-resourced communities and families, health promotion, prevention, and treatment are scarce and, in some instances, nonexistent (Jensen et al., 2017; Marmot et al., 2008;

Minh et al., 2017). One pathway to alternative outcomes involves advanced education and technical and vocational training and skills.

It is essential to better understand the historical and current dynamics that helped to create societal structures that proliferate and maintain poverty and poor health outcomes. The Home Owners' Loan Corporation, initiated in 1933, created descriptions of properties across the nation through the compilation of data organized by local real estate developers, lenders, and appraisers. From the generated data, a grading system was developed and later visualized on maps through a process called *redlining*. The name comes from the practice of drawing red lines around the perimeters of neighborhoods inhabited by marginalized and minority populations (e.g., immigrants and African, Asian, Jewish, Italian, Hispanic, and Native Americans).

As seen in Figure 20.2, the A grade represented neighborhoods that were categorized as low risk with good mortgage security. The D grade indicated that the area was inhabited by "hazardous, subversive, undesirable, low grade populations" (Federal Housing Administration, 1936). Due to the preordained assumption of high-risk of loan foreclosure, persons in the grade D redlined districts have been categorically blocked from obtaining home loans. These federally supported practices were the instruments used in the creation of a nation-wide system that prohibited or severely limited the capacity for people in some of the areas to receive public and private capital for mortgages and home ownership, while at the same time facilitating the process for native-born White Americans (Nardone et al., 2020; Powell, 2007).

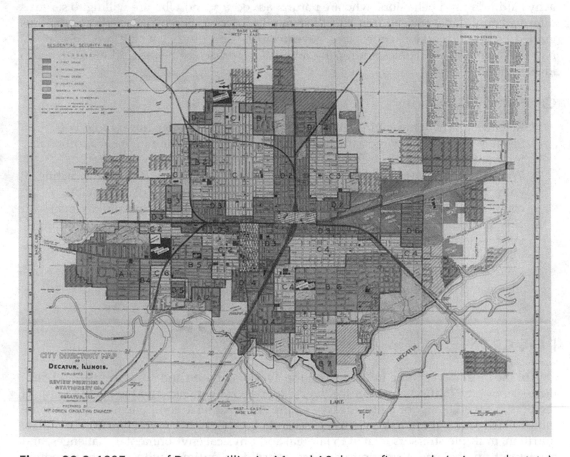

Figure 20.2 1937 map of Decatur, Illinois. A1 and A2 denote first-grade (prime real estate) neighborhoods, B1 to B7 are considered second-grade neighborhoods, C1 to C6 are third grade, and D1 to D6 are fourth grade.

Source: Nelson, R. K., Winling, L., Marciano, R. et al. (n.d.). *Mapping inequality.* richmond.edu.

BOX 20.2: Impact of Racial Zoning

- Inadequate public schools and low graduation rates.
- Schools and housing structures in violation of codes (e.g., lead-based paint, asbestos, inadequate electrical wiring, substandard air conditioning and heating systems).
- Highway and transportation structures that dissect neighborhoods and produce toxins.
- Proximity to toxic waste sites.
- Unsafe water sources.
- A lack of health facilities in communities.
- Absence of local grocery, clothing, and hardware stores.
- Unavailability of banking facilities, hospitals, clinics, pharmacies, and so forth.
- Limited tax-generating revenues from businesses and corporate structures.
- Isolation from other, more affluent neighborhoods.

Source: Adapted from by Bailey, Z. D., Krieger, N., Agénor, M., Graves, J., Linos, N., & Bassett, M. T. (2017). Structural racism and health inequities in the USA: Evidence and interventions. *Lancet*, *389*(10077), 1453-1463. https://doi.org/10.1016/S0140-6736(17)30569-X.

Mapping inequality should provide the backdrop for a more in-depth understanding of how the federal government and private agencies helped to create and sustain the intersectionality among the social determinants of health and the perils of health disparities as currently evidenced in the United States. For additional background on redlining, see "Resources for More In-Depth Information" at the end of this chapter. You are encouraged to examine the map and find your home in relation to other neighborhoods.

The structure of a system is influential in determining behavior (Powell, 2007). Despite the availability of funds for purchasing homes and building sustainable communities, such opportunities were denied to African American people and selected ethnic, minority, and immigrant groups. The federal government classified these communities as undesirable, hazardous, and high risk—the communities were redlined. Across the nation, redlining maps were developed and are evident to this day. Several long-term outcomes persist, including thwarted opportunities related to a lack of property-related accumulated wealth that can be transmitted from one generation to the next for those minority groups. Eminent domain and racial zoning helped to secure structural racism policies. True to their design and intent, the fateful, unjust laws and policies have been effective and may be evidenced across our nation.

Researchers have associated redlining with one of the most frequently diagnosed childhood health conditions, asthma—further evidence of the proliferation of health disparities among minority groups (Bailey et al., 2017; Nardone et al., 2020; Powell, 2007; Schwartz et al., 2021). Redlining is also associated with the presence of tobacco sales in historically underresourced neighborhoods (Schwartz et al., 2021), making cigarette smoking a potentially convenient, but undesirable, health-related behavior among many minority groups (Box 20.2; Assari et al., 2019; Case & Deaton, 2021a, 2021b; Fiocco et al., 2007; Ho & Elo, 2013; Horowitz, 2018; Park et al., 2019; Saito et al., 2018; Skalamera & Hummer, 2016; Zajacova & Lawrence, 2018).

EDUCATION

The impact of education is a powerful dynamic that influences the life course of the individual. Unfortunately, not all youth have access to a quality education (primarily those from minority and immigrant groups and some rural populations), and the outcomes can be devastating. Evidence suggests that there is a significant educational gap between more privileged and less privileged youth and their families (Flores, 2017; Horsford et al., 2019; Hursh, 2007; Junca, 2007). This trend has existed for centuries. Quality and relevant education provides

BOX 20.3: A Pound of Cure for Adverse Childhood Experiences

- Educate people, including health professionals, to conceptualize the causes of ACEs and who could help prevent them.

- Support community solutions and shift focus away from individual responsibilities.

- Reduce and eliminate the stigma that is embedded around help-seeking for parental problems, substance abuse, depression, suicidal thoughts, and physical dysfunction and disease (e.g., heart disease, respiratory problems, diabetes, obesity).

- Embrace culturally appropriate, safe, and enduring positive relationships and environments where people live, learn, play, and pray.

Source: Adapted from Centers for Disease Control and Prevention. (2019). Adverse childhood experiences (ACEs): Preventing early trauma to improve adult health. https://www.cdc.gov/vitalsigns/aces/pdf/vs-1105-aces-H.pdf.

a direct connection to higher paying jobs, more stable incomes, and access to resources necessary for optimizing personal, family, and community health outcomes (Assari et al., 2019; Case & Deaton, 2021a, 2021b; Fiocco et al., 2007; Horowitz, 2018; Park et al., 2019; Saito et al., 2018; Skalamera & Hummer, 2016; Zajacova & Lawrence, 2018). Stable families and communities are also likely results. The essentials for good health for all people include quality food, exercise facilities and walking paths, reliable and safe transportation, green outdoor spaces, access to health promotion and disease prevention facilities, a culturally competent workforce, and high-performing schools. Well-educated youth (and later adults) are more likely to experience less stress, fewer crises, enhanced social network systems, and interactions with others who offer bridges to expanded opportunities and career planning. For too many minority youths, a poor education confines and restricts them to a life of poverty and lost dreams (Chaudry & Wimer, 2016; Ghosh-Dastidar et al., 2014; Giurgescu et al., 2015; Shultz et al., 2021). See Box 20.3 for steps to mitigate the impact of ACEs.

It cannot be emphasized enough that, from among the social and economic disparities that exist in the United States and across the globe, education stands out (Assari et al., 2019; Case & Deaton, 2021a, 2021b; Fiocco et al., 2007; Flores, 2017; Horowitz, 2018; Marmot et al., 2008; Park et al., 2019; Saito et al., 2018; Skalamera & Hummer, 2016; Zajacova & Lawrence, 2018). Education is paramount in enabling the acquisition of knowledge and skill sets that translate into the security, empowerment, and control over one's own life that open the door to opportunities for inclusion in the fabric of a society (Marmot et al., 2008). Recall that disparities are caused, to a great degree, by inadequate childhood development. Societal disparities created by numerous systems—legal, eductional, health, and economic—that exclude some while providing privilege and advantage to others are the *root cause* of injustices in education. This inequity deprives individuals of being empowered and having control over the quality of their own lives (Assari et al., 2019; Case & Deaton, 2021a, 2021b; Currie & Moretti, 2003; Fiocco et al., 2007; Horowitz, 2018; Park et al., 2019; Saito et al., 2018; Skalamera & Hummer, 2016; Zajacova & Lawrence, 2018). For example, as mothers' education level increases, infant mortality decreases (Skalamera & Hummer, 2016; Zajacova & Lawrence, 2018). Children of parents who have completed some post-secondary education earn higher grade point averages in school (Assari et al., 2019). The value of education continues to bear dividends all along the life course. Whereas in the 1990s race was a major factor in determining life expectancy, as of 2018, higher education levels have become the most predictive factor of longer, healthier, more productive, and satisfying lives, regardless of race (Case & Deaton, 2021a; Currie & Moretti, 2003; Fiocco et al., 2007; Horowitz, 2018; Park et al., 2019; Saito et al., 2018; Skalamera & Hummer, 2016; Zajacova & Lawrence, 2018).

At the top of most lists for morbidity and mortality are American Indians and Alaska Natives, African Americans, and Hispanic Americans (Chaudry & Wimer, 2016; Donkin, 2014; Gary et al., 2018; Hardeman et al., 2018; Hess, 2020; Marmot et al., 2008; Matthew, 2018;

Reich, 2018; Satcher, 2020; Trent et al., 2019; Verlinde et al., 2012; WHO, 2021). Research suggests that, in the instance of African Americans and Native Americans, the color of the skin has very little to do with the devastating inequities that they have experienced for centuries. Rather, their status in society ordains the extent to which social disadvantage, restricted opportunities, and discrimination are emboldened into the fabric of everyday life in the United States (Marmot et al., 2008; Meyer et al., 2013). Yet people have little control over where they were born; under what conditions and political systems they live, learn, play, and pray; and how much education they acquire (Chaudry & Wimer, 2016; Hess, 2020; Marmot et al., 1991, 2008; Matthew, 2018; Reich, 2018; Satcher, 2020; Weiss-Laxer et al., 2020).

For generations, public and private education and health systems have helped to create and maintain methods by which poverty gets under the skin and produces burdens of health disparities that are disproportionately carried by minority groups (Assari et al., 2019; Case & Deaton, 2021a, 2021b; Fiocco et al., 2007; Horowitz, 2018; Park et al., 2019; Saito et al., 2018; Skalamera & Hummer, 2016; Zajacova & Lawrence, 2018). Laws and practices that help to determine the allocation of privilege and the distribution of goods and services are based on discrimination of racial/ethnic groups. Nurses, physicians, and other healthcare professionals have been recruited as active participants in the implementation of these inequitable laws, policies, and practices (Byrd & Clayton, 2000, 2001). Conversely, they are well-positioned to help unravel the multilevel and complex issues associated with the intersectionality between education and health outcomes across the life course.

NARRATIVE 20.2: JEWEL'S STORY

This narrative is based on the experience of a young girl who was transported to a facility for homeless youth by a law enforcement officer in the local community. The details are centered on clinical histories as reported by a nurse. A caseworker, social worker, and public-school liaison were also involved in planning and coordinating her care as guided by shelter policies.

When youth are in the custody of law enforcement personnel, the reason for the contact is varied. In this community, based on the youth's information and the officer's inferences and judgment, a decision may be made to transport any youth to a shelter for homeless children if one exists. Individuals transported to a shelter receive the designation of "being a dependent"; those admitted to a juvenile detention center carry the title of "juvenile delinquent." The outcomes for the youth can have profound variability and influence across the life course. The officer, in this instance, made a critical decision, which led to this young person being placed in a protective and facilitative environment.

Jewel (not her real name) is a 15-year-old female patient who lived in mid-America until she decided to run away from home. Her decision was a difficult one. She was an honor student and had plans to become a biologist focusing on climate change in the world's largest mangrove forest. She intended to conduct research in India and Bangladesh while studying in America's most prestigious universities.

Jewel thought that running away from home might help to make her dreams a reality and provide escape from the sexual abuse of her stepfather and the neglect and physical abuse that she attributed to her mother, who did not respond to Jewel's subtle but frequent comments about her stepfather's "interest" in her. The abuse had continued for about 2 years—Jewel was vague about the timeline.

After school one day, Jewel kept walking and ended up at a large truck stop in her community. She had been there before to use the restroom and get a quick bite to eat. One of the truckers had paid for her meal and admonished her that she should be returning home and staying in school. This time, things were different.

The trucker who paid for her meal invited her to travel with him to a lovely home in a sunny part of the nation. He purchased personal items for Jewel; she joined the man, and

(continued)

NARRATIVE 20.2: JEWEL'S STORY (*CONTINUED*)

they headed to the beautiful home as promised. After a few hours of travel, the man suggested that the two of them "snuggle" to stay warm and to get to know each other. They did. Snuggling happened again, but soon intimate sexual contact was added. This frightened Jewel. The trucker reassured her that he would protect her and keep her safe. The sexual activity increased in duration and intensity—sometimes two or three times a day or night.

Jewel noticed that "on the road" she would be introduced as the trucker's daughter or niece—she was well aware of the evident deception and began to become anxious, tearful, and eventually, depressed. She was smart and had to make another plan. "At the next truck stop," she told herself, "run away!" She did.

The police apprehended Jewel one night while she was walking down a deserted road. Frightened but relieved, she confided to the officer that she had nowhere to go and needed a safe place to rest. Jewel was taken to a facility* for youth who have run away from home and are homeless. The newly built facility was clean and well appointed. The staff was known to the officer, and Jewel began to feel somewhat safe. But what comes next?

An experienced nurse interviewed and admitted Jewel to the home, and a physical examination was also completed. Jewel was worried about the physical examination outcome and acknowledged to the nurse that she had "woozy" feelings in the mornings. She had shared these sensations with her mother, but no action had been taken. After several days at the home, Jewel learned that she was pregnant.

The devastating news created feelings of hopelessness and helplessness. This was not the life that Jewel had planned for and dreamed of for herself. She became suicidal and threatened to kill herself by taking pills, banging her head against the wall until she passed out, or cutting the large vein in her arm and slowly bleeding to death one night while others were sleeping.

Jewel was placed on suicide precautions, and the same intake nurse was designated as Jewel's primary care nurse during this crisis period. Safety was paramount. Plans included (a) encouraging Jewel to share her feelings of dread, despair, and hope; (b) providing comprehensive healthcare for Jewel and planning for the birth and long-term care of her child; (c) enrolling Jewel in high school classes and completing requirements for graduation; and (d) being placed in a therapeutic home while awaiting the birth of the infant.

Jewel had not yet decided whether to place the infant up for adoption or to keep the baby. It was apparent that her stepfather was the father of her child. She hated that thought and vowed never to go home again. She delivered the baby, placed the child in foster care, and completed high school with high honors.

Currently, Jewel is enrolled in a large flagship public university, studying biology. She and her son live in a modest apartment, and her academic work is superb—India and Bangladesh are still viable career dreams. She began to experience "splitting migraines" soon after the birth of her child and is receiving treatment for the condition. The interventions that Jewel received have been timely, humane, and continuous.

* The mission of the facility that helped Jewel is to provide evidence-based care to all individuals and address the root causes of the problems in the service of protecting those in need.

Discussion Questions

1. From statistical data, in addition to redlining laws and policies, identify three risk-related behaviors that are common among adolescents in your community. Explain how they could create antecedent factors that might be manifested in their adult lives and across the life course. What sources of information were used to construct your response?

2. Discuss the origins of mandatory reporting of child maltreatment and the responsibilities that health professionals and others have for following this law. Include in your discussion (a) the difficulties that families perceive they might encounter when reporting occurs, and (b) science-based statements about how poverty often helps to create ACEs in youth.
3. Develop an interactive seminar for parents and teachers in an underresourced school in your community that will engage them in a discussion about the relationships among education, health status, and overall well-being for themselves and future generations. What steps would you take when developing the seminar? What topics would you research about the community and parents/families when creating your dynamic seminar?

ADDITIONAL RESOURCES

ACEs and American Indian and Alaska Native Children

Excellent article that addresses these often overlooked minority groups:

Bell et al. (2021, March 22). Caring for American Indian and Alaska Native children and adolescents. *Pediatrics*, e2021050498. https://doi.org/10.1542/peds.2021-050498

ACEs Overview

For ACEs information in a nutshell:

Centers for Disease Control and Prevention. (2019, November). Adverse childhood experiences (ACEs): preventing early trauma to improve adult health. https://www.cdc.gov/vitalsigns/aces/pdf/vs-1105-aces-H.pdf.

ACEs Questionnaire

For a link to a brochure used in parenting fundamentals classes. It includes the ACEs scoring questionnaire:

Bensinger, K., & Community Counseling Centers of Chicago. (2014). *Parenting fundamentals: ACEs awareness for prevention-adverse childhood experiences.* C4's ACE booklet 11-14.pdf | PACEsConnection.

Building Better Communities

After examination of innovative practices being piloted throughout the nation, concrete solutions are offered for building social and economic equity:

PolicyLink and California Endowment. (2017). *Why place matters: Building a movement for healthy communities.* https://www.policylink.org/sites/default/files/WHYPLACEMATTERS_FINAL.PDF

Redlining Explained

For a 6-minute educational video on redlining:

Conover, A. (2017, October 4). *The disturbing history of the suburbs: Adam ruins everything* [Video]. YouTube. https://www.youtube.com/watch?v=ETR9qrVS17g

Redlining Maps

You can look up historical maps of your city. For interactive maps showing redlining of American cities during the New Deal Era (1930s):

Nelson, R. K., Winling, L., Marciano, R., Connolly, N., Ayers, N., University of Richmond Digital Scholarship Lab, Virginia Technical Institute, & University of Maryland. (2021). *Mapping inequality, American Panorama.* Mapping Inequality (richmond.edu).

Sexual Assault Nurse Examiner (SANE) Certification

One pathway toward becoming certified as a SANE requires being a registered nurse with at least 2 years of experience in critical care to complete an adult/adolescent SANE education program that includes 40 hours of continuing nursing education contact hours and 40 hours of an adult/adolescent SANE education program from an accredited provider. State requirements may vary. This website provides details:

International Association of Forensic Nursing. (2021). *SANE certification central.* https://www.forensicnurses.org/page/Certification

Violence Prevention Resources

This is a toolkit that has been developed by the CDC. It provides a goldmine of prevention resources covering the topics of child abuse and neglect, intimate partner violence, sexual violence, youth violence, suicide, and ACEs:

Centers for Disease Control and Prevention. (2020). *Technical packages for violence prevention.* https://www.cdc.gov/violenceprevention/communicationresources/pub/technical-packages.html

Further Resources

Braveman, P., & Gottlieb, L. (2014). The social determinants of health: It's time to consider the causes of the causes. *Public Health Reports, 129*(suppl 2), 19–31. https://doi.org/10.1177/00333549141291S206

Hedegaard, H., Miniño, A. M., & Warner, M. (2020, January). Drug overdose deaths in the United States, 1999–2018 (NCHS Data Brief No. 356). National Center for Health Statistics, U.S. Department of Health and Human Services. https://www.cdc.gov/nchs/data/databriefs/db356-h.pdf

Parmet, W. E., & Huer, J. L. (2018, July 22). Introduction to "diseases of despair: The role of policy and law" [symposium]. *Bill of Health.* https://blog.petrieflom.law.harvard.edu/2018/07/22/diseases-of-despair-the-role-of-policy-and-law/

Zeglin, R. J., Niemela, D. R. M., & Baynard, C. W. (2019). Deaths of despair in Florida: Assessing the role of social determinants of health. *Health Education & Behavior, 46*(2), 329–339. https://doi.org/10.1177/1090198118811888

REFERENCES

Alaggia, R., Collin-Vézina, D., & Lateef, R. (2019). Facilitators and barriers to child sexual abuse (CSA) disclosures: A research update (2000–2016). *Trauma, Violence & Abuse, 20*(2), 260–283. https://doi.org/10.1177/1524838017697312

Alvidrez, J., Castille, D., Laude-Sharp, M., Rosario, A., & Tabor, D. (2019). The national institute on minority health and health disparities research framework. *American Journal of Public Health, 109*(S1), S16–S20. https://doi.org/10.2105/AJPH.2018.304883

Annapragada, A. V., Donaruma-Kwoh, M. M., Annapragada, A. V., & Starosolski, Z. A. (2021). A natural language processing and deep learning approach to identify child abuse from pediatric electronic medical records. *PloS One, 16*(2), e0247404. https://doi.org/10.1371/journal.pone.0247404

Assari, S., Caldwell, C. H., & Bazargan, M. (2019). Association between parental educational attainment and youth outcomes and role of race/ethnicity. *JAMA Network Open, 2*(11), e1916018. https://doi.org/10.1001/jamanetworkopen.2019.16018

Bailey, Z. D., Krieger, N., Agénor, M., Graves, J., Linos, N., & Bassett, M. T. (2017). Structural racism and health inequities in the USA: Evidence and interventions. *Lancet, 389*(10077), 1453–1463. https://doi.org/10.1016/S0140-6736(17)30569-X

Byrd, W. M., & Clayton, L. A. (2000). An American health dilemma. In *The medical history of African Americans and the problem of race: Beginnings to 1900* (Vol. 1). Routledge.

Byrd, W. M., & Clayton, L. A. (2001). An American health dilemma. In *Race, medicine, and health care in the United States 1900–2000* (Vol. 2). Routledge.

Case, A., & Deaton, A. (2021a). Life expectancy in adulthood is falling for those without a BA degree, but as educational gaps have widened, racial gaps have narrowed. *Proceedings of the National Academy of Sciences, 118*(11), e2024777118. https://doi.org/10.1073/pnas.2024777118

Case, A., & Deaton, A. (2021b). *Deaths of despair and the future of capitalism* (K. Harper, Narr.) [Audiobook]. Princeton University Press.

Centers for Disease Control and Prevention. (2019, November). Adverse childhood experiences (ACEs): Preventing early trauma to improve adult health. https://www.cdc.gov/vitalsigns/aces/pdf/vs-1105-aces-H.pdf

Chandramani, A., Dussault, N., Parameswaran, R., Rodriguez, J., Novack, J., Ahn, J., Oyola, S., & Carter, K. (2020). A needs assessment and educational intervention addressing the care of sexual assault patients in the emergency department. *Journal of Forensic Nursing, 16*(2), 73–82. https://doi .org/10.1097/JFN.0000000000000290

Chaudry, A., & Wimer, C. (2016). Poverty is not just an indicator: The relationship between income, poverty, and child well-being. *Academic Pediatrics, 16*(3), S23–S29. https://doi.org/10.1016/ j.acap.2015.12.010

Commission on Social Determinants of Health. (2008). *Closing the gap in a generation: Health equity through action on the social determinants of health. Final Report of the Commission on Social Determinants of Health.* World Health Organization. https://www.who.int/social_determinants/final_report/ csdh_finalreport_2008.pdf

Currie, J., & Moretti, E. (2003). Mother's education and the intergenerational transmission of human capital: Evidence from college openings. *Quarterly Journal of Economics, 118*(4), 1495–1532. https:// doi.org/10.1162/003355303322552856

Deighton, S., Neville, A., Pusch, D., & Dobson, K. (2018). Biomarkers of adverse childhood experiences: A scoping review. *Psychiatry Research, 269,* 719–732. https://doi.org/10.1016/j. psychres.2018.08.097

Donkin, A. J. (2014). Social gradient. *Wiley Blackwell Encyclopedia of Health, Illness, Behavior, and Society,* 2172–2178. https://doi.org/10.1002/9781118410868.wbehibs530

Drake, B., & Jonson-Reid, M. (2015). Competing values and evidence: How do we evaluate mandated reporting and CPS response?. In B. Matthews & D. Bross (Eds.), Mandatory reporting raws and the identification of severe child abuse and neglect (Vol. 4, pp. 33–60). Springer.

Federal Housing Administration. (1936). Underwriting manual: Underwriting and valuation procedure under Title II of the National Housing Act. http://urbanoasis.org/projects/fha/ FHAUnderwritingManualPtI.html

Felitti, V. J. (2019). Origins of the ACE study. *American Journal of Preventive Medicine, 56*(6), 787–789. https://doi.org/10.1016/j.amepre.2019.02.011

Felitti, V. J., Anda, R. F., Nordenberg, D., Williamson, D. F., Spitz, A. M., Edwards, V., Koss, M. P., & Marks, J. S. (2019). Reprint of: Relationship of childhood abuse and household dysfunction to many of the leading causes of death in adults: The adverse childhood experiences (ACE) study. *American Journal of Preventive Medicine, 56*(6), 774–786. https://doi.org/10.1016/ j.amepre.2019.04.001

Fiocco, A. J., Joober, R., & Lupien, S. J. (2007). Education modulates reactivity to the trier social stress test in middle-aged adults. *Psychoneuroendocrinology, 32*(8–10), 1158–1163. https://doi .org/10.1016/j.psyneuen.2007.08.008

Flores, R. L. (2017). The rising gap between rich and poor: A look at the persistence of educational disparities in the United States and why we should worry. *Cogent Social Sciences, 3*(1), Article 1323698. https://doi.org/10.1080/23311886.2017.1323698

Gary, F. A., Yarandi, H., Evans, E., Still, C., Mickels, P., Hassan, M., Campbell, D., & Conic, R. (2018). Beck depression inventory-II: Factor analyses with three groups of midlife women of African descent in the Midwest, the South, and the U.S. Virgin Islands. *Issues in Mental Health Nursing, 39*(3), 233–243. https://doi.org/10.1080/01612840.2017.1373175

Ghebreyesus, T. A. (2020). Strengthening our resolve for primary health care. *Bulletin of the World Health Organization, 98*(11), 726–726A. https://doi.org/10.2471/BLT.20.279489

Ghosh-Dastidar, B., Cohen, D., Hunter, G., Zenk, S. N., Huang, C., Beckman, R., & Dubowitz, T. (2014). Distance to store, food prices, and obesity in urban food deserts. *American Journal of Preventive Medicine, 47*(5), 587–595. https://doi.org/10.1016/j.amepre.2014.07.005

Giurgescu, C., Misra, D. P., Sealy-Jefferson, S., Caldwell, C. H., Templin, T. N., Slaughter-Acey, J. C., & Osypuk, T. L. (2015). The impact of neighborhood quality, perceived stress, and social support on depressive symptoms during pregnancy in African American women. *Social Science & Medicine, 130,* 172–180. https://doi.org/10.1016/j.socscimed.2015.02.006

Greengard, J. (1964). The battered-child syndrome. *American Journal of Nursing, 64,* 98–100. https:// doi.org/10.1097/00000446-196464060-00024

Hardeman, R. R., Murphy, K. A., Karbeah, J. M., & Kozhimannil, K. B. (2018). Naming institutionalized racism in the public health literature: A systematic literature review. *Public Health Reports, 133*(3), 240–249. https://doi.org/10.1177/0033354918760574

Hassan, M. A., Gary, F. A., Lewin, L., Killion, C., & Totten, V. (2020). Age-related child sexual abuse experiences. *Western Journal of Nursing Research.* https://doi.org/10.1177/0193945920958723

Hassan, M., Gary, F. A., Hotz, R., Killion, C., & Vicken, T. (2015a). Young victims telling their stories of sexual abuse in the emergency department. *Issues in Mental Health Nursing, 36*(12), 944–952. https://doi.org/10.3109/01612840.2015.1063026

Hassan, M., Killion, C., Lewin, L., Totten, V., & Gary, F. (2015b). Gender-related sexual abuse experiences reported by children who were examined in an emergency department. *Archives of Psychiatric Nursing, 29*(3), 148–154. https://doi.org/10.1016/j.apnu.2015.01.006

Hayes, M. (1988). Book reviews: The battered child. *International Journal of Law, Policy and the Family, 2*(2), 237–238. https://doi.org/10.1093/lawfam/2.2.237

Helfer, M. E., Kempe, R. S., & Krugman, R. D. (Eds.). (1999). *The battered child*. University of Chicago Press.

Helfer, R. E. (1987). Commentary: Back to the future. *Child Abuse & Neglect, 11*, 11–14. https://doi.org/10.1016/0145-2134(87)90028-7

Hess, C. (2020). Residential segregation by race and ethnicity and the changing geography of neighborhood poverty. *Spatial Demography.* https://doi.org/10.1007/s40980-020-00066-3

Ho, J. Y., & Elo, I. T. (2013). The contribution of smoking to black-white differences in US mortality. *Demography, 50*(2), 545–568. https://doi.org/10.1007/s13524-012-0159-z

Horowitz, J. (2018). Relative education and the advantage of a college degree. *83*(4), 771–801. https://doi.org/10.1177/0003122418785371

Horsford, S. D., Scott, J. T., & Anderson, G. L. (2019). *The politics of education policy in an era of inequality: Possibilities for democratic schooling*. Routledge.

Hursh, D. (2007). Exacerbating inequality: The failed promise of the no child left behind act. *Race Ethnicity and Education, 10*(3), 295–308. https://doi.org/10.1080/13613320701503264

Jalongo, M. R. (2006). The story of Mary Ellen Wilson: Tracing the origins of child protection in America. *Early Childhood Education Journal, 34*(1), 1–4. https://doi.org/10.1007/s10643-006-0121-z

Jensen, S. K. G., Berens, A. E., & Nelson, III, C. A. (2017). Effects of poverty on interacting biological systems underlying child development. *Lancet Child & Adolescent Health, 1*(3), 225–239. https://doi.org/10.1016/S2352-4642(17)30024-X

Junca, H. (2007). Eight Americas: A new definition for "Americas"? *PLoS Medicine, 4*(1), e42. https://doi.org/10.1371/journal.pmed.0040042

Kalmakis, K. A., & Chandler, G. E. (2015). Health consequences of adverse childhood experiences: A systematic review. *Journal of the American Association of Nurse Practitioners, 27*(8), 457–465. https://doi.org/10.1002/2327-6924.12215

Kempe, C. H. (1975). Uncommon manifestations of the battered child syndrome. *American Journal of Diseases of Children, 129*(11), 1265–1265. https://doi.org/10.1001/archpedi.1975.02120480003001

Kempe, C. H., Silverman, F. N., Steele, B. F., Droegemueller, W., & Silver, H. K. (1962). The battered-child syndrome. *Journal of the American Medical Association, 181*, 17–24. https://doi.org/10.1001/jama.1962.03050270019004

Kempe, C. H., Silverman, F. N., Steele, B. F., Droegemueller, W., & Silver, H. K. (1985). The battered-child syndrome. Reprint. *Child Abuse & Neglect, 9*, 143–154. https://doi.org/10.1016/0145-2134(85)90005-5

Kiprop, V. (2018). Countries with universal health care. https://www.worldatlas.com/articles/countries-with-universal-health-care.html

Levesque, R. J. (2011). Encyclopedia of adolescence. Springer.

Lindenmeyer, K. (1997). A right to childhood: The U.S. Children's Bureau and child welfare, 1912–46. University of Illinois Press.

Marmot, M. G., Stansfeld, S., Patel, C., North, F., Head, J., White, I., Brunner, E., Feeney, A., & Smith, G. D. (1991). Health inequalities among British civil servants: The Whitehall II study. *Lancet, 337*(8754), 1387–1393. https://doi.org/10.1016/0140-6736(91)93068-K

Marmot, M., Friel, S., Bell, R., Houweling, T. A. J., & Taylor, S. (2008). Closing the gap in a generation: Health equity through action on the social determinants of health. *Lancet, 372*(9650), 1661–1669. https://doi.org/10.1016/S0140-6736(08)61690-6

Matthew, D. B. (2018). Just medicine: A cure for racial inequality in American health care. New York University Press.

McElvaney, R., Greene, S., & Hogan, D. (2012). Containing the secret of child sexual abuse. *Journal of Interpersonal Violence, 27*(6), 1155–1177. https://doi.org/10.1177/0886260511424503

Melton, G. B. (2005). Mandated reporting: A policy without reason. *Child Abuse & Neglect, 29*(1), 9–18. https://doi.org/10.1016/j.chiabu.2004.05.005

Meyer, P. A., Yoon, P. W., Kaufmann, R. B., & Centers for Disease Control and Prevention. (2013). Introduction: CDC health disparities and inequalities report–United States, 2013. *Morbidity and Mortality Weekly Report Supplements, 62*(3), 3–5. http://europepmc.org/abstract/MED/24264483

Miles, J., Espiritu, R. C., Horen, N., Sebian, J., & Waetzig, E. (2010). A public health approach to children's mental health: A conceptual framework. Georgetown University Center for Child and Human Development, National Technical Assistance Center for Children's Mental Health. https://gucchd.georgetown.edu/products/PublicHealthApproach.pdf

Miller, N. A., Kirk, A., Kaiser, M. J., & Glos, L. (2014). The relation between health insurance and healthcare disparities among adults with disabilities. *American Journal of Public Health, 104*(3), e85–e93. https://doi.org/10.2105/ajph.2013.301478

Minh, A., Muhajarine, N., Janus, M., Brownell, M., & Guhn, M. (2017). A review of neighborhood effects and early child development: How, where, and for whom, do neighborhoods matter? *Health & Place*, 46, 155–174. https://doi.org/10.1016/j.healthplace.2017.04.012

Murphy, A., Steele, M., Dube, S. R., Bate, J., Bonuck, K., Meissner, P., Goldman, H., & Steele, H. (2014). Adverse childhood experiences (ACEs) questionnaire and adult attachment interview (AAI): Implications for parent child relationships. *Child Abuse & Neglect*, 38(2), 224–233. https://doi.org/10.1016/j.chiabu.2013.09.004

Murray, K. O., & Gesiriech, S. (2004). A brief legislative history of the child welfare system. Pew Commission on Children in Foster Care. Legislative History_Background Binder.doc (pewtrusts.org)

Nardone, A., Casey, J. A., Morello-Frosch, R., Mujahid, M., Balmes, J. R., & Thakur, N. (2020). Associations between historical residential redlining and current age-adjusted rates of emergency department visits due to asthma across eight cities in California: An ecological study. *Lancet Planetary Health*, 4(1), e24–e31. https://doi.org/10.1016/S2542-5196(19)30241-4

National Children's Alliance. (2021). National statistics on child abuse. https://www.nationalchildrensalliance.org/media-room/national-statistics-on-child-abuse/

New York Society for the Prevention of Cruelty to Children. (n.d.). Who we are. https://www.lawhelpny.org/organization/new-york-society-for-the-prevention-of-cruelt

O'Keefe, V. M., Tucker, R. P., Cole, A. B., Hollingsworth, D. W., & Wingate, L. R. (2018). Understanding Indigenous suicide through a theoretical lens: A review of general, culturally based, and Indigenous frameworks. *Transcultural Psychiatry*, 55(6), 775–799. https://doi.org/10.1177/1363461518778937

Park, C. L., Clark, E. M., Schulz, E., Williams, B. R., Williams, R. M., & Holt, C. L. (2019). Unique contribution of education to behavioral and psychosocial antecedents of health in a national sample of African Americans. *Journal of Behavioral Medicine*, 42(5), 860–872. https://doi.org/10.1007/s10865-018-00009-w

Patton, G. C., Olsson, C. A., Skirbekk, V., Saffery, R., Wlodek, M. E., Azzopardi, P. S., Stonawski, M., Rasmussen, B., Spry, E., Francis, K., Bhutta, Z. A., Kasselbaum, N. J., Mokdad, A. H., Murray, C. J. L., Prentice, A. M., Reavley, N., Sheeham, P., Sweeny, K., Viner, R. M., & Sawyer, S. M. (2018). Adolescence and the next generation. *Nature*, 554(7693), 458–466. https://doi.org/10.1038/nature25759

Powell, J. A. (2007). Structural racism: Building upon the insights of John Calmore. *North Carolina Law Review*, 86, 791.

Reich, D. (2018, March 23). How genetics is changing our understanding of "race." New York Times. https://www.nytimes.com/2018/03/23/opinion/sunday/genetics-race.html

Romeo, R. D. (2017). The impact of stress on the structure of the adolescent brain: Implications for adolescent mental health. *Brain Research*, 1654, 185–191. http://doi.org/10.1016/j.brainres.2016.03.021

Rosa, M. J., Lee, A. G., & Wright, R. J. (2018). Evidence establishing a link between prenatal and early-life stress and asthma development. *Current Opinion in Allergy and Clinical Immunology*, 18(2), 148–158. https://doi.org/10.1097/ACI.0000000000000421

Saito, J., Shibanuma, A., Yasuoka, J., Kondo, N., Takag, D., Jimba, M. (2018). Education and indoor smoking among parents who smoke: The mediating role of perceived social norms of smoking. *BMC Public Health*, 18(1), 211. https://doi.org/10.1186/s12889-018-5082-9

Satcher, D. (2020). *My quest for health equity: Notes on learning while leading.* Johns Hopkins University Press.

Schuman, M. (2017, January). History of child labor in the United States—Part 1: Little children working. *Monthly Labor Review*, U.S. Bureau of Labor Statistics. https://doi.org/10.21916/mlr.2017.1

Schwartz, E., Onnen, N., Craigmile, P. F., & Roberts, M. E. (2021). The legacy of redlining: Associations between historical neighborhood mapping and contemporary tobacco retailer density in Ohio. *Health & Place*, 68, 102529. https://doi.org/10.1016/j.healthplace.2021.102529

Sciaraffa, M. A., Zeanah, P. D., & Zeanah, C. H. (2018). Understanding and promoting resilience in the context of adverse childhood experiences. *Early Childhood Education Journal*, 46(3), 343–353. https://doi.org/10.1007/s10643-017-0869-3

Shultz, J. M., Sullivan, L., & Galea, S. (2021). Public health: An introduction to the science and practice of population health. Springer.

Shvili, J. (2020, May 30). 10 countries without universal healthcare. WorldAtlas. https://www.worldatlas.com/articles/10-notable-countries-that-are-still-without-universal-healthcare.html

Skalamera, J., & Hummer, R. A. (2016). Educational attainment and the clustering of health-related behavior among U.S. young adults. *Preventive Medicine*, 84, 83–89. https://doi.org/10.1016/j.ypmed.2015.12.011

Tang, X., Wang, M.-T., Guo, J., & Salmela-Aro, K. (2019). Building grit: The longitudinal pathways between mindset, commitment, grit, and academic outcomes. *Journal of Youth and Adolescence, 48*(5), 850–863. https://doi.org/10.1007/s10964-019-00998-0

Tener, D. (2018). The secret of intrafamilial child sexual abuse: Who keeps it and how? *Journal of Child Sexual Abuse, 27*(1), 1–21. https://doi.org/10.1080/10538712.2017.1390715

Texas Department of Family and Protective Services. (2020). When and how to report child abuse. DFPS - When and How to Report Child Abuse (state.tx.us).

Trent, M., Dooley, D. G., & Dougé, J. (2019). The impact of racism on child and adolescent health. *Pediatrics, 144*(2). https://doi.org/10.1542/peds.2019-1765

van Delft, I., Finkenauer, C., De Schipper, J. C., Lamers-Winkelman, F., & Visser, M. M. (2015). The mediating role of secrecy in the development of psychopathology in sexually abused children. *Child Abuse & Neglect, 46*, 27–36. https://doi.org/10.1016/j.chiabu.2015.04.019

Verlinde, E., De Laender, N., De Maesschalck, S., Deveugele, M., & Willems, S. (2012). The social gradient in doctor-patient communication. *International Journal for Equity in Health, 11*(1), 1–14. https://doi.org/10.1186/1475-9276-11-12

Watkins, S. A. (1990). The Mary Ellen myth: correcting child welfare history. *Social Work, 35*(6), 500–503. https://doi.org/10.1093/sw/35.6.500

Weiss-Laxer, N. S., Crandall, A. -A., Hughes, M. E., & Riley, A. W. (2020). Families as a cornerstone in 21st century public health: Recommendations for research, education, policy, and practice. *Frontiers in Public Health, 8*, 503. https://doi.org/10.3389/fpubh.2020.00503

World Health Organization. (2021). Child maltreatment: Violence against children fact sheet. https://www.who.int/news-room/fact-sheets/detail/child-maltreatment

Youth.gov. (2021). Mental health: Promotion & prevention. https://youth.gov/youth-topics/youth-mental-health/mental-health-promotion-prevention

Zajacova, A., & Lawrence, E. M. (2018). The relationship between education and health: Reducing disparities through a contextual approach. *Annual Review of Public Health, 39*(1), 273–289. https://doi.org/10.1146/annurev-publhealth-031816-044628

Zarse, E. M., Neff, M. R., Yoder, R., Hulvershorn, L., Chambers, J. E., & Chambers, R. A. (2019). The adverse childhood experiences questionnaire: Two decades of research on childhood trauma as a primary cause of adult mental illness, addiction, and medical diseases. *Cogent Medicine, 6*(1), Article 1581447. https://doi.org/10.1080/2331205X.2019.1581447

CHAPTER 21

Disturbing Maternal and Child Health Outcomes Among Vulnerable Populations

Margaret D. Larkins-Pettigrew, Veronica E. Villalobos, Gaetan L. Pettigrew, and Christina L. Wilds

LEARNING OBJECTIVES

- Compare vulnerable populations using the Social Vulnerability Index.

- Analyze Black maternal, child, and infant morbidity and mortality in the United States highlighting the root causes of poor outcomes.

- Explain the political social, economic, environmental, health risk behaviors that influence outcomes for Black mothers, Black birthing people, and children resulting in the social determinants of life.

- Understand the effects of racial discrimination encountered by Black birthing women and Black birthing people and children.

- Describe the role of health inequities and how they emerge to influence maternal and infant health disparities, including the challenges of access to care and the resistance to accessing care.

- Demonstrate the influence of health systems and healthcare professionals on improving health outcomes in Black and other minoritized maternal and child health.

Note: Throughout this chapter, we strive to use inclusive language, while acknowledging that much of the research has been focused on birthing women. Birthing people is used in recognition that not all persons giving birth identify as women.

INTRODUCTION

Vulnerable populations are those populations challenged with normal day-to-day activities that would allow them to be part of a productive society (Centers for Disease Control and Prevention [CDC], 2021a; Institute of Medicine, 2003). These activities include the social determinants of health, namely: food insecurity, education, income, lack of transportation, safe housing, unemployment, and job insecurity. Including the political determinants of health, such as policies affecting social and environmental justice, broadens the communities that meet the societal definition of social vulnerability.

Social vulnerability is a dimension of vulnerability due to external stresses that impact human health. These stresses include everything from natural hazards or disasters to abuse, social exclusion, or a disease outbreak (CDC, 2021a). Communities affected by social vulnerability include individuals who are underresourced or economically disadvantaged; racial and ethnic minorities; the lesbian, gay, bisexual, transgender, queer or questioning, intersex, asexual, and pansexual and other sexual orientation (LGBTQIA+) populations; those who are uninsured or underinsured; and those who have chronic health conditions (Knickman et al., 2001). Maternal and child health issues are represented within these affected communities (Callaghan, 2018).

Disturbing maternal and child health outcomes among vulnerable populations exist in the lives of Black and other minoritized women and people, including Native Americans and Alaska Natives. These outcomes are most notable when birthing women and birthing people navigate the healthcare system for the health and well-being of themselves and their families. Our discussion focuses on many of the components outlined by the Social Vulnerability Index (CDC, 2021a; Flanagan et al., 2011). We examine evidence and data that show economically disadvantaged and advantaged Black and minoritized women in vulnerable populations are at higher risk of poor maternal and infant outcomes.

Social Vulnerability Index

The Social Vulnerability Index is an invaluable tool that assesses a community's needs in times of natural and man-made disasters (Flanagan et al., 2011). The index utilizes factors of social vulnerability that include poverty, lack of access to transportation, crowded housing, human suffering, and financial loss to determine the needs of affected communities, factors that plague the everyday lives of economically challenged Americans. The Social Vulnerability Index is now used in population health science to build programs using geospatial research and U.S. census data explicitly targeting the social determinants of health (Agency for Toxic Substances and Disease Registry, 2021). Unfortunately, this tool does not incorporate the challenges of structural racism that will continue to dismantle any effort to help vulnerable populations. For additional background on geospatial research as it relates to health, see "Geospatial Research, Analysis, and Services Program" in Resources for More In-Depth Information at the end of this chapter.

Revised evidence reveals that the risk of adverse perinatal outcomes can increase because of stress that occurs due to situational experiences of racial discrimination. Adverse perinatal outcomes include both preterm birth and infant death for Black birthing women and Black birthing people. In addition, maternal mortality ratios (MMRs) differ significantly because of factors (e.g., race, ethnicity, socioeconomic status, and geography) affecting birthing women and birthing people that result in their experiencing significantly higher MMRs than the national average (Maternal Health Task Force, n.d.). Data also suggest that Black and minoritized women and birthing people who are not poor have undesirable outcomes (Fishman et al., 2020). Shorter gestational lengths explain the high mortality rates for infants born to Black birthing women and Black birthing people of all educational achievement. Moreover, the National Longitudinal Study of Adolescent to Adult Health conducted a supplementary analysis of data, reflecting Black women with a college education present with similar disadvantages related to health, socioeconomic status, and psychosocial factors as White women with a high school degree or less (Fishman et al., 2020).

Maternal Outcomes

Maternal mortality continues to be a global issue, with the number of maternal deaths continuing to increase over many decades (World Health Organization [WHO], 2017). The United States is one of the richest, most highly resourced countries globally; however, it has the highest maternal mortality rate and the highest financial burden secondary to the healthcare of developed countries (Tikkanen et al., 2020). Maternal health must be a priority as it is women's and people's health, which can result in significant negative impacts on a country's workforce and, subsequently, its prosperity and economic survival (Miller & Belizán, 2015).

Hoyert and Minino (2020) provided a comprehensive fact sheet and informative reference outlining the state of maternal health in the United States that serves as a helpful tool. Therein, WHO's definition for maternal death is used to include women who die while pregnant, or within 42 days from the termination of a pregnancy, excluding only causes that are accidental or incidental (WHO, 2017). The MMR is defined as the number of maternal deaths per 100,000 live births. Hoyert and Minino (2020) show an approximately 3% increase in maternal deaths between 2018 and 2019 overall (17.4 vs. 20.1 deaths per 100,000 live births, respectively). Most notably, Hoyert and Minino observed significant increases in rates for non-Hispanic Black women compared to their non-Hispanic White and Hispanic counterparts. The 2019 MMR for non-Hispanic Black women was 44.0 deaths per 100,000 live births, which is 2.5 times the rate for non-Hispanic White women (17.9 per 100,000 live births) and 3.5 times the rate for Hispanic women (12.6 per 100,000 live births; Hoyert & Minino, 2020). Indeed, among maternal and child health indicators, mortality related to pregnancy presents significant racial disparities (Chang et al., 2003).

Data show that racial disparities in maternal and infant health continue. Improving maternal and infant health is key for preventing unnecessary illness and death and advancing overall population health. Recent research finds that as many as 60% of all maternal deaths in the United States are preventable and that increasing access to preconception, prenatal, and interconception care can reduce pregnancy-related complications. Healthy People 2030, which provides 10-year national health objectives, identifies the prevention of pregnancy complications and maternal deaths and improvement of women's health before, during, and after pregnancy as a public health goal (Artiga et al., 2020).

For mothers who survive the pregnancy and birthing process, a disparity exists in the rate of complications resulting in long-term chronic disease or illness. Black birthing women and Black birthing people carry a three- to fourfold risk for complications compared to their White counterparts. This has been a consistent finding and represents the most significant disparity among population metrics that aim to determine perinatal health outcomes (Callaghan, 2018; Saftlas et al., 2020).

Reducing rates of disparities in preterm birth and low birth weight and eliminating racial disparities in these measures have been the focus of national and local initiatives from clinicians and policymakers. Growing recognition of disparities has prompted efforts from clinical groups and public health officials to become more informed about and address their biases; practice shared decision-making; and listen to and act upon the concerns of pregnant and postpartum patients, particularly in urgent situations. In addition, several initiatives are underway through Medicaid to improve maternal and infant health and reduce disparities due to the substantial role the program plays in covering low-income children and pregnant women and, particularly, low-income children and pregnant women of color (Artiga et al., 2020).

To address the persistent maternal health crisis in America, congressional leaders have advocated for critically important policies such as 12-month postpartum Medicaid coverage, investments in rural maternal health, the promotion of a diverse perinatal workforce, and the implementation of implicit bias trainings. To build on this work, Congresswoman Alma Adams, Congresswoman Lauren Underwood, Vice President Kamala Harris (while she served as a U.S. Senator), and members of the Black maternal health caucus introduced the Black Maternal Health Momnibus Act. Composed of nine separate bills, the Black Maternal Health Momnibus Act of 2021 seeks to improve maternal health, especially among minoritized populations, by, among other things, addressing the social determinants of health; extending postpartum eligibility for the Special Supplemental Nutrition Program for Woman, Infants and Children (WIC); increasing access to maternity care through grants; changing and enhancing the collection of data; and developing quality measures. In so doing, the drafters hope to improve maternal health, and better understand the causes of the U.S. maternal health crisis and identify solutions. The Momnibus, has the potential to be transformative for Black maternal health because it goes beyond addressing maternal death and helps to advance maternal health equity. By centering Black women-led organizations in the process, this package takes a proactive approach to addressing many of the systematic public health challenges, workforce development issues, and everyday experiences of Black birthing persons before, during, and after pregnancy (Black Maternal Health Momnibus Act, 2021).

Causes of Maternal Deaths

Community-based care models, including group prenatal care and pregnancy medical homes, may improve maternal health outcomes. Equity-centered approaches to maternity care may help reduce the rising rate of maternal mortality among women of color (Zephyrin et al., 2021). Maternal death remains preventable when systems are in place to address unnecessary delays in maternal care. Some of the critical aspects that delay maternal care are: (a) lack of access to appropriately trained providers; (b) lack of transportation to appropriate health care facilities; and (c) lack of cultural competence in providers, which leads to unconscious bias and delays of proper care. First, women are often in places where no one readily available can recognize signs that a woman is in danger (Box 21.1). Community healthcare workers provide a prime example of local talent trained to recognize and find assistance during a medical emergency. Second, lack of access to transportation presents another obstacle that hinders women from reaching a qualified healthcare worker. Third, finding a medically and culturally competent provider presents another significant void,

BOX 21.1: Danger Signs and Symptoms During Pregnancy

- Bleeding
- Pre-eclampsia
- Severe nausea and vomiting
- Significant decline in the baby's activity level
- Contractions early in the third trimester
- Water breaks
- Persistent severe headache
- Abdominal pain
- Visual disturbances
- Swelling during the third trimester
- Flu-like symptoms

Source: Adapted from "Pregnancy Complications" by United States Department of Health and Human Services (DHHS), Office of Women's Health. (2019, April 19). https://www.womenshealth.gov/pregnancy/youre-pregnant-now-what/pregnancy-complications.

even in cities that have numerous medical facilities (Barnes-Josia et al., 1998; National Academies of Sciences, 2018).

For low-income birthing women, birthing people, and other minoritized communities, doulas (dedicated support persons for laboring women) are considered a beneficial source of support. One study found that Medicaid beneficiaries who receive support from doulas had lower cesarean section (C-section) rates and preterm births than other pregnant women enrolled in Medicaid. Likewise, a New York City community-based doula program that provides care to predominantly Black and Latinx neighborhoods reported similar findings, and a California study found that doulas may improve the experience of minoritized women by delivering care that is culturally appropriate and patient-centered (Zephyrin et al., 2021). Studies suggest that increased access to doula care, especially in underresourced communities, can improve a range of health outcomes for birthing mothers, birthing people, and babies. They can also decrease maternal care deserts, lower health care costs, reduce C-sections, decrease maternal anxiety and depression, and help improve communication between low-income, racially and/or ethnically diverse pregnant women and birthing people and their healthcare providers (March of Dimes, 2019).

In 2020, 861 women are reported to have died of maternal causes in the United States, which is a significant increase from 2019 when 754 women died due to said causes. In 2020, the maternal mortality rate was 23.8 deaths per 100,000 live births, compared to 20.1 in 2019. Considerable racial and ethnic disparities in pregnancy-related mortality exist. In 2020, non-Hispanic Black women's maternal mortality rate was 55.3 deaths per 100,000 live births, which was 2.9 times the rate for non-Hispanic White women (19.1 per 100,000 live births). These data reveal that, from 2019 to 2020, the observed increase for non-Hispanic Black women was significant (Hoyert, 2022). There was a statistically significant increase for non-Hispanic White, non-Hispanic Black, and Hispanic birthing women in the MMR from 2019 to 2020. Access to and quality of care, the prevalence of chronic disease, and structural racism are cited as potentially accounting for variability in the risk of death by race and ethnicity. The pregnancy-related mortality ratio is calculated using the Pregnancy Mortality Surveillance System (PMSS), defined as the death of a person while pregnant or within 1 year of the end of pregnancy where the cause is related to, or aggravated by, the pregnancy. According to the CDC, pregnancy-related mortality ratios remained stable in recent years. For additional background on maternal mortality, pregnancy-related mortality, and causes of pregnancy-related death in the United States and for reporting on the effects of the COVID-19 pandemic on pregnancy outcomes, see "Maternal Mortality Rates" and "COVID-19 and Pregnancy" in Resources for More In-Depth Information at the end of this chapter.

Infant and Child Mortality and Morbidity

The United States has not found any definite interventions to date that have effectively prevented or reduced infant mortality. However, there are ways to minimize risks, including, for example, coordinating care from preconception to delivery with a focus on the health of the child. Coordinated care presents benefits for the health and well-being of birthing women, birthing people, and children, and can improve pregnancy and child health outcomes in the future. In addition, community-based care, including pre- and postnatal home visits and paid or volunteer community health workers, has been shown to improve healthcare delivery and outcomes (Lassi et al., 2016). For additional background on programs designed to prevent infant mortality, see "National Institute for Children's Health Quality, 2021" "Healthy Babies are Worth the Wait," and "CenteringPregnancy" in Resources for More In-Depth Information at the end of this chapter.

Infant mortality is defined as the death of an infant before their first birthday. Infant mortality rate (IMR) is defined as the number of infant deaths per every 1,000 live births. An important marker of the overall health of a society is the IMR. In 2019, the IMR in the United States was 5.6 deaths per 1,000 live births. The 10 leading causes of infant death in 2019 included congenital malformations (21%), low birth weight (17%), unintentional injuries (6%), sudden infant death syndrome (6%), maternal complications (6%), umbilical cord and placental complications, bacterial sepsis of the newborn, respiratory distress of the newborn, diseases of the circulatory system, and necrotizing enterocolitis. These causes account for 67.1% of all infant deaths in the United States. Maternal complications, the third leading cause of infant mortality in 2018, became the fifth leading cause in 2019. Neonatal hemorrhage, the 10th leading cause of infant mortality in 2018, dropped from among the top leading causes of infant death in 2019 and was replaced by necrotizing enterocolitis in newborns. The IMR for low birth weight decreased 5.3% from 97.0 in 2018 to 91.9 in 2019. The IMR for unintentional injuries increased 9.7% from 30.8 in 2018 to 33.8 in 2019 and 19.0% from 7.9 to 9.4 for necrotizing enterocolitis of newborns. Mortality rates for other leading causes of infant death did not change significantly (Ely & Driscoll, 2021; Kochanek et al., 2020).

The mortality rate declined for infants of non-Hispanic White women in 2019 compared with 2018; declines in rates for the other race and Hispanic-origin groups were not significant. The 2019 infant mortality rate for infants of non-Hispanic Black women (10.62) was more than twice as high as that for infants of non-Hispanic White (4.49), non-Hispanic Asian (3.38), and Hispanic (5.03) women. Infants born very preterm (less than 28 weeks of gestation) had the highest mortality rate (374.46), 184 times as high as that for infants born at term (37 to 41 weeks of gestation; 2.03; Ely & Driscoll, 2021). More on infant mortality can be found under the heading "Infant Mortality" in Resources for More In-Depth Information at the end of this chapter.

Root Causes of Poor Outcomes

Clear guidelines on race and medicine do not exist, and although genetic evidence shows that race is not a reliable substitute for genetic difference, diagnostic algorithms and practice guidelines continue to use a patient's race or ethnicity for outputs. As such, physicians use algorithms for patient risk assessment and clinical decisions, which may yield algorithms that produce a type of race-based medicine (Vyas et al., 2020). See Chapter 13 for a discussion on race and healthcare.

Reported by Vyas et al. (2020), the vaginal birth after cesarean (VBAC) algorithm, a calculator that helps determine whether a person will have a successful vaginal birth following a C-section, provides for a lower likelihood of success for birthing women and birthing people who identify as Black or Hispanic. On the other hand, other variables, including marital status and insurance type, were correlated with success in the VBAC and were not incorporated into the algorithm. Although vaginal deliveries have known health benefits, physicians perform C-sections on non-White U.S. women at higher rates (Vyas et al., 2020).

There are significant challenges to achieving optimal maternal and child healthcare. Some barriers to optimizing maternal child health include federal, state, and local policies; institutional policies and practices; provider attitudes and behaviors; social determinants preventing access; and decision by patients to self-limit entry due to negative experiences or lack of cultural competence among providers. Though there are significant complex challenges as outlined, these interrelated challenges provide excellent opportunities to explore and direct resources that reduce barriers to healthcare (Vyas et al., 2020).

The coronavirus disease of 2019 (COVID-19) has uncovered disparities in healthcare worldwide. Even after nearly 1,000,000 deaths at the time of writing, the United States still struggles to directly find resources to help our most vulnerable and marginalized populations. Due to COVID-19, all birthing people experienced limited access to in-person visits, and restrictions were placed on who could support a birth. However, despite the many challenges created by the pandemic, some innovations occurred in care delivery, creating an opportunity to create health equity by expanding access to high-value maternity care through telehealth, virtual doula appointments, and training on self-advocacy (Kemmerer et al., 2021; Ludington-Hoe et al., 2021; for more on COVID-19-related birthing strategies, see "Kangaroo Care" in Resources for More In-Depth Information at the end of this chapter). Unfortunately, pregnant people are not receiving the COVID vaccination at the same rate as others due to misinformation and mistrust of physicians, healthcare providers, and the government. The American College of Obstetricians and Gynecologists (2021) has warned physicians that they risk serious disciplinary action, including losing their medical licenses, for promoting false vaccine information.

Many political decisions result in governmental policies at the local, state, and federal levels. These policies are then used by institutional entities, like hospitals, judicial systems, and social services to create models for evidence-based policies, practices, and procedures under the auspicious of best practice. When looking at policies that affect healthcare delivery systems, it becomes evident that specific policies can impact real-time healthcare delivery, directly resulting in decisions contributing to poor outcomes, including lack of healthcare access. Layered upon these determinants is provider bias, which at times results in patients not accessing care and leading to poor healthcare outcomes (Robinson et al., 2021).

According to Baciu et al. (2017), health inequity results from two clusters of root causes. First, systemic mechanisms—intrapersonal, interpersonal, and institutional—organize power and resources differentially across identities, such as race, gender, LGBTQIA+ status, socioeconomic status, and other dimensions. Second, goods, services, and societal attention are unequally allocated to the underresourced. This unequal allocation creates health and quality of life risks referred to as the social determinants of health (Baciu et al., 2017).

The Urban Institute, a nonprofit organization focused on developing evidence-based solutions to improve the well-being of people and communities, estimates that 12.3% (40 million people) of the total U.S. population had annual family resources below the poverty threshold in 2017, compared to 13.7% (approximately one in seven Americans) in 2021 (Giannarelli et al., 2021). The official poverty measure indicates that 11.6 million children—16% of all children nationwide—lived in poverty in 2020. This total has increased by more than 1 million children since 2019. The data also reveal that poverty rates remain disproportionately high for children of color. Nationally, Black (28%), American Indian (25%), and Hispanic (23%) children are more likely to grow up poor when compared to their non-Hispanic White (10%) and Asian and Pacific Islander (9%) peers (Annie E. Casey Foundation, 2021).

Poverty and other social determinants of health have been found to lead to childhood health disparities and adverse health outcomes (Gitterman et al., 2016). Poverty impacts a range of circumstances during pregnancy, such as birth weight and infant mortality, as well as during childhood, such as language development, chronic illness, environmental exposure, nutrition, and injury (McLaughlin & Rank, 2018). Recent cost measurement analyses indicate that the annual aggregate cost of child poverty (calculated by anticipated lost productivity and increased social expenditure) in the United States is $1.0298 trillion annually, which is 5.4% of the gross domestic product. For every dollar spent on reducing childhood poverty, the United States would save $7.00 (McLaughlin & Rank, 2018).

Research further reveals that lower-socioeconomic status women and pregnant people experience barriers to prenatal care that are associated with medical and behavioral risk factors that contribute to preterm birth and other poor outcomes. Examples of barriers may include the inability to pay for services or not seeking care in a timely fashion because of prior negative experiences. In addition, some of the causes of preterm birth are more common in poor women. These include chronic hypertension, diabetes, and obesity, which are associated with pre-eclampsia. Nagahawatte and Goldenberg (2008) explained that some of these differences in pregnancy outcomes for lower-socioeconomic women and people can be accounted for by coupling later preventive/treatment health services with a heavier disease burden. The conditions that exist due to poverty continue to adversely impact pregnant women and pregnant people.

Other Factors Contributing to Poor Outcomes for Mothers and Babies

Unsafe Sleep

While a nationwide push to get babies to sleep on their backs initially produced steep declines in unexplained and sleep-related infant deaths, U.S. progress against these fatalities has been minimal in recent years. Sudden infant death syndrome (SIDS) has become much less common in recent decades. Doctors, nurses, and other health providers have urged parents to put infants to sleep on their backs without blankets or additional soft bedding and toys that could pose a suffocation risk. According to the American Academy of Pediatrics, SIDS remains a leading cause of infant mortality. However, the role of sudden unexpected infant death risk reduction programs, demographic changes, tobacco use, and emerging issues, such as increasing opioid use, deserves further investigation (Rapaport, 2018).

Placing babies on their backs at all sleep times, including during naps and at night, is the standard recommendation for safe sleep. About 3,500 babies in the United States are lost to sleep-related deaths each year; these rates are higher than in most other industrialized countries. Placing babies on their side or stomachs to sleep was more common among non-Hispanic Black mothers younger than 25 or those who have 12 or fewer years of education. The percentage of mothers who reported placing their baby on their side or stomach to sleep varied by state, ranging from 12.2% in Wisconsin to 33.8% in Louisiana (Bombard et al., 2018). Within the 32 states included in the analysis by Bombard et al. (2018):

◆ about one in five mothers (21.6%) described placing their baby to sleep on their side or stomach
◆ more than half of mothers (61.4%) reported any bed sharing with their baby
◆ two in five mothers (38.5%) related using any soft bedding in baby's sleep area

The promotion of safe sleep approaches is important for all parents (Bombard et al., 2018) and includes:

◆ using a firm sleep surface, such as a safety-approved mattress and crib
◆ keeping soft objects and loose bedding out of baby's sleep area
◆ sharing a room with baby, but not the same bed
◆ avoiding exposure to smoke, alcohol, and illicit drugs
◆ use of a pacifier

Prematurity

Preterm birth is when a baby is born before 37 weeks of pregnancy have been completed. Prematurity is one of the leading causes of death in all babies but is highest among Black neonates. Neonates born premature add another dimension of challenges mothers, parents and families must manage. There are also long-term health effects of premature birth (CDC, 2021b).

Prematurity can be prevented or reduced; however, experts have not determined why some babies are born prematurely. Although risk factors may increase the chance of a preterm birth, birthing women and birthing people with no risk factors can still have a premature birth. Risk factors for preterm birth include:

◆ the delivery of a preterm baby in the past
◆ being pregnant with multiples
◆ tobacco use and substance abuse
◆ failure to space pregnancies (i.e., less than 18 months between pregnancies; CDC, 2021b)

In 2019, preterm birth affected one of every 10 infants born in the United States. There was a decrease in preterm birth rates between 2007 and 2014. According to the CDC, this is primarily due to declines in the number of births to teens and young mothers. Unfortunately, since 2014, the preterm birth rate has continued to rise after nearly a decade, according to the annual premature birth report card from March of Dimes. In 2017, the early rate was up slightly from 2016, when it was 9.85%. The report card draws from CDC data. The difference may seem small, but it means about 3,000 more babies were born prematurely. Since 2014, cumulatively, that is 27,000 babies (Chatterjee, 2018). The year 2019 marked the fifth straight year the preterm birth rate has increased. While it is not certain what is driving the rise in premature birth rates, social and economic factors play a significant role. For example, unequal access to maternal care and high poverty rates increase a mother's risk of delivering prematurely (Chatterjee, 2018).

Over the last few years, racial disparities in premature birth rates have gotten worse, according to the March of Dimes report. Like maternal mortality, preterm birth also demonstrated differences along racial and ethnic lines. For example, in 2020, one in 10 infants born in the United States was a preterm birth. Although preterm birth rates declined .1% in 2020 (from 10.2% in 2019 to 10.1% in 2020), preterm birth rates remained the same for racial and ethnic women and birthing people. In 2020, Black women (14.4%) had 50% higher preterm births compared to White or Hispanic women (9.1% and 9.8% respectively; CDC, 2021b). Racism and structural discrimination, rather than race, influence Black women's risk for premature delivery. Research has shown that chronic stress from racism is associated with a higher risk of premature birth among Black birthing women and Black birthing people, putting them at risk of infant death (CDC, 2021b).

Infertility

Patients and providers rarely discuss the disease of infertility in minoritized populations. Indeed, minoritized patients experience barriers when they seek infertility treatment due to a range of issues, including, but not limited to, infertility treatment costs and lack of medical insurance. Evidence reveals that minoritized patients are much less likely to seek infertility treatment, with data reflecting that Black and Hispanic birthing women and Black and Hispanic birthing people are underrepresented in the infertility clinic setting (Insogna & Ginsburg, 2018). Data further reflect that Black birthing women and Black birthing people take an average of 4.3 years to seek infertility treatment compared to 3.3 years for their White counterparts. Notably, a Department of Defense study showed that addressing the cost of assisted reproduction technologies (ART) and equalizing access increased Black birthing women's use of ART. Of note, minoritized women have poorer ART outcomes (Insogna & Ginsburg, 2018).

Davis (2019) discussed the complexity and intersection of infertility and race. She delineated the dimensions of obstetric racism, which include diagnostic lapse, neglect, dismissiveness, and disrespect, which can intentionally cause pain and, in some instances, lead to coercion. Davis (2019) also stated that obstetric racism lies at the intersection of obstetric violence and medical racism. Obstetric violence is a form of gender-based violence experienced by people giving birth who are subjected to acts of violence that result in their being subordinated because they are obstetric patients. The term suggests that institutional violence and violence against birthing women and birthing people coalesce during pregnancy, childbirth, and postpartum. Obstetric violence includes dehumanizing treatment and medical abuse such as birth trauma or violations experienced during childbearing. It expresses the explicitly harmful consequences caused by medical professionals when they exert reproductive dominance over women. Obstetric racism is a threat to maternal and parental life and neonatal outcomes. It includes, but is not limited to, critical lapses in diagnosis, being neglectful, dismissive, or disrespectful, causing pain, and engaging in medical abuse through coercion to perform procedures or performing procedures without consent. This construct emerges specifically in reproductive care and places Black birthing women and Black birthing people and their infants at risk.

In addition, Davis (2020) added three dimensions and complexities minoritized peoples face when accessing ART. These include degradation ceremonies, medical abuse, and racial reconnaissance:

Ceremonies of Degradation

This is defined as the many ways that antagonize and deploy the burden of embarrassment, humiliation, shame, or holding someone emotionally hostage. Degradation is possible because the person(s) doing the degrading has power over the patient. However, such ceremonies can quickly be translated into a scene of subjection, a performance that results from domination. It is how Black people are sometimes coerced into presenting their Black selves to appear as nonthreatening as possible.

Racial Reconnaissance

Birthing mothers and birthing persons embark on a racial reconnaissance investigation to find a clinic or provider that would meet their needs. Hopefully, they would not have to be treated as racialized. Consider the experience of Angela, a Black woman pursuing ART to conceive. She believed that being Black led to the inattention of the in vitro fertilization coordinator. She wondered if maybe the coordinator did not think Angela deserved to conceive because she was Black. However, that can happen with racism: If something is connected to racism, the lack of certainty is just as disturbing as when one is sure. The fact that Angela thought race played a part in not having her calls returned led her to embark on a racial reconnaissance investigation to find a clinic that would meet her needs, where she hoped she would not have to be burdened by thinking that racism factored into her encounters. Ultimately, Angela changed clinics, locating one that was almost 300 miles from her home.

The interpretations of those encounters reveal that ART access does not preclude crisis. Adverse birth outcomes represent several crises that Black birthing women and Black birthing people experience in reproduction. However, the focus can be shifted to adverse conception processes when utilizing ART. When the issues of ART and race are framed in terms of inaccessibility and unaffordability, there is an underlying presumption that accessibility and affordability will produce positive results. Of course, the provisional nature of infertility treatment affects all women seeking ART (Davis, 2020).

Racial Discrimination: Intersectionality

A multicentered study resulted in findings showing a significant relationship between racial discrimination, low birth weight, preterm birth, small for gestational age, and maternal mortality (Braveman et al., 2021). Of 33 hypothesized causes, racism was the only factor identified that directly or indirectly could explain the racial disparities in the plausible causes of preterm birth. This can be demonstrated by examining the path of Serena Williams as she navigated pregnancy and the birthing process.

Serena Williams, considered by many to be the greatest tennis player of all time, provides a frightening example of the disparities experienced by Black women within the healthcare system. Williams, who was in phenomenal physical shape, had competed in professional tennis matches early in her pregnancy, and had excellent prenatal care, gave birth to her first child in 2017 by C-section. Everything with the procedure appeared to go well initially, but soon after delivery, Williams began experiencing shortness of breath. She knew something was wrong because she had a history of blood clots and was aware of the signs of pulmonary embolism. Although Williams informed her nurse that she was having a medical emergency, her concerns were ignored, and she had to insist on the doctor running tests. Initially, the doctor performed an ultrasound on her legs to determine whether she had a deep venous thrombosis, but none were revealed. Williams advocated for more testing given her ongoing symptoms and underwent a computed tomography (CT) scan of her chest and abdomen, which showed several small blood clots in her lungs, as well as a hematoma in her abdomen at the site of the C-section. Williams required two surgeries in the next 6 days before being discharged from the hospital. As an athlete at the top of her game and as a celebrity, she seemingly had a healthy pregnancy and uncomplicated delivery, and yet she was nearly denied the medical care she needed (Salam, 2018).

According to the CDC (2019) about 700 women die each year in the United States due to pregnancy or delivery complications. The risk of pregnancy-related death is three to four times higher for Black women as for White women. Crenshaw (1989) coined the term "intersectionality" to describe the double bind of simultaneous racial and gender prejudice. Intersectionality is the complex, cumulative way in which the effects of multiple forms of discrimination (such as racism, sexism, and classism) combine, overlap, or intersect, especially in the experiences of minoritized individuals or groups. Crenshaw's motivation for expanding our vocabulary was to foster a deeper understanding of discrimination to prompt us to consider the multiple types of discrimination a person can experience to understand their whole societal experience (Crenshaw, 1989).

Though first used as a legal theory, intersectionality has expanded our understanding of the unique discrimination encountered in the healthcare setting; coupling this with political determinants of health allows us to understand better the complexities experienced by minoritized women and people within healthcare systems. One can easily deduce that Black birthing women and Black birthing people must contend with sexism and racism and, at times, assumptions about their socioeconomic status, which has historically led to their experiences being minimized or ignored (Bridges, 2018; Hostetter & Klein, 2021a). Intersectionality in the healthcare system has a particularly troubling result given the precedent of institutionalized racism and bias (Braveman et al., 2021; Hostetter & Klein, 2021a). This results in Black birthing women and Black birthing people (and men) lacking trust in healthcare providers and preferring to seek alternative approaches for staying healthy (Campbell, 2009; Hostetter & Klein, 2021b). Black women's attitudes toward healthcare are more suspicious, and research reflects that they delay seeking medical treatment for longer, secondary to repeated negative experiences (Mijal, 2019). Racism and sexism combined with systemic discrimination have resulted in Black women and people continuing to experience marginalization even within efforts that seek to aid them (Mijal, 2019). Several approaches are being used within the Black community that show improved healthcare outcomes, including treating patients as experts (e.g., Questions to Guide Discussions During Trust-Building Prenatal Visits); inviting trusted community leaders to deliver important messages; building relationships outside of examination rooms; and uncovering causes of institutional racism (Hostetter & Klein, 2021b).

Considering the contribution of healthcare systems to this marginalization, healthcare professionals are often unaware of their prejudice, which is what makes this discrimination so threatening. Like all individuals, healthcare providers have implicit or unconscious biases. However, in the healthcare setting, the tendency can demonstrate positive attitudes toward Whites and negative attitudes toward minoritized people (Hall et al., 2015). These attitudes can have devastating consequences because implicit bias is related to patient/ provider interactions, treatment decisions, adherence, and patient health outcomes. Data examining implicit bias found that healthcare professionals tended to possess low to moderate levels of negative associations with Black Americans. Healthcare professionals associated Black Americans with being less cooperative, less compliant, and less responsible in medical decision-making (Hall et al., 2015). Though many of these negative attitudes and assumptions are commonly tied to economically challenged women, research reveals these troubling, negative attitudes and beliefs impact the care that Black women and other minoritized women are receiving during pregnancy and delivery (Salam, 2018).

In addition, a 2016 analysis found that Black college-educated mothers who gave birth in New York City hospitals were more likely to suffer severe complications during pregnancy and childbirth than uneducated White mothers, misattributed solely to poverty (New York City Department of Health and Mental Hygiene, 2016; Salam, 2018). While a college education decreases the mortality ratio for White mothers, Black mothers with a college education are at a 60% greater risk for a maternal death compared to White or Hispanic mothers or birthing people with less than a high school education (Declercq & Zephyrin, 2020). Maternal deaths across all education levels are higher among Black birthing mothers and Black birthing people, as compared to White and Hispanic birthing mothers and birthing people with less education. For additional background on maternal death by race and education, see "Maternal Mortality Rates" in Resources for More In-Depth Information at the end of this chapter.

A study of Indigenous, Hispanic, and Black birthing women revealed that these minoritized women reported mistreatment (e.g., shouting, scolding, ignoring, or refusing requests for help) during their pregnancy at significantly higher rates. Providing care with cultural humility can lead to significant improvements in Black infant mortality as revealed by a study of hospital births assisted by Black physicians in Florida (Artiga et al., 2020). Actions can mitigate the impacts of implicit bias on Black birthing women and Black birthing people and other minoritized people. The Institute of Medicine (2003) report explained that providers need to be educated about the disparities experienced by minoritized people. Physicians who have come to realize their own biases have had success in actively controlling their thought processes and changing how they address patients and their care (Cohen, 2009). For these reasons, all healthcare professionals should receive training on an ongoing basis regarding the biases we all have based on gender (Govender & Penn-Kekana, 2008) and race (Mijal, 2019) to mitigate the effects implicit biases have on the quality of care that patients receive.

When providers are trained and become aware of implicit bias and how it presents during individual interactions, they are better able to redirect responses and provide more equitable care. Strategies providers can use to reduce implicit bias during individual interactions include:

- **Stereotype replacement:** recognizing that a response is based on stereotype and consciously adjusting the response
- **Counterstereotypic imaging:** imagining the individual as the opposite of the stereotype
- **Individuation:** seeing the person as an individual rather than a stereotype (e.g., learning about their personal history and the context that brought them to the doctor's office or health center)
- **Perspective-taking:** putting yourself in the other person's shoes
- **Increasing opportunities for contact with individuals from diverse groups:** expanding one's network of friends and colleagues or attending events where people of other racial and ethnic groups, gender identities, sexual orientation, and other groups may be present
- **Partnership building:** reframing the interaction with the patient as one between collaborating equals, rather than between a high-status person and a low-status person (Institute for Healthcare Improvement, 2017)

In addition, practical guidelines for healthcare providers to combat implicit bias in healthcare include:

- having a basic understanding of your patients' cultures
- avoiding stereotyping patients; individuate them
- understanding and respecting the tremendous power of unconscious bias
- recognizing situations that magnify stereotyping and bias
- knowing the National Culturally and Linguistically Appropriate Services (CLAS) standards
- doing a "teach back." Teach back is a method to confirm patient understanding of healthcare instructions associated with improved adherence, quality, and patient safety
- assiduously practicing evidence-based medicine (Institute for Healthcare Improvement, 2017)

Health Systems and Clinicians

In the past few years, amid a pandemic that has taken a disproportionate toll on Black and brown people and a national reckoning on racial justice, leaders from several U.S. health systems have named racism as a public health threat. They have pledged to identify and reverse racist policies and practices in their institutions. Specifically identifying racism as the threat and creating an urgency to implementing solutions is what sets these efforts apart from earlier health equity initiatives (Hostetter & Klein, 2021b).

For-profit and not-for-profit health systems all share a common thread of commitment to quality healthcare. But there are some differences, too. In theory, all large or small healthcare facilities and their providers have dedicated their workforce and resources to provide preventive health and wellness, treat acute and chronic diseases, and provide opportunities for lifelong productivity and prosperity for all they serve. Many health systems continue to fall short of providing accessible, affordable, and equitable care as they strive to stay competitive in a system that promotes financial growth, sometimes at the cost of quality comprehensive care. In recent times, the issues of race, minoritized populations, and health disparities have come front and center, especially in light of the COVID-19 pandemic. Health systems and health policy experts highlight the burden minoritized populations, including immigrants and refugees, place on the health care system. A complex and multi-factorial construct of structural racism challenges these populations with access and treatment (Crear-Perry et al., 2021; Riley, 2012). Access to healthcare focuses on multiple challenges vulnerable women and children experience that frequently derail entire families. Health systems that continue to struggle with systemic structural racism have also seen behaviors in well-meaning clinicians that at times result in poor outcomes (Riley, 2012). For example, cardiovascular disease, obstetric, and pediatric care are the primary areas where clinical treatment by health systems and clinicians has been associated with preventable outcomes (Riley, 2012). Health systems, clinicians, and support staff must be held accountable to acknowledge and embrace sustainable programs that address their contributions to creating culturally insensitive healthcare, inequities, and resultant heath disparities (Riley, 2012).

The Institute for Healthcare Improvement conducted a poll of 500 U.S. healthcare professionals in July 2021, and health equity emerged as a top priority for 58% of organizations, up from 25% in 2019. Respondents identified various barriers to health equity, including the lack of relevant, consistent data about patients and the lack of dedicated staff or other resources (Hostetter & Klein, 2021b). With health equity an even greater priority, academic medical centers are focusing on those things they can control within their systems, including the patient's experience, hiring and promotion practices, inclusion and engagement in the workplace, and community investments.

CASE STUDY 21.1: PREGNANT, UNMARRIED, UNINSURED, AND NOT WHITE

Jennifer is a 24-year-old who is 6 weeks pregnant by a sure menstrual cycle. She is uninsured and unemployed, living in public housing in a one-bedroom unit with her two small children. Jennifer dropped out of high school at age 16 when she became pregnant with her first child. At that time, she moved into her boyfriend's home that he shared with his mother. Her children have different fathers, and her current boyfriend is the father of the child with which she is pregnant. Her experience with the first child was not ideal. She believed a White male doctor at the free clinic was disrespectful and dismissive because she was an uninsured, unwed, teenage mother. Being a Black single parent, she is again fearful that she will not receive the care to have a positive pregnancy outcome. Jennifer is concerned that she is unable to navigate a safe, personalized birthing experience through the postpartum period.

Case Study Discussion Questions

Following is a list of questions a clinician might ask Jennifer about her support system, and what she needs to have a healthy pregnancy and delivery and fourth trimester support. Why is each important? What would you add to the list?

(continued)

CASE STUDY 21.1: PREGNANT, UNMARRIED, UNINSURED, AND NOT WHITE (*CONTINUED*)

◆ Are you all alone in the process or do you have a support system to assist you: a partner, family members, or friends?
◆ Do you have adequate housing?
◆ Do you have daycare for your children?
◆ Have you enrolled in Medicaid for yourself or CHIP (Children's Health Insurance Program) for your children?
◆ Would you like to be connected to a doula or midwife during your pregnancy?
◆ What can we do to make you feel safe?
◆ Do you have reliable transportation to attend follow-up OB/GYN appointments?
◆ Are there other interventions (including job training and education) that could assist you?
◆ Do you have a medical home where you receive routine care?
◆ Do you need someone to just listen?

Strategies for a Good Pregnancy

The pregnancy experience begins before the actual implantation of the ovum, which starts the beautiful creation of a living and breathing human being in a matter of 9 months. This miracle is not without unpredictable stressors and may impact the joyful anticipation of a newborn. There are several recommendations to minimize these stressors, but the five top strategies that could assist in making this experience a safe and personalized one include:

1. Intentional investment in the prenatal period.
2. Understanding the pregnancy course including risks and benefits.
3. Securing a clinician who will act as a medical partner in decision-making and include a doula or community health worker who will act as an additional knowledgeable support person by relieving fears and concerns before, during, and after giving birth.
4. Engaging in a centering health program (in-person or virtually).
5. Continuing utilization of support individuals and services for a minimum of 1 year after giving birth.

Intentional Investment in the Prenatal Period

First, one should develop a support system or interventions to create a positive pregnancy and birth experience. This would present an opportunity to ensure resources are made available to the patient to help achieve successful birth outcomes. Pregnancy is described as a normal physiological process that exerts significant abnormal stressors on a women's body as she supplies protection and needed nutrients to her unborn child. The prenatal period is the optimal time to become familiar with the birthing process while preparing your body, mind, soul, and family for this planned event. This requires more than prenatal vitamins, physical wellness, and gathering needed genetic information. The decision focused on planning and timing is critical. More than in any previous time in history, it has become increasingly possible to control fertility and conception. Pregnancy benefits from preparation that includes the future mother's psychological/emotional, and social wellness.

An unintended pregnancy is either unwanted (occurring when no children are desired) or mistimed (happening at a different time than expected). In the United States, 30.6% of pregnancies were unintended. Unintended pregnancies may pose health risks to the mother and baby, resulting from delayed or lack of prenatal care. Births resulting from unintended pregnancies are associated with adverse health outcomes for mother and baby, including low birth weight, shorter duration of breastfeeding, increased risk of postpartum depression and parental stress, and physical or psychological abuse.

Public insurance programs such as Medicaid pay for 68% of unplanned births, compared with 38% of planned births. In addition, Healthy People 2030 has set the goals of increasing the effective use of birth control and decreasing unintended pregnancies from 43.0% to 35.6% (United Health Foundation, 2022). Estimates reveal that, in 2018, the immediate direct medical cost of unintended pregnancy was $5.5 billion, representing an increase from $4.6 billion in 2011. This increase came about even as unintended pregnancy rates declined. Moreover, a 2014 study found that publicly supported family-planning programs (e.g., Title X Family Planning program, federally qualified health center services) led to a net annual federal and state government savings of $13.6 billion. These savings were primarily due to avoided medical costs from prevented unplanned pregnancies (National Conference of State Legislatures, 2021).

Research has been conducted investigating the mother's psychological wellness, which often manifests itself in the postpartum period but can be a constant challenge during pregnancy. Mental health is essential to be prepared for the pregnancy, and mood swings and previous history or current manifestations of mental illness many be exacerbated during pregnancy. It is necessary to seek and maintain mental health management and support before pregnancy. Women with histories of psychiatric illness, or first onset of psychiatric illness while pregnant, must work closely with healthcare providers on treatment plans and the decision to use psychotropic medications during pregnancy (Massachusetts General Hospital, 2018).

Understand the Pregnancy Course, Including Risks and Benefits

Regular and scheduled prenatal visits are highly beneficial to a successful pregnancy. Although pregnancy is considered a normal process, entering this phase of motherhood should be approached with a broad foundation of knowledge of both the risks and benefits. Because the symptoms and complications of pregnancy can range from mild to severe, birthing women and birthing people may find it difficult to determine which symptoms are atypical. Problems experienced during pregnancy may be physical and/or mental impairments that can affect the health of the birthing mother or birthing parent or the baby. While some problems may be mild, others may prove harmful to the birthing mother or birthing parent and their baby (CDC, 2020).

Morning sickness, back pain, constipation, and mood swings are common complaints echoed by pregnant women. These are normal discomforts that the changes and fluctuations of hormones bring to this experience. These hormonal changes also give women protection against ovarian and breast cancer development. Intimacy, sex, and orgasms may be more enjoyable as well. In addition to providing the developing baby's nutrition, many moms reduce habits not conducive to pregnancy and take better care of their bodies. These are many of the expected changes, but other risks are essential to understand. Preterm labor, preterm delivery, hypertensive disease, pre-eclampsia, and diabetes are common pregnancy complications, especially for vulnerable populations (Nagahawatte & Goldenberg, 2008). During labor and delivery, the risk of C-section delivery, intrapartum and postpartum hemorrhage, and anesthesia complications are potential risks that providers should discuss.

Secure a Support Team

It is of immense value to secure a clinician who will act as a medical partner in decision-making and include a doula or community health worker who will serve as an additional knowledgeable support. The care that women receive before, during, and after the birth of a child can limit the anxiety that usually accompanies this anticipation. Selecting a caregiver is one of the most important decisions a mother can make. A partnership with a clinician that will listen, advise, and always treat a mother with dignity and respect should never be compromised. Including a doula or community health worker could become a valuable asset to any mother. These individuals give mothers an added layer of protection by understanding their communities' cultural, socioeconomic, and political strengths and weaknesses. Doulas give women a voice when they are fearful, in pain, and too weak to use their own voices. Sometimes they are frightened, too! They can bring comfort to the entire family. Developing a birth plan that is safe, evidence-based, and reflects a mother's wishes can be developed jointly with her clinical team.

Available literature discusses how increasing access to doula care, especially in under-resourced communities, may improve birth outcomes, enhance the experience of care, and lower costs by reducing nonbeneficial and unwanted medical interventions (March of Dimes, 2019). For example, a doula support program in New York City found that among almost 500 infants born to non-Hispanic Black women over a 5-year period (2010–2015), doula-supported women had lower rates of preterm birth and low birthweight. The program served women in a neighborhood with the highest rates of infant mortality, prematurity, and low birthweight in New York City. Program participants also felt highly valued and felt thought they had a voice in consequential childbirth decisions. A study that compared outcomes for doula-supported Medicaid recipients with a national sample of similar women who did not receive doula care found lower C-section and preterm birth rates for doula-supported births among subgroups including Black women. These findings suggested doulas have the potential to reduce persistent racial/ethnic disparities in outcomes (March of Dimes, 2019). A focus group of low-income pregnant women found that access to doulas can mitigate the effects of social determinants of health by addressing health literacy and social support needs. For example, doulas can help improve communication between low-income, racially/ethnically diverse pregnant women and their healthcare providers (March of Dimes, 2019).

As with doulas, there is evidence to suggest that socially and financially disadvantaged women may thrive in midwifery models of care across all birth settings. The woman-centered philosophy of care that characterizes these models affirms agency among women of color. Group prenatal care models offer needed social support. These models mitigate the harmful impact of medical models that have historically failed to trust the competence and capabilities of women, particularly Black women, including the experiences of disregard and disrespect described by many Black women in traditional care (National Academies of Sciences, 2020).

However, the available evidence is inadequate to determine health outcomes among women of color associated with hospital births that follow the midwifery model of care. Until more data are available to guide policy, there may be meaningful opportunities to integrate midwifery models of care and doulas for labor support into hospital-based delivery settings. Doing so would enable women of color, particularly those with high medical, social, or obstetric risk factors, to still garner the benefits of woman-centered midwifery models of care and labor support (National Academies of Sciences, 2020).

Engage in a Centering Health Program (In-Person or Virtually)

The centering pregnancy model has demonstrated that group care has improved pregnancy outcomes for mothers and babies. Bringing women together to perform risk assessments, educate them on how to practice self-care, and give support as part of wrap-around clinical care. This method of pregnancy care brings patients out of the exam room into a unique group. The psychology of this care model is focused on decreasing stress and anxiety through meditation, mindfulness, yoga, and dance. For more on centering pregnancy, see "Centering Health Care Institute" in Resources for More In-Depth Information at the end of this chapter.

Continue With Support Services for a Minimum of 1 Year After Giving Birth

New motherhood is a taxing time. The postpartum period may sometimes be the most stressful time of the pregnancy journey. New mothers are at the most risk, especially where there are complications during pregnancy or delivery. This is the period that traditionally extends through 6 weeks after delivery. It has been demonstrated that women need more support well beyond 6 weeks. This is especially critical for underresourced mothers who find it more challenging to secure needed support for this period. A newborn is demanding, and mothers return home to continue mothering with a body and mind that have been drained. The birthing experience requires a tremendous amount of energy. Lack of sleep, in conjunction with the demands of a newborn, can lead to significant stress, anxiety, and depression. Support through this period is critical. Postpartum support can take many forms, including medical support (obstetricians, primary care, lactation specialists, nurses, and social workers) and social support (friends, family, and neighbors; Glover, 2020).

CASE STUDY 21.2: PERSISTENT MISCARRIAGE ANXIETY

Tasha, age 32, is married and the mother of two children. She is currently 7 months pregnant with her third child. She is a school district superintendent, and her husband is a tenured university professor. They both earned doctorate degrees, and each earns a six-figure salary. The family lives in an upper-middle class neighborhood and has a great support system that includes extended family and a network of friends. They are financially secure, have health insurance and a choice of medical providers. Unfortunately, Tasha's previous pregnancy ended in a miscarriage at 7 months. At that time, Tasha had repeatedly told her OB/GYN that something did not feel normal; she was experiencing severe pain. She had been told not to worry; it was just the baby. However, there had been a problem: pre-eclampsia. Now that Tasha is almost ready to give birth, she is terrified of something happening with this pregnancy, too. The new OB/GYN has reassured her that are no issues as this has been a healthy pregnancy. However, Tasha is still doubtful and is completely stressed about miscarrying again.

Discussion Questions for Persistent Miscarriage Anxiety

What follows are questions a clinician should ask Tasha in the interest of reducing stress and anxiety. After each, list two or three concrete suggestions or questions you would use as a follow-up to help Tasha arrive at a satisfactory plan of action or support, assuming that Tasha is seeking help within your healthcare facility and the local community.

1. How can we best help you plan for a successful pregnancy?
2. Is there something in particular that I can do to alleviate your concerns?
3. How does your network support you?
4. How can we help you with anxiety; would you consider prescription medication or a therapist?
5. Would you like a doula, midwife, or some other assistance before or during delivery to support you?
6. Can I connect you to a support group?

The Transformation Toward Social Justice and Equity

Starting the journey toward health equity for the most vulnerable is complex. Health systems providing maternal and infant care and treatment to underrepresented populations must find a way to address disparate care by governing through a social justice lens. Health systems have a unique opportunity to lead the way in demonstrating the transformational impact that antiracism, antisexism, antiminority, inclusion, and diversity have on innovation, collaboration, and global healthcare results. Systemness can facilitate an organization's ability to evolve into a "connected care community" that is more agile and virtually integrated (Jones, 2018; details can be found under the heading "Systemness" in Resources for More In-Depth Information at the end of this chapter).

Leaders, practitioners, researchers, and variegated caregivers from diverse disciplines can come together to form a transformational team that is focused on dismantling racism followed by other "isms" to ensure the quality of care for patients, employees, and the communities they serve. Such a team should focus on behaviors that prevent optimal care to oppressed persons, including policies that affect maternal and child healthcare for minoritized women and children. While complex and significant challenges may exist within said policies, a transformation team, made up of senior leaders, could be charged with identifying and exploring natural resources that can reduce barriers to healthcare for specific populations (Vyas et al., 2020).

According to Braveman et al. (2021), targeted education on the significant relationship between racial discrimination, low birth weight, preterm birth and early gestational age, and maternal mortality can be emphasized by a transformation team. The work would be accomplished by fostering exhaustive research-based strategies to inform and create policy, innovation, data-driven education and advocacy campaigns, and narrative-change initiatives. Transformation teams accomplish their work by forming and leveraging subcommittees which work independently. Subcommittees are responsible for supporting improvements in focus areas, such as maternal morbidity and infant mortality and improving maternal and child health outcomes through an antiracism lens. It is through communication that a transformation team creates the systemness required to change and/or improve complex health systems, create transparency, share accountability, improve health outcomes, and address racism.

CONCLUSION

Poverty, lack of access to care, decisions to not access care, and continued poor outcomes have multifactorial root causes. Although structural racism is cited as a significant contributor to the state of our economic wealth gap, which results in much of the poverty, it is not this alone that causes us to exhibit behaviors that are human but inhumane. Social determinants of health have resulted in challenges for all minoritized populations, but it is in the hospital's systems and other settings that we find disheartening attitudes that have resulted in behaviors that do not result in optimal care. We are at a tipping point, for the sake of humanity in the United States and globally, especially regarding healthcare, to embrace the most vulnerable as valued individuals who bring expertise and productivity to society. As clinicians and hospital systems leaders, we declare no room for hate in a healing place. We have enough data to move us forward, developing sustainable movements and programs that offer equity in opportunity to all while dispelling the myth of a zero-sum game. This is where we must start.

Discussion Questions

1. Using the Social Vulnerability Index, delineate how you might use the measure to assist with identifying health issues and making a comprehensive plan of care for women of childbearing age and those who are pregnant.
2. Utilizing Healthy People 2030, review the section on maternal and child care, and identify two goals and approaches that you think would help in addressing and eliminating the health disparities among birthing women.
3. When focusing on the socioeconomic status of women, discuss how this factor can impact the health and well-being of birthing women and their health outcomes. Propose a short- and long-term plan of action that could assist women in your practice who are vulnerable because of their economic status.
4. What are three barriers encountered by ethnic/minority women that hinder their participation in quality healthcare that you can identify in your practice, research, and policy activities?
5. Define health inequities and health equities. Write a brief case study that highlights these two concepts in your practice, research, teaching, and policy work.

ADDITIONAL RESOURCES

CenteringPregnancy decreases the rate of preterm and low-weight babies, increases breastfeeding rates, and leads to better pregnancy spacing. In CenteringParenting family-centered well-childcare, there is better attendance at recommended visits and improved immunization rates. CenteringPregnancy has been shown to nearly eliminate racial disparities in preterm birth. Black birthing women and Black birthing people, who are at higher risk for preterm birth in the Unites States, experience a lower risk of preterm birth when enrolled in CenteringPregnancy than in traditional care.

Centering Health Care Institute. (2021). *CenteringPregnancy*. https://centeringhealth care .org/what-we-do/centering-pregnancy

Geospatial Research, Analysis, and Services Program (GRASP). Use this site to explore the relationship between where a person lives and their quality of life. Follow the links to delve into topics of interest.

Agency for Toxic Substances and Disease Registry. (2021). *Place and health: The places of our lives affect the quality of our health*. https://www.atsdr.cdc.gov/placeandhealth/

Health Equity. Healthcare professionals have expressed an interest in prioritizing healthy equity and workforce diversity. Theis site depicts, among other things, that the top two barriers were inconsistent collection of data and lack of staff support:

Hostetter, M., & Klein, S. (2021b, October 18). *Confronting racism in health care: Moving from proclamations to new practices*. The Commonwealth Fund. https://doi.org/10.26099/kn6g-aa68

Healthy Babies are Worth the Wait. The March of Dimes awarded a grant to this community pilot program in Kentucky. The pilot program educated pregnant people, providers, and the community on preterm risk factors and how to reduce preterm births. Singleton births declined through the Kentucky program, and San Bernardino County designed their program using the same successful strategy.

Let's Get Healthy California. (2016). *Innovation challenges: Healthy babies are worth the wait*. https:// letsgethealthy.ca.gov/innovation-challenge/healthy-babies-are-worth-the-wait-community -program/

Infant Mortality. Statistics are presented based on data from the 2019 period linked birth/infant death file. There has been a miniscule decrease in infant mortality in the United States in recent times. A breakdown of the four most common causes for 2019 were sudden infant death syndrome (37%), accidental suffocation (28%), unknown causes (35%), and combined sudden unexpected infant death (SUID) rate. Graphics illustrate trends in unexpected infant death by cause, including unsafe sleep:

Centers for Disease Control and Prevention. (2021c). *Sudden unexpected infant death and sudden infant death syndrome*. https://www.cdc.gov/sids/data.htm

Ely, D. M., & Driscoll, A. K. (2021). *Infant mortality in the United States, 2019: Data from the period linked birth/infant death file*. National Vital Statistics Reports. https://www.cdc.gov/nchs/data/nvsr/ nvsr70/nvsr70-14.pdf

Kangaroo Care. This article provides an analysis of strategies that were recommended during the COVID-19 pandemic:

Ludington-Hoe, S. M., Lotas, M., & D'Apolito, K. (2021). Skin-to-skin contact (kangaroo care) during the COVID-19 pandemic. *Neonatal Network, 40*(3), 161–174. https://doi.org/10.1891/11-T-748

Maternal Mortality Rates. These sites depict trends in pregnancy-related mortality and causes of pregnancy-related death in the United States from 1987 to 2017:

Centers for Disease Control and Prevention. (2020, November 25). *Pregnancy mortality surveillance system*. https://www.cdc.gov/reproductivehealth/maternal-mortality/pregnancy-mortality -surveillance-system.htm#trends

Declercq, E., & Zephyrin, L. (2020). *Maternal mortality in the United States: A primer* [Issue Brief]. The Commonwealth Fund. https://www.commonwealthfund.org/publications/ issue-brief-report/2020/dec/maternal-mortality-united-states-primer

Hoyert, D. L. (2022, February 23). Maternal mortality rates in the United States, 2020. *NCHS Health E-Stats*. https://doi.org/10.15620/cdc:113967

National Institute for Children's Health Quality (NICHQ). This new e-toolkit to address infant mortality has packaged evidence-based practices and lessons learned from implementing six key strategies for reducing infant mortality rates into an easy-to-use e-toolkit. The NICHQ-led Collaborative Improvement and Innovation Network to Reduce Infant Morality (Infant Mortality CoIIN) has engaged teams from around the United States to improve health outcomes for every mom and every baby.

National Institute for Children's Health Quality. (2021). *New toolkit for addressing infant mortality.* https://www.nichq.org/insight/new-toolkit-addressing-infant-mortality

COVID-19 and Pregnancy. This article provides an extensive review of the impact of COVID-19 infection on pregnant patients:

Di Mascio, D., Khalil, A., Saccone, G., Rizzo, G., Buca, D., Liberati, M., Vecchiet, J., Nappi, L., Scambia, G, Berghella, V., & D'Antonio, F. (2020). Outcome of coronavirus spectrum infections (SARS, MERS, COVID-19) during pregnancy: A systematic review and meta-analysis. *American Journal of Obstetrics & Gynecology MFM, 2*(2), 100107. https://doi.org/10.1016/j.ajogmf.2020.100107

Systemness. This strategy can facilitate an organization's ability to evolve into a "connected care community" that is more agile and virtually integrated, and more fully prepared to demonstrate new and sustainable ways to solve health problems and advance its health equity agenda:

Jones, B. (2018). *Cheat sheet: Systemness in health care.* Advisory Board. https://www.advisory.com/Topics/Providers-outside-the-US/2018/06/Systemness-Cheat-Sheet

REFERENCES

Agency for Toxic Substances and Disease Registry. (2021). Place and health: The places of our lives affect the quality of our health. https://www.atsdr.cdc.gov/placeandhealth/

American College of Obstetricians and Gynecologists. (2021, October 8). COVID-19 vaccination, pregnancy, and medical misinformation: How you can help. https://www.acog.org/news/news-articles/2021/10/covid-19-vaccination-pregnancy-medical-misinformation-how-you-can-help

Annie E. Casey Foundation. (2021, September 20). New child poverty data illustrate the powerful impact of America's safety net programs. https://www.aecf.org/blog/new-child-poverty-data-illustrates-the-powerful-impact-of-americas-safety-net-programs

Artiga, S., Pham, O., Orgera, K., & Ranji, U. (2020). Racial disparities in maternal and infant health: An overview [Issue Brief]. https://www.kff.org/report-section/racial-disparities-in-maternal-and-infant-health-an-overview-issue-brief/

Baciu, A., Negussie, Y., Gellerc, A., & Weinstein, J. N. (Eds.). (2017). Communities in action: Pathways to health equity. National Academies Press. https://doi.org/10.17226/24624

Barnes-Josiah, D., Myntti, C., & Augustin, A. (1998). The "three delays" as a framework for examining maternal mortality in Haiti. *Social Science & Medicine, 46*(8), 981–993. https://doi.org/10.1016/S0277-9536(97)10018-1

Black Maternal Health Momnibus Act. (2021). Black Maternal Health Momnibus Act of 2021, H.R. 959, 117th Cong. https://www.congress.gov/bill/117th-congress/house-bill/959/text

Bombard, J. M., Kortsmit, K., Warner, L., Shapiro-Mendoza, C. K., Cox, S., Kroelinger, C. D., Parks, S. E., Lee, D. L., D'Angelo, D. V., Smith, R. A., Burley, K., Murrow, B., Olson, C. K., Shulman, H. B., Harrison, L., Cottengim, C., & Barfield, W. D. (2018). Vital Signs: Trends and disparities in infant safe sleep practices — United States, 2009–2015. *Morbidity and Mortality Weekly Report, 1.* https://www.cdc.gov/mmwr/volumes/67/wr/pdfs/mm6701e1-H.pdf

Braveman, P., Dominguez, T. P., Burke, W., Dolan, S. M., Stevenson, D. K., Jackson, F. M., Collins, J. W. Jr., Driscoll, D. A., Haley, T., Acker, J., Shaw, G. M., McCabe, E. R. B., Hay, W. W. Jr., Thornburg, K., Acevedo-Garcia, D., Cordero, J. F., Wise, P. H., Legaz, G., Rashied-Henry, K., … Waddell, L. (2021). Explaining the Black-White disparity in preterm birth: A consensus statement from a multi-disciplinary scientific work group convened by the March of Dimes. *Frontiers in Reproductive Health, 3,* 684207. https://doi.org/10.3389/frph.2021.684207

Bridges, K. M. (2018, November 18). Implicit bias and racial disparities in health care. *Human Rights, 43*(3), 19–21. https://www.americanbar.org/groups/crsj/publications/human_rights_magazine_home/the-state-of-healthcare-in-the-united-states/racial-disparities-in-health-care/

Callaghan, W. (2018). Maternal deaths in the United States: Understanding the data and moving forward. https://www.health.ny.gov/community/adults/women/task_force_maternal_mortality/docs/meeting1/callaghan_ny_mmtf.pdf

Campbell, M. (2009). Perceptions of personal health of contemporary Black women. In Y. Wesley (Ed.), *Black women's health: Challenges and opportunities* (pp. 131–146). Nova Science Publishers, Inc.

Centers for Disease Control and Prevention. (2019, September 18). Pregnancy-related deaths. https://www.cdc.gov/reproductivehealth/maternalinfanthealth/pregnancy-relatedmortality.htm

Centers for Disease Control and Prevention. (2020). Pregnancy complications. https://www.cdc.gov/reproductivehealth/maternalinfanthealth/pregnancy-complications.html

Centers for Disease Control and Prevention. (2021a). CDC/ATSDR Social Vulnerability Index fact sheet [Fact Sheet]. https://www.atsdr.cdc.gov/placeandhealth/svi/index.html

Centers for Disease Control and Prevention. (2021b). Reproductive health: Preterm birth. https://www.cdc.gov/reproductivehealth/maternalinfanthealth/pretermbirth.htm

Chang, J., Elam-Evans, L. D., Berg, C. J., Herndon, J., Flowers, L., Seed, K. A., & Syverson, C. J. (2003). Pregnancy-related mortality surveillance—United States, 1991–1999. *Morbidity and Mortality Weekly Report*, 2. https://www.cdc.gov/mmwr/preview/mmwrhtml/ss5202a1.htm

Chatterjee, R. (2018, November 1). *Premature birth rates rise again, but few states are turning things around*. NPR. https://www.npr.org/sections/health-shots/2018/11/01/662683176/premature-birth-rates-rise-again-but-a-few-states-are-turning-things-around

Cohen, D. (2009). Genetics and the health of African American women: Finding the cure for disease and the cure for social ills. In Y. Wesley (Ed.), *Black women's health: Challenges and opportunities* (pp. 57–78). Nova Science Publishers, Inc.

Crear-Perry, J., Correa-de-Araujo, R., Lewis Johnson, T., McLemore, M. R., Neilson, E., & Wallace, M. (2021). Social and structural determinants of health inequities in maternal health. *Journal of Women's Health*, 30(2), 230–235. http://doi.org/10.1089/jwh.2020.8882

Crenshaw, K. (1989) Demarginalizing the intersection of race and sex: A Black feminist critique of antidiscrimination doctrine, feminist theory and antiracist politics. *University of Chicago Legal Forum*, 1989(1/8). https://chicagounbound.uchicago.edu/uclf/vol1989/iss1/8

Davis, D. A. (2019). Obstetric racism: The racial politics of pregnancy, labor, and birthing. *Medical Anthropology*, 38(7), 560–573. https://doi.org/10.1080/01459740.2018.1549389

Davis, D. A. (2020). Reproducing while Black: The crisis of Black maternal health, obstetric racism and assisted reproductive technology. *Reproductive Biomedicine & Society Online*, 11, 56–64. https://doi.org/10.1016/j.rbms.2020.10.001

Declercq, E., & Zephyrin, L. (2020). Maternal mortality in the United States: A primer [Issue Brief]. The Commonwealth Fund. https://www.commonwealthfund.org/publications/issue-brief-report/2020/dec/maternal-mortality-united-states-primer

Ely, D. M., & Driscoll, A. K. (2021). Infant mortality in the United States, 2019: Data from the period linked birth/infant death file. National Vital Statistics Reports. https://www.cdc.gov/nchs/data/nvsr/nvsr70/nvsr70-14.pdf

Fishman, S. H., Hummer, R. A., Sierra, G., Hargrove, T., Powers, D. A., & Rogers, R. G. (2020). Race/ethnicity, maternal educational attainment, and infant mortality in the United States. *Biodemography and Social Biology*, 66(1), 1–26. https://doi.org/10.1080/19485565.2020.1793659

Flanagan, B., Gregory, E., Hallisey, E., Heitgerd, J., & Lewis, B. (2011). A social vulnerability index for disaster management. *Journal of Homeland Security and Emergency Management*, 8(1), 0000102202154773551792. https://doi.org/10.2202/1547-7355.1792

Giannarelli, L., Wheaton, L., & Shantz, K. (2021). 2021 Poverty projections: One in seven Americans are projected to have resources below the poverty level in 2021 [Issue Brief]. Urban Institute. https://www.urban.org/sites/default/files/publication/103656/2021-poverty-projections_1.pdf

Gitterman, B. A., Flanagan, P. J., Cotton, W. H., Dilley, K. J., Duffee, J. H., Green, A. E., Keane, V. A., Krugman, S. D., Linton, J. M., McKelvey, C. D., Nelson, J. L., & the American Academy of Pediatrics AAP Council on Community Pediatrics. (2016). Poverty and child health in the United States. *Pediatrics*, 137(4), e20160339. https://doi.org/10.1542/peds.2016-0339

Glover, A. (2020, October). Five reasons why you need a postpartum support network. American College of Obstetricians and Gynecologists. https://www.acog.org/womens-health/experts-and-stories/the-latest/5-reasons-why-you-need-a-postpartum-support-network

Govender, V., & Penn-Kekana, L. (2008). Gender biases and discrimination: A review of health care interpersonal interactions. *Global Public Health*, 3(suppl 1), 90–103. https://doi.org/10.1080/17441690801892208

Hall, W. J., Chapman, M. V., Lee, K. M., Merino, Y. M., Thomas, T. W., Payne, B. K., Eng, E., Day, S. H., & Coyne-Beasley, T. (2015). Implicit racial/ethnic bias among health care professionals and its influence on health care outcomes: A systematic review. *American Journal of Public Health*, 105(12), e60–e76. https://doi.org/10.2105%2FAJPH.2015.302903

Hostetter, M., & Klein, S. (2021a, 14 January). Understanding and ameliorating medical mistrust among Black Americans. The Commonwealth Fund. https://www.commonwealthfund.org/publications/newsletter-article/2021/jan/medical-mistrust-among-Black-americans

Hostetter, M., & Klein, S. (2021b, October 18). Confronting racism in health care: Moving from proclamations to new practices. The Commonwealth Fund. https://doi.org/10.26099/kn6g-aa68

Hoyert, D. L. (2022, February 23). Maternal mortality rates in the United States, 2020. NCHS Health E-Stats. https://doi.org/10.15620/cdc:113967

Hoyert, D., & Minino, A. (2020). Maternal mortality in the United States: Changes in coding, publication, and data release, 2018. *National Vital Statistics Reports, 69*(2), 1–18.

Insogna, I. G., & Ginsburg, E. S. (2018). Infertility, inequality, and how lack of insurance coverage compromises reproductive Autonomy. *AMA Journal of Ethics, 20*(12), E1152–E1159. https://doi.org/10.1001/amajethics.2018.1152

Institute for Healthcare Improvement. (2017, September 28). How to reduce implicit bias. http://www.ihi.org/communities/blogs/how-to-reduce-implicit-bias

Institute of Medicine. (2003). Unequal treatment: Confronting racial and ethnic disparities in health care. https://doi.org/10.17226/10260

Jones, B. (2018). Cheat sheet: Systemness in health care. Advisory Board. https://www.advisory.com/Topics/Providers-outside-the-US/2018/06/Systemness-Cheat-Sheet

Kemmerer, A., Zook, M., & Traylor, J. (2021, May 6). Maternity care innovations during COVID-19: Short-term solutions, long-term potential. https://www.commonwealthfund.org/blog/2021/maternity-care-innovations-during-covid-19-short-term-solutions-long-term-potential

Knickman, J., Bethel, C., Fiorillo, J., & Lansky, D. (2001). A portrait of the chronically ill in America, 2001. Robert Wood Johnson Foundation. https://folio.iupui.edu/bitstream/handle/10244/775/ChronicIllnessChartbook2001.pdf?sequence=1

Kochanek, K. D., Xu, J., & Arias, E. (2020, December). Mortality in the United States, 2019 (Data Brief No. 395). National Center for Health Statistics. https://www.cdc.gov/nchs/data/databriefs/db395-H.pdf

Lassi, Z. S., Kumar, R., & Bhutta, Z. A. (2016). Community-based care to improve maternal, newborn, and child health. In R. E. Black, R. Laxminarayan, M. Temmerman, & N. Walker (Eds.), Reproductive, maternal, newborn, and child health: Disease control priorities (3rd ed., pp. 263–284). International Bank for Reconstruction and Development/The World Bank. https://www.ncbi.nlm.nih.gov/books/NBK361898/

Ludington-Hoe, S. M., Lotas, M., D'Apolito, K. (2021). Skin-to-skin contact (kangaroo care) during the COVID-19 pandemic. *Neonatal Network, 40*(3), 161–174. https://doi.org/10.1891/11-T-748

March of Dimes. (2019, January 30). Position statement: Doulas and birth outcomes. https://www.marchofdimes.org/materials/Doulas%20and%20birth%20outcomes%20position%20statement%20final%20January%2030%20PM.pdf

Massachusetts General Hospital Center for Women's Mental Health. (2018). Psychiatric disorders during pregnancy. https://womensmentalhealth.org/specialty-clinics/psychiatric-disorders-during-pregnancy/

Maternal Health Task Force. (n.d.). Maternal health in the United States: Resources: *The role of the MHTF*. https://www.mhtf.org/topics/maternal-health-in-the-united-states/#Resources

McLaughlin, M., & Rank, M. R. (2018). Estimating the economic cost of childhood poverty in the United States. *Social Work Research, 42*(2), 73–83. https://doi.org/10.1093/swr/svy007

Mijal, K. (2019). Intersectionality and maternal mortality: African American women and health care bias [Global Honors thesis, The University of Washington, Tacoma]. University of Washington Tacoma Digital Commons. https://digitalcommons.tacoma.uw.edu/gh_theses/66

Miller, S., & Belizán, J. M. (2015). The true cost of maternal death: Individual tragedy impacts family, community and nations. *Reproductive Health, 12*(56), 1–4. https://doi.org/10.1186/s12978-015-0046-3

Nagahawatte, N. T., & Goldenberg, R. L. (2008). Poverty, maternal health, and adverse pregnancy outcomes. *Annals of the New York Academy of Sciences, 1136*(1), 80–85. https://doi.org/10.1196/annals.1425.016

National Academies of Sciences, Engineering, and Medicine. (2018). Health-care utilization as a proxy in disability determination. https://doi.org/10.17226/24969

National Academies of Sciences, Engineering, and Medicine. (2020). Birth settings in America: Outcomes, quality, access, and choice. https://doi.org/10.17226/25636

National Conference of State Legislatures. (2021). Preventing unplanned pregnancy: Overview. https://www.ncsl.org/research/health/preventing-unplanned-pregnancy.aspx

National Institute for Children's Health Quality. (2021). New toolkit for addressing infant mortality. https://www.nichq.org/insight/new-toolkit-addressing-infant-mortality

New York City Department of Health and Mental Hygiene. (2016). Severe maternal morbidity in New York City, 2008–2012. https://www1.nyc.gov/assets/doh/downloads/pdf/data/maternal-morbidity-report-08-12.pdf

Rapaport, L. (2018, February 12). U.S. progress against sleep-related infant deaths is stalling. Reuters Health. https://www.reuters.com/article/idUSKBN1FW29R

Riley, W. J. (2012). Health disparities: Gaps in access, quality and affordability of medical care. *Transactions of the American Clinical and Climatological Association, 123,* 167–174. https://www.ncbi.nlm.nih.gov/pmc/articles/PMC3540621/

Robinson, E. J., Embí, P. J., Raju, R., & Yu, Y. (2021, August 16). AHRQ Views: Blog posts from AHRQ leaders: A call for action to achieve health equity. https://www.ahrq.gov/news/blog/ahrqviews/achieve-health-equity.html

Saftlas, A., Koonin, L., & Atrash, H. (2020). Racial disparity in pregnancy-related mortality associated with livebirth: Can established risk factors explain it? *American Journal of Epidemiology, 152*(5), 413–419. https://doi.org/10.1093/aje/152.5.413

Salam, M. (2018, January 11). For Serena Williams, childbirth was a harrowing ordeal. She's not alone. The New York Times. https://www.nytimes.com/2018/01/11/sports/tennis/serena-williams-baby-vogue.html

Tikkanen, R., Gunja, M., FitzGerald, L., & Zephyrin, L. (2020). Maternal mortality and maternity care in the United States compared to 10 other developed countries [Issue Brief]. The Commonwealth Fund. https://doi.org/10.26099/411v-9255

United Health Foundation. (2022). Health of women and children: Unintended pregnancy. https://www.americashealthrankings.org/explore/health-of-women-and-children/measure/unintended_pregnancy/state/ALL

Vyas, D. A., Eisenstein, L. G., & Jones, D. S. (2020). Hidden in plain sight—Reconsidering the use of race correction in clinical algorithms. *New England Journal of Medicine, 383*(9), 874–882. https://doi.org/10.1056/NEJMms2004740

World Health Organization. (2017). Indicator metadata registry list, maternal health. https://www.who.int/data/gho/indicator-metadata-registry/imr-details/4622

Zephyrin, L., Seervai, S., Lewis, C., & Katon, J. G. (2021, March 4). Community-based models to improve maternal health outcomes and promote health equity [Issue Brief].

CHAPTER 22

Lead Poisoning in Children: The Burden of Illness in Marginalized Populations

Marilyn J. Lotas, Robin Brown, and Alexis A. Lotas

LEARNING OBJECTIVES

- Understand the Centers for Disease Control and Prevention (CDC) definition of lead poisoning and how it is determined.

- Analyze two separate metrics for the measurement of lead in the body.

- Describe the scope of the lead problem globally and in the United States.

- Identify three common sources of lead in the environment.

- Identify four symptoms of lead poisoning in children.

- Identify two strategies used to treat children diagnosed with lead poisoning.

- Analyze the individual, family, and societal costs of lead poisoning in children.

- Identify one action that can be taken to reduce the incidence of lead poisoning in children of marginalized populations.

INTRODUCTION

Childhood lead poisoning, also known as *plumbism*, is a 100% preventable condition that has devastating consequences for the children who are impacted by it (Centers for Disease Control and Prevention [CDC], 2018). The incidence of lead poisoning in children has dropped dramatically in the United States since the 1950s and represents a national public health success story. However, lead poisoning continues to impact children, in both rural and urban areas with high levels of poverty, aging housing stock, contaminated environments, and, often but not always, minority communities (Akkus & Ozddenerol, 2014; LeBron et al., 2019; Neuwirth, 2018). This chapter (a) defines lead poisoning and how the reportable level is determined; (b) analyzes two metrics for measurement of lead in the body; (c) describes the scope of the lead problem globally and in the United States; (d) identifies common sources of lead exposure globally and in the Unite States; (e) describes common effects of lead poisoning in children; (f) describes the current treatments for lead poisoning; (g) describes the emotional and socioeconomic cost to individuals, families, and society; and (h) makes recommendations for public health policy.

DEFINITION OF LEAD POISONING AND MEASUREMENT OF BODY LEAD LEVELS

Lead poisoning is defined by the CDC as blood lead levels (BLLs) above the 97.5 percentile of those test results reported to the CDC by individual states (cdc.gov/lead surveillance/). Since the mid-20th century, the CDC has established what it considers the BLL of concern. As shown in Figure 22.1, this level has dropped from 60 mcg/dL in 1950 to a 5 mcg/dL limit established in 2012 (CDC, 2021a).

However, the CDC has determined since that time that no level of lead is safe for children. Children with lead levels well below the reportable blood level reference value (BLRV) have demonstrated deficits in cognitive functioning and fine motor skills, decreased visual-motor integration, and an increase in "acting out" behaviors (Neuwirth, 2018). Adding to the concern, Hauptman et al. (2021), in a 2018 to 2020 survey of 1,141,411 children ages 0 to 6 years, found that more than 50% of the children had detectable BLLs. These children had BLLs below 5 mcg/dL (the reportable level prior to May 2021) and therefore would not be reflected in the routine surveillance data submitted to the CDC by the states, but they still are likely to have some negative effects from lead exposure. Currently, the annually reported childhood BLLs have dropped, and the 97th percentile is lower. In May 2021, the CDC updated its BLRV from 5 mcg/dL to 3.5 mcg/dL in response to the Lead Exposure Prevention and Advisory Committee (LEPAC) recommendation made on May 14, 2021 (CDC, 2021b).

Methods of Measurement

While BLLs are the standard test used for the diagnosis of lead poisoning, a second measure of lead poisoning, bone lead levels, is less commonly used, but provides additional, valuable information about the potential for lead-related damage to the child. BLLs provide a description of the child's current lead exposure, within approximately 30 days (Neuwirth,

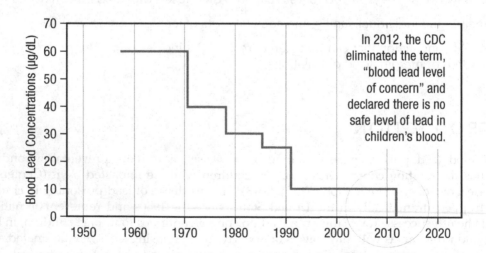

Figure 22.1 Blood lead levels considered harmful by the Centers for Disease Control and Prevention, 1950 to 2012.

Source: CDC Lead Poisoning Infographic: Safe Homes Report. www.safehomesreport.com.

2018). Measurement of bone lead levels is much more complex than obtaining a BLL but provides a measure of the child's longitudinal lead history and potential for early and ongoing lead damage. Lead stored in the bones has a half-life of up to 30 years and, during stressful conditions such as a major illness, stressful environment, or pregnancy, may move back into the bloodstream (Neuwirth, 2018). Thus, while the BLLs may be very low, the longitudinal history of lead exposure in the bones can demonstrate the probable longitudinal lead damage to the child and the potential for future damage if the lead returns to the bloodstream (Neuwirth, 2018). Also, since the initial physical damage of lead is still present in the child, as well as the effects of that damage, the longitudinal lead history is a valuable additional tool for understanding the effects of lead poisoning on children. In spite of its usefulness, it is not routinely used to identify elevated lead levels due to the cost, the time it takes to do it, and the invasiveness of the procedure compared with a blood test (Neuwirth, 2018).

SCOPE OF THE LEAD PROBLEM GLOBALLY AND IN THE UNITED STATES

Lead is a heavy metal and widely present in the environment. While lead was known and commonly used as early as 4,000 BCE and the symptoms of lead poisoning were described in early medical writings, it was not until the first century CE that the connection between lead and the symptoms of lead poisoning were clearly identified (Hernberg, 2000). Some of the properties of lead that have contributed to its wide usage are: (a) In the past, its sweet taste led to its usage in food and wine; (b) because of its high resistance to corrosion, until recently it was commonly used in water pipes; and (c) because it does not transmit radiation, it is used in protective insulation around nuclear plants and x-ray equipment and in transferring radioactive material (Gottesfeld & Pokhrel, 2011).

Scope of the Lead Problem Globally

Lead is widely and naturally distributed in every part of the world, in soil, water, and plants (Needleman, 1999). The World Health Organization (WHO) has identified lead as one of 10 toxic substances of major public health concern and has urged action by member states to protect the health of workers, children, and those of reproductive age (United Nations Children's Fund & Pure Earth, 2020; WHO, 2020). The health problems caused by lead have been documented on every continent and across a wide range of levels of exposure. The Institute for Health Metrics and Evaluation (IHME), an independent global research center at the University of Washington in Seattle, evaluated the burden of disease related to lead poisoning and estimated that in 2019, lead exposure accounted for 900,000 deaths worldwide and 21.7 million years of healthy life lost, with the highest burden of lead-related disease occurring in low- to middle-income countries (WHO, 2020).

The sources of lead vary regionally, but some significant sources are common to most areas of the world. More than three quarters of global lead consumption is related to the manufacturing of lead-acid batteries for motor vehicles and to the unsafe recycling of used lead-acid batteries (WHO, 2020), but leaded gasoline in motor vehicles has spread lead throughout the world and increased exposure significantly. Despite the incidence of severe illness and death of workers working with leaded gasoline, its production and widespread use continued throughout most of the 20th century (Needleman, 1999). As of July 2021, however, leaded fuel for vehicles is no longer sold anywhere globally, removing a major source of lead exposure.

Leaded paint was identified as another significant source of lead exposure. In 1914, lead in paint was banned in Australia, the same year that the diagnosis of lead poisoning was first recognized in the United States and 64 years before the United States banned leaded paint in 1978 (Needleman, 1999). Since leaded paint continues to be a major source of exposure in many countries, WHO has partnered with the United Nations Environment Program to form the Global Alliance to Eliminate Lead Paint and with the Global Environmental Facility, which aims to support at least 40 countries in enacting laws banning lead paint. However, at this time, only 41% of countries have enacted laws controlling the manufacture and use of leaded paint (Global Alliance to Eliminate Lead Paint, 2020).

A recent report from the IHME found that worldwide, 34% of children age 5 years or younger, almost 800 million children globally, had BLLs of 5 mcg/dL or higher. This is a previously unknown, massive scale of lead exposure in children and an equally massive number of children with unidentified and untreated lead-related damage. Almost half of the affected children are in South Asia (UNICEF press release, July 2020). Again, low- to middle-income countries are hardest hit. The report states that the informal and substandard recycling of lead-acid batteries is a leading contributor to lead poisoning in these countries. It is estimated that 50% of lead-acid batteries are unsafely recycled (WHO, 2017). Childhood lead exposure globally is estimated to cost almost $1 trillion, due to the lifetime lost economic potential of these children and the increased cost of healthcare for them.

Scope of the Lead Problem in the United States

In the mid-20th century, the magnitude of the health and social effects of lead became fully recognized in the United States (Mielke et al., 2022). In the second half of the 20th century, concern began to focus on lead sources in the environment, such as leaded gasoline, leaded paint, industrial waste containing lead, and lead-contaminated drinking water (Mielke et al., 2022). In response to that concern, a series of laws were enacted to protect the environment from lead contamination and the population from lead exposure. In 1978, the Lead-Based Paint Poisoning Prevention Act was passed, banning lead-based paint in the United States. In 1986, lead plumbing was banned in the United States; in 1988, legislation was passed that virtually banned the use of leaded gasoline; and in 1996, the ban on almost all leaded gasoline went into effect (cdc.gov/nceh/lead). From 1976, before these laws were enacted, through 2014, both the estimated percentage of children diagnosed with elevated BLLs and the average BLL found in children ages 1 to 5 years dramatically dropped. At the same time, the incidence of neurodevelopmental issues associated with lead exposure declined (Figure 22.2).

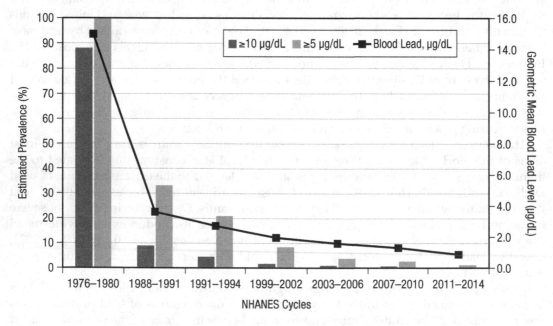

Figure 22.2 Blood levels in children ages 1 to 5 years, 1976 to 2014.
Source: U.S. National Health and Nutrition Examination Survey.

This represented a major public health success story, but one that did not extend equally to all communities in the United States.

In large urban communities and rural communities experiencing high levels of poverty and with a significant percentage of homes built before 1978, comparatively high BLLs continue to be found, particularly in children (Ettinger et al., 2019). These areas, often home to Black, Indigenous, and people of color (BIPOC) communities, have been systematically disadvantaged over decades through practices such as redlining (see Chapter 20), limited city services, limited access to healthcare, limited economic opportunities, lack of enforcement of environmental protection laws, limited power to positively impact their communities, and, over time, the cumulative effects of underfunded schools. Often these communities have disproportionately been the sites for industrial waste disposal. Although environmental protection laws were passed, they were not always rigorously enforced, especially in lower-income neighborhoods. As a result, both African American and Native American communities and those living below the poverty line continue to be vulnerable to lead exposure and the effects of lead poisoning (Neuwirth, 2018). In the United States, the non-Hispanic Black population has more than twice the percentage of children diagnosed with lead poisoning than the White population, and those living below the poverty line have approximately four times as many children diagnosed with lead poisoning as those living above the poverty line (Figure 22.3; CDC, 2019).

As a result of the continuing decline in the incidence of childhood lead poisoning, relatively little public attention was focused on the lead problem until the Flint water crisis in 2015 (see Chapter 5). The tragedy in Flint renewed national concern, specifically about the quality of water available in some communities, and more generally about the larger issue of lead exposure and poisoning in children. For many communities, childhood lead poisoning remains a problem. What began as a public health issue is now also a major social and environmental justice issue (Ettinger et al., 2019; Whitehead & Buchanan, 2019). Based on CDC lead surveillance data, 87,144 children were identified with elevated BLLs in 2018 with only 17.6% of eligible children tested (cdc.gov. lead surveillance data, 2018). The actual number of children affected by lead in the United States in 2018 could be more than 496,000. The child, family, and social costs of lead poisoning in the United States are discussed later in the chapter.

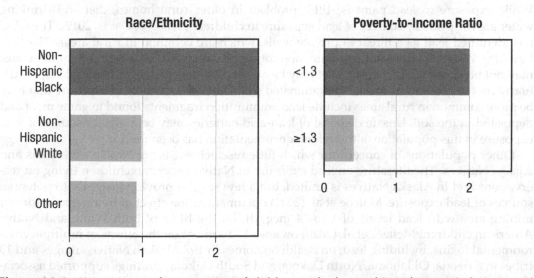

Figure 22.3 Comparison of percentage of children with elevated BLLs by race/ethnicity and poverty level.

Source: National Health and Nutrition Examination Survey (NHANES), https://www.cdc.gov/nceh/lead/data/healthy-people-objectives.htm.

COMMON SOURCES OF LEAD

Children are vulnerable to lead exposure from a variety of sources. Lead can be ingested, inhaled, absorbed through the skin, passed through the blood/brain barrier, and transmitted through the placenta to an unborn child (Manisalidis et al., 2020). Lead was widely used in paint, leaded gasoline, and water pipes, and, while lead from those sources has now been banned for decades, it remains in the environment. The manufacture of lead-acid batteries and unsafe disposal of them is an ongoing source of exposure in the United States and globally. In addition, there are some differences in the most common sources of exposure in urban versus rural settings.

Lead in Urban Settings

In urban settings, lead-based paint is still found in housing built before 1978, when leaded paint was banned. Lead paint, lead paint-contaminated house dust, and lead-contaminated soil account for 70% of lead exposure in the United States (Mayans, 2019). Lead-based paint represents a hazard, particularly for small children who demonstrate hand-to-mouth behaviors. The risks are that they may eat lead paint chips and that the dust from the paint may contaminate a child's hands and be conveyed to the mouth directly or be conveyed to food and then consumed. Paint dust may also be inhaled. The lead in contaminated soil results from the demolition or remodeling of buildings built before 1978, from industrial waste, and from the residual lead from car emissions of leaded gasoline before the 1988 ban on lead as a gasoline additive (Mayans, 2019).

In urban settings, a lesser percentage of lead exposure (under 30%) is from drinking water (Mayans, 2019). However, in some communities, as much as 50% of water pipes are still lead-based. Particularly, houses built before 1986, when lead plumbing was banned, may still have lead-based plumbing. To prevent lead from being leached from the pipes, a chemical such as orthophosphate may be added to the water, even when it tests free from lead as the water leaves the pumping station (Federal Register, 2019). However, if the pipes are broken or damaged or there is a sudden large change in water pressure, lead may still be leached into the water.

Lead in Rural Settings

While exposure to lead paint is still a problem in older rural homes, diet and drinking water are the primary sources of lead exposure in children (Aelion & Davis, 2019). The CDC has identified lead as a threat in private wells, which are common in rural areas. The Safe Drinking Water Act does not mandate monitoring private wells, so the quality of the water may not be known (CDC, 2019). Diet may be affected by vegetables containing lead, particularly root vegetables from lead-contaminated soil. Other sources of lead exposure that may be more common in rural areas include lead ammunition fragments found in game meat and deposited in the soil. Unsafe disposal of lead-acid batteries may be a greater source of lead exposure in this population, although no documentation has been found.

Other populations of concern for which little research exists are Native Americans and Alaska Natives. The literature on lead exposure in Native American children living on reservations and in Alaska Natives is limited, but a few studies provide insight into potential sources of lead exposure. Malcoe et al. (2002) documented the effect of living near a former mining area with lead levels of 1 to 24 mcg/dL on the BLLs of both White and Native American children. Meltzer et al. (2020) reviewed 31 articles on the effects of multiple environmental toxins, including lead, on health outcomes in 197 Alaskan Native villages and 13 tribes in Arizona, Oklahoma, North Dakota, and South Dakota. Findings supported associations between toxicant exposure and various chronic illnesses, but no definitive findings on lead were reported. Harris and Harper (2001) explored the possible relationship of lifestyle and diets to lead exposure among Native Americans but found no conclusive relationship.

Bressler et al. (2019) reported research on sources of lead exposure in Alaskan children, including Alaskan Natives, from 2011 to 2018. All children with BLLs of 10 mcg/dL in 2011 were reviewed, and all children with BLLs of 5 mcg/dL or higher during the 2012 to 2018 period were reviewed. Follow-up calls were made to the families of the children, asking them to identify possible sources of lead exposure. The most common source identified was parent occupation, including mining and work with airplanes, cars, or firearms (54%); other sources included consumption of game meat hunted with lead ammunition (50%), pre-1978 housing (38%), and pica (eating or mouthing of non-nutritive substances; 27%). It is notable that contaminated drinking water was not included in the list. The limitation in the study was that the interviews were conducted by telephone, so no confirmatory evidence was collected about lead sources.

The limited accessibility of Alaskan communities has prevented the kind of site visits to identify lead exposure sources commonly done in most states in the United States. One concern related to the impact of exposure to lead ammunition is that for many Native Alaskans, hunting and fishing provide a significant part of their protein intake, which increases their vulnerability to exposure to lead ammunition. One study of lead shot contribution to the BLLs of Canada's First Nation people compared BLLs before and after hunting with shotguns and eating game meat. Findings included a significant increase ($p < 0.05$) in some lead (Pb) isotopes after hunting and eating game meat. It was also suggested that the process of hunting and handling a shotgun was an important route of lead exposure even without the inclusion of eating game meat (Tsuji et al., 2008). The issue of lead exposure and health impacts on Native Americans and Alaskan Natives is an area of needed study at this time. Some of the reported findings are suggestive, but none provides a clear picture of the risk factors for lead exposure in these populations.

ACTION AND EFFECTS OF LEAD IN THE BODY

Lead has a major impact on the entire body but has a particularly devastating effect on the nervous system. The mechanisms by which lead affects the body, including the nervous system, are not fully understood. However, lead has an affinity for calcium-binding sites, which allows it to pass the blood-brain barrier and enter the brain as a substitute for a calcium ion (Neuwirth, 2018). Once it has passed through the blood-brain barrier, damage to the nervous system can be severe. Research links elevated BLLs with lower cognitive functioning, lower academic achievement, evidence of attention deficit/hyperactivity disorder (ADHD), speech and hearing problems, and short stature. Children up to age 6 years are particularly vulnerable to the effects of lead due to the rapid growth of the brain and nervous system throughout this period and beyond (Neuwirth, 2018). The earlier in the child's development the exposure occurs, the more pervasive the damage, and, once the damage is done, the effects are long-standing. Once the damage occurs, it cannot be undone, but with early identification and remediation, the effects may be mitigated.

Several studies have documented a significant relationship between early lead exposure and later criminal activity, firearm use, and violent crime (Emer et al., 2020; Haynes et al., 2011; Hoover et al., 2021; Taylor et al., 2016). In one classic early case-control study comparing the bone lead levels of 194 adjudicated delinquents, ages 12 to 18 years, with a control group of 147 adolescents ages 12 to 18 years with no criminal record, it was found that the adjudicated delinquent group was four times likelier to have significantly elevated bone lead levels than the control group (Needleman et al., 2002). As previously discussed, bone lead levels are a measure of long-term exposure to lead, and such exposure indicates a strong probability of chronic, irreparable damage to the nervous system (Needleman et al., 2002). A second classic study (Wright et al., 2008) identified over 350 pregnant persons with elevated BLLs. The behavioral progress of the infants of these people was then followed through adolescence and into early adulthood. A significant relationship was found between prenatal exposure to lead and total arrests in these children, including arrests for violent crime.

Growing concern is focused on the effects of prenatal lead exposure on the developing fetus (Segal & Giudice, 2019; Silver et al., 2016; Thomason et al., 2019). The effects are related to both the dosage of lead and the developmental stage of the fetus, with the most pervasive damage occurring in the first trimester of pregnancy. Also, an increased risk of miscarriage or fetal death has been found to be associated with pregnant persons living in areas with lead-contaminated drinking water (Edwards, 2014). Additionally, while pre-eclampsia in pregnancy has not been thought to be associated with an increase in BLLs, a meta-analysis of studies of pre-eclampsia and BLLs (Poropat et al., 2018) found a significant relationship between the two. Poropat et al. (2018) identified a total of 2,089 articles, reviewed 46 articles, and selected 11 for analysis. The studies selected were from eight countries worldwide, with different risks for bias. Poropat et al. (2018) found that an increase in BLLs of 1 mcg/dL was associated with a 1.6% increase in the incidence of pre-eclampsia. While other individual studies have contradictory results, this well-controlled meta-analysis suggests that lead may be a risk factor for pre-eclampsia and that BLLs should be monitored carefully during pregnancy, including in the United States.

The fact that lead stored in the bones may be released into the bloodstream in times of illness or stress may be particularly concerning for persons living below the poverty line, for populations suffering high levels of chronic stress, and for persons working in high-stress environments, such as healthcare professionals in the era of COVID.

Finally, increased BLLs in children have been associated with short stature as the child develops. Burns et al. (2017) studied 481 Russian boys from ages 8 through 18 years. The children were assessed annually for BLLs and growth. Boys with BLLs of 5 mcg/dL or higher were found to be significantly (0.001) shorter in stature through age 18 than boys with BLLs below 5 mcg/dL. A second study reported on 1,153 women and their infants in Bangladesh. Bangladesh is a developing country that is particularly vulnerable to high levels of lead exposure due to both its poorly regulated environmental protection laws and its high levels of malnutrition. BLLs were measured from umbilical cord blood at the delivery of infants to determine prenatal exposure and at 20 and 40 months of age. A positive correlation was found between elevated BLLs at 20 and 40 months of age and short stature using the WHO Child Growth Standards for measurement (Gleason et al., 2016).

TREATMENT OF ELEVATED BLOOD LEAD LEVELS

Treatment for elevated BLLs includes (a) anticipatory guidance of the family on the dangers of lead, where it can be found, and how to protect their children from it; (b) identification of specific sources of lead exposure for an affected child and elimination of the sources; (c) regular healthcare and developmental assessments; (d) regular testing for BLLs, minimally once a year and more often as clinical status dictates; (e) nutritional guidance, including a healthy diet, checking of iron levels, and possible calcium and iron supplements; and (f) consideration of chelation therapy at 45 mcg/dL with caution, guidance, and consultation.

INDIVIDUAL, FAMILY, AND SOCIETAL COSTS OF LEAD POISONING IN THE UNITED STATES

Cost to Child and Family

The cost of lead poisoning to the child and family is high. For the child, the struggle to learn and the identification of being different and socially difficult may result in lowered self-esteem and a lowered sense of self-efficacy. Long-term effects may include chronic illness, limited earning ability, and a higher risk of incarceration. For the family, the lack of knowledge about lead sources and effects may result in confusion and guilt for "allowing" this to happen to the child. The stress of caring for the child may be high, and the fear about the child's future is real. Some of the costs to the family are illustrated in Case Study 22.1.

CASE STUDY 22.1: A MOTHER'S STORY, BY ROBIN BROWN, DIRECTOR OF CONCERNED CITIZENS ORGANIZED AGAINST LEAD (CCOAL)

My story began when my 4-year-old daughter's doctor called and said to take her the hospital immediately and she would be directly admitted. She'd had a checkup and routine blood work, but my daughter had no illness. I was so scared and confused, but I did what he said. I thought that when we got to the hospital, she would be healed of whatever was wrong. I didn't know that she had a blood lead level of 70, which could be fatal. For 5 days, I stayed in the room 24 hours a day while my daughter was there. My daughter was getting chelation therapy. The treatment lasts 5 days. It's not a cure. But at the time, I didn't know that. Unfortunately, after her chelation, her lead went from 70 mcg/dL to 27 but 2 hours later went back up to 35, and she had to have another round of chelation. I was horrified and thought we couldn't do it. But we had to for my daughter's sake. They said we could do the second round at home, but first our home had to be inspected for lead. No one talked to me about lead poisoning while we were in the hospital. No pamphlet, no information, no nothing. So, I asked the lead inspector who came to my house all of my questions. When I understood, I flipped. The healthcare system failed my family. We never got proper information about what lead poisoning is, what it does, what the symptoms are, how to manage it, what to do with your child, none of that. But the lead inspector gave me the name of a young woman who worked with lead, and she helped me with my daughter. I made up my mind that whatever lead took out of my child, I would put back in. So I did the following:

◆ I made up number games; we would count the sidewalk blocks and different color houses.
◆ I taught her content from the grade higher than where she was. I did this until she got out of junior high.
◆ I worked with her teachers to help them understand about lead. When my daughter became disruptive, they would call me instead of sending her to the office. My daughter and I would talk and I helped her to refocus. I received these calls every day from preschool to the 11th grade. They were heart-wrenching.

It was hard on both of us. My life was organized around helping my daughter. But I did what I had to do. When anyone said my daughter can't learn, I said she will learn differently, but she will learn. And she did.

Discussion Questions

1. What is the major deficit Ms. Brown identified in the care her daughter received, and what are two strategies that would begin to address that?
2. If you were to design a community education program about lead, what are three components you would include?
3. Ms. Brown maintained an active role in her daughter's education. What are the most important strategies she used?
4. What advice would you give a parent whose child was diagnosed with lead poisoning?

Cost to Society

The cost of lead poisoning to society is equally high. The Pew Foundation, through its Partnership for America's Economic Success initiative, has calculated the lifetime economic cost of childhood lead exposure to American society by birth cohort (Pew Center on the States, 2010). All children born in a given calendar year and diagnosed with lead poisoning are considered one cohort. The calculations include health care, IQ and lifetime earning losses, special education costs related to ADHD, and behavioral problems and crime. The costs per cohort were estimated over 10 cohorts. Because the number of children in each cohort varies, costs are presented as variable estimates. The cost of healthcare is estimated to be between $10.8 and $53.1 million. The cost of loss of IQ and lifetime earning losses are estimated to be between $190 and $268 billion. The cost of special education for ADHD is estimated to be between $297 and $413 million. Finally, the cost of behavioral problems, including criminal behavior and incarceration, is estimated to exceed $1.7 billion. Thus, the total estimated cost of childhood lead poisoning to society is estimated to be approximately $192 to $270 billion over the lifetime of each cohort.

The cost of prevention was also calculated. Since 70% of childhood lead poisoning is related to lead-based paint, the estimated cost of lead hazard control in the Pew Foundation report includes only the cost of abatement of lead in homes and other buildings, such as schools that are contaminated with lead-based paint. Other sources of lead contamination, such as contaminated water or industrial waste, are not included. The cost of lead-based paint abatement for the United States is estimated to be between $1.2 and $11 billion. It is estimated that every $1 spent on lead hazard control (prevention) would save $17 in tax-payer costs to deal with the effects of childhood lead poisoning. Because these data are from 2010, data from 2021 are likely to be different. However, CDC surveillance data for 2018 found that 87,144 children younger than 6 years had BLLs above 5 mcg/dL, with only 17.6% of eligible children tested nationally. Six states submitted no report to the CDC, nine states reported that fewer than 10% of eligible children were tested, and only one state out of 50 reported having tested more than a third of the eligible children (cdc.gov/lead surveillance, 2018). With these statistics, and given the rising cost of healthcare and educational costs, the current number of children identified with lead poisoning and the cost of treating them are unlikely to be less than described in the Pew report (Pew Center on the States, 2010).

RECOMMENDATIONS FOR REDUCING CHILDHOOD LEAD POISONING

Roles for nurses and other health professionals in reducing childhood lead poisoning, in addition to direct care provision, include advocacy, education, community partnerships, and support. The following recommendations highlight the importance of and opportunities for these strategies. It should be noted that these recommendations are not presented in the order of importance. While primary prevention is essential for reducing the incidence of lead poisoning, the children who are currently being exposed need to be identified and treated, and comprehensive community programs are essential.

Primary prevention of lead poisoning in children begins with eliminating the sources of lead where children live, play, and learn. The following recommendations are related to primary prevention, the elimination of lead in the child's daily environment, and the focus on advocacy.

Recommendations for Government

1. The federal government's role in providing resources to combat lead should be increased through the U.S Department of Housing and Urban Development (HUD) for the comprehensive abatement of lead-contaminated housing; more stringent

enforcement of Environmental Protection Agency (EPA) regulations regarding lead; and continued national surveillance and reporting mechanisms through the CDC. These data can inform and support the development of health policy.

2. State and local governments and school boards should mandate an assessment of lead in all schools built before 1978, and perform abatement and re-evaluation as necessary.

3. State and local governments and school boards should mandate regular testing of all water sources in schools on an annual basis. Where lead is found to be present in the water, the contaminated sources should be closed until the source of the lead can be identified and eliminated. Uncontaminated water from other sources should be made available to children until the school's water is free from lead (Neuwirth, 2018).

Rationale

All of these recommendations are strategies for the primary prevention of childhood lead poisoning and are recommended by the American Academy of Pediatrics (AAP): Council on Environmental Health (CEH; 2021). While the initial expenses may seem high, the Pew Foundation estimates that $1 in prevention saves $17 in treatment cost to the taxpayer, providing a compelling argument for the commitment of federal, state, and local resources.

Recommendations for Improving Testing Percentages: Secondary Prevention

One of the issues that most dramatically and negatively affects the continuing crisis in childhood lead poisoning is the lack of systematic testing of children up to age 72 months (secondary prevention). As noted earlier, only 17.6% of eligible children were tested in the United States in 2018. These steps are secondary prevention. Early identification allows early intervention to minimize the damage. Recommendations to increase the percentage of children who are tested for BLLs include (American Academy of Pediatrics & Council on Environmental Health, 2016):

1. All pregnant or lactating persons should be tested for BLLs.
2. All children should be tested for BLLs between age 12 and 24 months, regardless of insurance status.

Rationale

Maternal blood lead is known to pass through to the fetus and is present in breast milk. Early exposure to lead can have particularly devastating effects on the fetus or child up to age 24 months. Therefore, it is imperative that BLLs of pregnant and lactating persons and BLLs of children age 12 to 24 months are identified so that early intervention to protect the child can begin. Although Medicaid mandates that all children should be tested for BLLs at 12 and 24 months of age, in Ohio, for example, only 59% of children are actually tested (cdc.gov/lead/surveillance, 2018).

1. Increase the opportunities for children to be tested for BLLs by taking the point of service (testing) to the sites where children live, play, and learn.

Rationale

Churches, schools, school nurses, school-based clinics, and neighborhood clinics all represent opportunities to improve access to health services by moving the point of delivery close to the child rather than requiring the family to take the child to a clinical site that may be a significant distance from them. The need to go to a clinic site to access healthcare for a child may require travel time, often by bus and with other children, and may require the parent to take time off from work, with a loss of income for the day. This can be a substantive barrier for families in accessing healthcare. One project providing lead testing in schools for children ages 3 to 6 years was able to test 70% to 90% of eligible children in most schools after having obtained parental consent (Lotas, not published). This was a three- to fourfold increase in the percentage of children tested from the state-reported testing percentage of 18% to 20% annually from 2015 to 2018, the last year for which complete data are available (cdc.gov/surveillance data, 2018). Establishing regular lead testing in schools can be achieved by (a) increasing the number of school nurses to make it possible for them to do more comprehensive health screening, including lead testing; (b) partnering with a local hospital to establish school-based clinics to provide health services, including lead testing; and (c) partnering with area healthcare professional schools to provide lead testing services.

1. State and local governments and school boards should consider mandating annual lead tests for children enrolled in schools as they currently mandate recommended vaccines for childhood diseases.

Rationale

Lead poisoning is a public health issue with major costs to affected children and families and a major financial burden to society. Because of the extreme burden of lead poisoning on affected children, families, and society, and because it is an issue of social justice and the result of decades of neglect and structural racism, an intensive community-based approach is essential.

Recommendations for Public Education and Parent Empowerment

As Case Study 22.1 illustrates, the lack of information about lead poisoning; its causes, symptoms, and treatment; and steps to protect children from lead exposure are significant barriers to the elimination of the illness and its early identification and treatment. The lack of information also increases the difficulty and stress families experience when a child is identified with elevated BLLs. Education improves the chances of both primary and secondary prevention (Markowitz, 2021; Neuwirth, 2018). The recommendation is:

1. Implement a comprehensive educational outreach to families through partnerships with community groups, community leaders, and activists who are known and trusted in the community.

Rationale

The lack of information is compounded by the well-documented and justified mistrust of the healthcare system in BIPOC communities. It is essential that families be empowered to protect and care for their children by providing them with information and resources in ways that effectively communicate with them and minimize the concern and mistrust they may experience. The importance of strong community partnerships cannot be overemphasized. Case Study 22.2 describes the development and implementation of a grassroots organization that actively educates and supports families in addressing lead-related issues.

CASE STUDY 22.2: BIRTH OF A MOVEMENT, BY ROBIN BROWN, DIRECTOR OF CCOAL

For 5 years, my daughter and I worked on lead advocacy. Then my daughter said, "We need to do more," and we started the work that became Concerned Citizens Organized Against Lead (CCOAL). We surveyed the parents of lead-poisoned children and asked them what they needed to know and what they didn't have when their children became poisoned. What they said was, "If I'd been educated about lead, I could have prevented this happening to my child."

(continued)

CASE STUDY 22.2: BIRTH OF A MOVEMENT, BY ROBIN BROWN, DIRECTOR OF CCOAL (*CONTINUED*)

So, we created a curriculum that talked about all the things parents wanted to know. We created pamphlets, which we gave out, and did a public service announcement on the radio. With our curriculum we started working one block at a time, going door to door passing out our pamphlets to recruit interested people for our education program. We gave four sessions on the issue of lead. From that, we inspired 20 people who wanted to work with us, and with this group of community partners we were able to branch out and cover more neighborhoods. Eventually, we had over 200 community members in CCOAL. They canvassed the streets, put up posters, passed out pamphlets, and passed out lead hazard kits. We put materials in schools also because we knew we needed to be in the schools. Our outreach strategies included the following:

◆ We maintained our ongoing education program.
◆ We developed a curriculum for the schools. We identified 20 students and we would end up with 12, which was our target number. We educated them about lead and they talked to and taught their classmates. We held contests, gave prizes, and hung posters. It was a phenomenon.
◆ We focused on pediatric clinics and prenatal clinics in the area so we could talk to mothers and pregnant women about the dangers of lead to the young child and to the fetus. We would set up a table in the waiting room with our materials and engage patients in conversation while they waited.
◆ We started a hardware store initiative. We put pamphlets in the stores and when people bought a can of paint, a paint stick, or whatever, they would get a pamphlet.

It's been 15 years and we aren't done by a long shot. But CCOAL is still growing, and we are still working.

Discussion Questions

1. The CCOAL initiative surveyed parents of lead-poisoned children to develop their curriculum. What other sources might provide valuable information?
2. If you were developing a lead poisoning prevention program for schools, what would you include?
3. Why would conversations with pregnant patients be particularly effective?
4. The CCOAL Institutes worked with hardware stores to get their message out. What are some other venues you might include to reach the community with your message?

CONCLUSIONS

Lead poisoning is a 100% preventable condition that remains a public health issue and an issue of environmental and social justice and has major costs to individuals, families, and society. While lead poisoning has been dramatically reduced or eliminated in many areas of the United States, communities with elevated levels of poverty and, often, a minority population continue to be affected by this problem, with devastating and long-term effects on the children. A complex of variables impacts this issue, including the continued presence of environmental lead in places where children live, learn, and play without a well-organized and effective program of abatement and the continuing effects of poverty, reduced opportunity, differential enforcement of environmental protection laws, underfunded schools, and barriers to accessing healthcare.

Healthcare professionals, including nurses, are well positioned to strongly advocate for the changes necessary to overcome lead poisoning risk to children in their communities. This may include advocating for more and sustained governmental resources for abatement and mandates for lead screening. In partnership with other healthcare professionals, nurses have a particular role in developing strategies for increasing the percentage of children tested for BLLs, removing the barriers to accessing healthcare, and developing programs of community outreach with education, support, and resources. Lead poisoning can be eradicated from communities with a concentrated, collaborative strategy that includes governments, communities, and nurses as part of interprofessional healthcare provider teams.

DISCUSSION QUESTIONS

1. Describe three of the most important impacts of lead poisoning on a child.
2. What is the most dangerous time for a child to be exposed to lead, and why?
3. What are the barriers to accessing healthcare that may make it more difficult for families to receive care for their children, and how can they be overcome?
4. What are the major components of society's cost in relation to lead poisoning?
5. Why is lead poisoning considered an issue of social justice?

ADDITIONAL RESOURCES

Environmental Protection Agency. (2019). Proposed rules. *Federal Register, 84*(219), 61684–61774. https://www.govinfo.gov/content/pkg/FR-2019-11-13/pdf/2019-22705.pdf
Federal Register/Vol. 84, Number 219/Wednesday, 13. (2019). Proposed rules. https://www .govinfo.gov/content/pkg/FR-2019-11-13/pdf/2019-22705.pdf

REFERENCES

Aelion, C., & Davis, H. (2019). Blood lead levels in children in urban and rural areas: Using multilevel modeling to investigate impacts of gender, race, poverty and the environment. *Science of the Total Environment*. https://doi.org/10.1016/j.scitotenv.2019.133783
Akkus, C., & Ozddenerrol, E. (2014). Exploring childhood lead exposure through GIS: A review of the recent literature. *International Journal of Environmental Research and Public Health, 11*, 6314–6334. https://doi.org/10.3390/ijerph11066314
American Academy of Pediatrics & Council on Environmental Health. (2016). Prevention of childhood lead toxicity. *Pediatrics, 138*(1). https://doi.org/10.1542/peds.2016-1493
Bressler, J., Yoder, S., Cooper, S., & McLaughlin, J. (2019). Blood lead surveillance and exposure sources among Alaska children. *Journal of Public Health Management & Practice, 5*(suppl 1), S71–S75. https://doi.org/10.1097/PHH.0000000000000877
Burns, J., Williams, P., Leed, M., Revich, B., Sergeyev, O., Hauser, R., Hauser, S., & Korricka, S. (2017). Peripubertal blood lead levels and growth among Russian boys. *Environment International, 106*, 53–59. https://doi.org/10.1016/j.envint.2017.05.023
Centers for Disease Control and Prevention. (2018). Childhood lead poisoning prevention: Sources of lead exposure. https://www.cdc.gov/nceh/lead/prevention/sources.htm
Centers for Disease Control and Prevention. (2019). Ground water corrosivity and lead in private wells. https://www.cdc.gov/nceh/ehs/safe-watch/corrosive-groundwater.html
Centers for Disease Control and Prevention. (2021a, December 1). Childhood lead poisoning prevention CDC. https://www.cdc.gov/nceh/lead/default.htm
Centers for Disease Control and Prevention. (2021b, May, 14). Lead Exposure Prevention and Advisory Committee (LEPAC). https://www.cdc.gov/nceh/lead/default.htm
Edwards, M. (2014). Fetal death and reduced birth rates associated with exposure to lead-contaminated drinking water. *Environmental Sce Technology, 48*(1), 739–746. https://doi.org/10.1021/es4034952
Emer, L., Kalkbrenner, A., O'Brien, M., Yan, A., Cisler, R., & Weinhardt, L. (2020). Association of childhood blood lead levels with firearm violence perpetration and victimization in Milwaukee. *Environmental Research*. https://doi.org/10.1016/j.envres.2019.108822
Ettinger, A., Ruckart, P., & Dignam, T. (2019). Lead poisoning prevention: The unfinished agenda. *Journal of Public Health Management and Practice, 25*(suppl 1). https://doi.org/10.1097/PHH.0000000000000902

Gleason, K., Valeri, L., Shankar, A., Sharif Ibne Hasan, M., Quamruzzaman, Q., Rodrigues, E., Christiani, D., Wright, R., Bellinger, D., & Mazumdar, M. (2016). Stunting is associated with blood lead concentration among Bangladeshi children aged 2–3 years. *Environmental Health*, *15*, 103. https://doi.org/10.1186/s12940-016-0190-4

Global Alliance to Eliminate Lead Paint. (2020, December 31). 2020 update on the global status of the legal limits of lead in paint. https://www.unep.org/resources/report/2020-update-global-status-legal-limits-lead-paint

Gottesfeld, P., & Pokhrel, A. K. (2011). Review: Lead exposure in battery manufacturing and recycling in developing countries and among children in nearby communities. *Journal of Occupational and Environmental Hygiene*, *8*(9), 520–532. https://doi.org/10.1080/15459624.2011.601710

Harris, S., & Harper, B. (2001). Lifestyles, diets and native American exposure factors related to possible lead exposure and toxicity. *Environmental Research*, *86*(2), 140–148. https://doi.org/10.1006/enrs.2001.4250

Hauptman, M., Niles, J., & Gudin, J. (2021). Individual and community-level factors associated with detectable and elevated blood lead levels in U.S. children, results from a national clinic laboratory. *Journal of the American Medical Association Pediatrics*, *175*(12), 1252–1260. https://doi.org/10.1001/jamapediatrics.2021.3518

Haynes, E., Chen, A., Ryan, P., Succop, P., & Dietrich, K. (2011). Exposure to airborne metals and particulate matter and risk for youth adjudicated criminal activity. *Environmental Research*, *111*(8), 1–13. https://doi.org/10.1016/j.envres.2011.08.008

Hernberg, S. (2000). Lead poisoning in a historical perspective. *American Journal of Industrial Medicine*, *38*: 244–254.

Hoover, C., Hoover, G., & Specht, A. (2021). Firearm licenses associated with elevated pediatric blood lead levels in Massachusetts. *Environmental Research*, *202*, 111642. https://doi.org/10.1016/j.envres.2021.111642

LeBron, A., Torres, I., Valencia, E., Dominguez, M., Garcia-Sanchez, D., Logue, M., & Wu, J. (2019). The state of public health lead policies: Implications for urban health inequities and recommendations for health equity. *International Journal of Environmental Research in Public Health*, *16*(6). https://doi.org/10.3390/jierph16061064

Malcoe, L., Lynch, R., Keger, M., & Skaggs, V. (2002). Lead sources, behaviors, and socioeconomic factors in relation to blood lead of native American and white children: A community-based assessment of a former mining area. *Environmental Health Perspectives*, *110*(suppl 2), 221–231. https://doi.org/10.1289/ehp.02110s2221

Manisalidis, I., Stavropoulou, E., Stavropoulous, A., & Berzirtzoglou, E. (2020). Environmental and health impacts of air pollution: A review. *Frontiers in Public Health*, https://doi.org/10.3389/fpubh.2020.00014

Markowitz, M. (2021). Lead poisoning: An update. *Pediatric Review*, *42*(6), 302–315. https://doi.org/10.1542/pir.2020-0026

Mayans, L. (2019). Lead poisoning in children. American Academy of Family Physicians. www.aapf.org/afp

Meltzer, G., Watkins, B., Vieira, D., Zelikoff, J., & Bodin-Albala, B. (2020). A systematic review of environmental health outcomes in selected native American and Alaskan native populations. *Journal of Racial and Ethnic Health Disparities*, *7*(4), 698–739. https://doi.org/10.1007/s40615-020-00700-2

Mielke, H. W., Gonzales, C. R., Powell, E. T., & Egendorf, S. P. (2022). Lead in air, soil, and blood: Pb poisoning in a changing world. *International Journal of Environmental Research and Public Health*, *19*(15), 9500. https://doi.org/10.3390/ijerph19159500

Needleman, H. (1999). History of lead in the world. Unpublished Manuscript.

Needleman, H., McFarland, C., Ness, R., Fienberg, S., & Tobin, M. (2002). Bone lead levels in adjudicated delinquents: A case control study. *Neurotoxicology and Teratology*, *24*(6), 711–717. https://doi.org/10.1016/s0892-0362(02000269-6

Neuwirth, L. (2018). Resurgent lead poisoning and renewed public attention towards environmental social justice issues: A review of current efforts and call to revitalize primary and secondary lead poisoning prevention for pregnant women, lactating mothers, and children within the U.S. *International Journal of Occupational and Environmental Health*, *24*(3–4), 86–100. https://doi.org/10.1080/10773525.2018.1507291

Pew Center on the States. (2010). Cutting lead poisoning and public costs. Pew Charitable Trusts, Issue Brief #14, www.partnershipforsuccess.org

Poropat, A., Laidlaw, M., Lamphear, B., Ball, A., & Mielke, H. (2018). Blood lead and preeclampsia: A meta-analysis and review of implications. *Environmental Research*, *160*, 12–19. https://doi.org/10.1016/j.envres.2017.09.014

Segal, T., & Giudice, L. (2019, October). Before the beginning: Environmental exposures and reproductive and obstetrical outcomes. *Fertility and Sterility*, *112*(4), 614–621. https://doi.org/10.1016/j.fertnstert.2019.08.001

Silver, M., Li, X., Lui, Y., Li, M., Mai, X., Kaciroti, N., Kileny, P., Tardif, T., Meeker, J., & Lozoff, B. (2016). Low-level prenatal lead exposure and infant sensory function. *Environmental Health, 15*, 65. https://doi.org/10.1186/s12940-016-0148-6

Taylor, M., Forbes, M., Opeskin, B., Parr, N., & Lamphear, B. (2016). The relationship between atmospheric lead emissions and aggressive crime: An ecological study. *Environmental Health, 15*, 23. https://doi.org/10.1186/s12940-016-0122-3

Thomason, M., Hect, J., Rauh, V., Trentacosta, C., Wheelock, M., Eggebrecht, A., Espinoza-Heredia, C., & Burt, S. (2019). Prenatal lead exposure impacts cross-hemispheric and long-range connectivity in the human fetal brain. *Neuroimage, 1*(191), 186–192. https://doi.org/10.1016/j.neuroimage.2019.02.017

Tsuji, L. J., Wainman, B. C., Martin, I. D., Weber, J. P., Sutherland, C., Liberda, E. N., & Nieboer, E. (2008). Elevated blood-lead levels in first nation people of Northern Ontario, Canada: Policy implications. *Bulletin of Environmental Contaminations and Toxicology, 80*(1), 14–18. https://doi.org/10.1007/s00128-007-9281-9

United Nations Children's Fund & Pure Earth. (2020, July). The toxic truth: Children's exposure to lead pollution undermines a generation of future potential. Joint Report. https://www.unicef.org/reports/toxic-truth-childrens-exposure-to-lead-pollution-2020

Whitehead, L., & Buchanan, S. (2019). Childhood lead poisoning: A perpetual environmental justice issue? *Journal of Public Health Management and Practice, 25*(suppl 1), S115–S120. https://doi.org/10.1097/PHH.0000000000000891

World Health Organization. (2017). Recycling used lead acid batteries: Health considerations. World Health Organization. License: CC BY-NC-SA 3.0 IGO. https://apps.who.int/iris/bitstream/handle/10665/259447/9789241512855-eng.pdf;sequence=1

World Health Organization. (2020, December 31). 2020 update on the global status of the legal limit of lead in paint. https://www.unep.org/resources/report/2020-update-global-status-legal-limits-lead-paint

Wright, J., Dietrich, K., Ris, M., Hornung, R., Wessel, S., Lamphear, B., Ho, M., & Rae, M. (2008). Assocpiation of prenatal and childhood blood lead concentrations with criminal arrests in early adulthood. *PLos Medicine, 5*(5), e101. www.plosmedicine.org

CHAPTER 23

Socioeconomic Determinants and Cancer Disparity

Amy Y. Zhang and Erika S. Trapl

LEARNING OBJECTIVES

- Provide an overview of current cancer disparity trends (incidence and death rate) across racial and ethnic groups in the United States.

- Examine cancer disparity across the socioeconomic spectrum including age, gender, education, income, insurance status, and urban/rural residence.

- Evaluate cancer disparity during the COVID-19 pandemic and its correlation with socioeconomic factors such as living conditions, neighborhood environment, and access to healthcare services.

- Analyze socioeconomic determinants of health outcomes through an in-depth glimpse at two cancer cases.

- Identify the interpersonal, organizational, and policy practices that contribute to cancer prevention behaviors, including tobacco use and cancer screenings.

INTRODUCTION

Like many other chronic health conditions, cancer has both biological and sociological factors that contribute to its development as well as its detection, treatment, and survival. In this chapter, we provide an overview of cancer statistics as well as highlight populations that are disproportionately burdened by cancer diagnoses and mortality. We highlight how factors at various levels of the social-ecological model (introduced in Chapter 1) facilitate and exacerbate cancer disparities.

We open the chapter from the perspective of strategies that have been proposed to promote worldwide relief from the burdens of cancer and other noncommunicable diseases (NCDs). From there, the spotlight shifts to the United States and the goals and objectives designed to benefit the health of the nation, including improved diagnosis and treatment of cancer. This leads to a broad discussion of current disparities in cancer outcomes across racial and ethnic identity populations. Next, we highlight the role of other population characteristics and social determinants in cancer disparities, including age, gender, socioeconomic status, education, and geography. Delving deeper, we provide two specific examples, prostate cancer and tobacco use, highlighting how systems and policy have contributed to significant disparities among minoritized populations. Finally, we discuss how the recent COVID-19 pandemic impacted cancer screening and cancer treatment, with unique insight into the effects of the COVID-19 pandemic and cancer on mental health. The chapter concludes with two narratives based upon true-life stories to impart a deeper understanding of subjective experiences of cancer.

THE BURDEN OF CANCER ACROSS THE WORLD COMMUNITY: AN EYE ON PREVENTION

The World Health Organization (WHO) has determined that the most impactful and cost-saving long-term approach to reducing and eliminating cancer requires placing a focus on cancer prevention. WHO does its work through collaboration with member states to help them galvanize their policies and program initiatives that (a) enhance awareness, (b) lessen exposure to cancer-related risks, and (c) ensure that people have access to accurate and relevant information necessary to improve their overall lifestyles (WHO, 2022). The *WHO Global Action Plan for the Prevention and Control of NCDs 2013 to 2020* has been developed to assist citizens, healthcare professionals, and policymakers worldwide as they grapple with the serious immediate and long-term consequences of cancer and other NCDs (WHO, 2013). The strategies that have been proposed are aimed at effectuating significant reductions in risk factors and morbidity and mortality by the year 2025 (WHO, 2021). These guidelines are reflected in the *Healthy People 2030 Goals* that have been promulgated in the United States (Office of Disease Prevention and Health Promotion, 2022a).

HEALTHY PEOPLE 2030: THE UNITED STATES

Healthy People 2030 lays down strategies that will create policy changes to foster more beneficial outcomes for the health of the American people over the next 10 years. Its 355 measurable development and research objectives focus on health conditions, health behaviors, populations, settings and systems, and the social determinants of health. For cancer, the goal is to reduce new cases of cancer and cancer-related illness, disability, and death (Office of Disease Prevention and Health Promotion, 2022b).

RECENT TRENDS OF CANCER DISPARITY OUTCOMES

By estimation, 1.9 million people were anticipated to be diagnosed with cancer, and 601,000 were projected to die of this disease in the United States in 2022 (American Cancer Society [ACS], 2022a). The disparity continues to exist across racial and ethnic groups despite a continuing decline in overall cancer incidence and mortality. For African American people, 111,990 men and 112,090 women were expected to be newly diagnosed in 2022 (ACS, 2022b). When all cancers are combined, African American men have the highest rate of new cancer diagnoses, most commonly in the categories of prostate, lung, bronchus, and colorectal cancers (National Cancer Institute [NCI], 2022a). The incidence rates for Kaposi's sarcoma are four times higher in African American people than in others (ACS, 2022b). Asians and Pacific Islanders have the highest incident rates for liver and stomach cancers, although they have the lowest overall cancer incidence compared to others (ACS, 2022a). For American Indians and Alaska Natives, incidence rates of lung, colorectal, and kidney cancers are higher than among White individuals (ACS, 2022a;

Suran, 2022). Cancer risk and disparities among American Indians and Alaska Natives vary substantially by location or region (ACS, 2022a). For Hispanic and Latino people, the overall rates for the most common cancers are lower; however, they have the highest rates for cancers associated with infectious agents (e.g., HIV). In fact, cervical cancer incidence rates are nearly 30% higher among Hispanic people than among White people (ACS, 2022a).

In 2020, 46.9 million Americans self-identified as Black or African American, counting for 14.2% of the total U.S. population and the third largest racial/ethnic group in the United States (ACS, 2022b). They have the lowest survival rate than any other racial or ethnic group for most cancers (DeSantis et al., 2019b); the cancer mortality rate is 19% higher in Black men and 12% higher in Black women than White men and women. Among Black people, the death rates for stomach and prostate cancers and myeloma are more than double that of White people (ACS, 2022b). Despite breast cancer incidence being 4% lower among Black women than White women, the mortality rate is 41% higher among Black women (Suran, 2022). American Indians and Alaska Natives have lower 5-year relative survival rates than Whites for most cancer types, often due to cancer diagnosis at a later stage. For example, the 5-year survival for stomach cancer is 19% among American Indians and Alaska Natives as compared to 32% among Whites (ACS, 2022a).

CANCER DISPARITY ACROSS THE SOCIOECONOMIC SPECTRUM

WHO (n.d.) has defined the social determinants of health as the "conditions in which people are born, grow, work, live and age, and the wider set of forces and systems shaping the conditions of daily life" (para. 1). Cancer disparity exists across these socioeconomic divides.

Patients with cancer at age 85 or older have the lowest relative survival compared to any other age group. Patients in this group are often diagnosed at an advanced stage and are less likely to receive surgical treatment. For example, breast and colorectal cancers are 10% less likely to be diagnosed in a local stage in this group than in those aged 65 to 84 (DeSantis et al., 2019a). In 2022, men were expected to have more new cancer cases than women (983,160 and 934,870, respectively) and more cancer deaths (322,090 and 287,270, respectively; ACS, 2022a). Data have shown that people with a higher level of education were less likely to die of colorectal cancer before age 65 than those with less education (NCI, 2022b). In 2016, for example, men with lung cancer who had 12 years or less of education had death rates that were 4.6 times higher than that of men who were college educated (ACS, 2022a).

Poverty significantly determines a person's living conditions and access to care, which is reflected in cancer outcomes. According to the 2020 U.S. Census, 20% of Black and 17% of Hispanic/Latino populations lived below the federal poverty line, but only 8% of non-Hispanic White and Asian populations did so (ACS, 2022a). During the same period of time, 10% of Black and 19% of Hispanic/Latino populations were uninsured, compared to 6% to 7% of Whites and Asians (ACS, 2022a). Unfortunately, people without health insurance are more likely to be diagnosed with advanced cancer or die of cancer than those who are insured (Suran, 2022). It is not surprising that, when compared with more affluent communities, high-poverty communities have a higher percentage of colorectal, female breast, cervical, and prostate cancer diagnoses in a distant stage rather than a local stage; all these cancers are highly preventable through routine cancer screening, which is commonly covered by insurance (Kish et al., 2014; NCI, 2022a). When all cancers are combined, those living in poorer communities have a 13% higher rate of cancer death in men and 3% in women than those living in more affluent communities (NCI, 2022a).

Data from recent years have shown that rural areas have worse cancer outcomes than urban and suburban areas. According to the Centers for Disease Control and Prevention

(CDC), from 2006 to 2015, the declination of overall cancer mortality rates was slower in nonmetropolitan (rural) counties than in urban counties (Henley et al., 2017). Data from the NCI of the National Institutes of Health have shown that people living in rural Appalachia have much higher incidence rates of colorectal, lung, and cervical cancers than those living in urban areas (NCI, 2022b). Rural residents are more likely to have less education, lower income, higher unemployment rates, and less health insurance coverage than their urban counterparts (Henley & Jemal, 2018; Kish et al., 2014). The elevated cancer mortality in rural areas has been explained in part by higher poverty rates and barriers to healthcare access (Blake & Green Parker, 2020; Henley et al., 2017; James et al., 2017). For example, one study reported that half (50.5%) of 1,359 surveyed rural cancer survivors reported financial problems due to cancer as opposed to 38.8% of urban cancer survivors, a difference that is statistically significant (Zahnd et al., 2019). Another study reported that only 3.1% of medical oncologists worked in rural areas (which comprise 19.3% of the U.S. population); 70% of rural counties in the United States had no medical oncologists in 2014 (Kirkwood et al., 2014). This lack of a workforce in rural areas seriously restricts patient access to quality cancer care. Behavioral risk factors were also examined for the understanding of rural/urban differences in cancer mobility. A study of the North American Association of Central Cancer Registries' public use dataset, which includes population-based cancer incidence data from 46 states representing 93% of the U.S. population, reported that higher incidence rates of colorectal, cervical, and lung cancers in the rural over urban areas are associated with modifiable risks of the human papilloma virus (HPV) and tobacco use (Zahnd et al., 2018).

Prostate Cancer Disparities Among African American Men

In 2022, it was anticipated that over 268,000 new cases of prostate cancer would be diagnosed; one out of eight men will be diagnosed with prostate cancer in their lifetime (ACS, 2022a). The average age of diagnosis is 66 years. One out of 41 men will die from prostate cancer, leading to about 34,500 deaths per year, accounting for 11% of all cancer deaths. Prostate cancer mortality among non-Hispanic Black men is more than twice that of any other racial or ethnic group.

Currently, there are no known primary prevention strategies for prostate cancer. Known risk factors include increasing age, a family history of prostate cancer, and African ancestry (typically simplified as Black race). In fact, African American men tend to be diagnosed with prostate cancer at a younger age than men of other racial/ethnic categories. Many cancers rely on secondary prevention strategies, such as cancer screenings, as cancers caught in earlier stages are more treatable and have better survival outcomes.

Prostate-specific antigen (PSA) is a protein produced by the cells of the prostate, and levels of PSA can be detected in the blood using a simple blood test. When a man has prostate cancer, his PSA levels increase; however, there are other factors that may contribute to a higher-than-normal PSA level, such as another prostate-related health condition (e.g., prostatitis) or a behavior (e.g., riding a bike or having had sex recently). Thus, the PSA test can screen for prostate cancer, but subsequent diagnostic testing is needed to confirm a diagnosis. PSA tests are typically ordered by primary care providers during routine annual wellness visits.

Unfortunately, there has been inconsistency on whether a PSA test should be recommended. The U.S. Preventive Services Task Force (USPSTF) is a volunteer panel of experts that reviews existing peer-reviewed literature to make evidence-based recommendations about clinical services, such as screenings. These recommendations often influence clinical practice guidelines. In 2012, the USPSTF gave a "D" grade, resulting in a recommendation against prostate cancer screening (Moyer et al., 2012). As a result, prostate cancer screening declined from 29.9% in 2012 to 20.4% in 2018, with the decline being greater among non-Hispanic Black men when compared to non-Hispanic White men (Kensler et al., 2021).

In 2018, the USPSTF gave prostate cancer screening a "C" grade, suggesting that providers "offer or provide this service for selected patients depending on individual circumstances" among men between the ages of 55 to 70 (USPSTF, 2018). This recommendation was based on data from three large randomized clinical trials. Despite existing knowledge that African American men develop prostate cancer at an earlier age, and despite existing data indicating that African American men have disproportionately high incidence and mortality, citing insufficient evidence, the USPSTF refrained from any recommendations specific to African American men.

The ACS (2021) has put forward alternative recommendations for prostate cancer screening. They suggest that prostate cancer screening should begin at age 50 for men at average risk; at age 45 for men at elevated risk, including African American men and men who have a first-degree relative diagnosed with prostate cancer at less than 65 years of age; and at age 40 for men at even higher risk, such as those with more than one first-degree relative diagnosed with prostate cancer at less than 65 years (ACS, 2021). This may increase the likelihood that African American men will begin PSA testing at an earlier age, thereby facilitating the diagnosis of prostate cancer at an earlier and more treatable stage.

Regardless of the recommendation, it is important to remember that these recommendations are meant to be interpreted by and integrated into practice by healthcare providers and healthcare systems. It is unlikely that the details of these recommendations are reaching individuals in a way that is easy to understand. Thus, healthcare providers are directly influencing who may be offered prostate cancer screening and may be inadvertently contributing to delayed screening and a later stage of diagnosis among African American men. Of further concern is the underutilization of primary care by African American men, and thus the missed opportunity for preventive healthcare services, including cancer screenings.

Access to healthcare, structural racism, and bias within the healthcare system have also been shown to contribute to the disparity in mortality experienced by African American men. As previously mentioned, non-Hispanic African American men experience prostate cancer mortality at over twice the rate of other racial and ethnic groups in the United States.

BOX 23.1: Colorectal Cancer

The second leading cause of death in the United States.

- It affects men and women.
- Screening can identify cancer at an early stage.
- Early treatment saves lives.

Colonoscopy is less likely among:

- Men
- Hispanics
- American Indian and Alaska Natives
- People 50 to 64 years old
- Rural residents
- People of lower socioeconomic levels
- Individuals who are less educated
- Those with limited health literacy

Note: Adapted from Centers for Disease Control and Prevention. (2022, February 15). Colorectal Cancer Control Program (CRCCP)–guide to community preventive services: highlights from the field [Video]. www.cdc.gov/cancer/crccp/about.htm.

Some researchers have assumed that incidence and mortality were related to ancestry given the high rates of prostate cancer in African and Afro-Caribbean countries. However, a comparison of non-Hispanic White and non-Hispanic African American men receiving care through the Veterans Health Administration revealed that neither group was more likely to experience a delay in prostate cancer diagnosis and care; neither group was more likely to experience an advanced stage diagnosis; and neither was more likely to die from prostate cancer (Riviere et al., 2020). This research highlights the importance of equitable care in reducing racial and ethnic cancer disparities.

Tobacco Use Disparities Contribute to Cancer Disparities

Smoking contributes to more than 480,000 deaths annually, including the deaths of 41,000 individuals who were exposed to secondhand smoke; over a third of these deaths are due to tobacco-related cancers (U.S. Department of Health and Human Services [DHHS], Office of the Surgeon General, 2014). Tobacco use remains the leading preventable cause of cancer death and death overall in the United States. Smoking is a risk factor for 13 unique cancers (i.e., lung, larynx, mouth, esophagus, throat, bladder, kidney, liver, stomach, pancreas, colon and rectum, cervix, and acute myeloid leukemia; DHHS, Office of the Surgeon General, 2014). There have been significant declines in tobacco use over the past several decades due to public health actions that contributed both to reducing the number of new smokers (prevention) and helping current smokers to quit (cessation). However, benefits from these efforts have not been equitable, and smoking is most common among marginalized populations, with disparities observed by race, ethnicity, socioeconomic status, educational attainment, sexual orientation, and geographic region (Cornelius et al., 2020).

Tobacco industry tactics have contributed to the current tobacco use disparities (Gardiner, 2004). For example, there is a long history of the tobacco industry targeting African Americans with increased advertising, particularly promotion of menthol cigarettes. Roughly 85% of African American smokers use menthol cigarettes, compared to 29% of White smokers (Mills et al., 2018). The Family Smoking Prevention and Tobacco Control Act was passed in 2009 and established the Center for Tobacco Products within the U.S. Food and Drug Administration. As part of this action, flavored cigarettes were banned based on the public health harms and appeal of flavored tobacco, yet menthol cigarettes were excluded from this ban. Ongoing research on the use of menthol has shown that menthol flavoring makes cigarettes easier to smoke and may make harmful chemicals easier for the body to absorb. Notably, 91% of the decline in cigarette use since 2009 has been due to a decline in nonmenthol cigarette use (Delnevo et al., 2020), indicating that African Americans may not have benefited equitably from tobacco control efforts driving smoking declines. The African American Tobacco Control Leadership Council has been advocating for tobacco control policies, such as a menthol ban, since 2008, raising awareness and providing support to local jurisdictions and states willing to advance menthol bans in their communities while awaiting federal decisions from the Center for Tobacco Products. Despite the Center for Tobacco Products putting forward its first Advanced Notice of Proposed Rule Making related to the regulation of menthol in 2013, no action has been taken as of 2022. In 2018, a proposal was announced for the regulation of flavors in tobacco. In January of 2022, the Center for Tobacco Products indicated their intent to propose two new tobacco standards, including one to prohibit menthol as a characterizing flavor in cigarettes.

African Americans have also been disproportionately targeted by the tobacco industry with advertising to promote the use of cheap cigar products, such as cigarillos and little cigars, which have been on the market for over 40 years. Overwhelmingly, these products come in flavors that appeal to youth, and the targeted marketing has led to significantly greater use of these products by African American youth compared to their White counterparts. In addition to prohibiting menthol cigarettes, the Center for Tobacco Products also announced in January of 2022 that they will advance a tobacco standard to prohibit all flavors in cigars. As of the completion of this chapter (March 2022), no standards have been advanced.

Contrast this experience with that of e-cigarettes, which came onto the U.S. market around 2007. E-cigarettes, also referred to as electronic nicotine devices (ENDS), became immensely popular, and much of this popularity has been attributed to the hundreds of flavors on the market, such as mango, cotton candy, or gummy bear. The youth quickly adopted ENDS, and in 2018, the U.S. Surgeon General declared vaping an epidemic. At the same time, three White women organized Parents Against Vaping e-Cigarettes (PAVe) and advocated against e-cigarettes. By January 2020, then-President Trump enacted legislation to ban the sale of fruit-, mint-, and dessert-flavored pods for refillable cartridge-based ENDS (excluding tobacco and menthol flavors).

Tobacco companies have targeted other marginalized populations, contributing to their disproportionate use of tobacco products. The tobacco industry has used targeted marketing tactics, including sponsorship, bar promotions, giveaways, and advertisements, to appeal to sexual- and gender minority individuals, who smoke cigarettes at rates higher than their straight and cis-gender counterparts. In low-income neighborhoods, researchers have found a higher density of tobacco retailers compared to higher-income neighborhoods, potentially contributing to the higher rates of smoking among lower-income individuals. Hispanics have been targeted through branding, advertisements in Hispanic publications, and financial support of political organizations and cultural events. American Indian and Alaska Native communities have the highest rates of cigarette smoking among racial and ethnic groups and have also been targeted by the tobacco industry through the industry's manipulation of symbols and names with special meaning to their demographics.

Cancer Disparity During the COVID-19 Pandemic

Cancer patients tend to be older and have more comorbidity and compromised immunity, hence a higher risk for COVID-19 infection and consequent life-threatening conditions (DeSantis et al., 2019a). They have been more likely to be diagnosed with and die from COVID-19 than people without cancer (Yang et al., 2021). A retrospective case-control study, which analyzed electronic health records of 73.4 million patients from 360 hospitals across 50 states, has shown that, as of August 2020, patients with a cancer diagnosis had a significantly increased risk for COVID-19 infection than those without cancer, and the risk was 7 to 12 times higher among patients with leukemia, non-Hodgkin lymphoma, or lung cancer. Patients diagnosed with cancer and COVID-19 were hospitalized or died nearly two times more than patients having COVID-19 infection without cancer or three times more than patients having cancer without COVID-19 infection. African American cancer patients, particularly those with breast, prostate, colorectal, and lung cancer, had a significantly higher risk for COVID-19 infection than White cancer patients (Wang et al., 2021). A similar observation of the increased risk for COVID-19 infection among Black and Hispanic cancer patients living in New York and Boston and from the U.S. Veterans Affairs Healthcare System was also reported (Fillmore et al., 2021; Schmidt et al., 2020). One study showed that COVID-19 infection cases were double among African American cancer patients and four times higher in Hispanic cancer patients than in White cancer patients (Potter et al., 2020).

The heightened cancer disparity during the COVID-19 pandemic has been explained by a variety of contributing factors, most notably socioeconomic factors such as a lack of financial resources (e.g., medical supplies or housing), a lack of access to quality healthcare (e.g., transportation or insurance), low health literacy, high comorbidities, poor social support, and detrimental lifestyle factors (Erhunmwunsee et al., 2021; Newman et al., 2021). The needs for remaining in the workforce and associated risks for coronavirus exposure were also noted. Among those at substantial risk for severe COVID-19 illness, when compared with Whites, African American people were found to be 1.6 times more likely to live with a family member working in the healthcare sector, and nearly 18% more Hispanic people lived with someone whose only option was to go out of the home to work (Selden & Berdahl, 2020).

A cross-sectional survey study of cancer patients shed light on the observed cancer disparity during the COVID-19 pandemic. This study surveyed 322 patients who received a cancer diagnosis between January 2019 and January 2020 and were undergoing cancer treatments. These patients included 40 African Americans and 282 Whites, of whom 215 lived in urban or suburban areas and 67 lived in nonmetropolitan/rural areas. The survey was conducted online electronically in a Midwestern city between late November 2020 and March 2021 during the height of the COVID-19 pandemic. It aimed to assess physical and mental health outcomes across three groups of Black, metropolitan White, and nonmetropolitan White cancer patients (Zhang et al., 2022).

One of the main findings of this study was that living conditions matter to the health outcomes of cancer patients. The study participants who had been feeling too lonely or too crowded in their living space reported significantly poorer global health status and felt significantly more irritable and depressed than other participants. Under the stay-at-home order, feeling lonely may imply living alone and/or living without usual connection with others; similarly, feeling crowded at home may imply a limited personal space and/or inability to get out. Both living conditions were associated with an increase in stress hormones (Adegoke, 2014; Drake et al., 2015; Gove et al., 1979). Feeling lonely correlates with increasing cortisol during the day and excessive cortisol weakens immunological function (Doane & Adam, 2010). This situation was especially dire for the study participants because their immunological function was already compromised during cancer treatments. Poor living conditions might have profoundly affected their physical and mental health. Moreover, the study participants that maintained exercises at least 5 days a week reported significantly better global health status. African American participants exercised significantly less, however, as they considered their neighborhoods unsafe for exercise twice as much as did the White participants (Zhang et al., 2022). Their living environment restricted the maintenance of daily exercises, an important health-enhancement revenue. Physical environment and living conditions played a vital role in the quality of life and health outcomes of these cancer patients during the pandemic.

Another finding from this study was that access to healthcare matters dearly to participants' health, especially mental health. Those study participants who had Medicaid experienced significantly greater depression than the participants who had Medicare, who, in turn, felt significantly more irritable than the participants that had private insurance or Obamacare. Socioeconomic status determines a person's medical insurance and obviously has marked their mental health status as well. Further, the study participants experiencing difficulties in getting needed medications reported feeling significantly more irritable and depressed than the other participants, and so did the participants that were less satisfied with telehealth appointments for meeting general medical needs (Zhang et al., 2022).

Importantly, the disparity was found most pronounced in the mental health outcomes. In this study, African American participants reported feeling irritable at a significantly higher level than did the White participants, which increases the risk for depression (Zhang et al., 2021). Moreover, African American participants who felt lonely, reported feeling significantly more irritable and depressed than not only the White participants but also other African Americans who did not report feeling lonely. Similarly, the participants who had a low income of $25,000 or less and felt lonely, reported feeling significantly more depressed than the participants who had more income or the participants who had a similar low income but did not feel lonely. These findings show that African American and low-income cancer patients were most vulnerable to the pandemic's detrimental impacts. The observed disparity in mental health outcomes may well be the tip of the iceberg because mental health declination can eventually affect physical and overall health as the pandemic continues. The following report of a cancer patient's journey demonstrates this point clearly.

NARRATIVE 23.1: MS. KAHANANUL'S CATASTROPHE: OUT-OF-POCKET EXPENSES

Upon receiving a diagnosis of colon cancer, Ms. Kahananul was stunned. She had always been careful with her health and had gotten regular check-ups. She hid the information from her colleagues at work and resolved not to share the diagnosis with her family. She feared that the disease could be contagious, just as her family had experienced with COVID—her Aunt Aria had gotten such a severe case of it that she required hospitalization. She survived, stayed strong, and believed in her culture and traditional practices, but the ordeal left the family in debt and a profound fear of hospitals and healthcare providers.

Ms. Kahananul worked at a private home to care for a widowed man with lung cancer. She transported him to his daily radiation treatments for more than a month. Keeping her secret was of utmost importance. Even before initiating her chemotherapy treatments, she began wearing a wig. She never complained about feeling tired. In her efforts to dissuade any notion that she was unhealthy or unfit to perform, she worked long hours and struggled to prepare tasty menus for the gentleman.

Despite having top-tier health insurance, Ms. Kahananul's policy would not pay for the type of medications her doctor ordered to treat her cancer. Other procedures deemed necessary for her optimal care were also rejected for coverage. Paying for her cancer treatments out-of-pocket nearly exhausted all her life's savings and provoked a sense of helplessness.

Ms. Kahananul struggled at work. Her weight loss was evident and no longer voluntary. Her healthcare providers did not readily recognize her downhill spiral trajectory as the sense of hopelessness became ever more challenging to control. She did not seek help, thinking the depression, sleeplessness, and helplessness were related to the chemotherapy and her trying to "fight off cancer"—just like her Aunt Aria had done with the pandemic. Fortunately, her colon cancer was beginning to respond to treatments, and clinical data showed an improvement. Also, she associated her low energy status with the therapeutic benefit of chemotherapy and would endure her health condition. She began to self-medicate with alcohol while the depression, helplessness, and hopelessness deepened.

One evening, Ms. Kahananul accidentally over-medicated herself with alcohol and sleeping pills. After about 2 days of absence from work, her employer—the gentleman—notified Aunt Aria, her next of kin, about Ms. Kahananul's untimely death. She was shocked and grieving profoundly; her family had her body shipped back home to Hawaii.

Discussion Questions

1. What impact do you think Aunt Aria's illness had on Ms. Kahananul and how she managed her illness?
2. What are your thoughts about why Ms. Kahananul kept her diagnosis and treatment of cancer a secret from her family and her employer—the gentlemen—even though she supported, transported, and nurtured him daily?
3. Should the healthcare providers have known more about Ms. Kahananul's emotional state and perceptions of her condition? Could this have prevented the downward spiral she experienced? What clues to action may have been missed? Be specific and provide an informed rationale.
   a. Do you think you are culturally competent to address the healthcare needs of people from cultures other than your own?
   b. How did you develop your knowledge and skillsets that led to your sense of competency?
4. What are best practices for assessing and managing physical symptoms and mood states such as sleep problems, depression, hopelessness, stressors associated with insurance issues, lack of access to essential treatment, and others?

(continued)

NARRATIVE 23.1: MS. KAHANANUL'S CATASTROPHE: OUT-OF-POCKET EXPENSES (*CONTINUED*)

5. How would you design an interdisciplinary plan for Ms. Kahananul's culturally sensitive care and address the short- and long-term issues associated with cancer care, including the fear of death associated with the disease among people in many cultures?
6. Should the healthcare team follow up with Ms. Kahananul's family in Hawaii? Why? Why not? Please explain your position.
7. Do you think Ms. Kahananul might have been interested in participating in a clinical trial that is often available to patients and supported by the NCI, a federal agency?
8. Write a brief statement about how you think persons get recruited to clinical trials in your community. Are there any clinical trials occurring in the health system(s) where you work and receive healthcare? What is the focus of the research?

CASE STUDY 23.1: "WHAT IF" SYNDROME: DEVOTION TO DUTY AND FAMILY

Mr. Amaris Yusuf, a 30-year-old man, is devoted to his wife, children, and extended family. They live in a multigenerational home, where he has a leadership role in caring for all members, including providing for their overall well-being. As a young boy, he had been encouraged by his family and friends to have strong faith, be devoted to his family, and take a good wife who would love him and his children. Mr. Yusuf was an accomplished engineer and well respected in his community. When he began to have spells of lightheadedness, headaches, nausea, weight loss, and fatigue, he attributed it to his long work hours and being intensely dutiful and responsive to his family's needs, just as he had been taught since childhood. Mr. Yusuf checked with his primary physician and nurse practitioner, and they referred him for further testing—the outcome was a diagnosis of leukemia. In disbelief, Mr. Yusuf agonized within himself, "I have strong faith; I have done what a man should do for his family...How could this fate come to me?!" After his initial shock and silent outcry were over, he made a plan for his care, which did not include the physician and nurse practitioner—and when contacted by the two of them, Yusuf commented, "I can handle this. I will do just fine. Thank you." Upon careful consultation with his family and close friends, Mr. Yusuf decided that his self-care regimen would include:

◆ Pray daily and be thankful for his many blessings.
◆ Drink six bottles of mineral water a day.
◆ Eat a traditional diet that consists of, for example, hummus, olives, tabbouleh, zbadi (yogurt), local fruit, and lamb burgers.
◆ Get more rest and work fewer hours.
◆ Have family prayers with tea every night.
◆ Walk a mile each day.
◆ Reduce and eventually eliminate cigarette smoking.

Initially, Mr. Yusuf did feel somewhat better; he was elated to find that he was disciplined enough to adhere to his self-care regimen. His family and friends were committed to his overall care plan for improving his health status. Over time—about 6 months into the regimen, his health status worsened: The weight loss continued, nausea and vomiting increased in frequency and duration, and his fatigue level interfered with all his activities of daily living, including his work, which was being questioned by others at his company.

(continued)

CASE STUDY 23.1: "WHAT IF" SYNDROME: DEVOTION TO DUTY AND FAMILY (*CONTINUED*)

After family consultation, Mr. Yusuf was encouraged to consult his healthcare team, but his adamant response was, "I can handle this. I will be fine...." He was mortally terrified to make that contact; he thought he would be rejected, scorned, shamed, and disrespected for his "ignorant decision by an educated and respected man about his health." Mr. Yusuf prayed for courage and acceptance. He confided to his family about "being able to see death." He and his family ultimately decided that he must return to the hospital and seek care. Five family members accompanied him in anticipation of a horrible and devasting conversation with the physician and nurse.

When Mr. Yusuf and his family arrived at the clinic, the nurse practitioner was notified. He immediately went to the lobby to greet Mr. Yusuf. Upon seeing he was not alone, the nurse commented, "Mr. Yusuf! It is so wonderful to see you and your family! We have been waiting for you, and we are prepared to help you. Come on in—yes—come on in—I will notify your physician and let him know you are here." The nurse practitioner got a wheelchair for Mr. Yusuf and assisted him and the family into a private room at the clinic. Mr. Yusuf and the family spontaneously began uttering prayers of thanksgiving. After the prayers were completed, beverages and snacks were offered to the family. Mr. Yusuf accepted a cup of warm water.

Conversations about the mutual relief and happiness of reconnecting with the physician and nurse practitioner flowed naturally into the history and assessment process. By Mr. Yusuf's preference, the family remained with him, providing valuable input. A short- and long-term plan of care was developed. The first step was to hospitalize Mr. Yusuf and focus on his immediate clinical health needs, involving attention to dehydration, nutritional status, fatigue, and mobility. The hospitalization extended over several weeks, and the family visited for long hours each day. His insurance covered all aspects of his care. Mr. Yusuf was discharged to his home with a plan of care; this included elements of his previous self-care regimen, but with the addition of evidence-based interventions to treat leukemia.

At the last clinic visit, Mr. Yusuf was following all aspects of the self-care regimen, and he had returned to work and other community activities. His reflection on his illness frequently includes remarks: "What if I had not returned to the clinic? What if the physician and nurse practitioner had scared and embarrassed me? What if I had been rejected and disrespected? What if they thought I was too sick to be helped, admonishing me that I had refused my only healthcare opportunity? What if I had no insurance? What if I did not have a supportive family? What if I had low or no education? What if I had no money? What if I had no transportation to the hospital? What if I had continued to 'see death'...I was so close to giving up. Am I a good enough man?"

Discussion Questions

1. As a healthcare provider, think about Mr. Yusuf's comments and plan how you might respond to each. What are the potential positive and negative aspects of such frequent reflections?

2. Should there be other supports and interventions offered to Mr. Yusuf and, perhaps, his family? Identify three action steps with rationale. List a minimum of four support materials (e.g., brochures, videos, music) that might be helpful to Mr. Yusuf and his family. Please share a brief rationale for selecting the materials that you have chosen. Document your work with evidence-based research and clinical practice publications.

DISCUSSION QUESTIONS

1. Describe recent trends in cancer disparity outcomes and delineate at least three reasons why you think these trends are evident among populations across the global and national communities.
2. Using the social determinants of health framework, focus on two factors—education and socioeconomic status—and discuss the intersectionality between them and health outcomes in the global and local communities.
3. What are three key points to remember regarding the relationship between COVID-19, cancer disparities, and health outcomes among vulnerable populations. As a health professional, delineate a short- and long-term approach to addressing the issues you identify.
4. How does health policy influence healthcare across three domains: the patient and family, the provider, and the system?
   a. **Which domain do you focus on in your practice, research, and educational activities?**
   b. Do you think that policy changes could influence better health outcomes in cancer disparities? What are the barriers to change?
   c. What are the facilitators that support change? Be specific and document your responses.

CONCLUSION

In this chapter, we have discussed the disproportionate cancer burdens experienced by minority populations and, more importantly, the contributions of socioeconomic factors to cancer disparity in American society. The chapter highlights issues related to prostate cancer screening, tobacco consumption, and the COVID-19 pandemic. Two person-centered narratives underscored patient experiences, followed by questions designed to provoke critical thinking and improve patient outcomes. Key elements of the socioeconomic determinants of health suggest that individual behavioral choices, though responsible, in part, for personal health, are determined by economic and social conditions—that is, an individual's human and material resources are potent determinants of health outcomes (Bartley, 2003; Marmot & Wilkinson, 2005; Townsend et al., 1992). This chapter has clearly illustrated the role of socioeconomic determinants in the morbidity and mortality of cancer.

First, poverty and income matter significantly and help to predict health outcomes of individuals with cancer. Many of these individuals had no control over their living conditions—whether living lonely lives or disconnected from family and friends, to being in crowded places and spaces. Some of them cannot exercise or take walks through woody trails or parks because of an abiding concern for their safety. Still, many have experienced worsening physical and mental health conditions during the pandemic, and some are still in the recovery stages. The physical environment also helps create a direct and profound influence on the overall health status of people with cancer.

Second, policies and practices of governments, organizations, and societies, which stem from socioeconomic and political realities, help shape risk behaviors for cancer. For example, when a minority group of people is ignored in health policy regulations (i.e., PSA screening) or targeted for a profiting purpose that increases cancer risks (i.e., tobacco use), the loss of life to cancer is potentially inevitable.

Lastly, stresses and mental health challenges generated from long-term socioeconomic structures, societal biases, and racism diminish health outcomes linked to health promotion, disease prevention, and prompt treatment that focuses on the individual's holistic healthcare needs. For instance, despite her positive physiological response to cancer treatment, Ms. Kahananul died of a drug overdose. Yet, social support from family and healthcare providers helped combat these obstacles and improved Mr. Yusuf's chance of survival and longevity.

The lessons to be learned from these cases are impactful. For all health professionals and others who participate in making policies and implementation, it is essential to recall that helping individuals with cancer and those at risk could benefit from empathy and support, knowledge about their illness condition, and enhanced health literacy. Lifestyle issues, the importance of adhering to a treatment regimen, and continuous individual assessment help strengthen patient/provider communications and trust and improve health outcomes. When working in any setting, healthcare providers should query the patients about their sense of safety, access to support persons and resources, lifestyle patterns and concerns, life stressors, and so forth. Understanding the person's belief system is reflected in their daily decision-making and reality testing. To achieve health equity in cancer care outcomes, all members of our society, especially health professionals, will have to invest more effort in combating inequality in every aspect of society's socioeconomic structures. Advocacy for the voiceless, the marginalized, and the most vulnerable—children, the elderly, the mentally ill, and the poor—are essential next steps.

ADDITIONAL RESOURCES

This section provides additional resources that provide a wealth of information for those who have specific interests in cancer.

This is a tremendously valuable resource for world population statistics dealing with every kind of human problem, cancer being just one among others such as climate change, war, poverty, and hunger. It includes links to numerous graphics, many of which are interactive. All are free to use and duplicate for any purpose—see for yourself on their website (https://ourworldindata.org/about) under the heading "Our World in Data Is a Public Good."

Roser, M., & Ritchie, H. (2015). *Cancer*. https://ourworldindata.org/cancer

The information in this publication was derived from projections based on data collected from 2004 to 2018. It includes informative charts and graphs that describe numerous types of cancer among various demographics along with discussion pages:

American Cancer Society. (2022). *Cancer facts & figures, 2022.* www.cancer.org/content/dam/cancer -org/research/cancer-facts-and-statistics/annual-cancer-facts-and-figures/2022/2022-cancer-facts -and-figures.pdf

The graphics on this site focus on cancer death statistics by sex, age, cancer type, and state of residence:

Centers for Disease Control and Prevention. (2022). *An update on cancer deaths in the United States.* www.cdc.gov/cancer/dcpc/research/update-on-cancer-deaths/index.htm

Numerous types of cancer statistics are available via links in the ribbon across the top of the page, such as information on new cancer cases and death counts in each state, survival trends, screening statistics, and more. The charts and figures offered in the links are live, so it is possible to access data for each state in a variety of different formats:

Centers for Disease Control and Prevention. (2021). *Cancer data and statistics.* www.cdc.gov/cancer/ dcpc/data/index.htm

This toolkit is designed as a guide for those who are involved in cancer prevention and control programs, whether you are designing such a program or responsible for evaluating program outcomes:

Centers for Disease Control and Prevention. (2010). *Comprehensive cancer control branch program evaluation toolkit.* www.cdc.gov/cancer/ncccp/pdf/CCC_Program_Evaluation_Toolkit.pdf

Here you will find brief descriptions along with links to fulsome information about programs the Centers for Disease Control and Prevention sponsors to promote health equity:

National Center for Chronic Disease Prevention and Health Promotion. (2021, September 15). *Social determinants of health: Achieving health equity by addressing the social determinants of health.* www.cdc .gov/chronicdisease/programs-impact/sdoh.htm

For those who work with senior citizens, or who anticipate becoming one, this article follows 413 elderly persons to discover how social loneliness and emotional loneliness correlate with mortality:

O'Súilleabháin, P. S., Gallagher, S., & Steptoe, A. (2019). Loneliness, living alone, and all-cause mortality: The role of emotional and social loneliness in the elderly during 19 years of follow-up. *Psychosomatic Medicine, 81*(6), 521–526. https://doi.org/10.1097/PSY.0000000000000710

REFERENCES

Adegoke, A. A. (2014). Perceived effects of overcrowding on the physical and psychological health of hostel occupants in Nigeria. *IOSR Journal of Humanities and Social Science, 19*(9), 1–9. https://doi.org/10.9790/0837-19980109

American Cancer Society. (2021). American cancer society recommendations for prostate cancer early detection. https://www.cancer.org/cancer/prostate-cancer/detection-diagnosis-staging/acs-recommendations.html

American Cancer Society. (2022a). Cancer facts & figures 2022. https://www.cancer.org/research/cancer-facts-statistics/all-cancer-facts-figures/cancer-facts-figures-2022.html

American Cancer Society. (2022b). Cancer facts & figures for African Americans 2022–2024. American Cancer Society. https://www.cancer.org/content/dam/cancer-org/research/cancer-facts-and-statistics/cancer-facts-and-figures-for-african-americans/2022-2024-cff-aa.pdf

Bartley, M. (2003). *Understanding health inequalities*. Polity Press.

Blake, K. D., & Green Parker, M. (2020). Social and behavioral intervention research to address modifiable risk factors for cancer in rural populations. https://cancercontrol.cancer.gov/brp/events/12-2020-social-behavioral

Cornelius, M. E., Wang, T. W., Jamal, A., Loretan, C. G., & Neff, L. J. (2020). Tobacco product use among adults–United States, 2019. *Morbidity and Mortality Weekly Reports, 2020*(69), 1736–1742. https://doi.org/10.15585/mmwr.mm6946a4

Delnevo, C. D., Giovenco, D. P., & Villanti, A. C. (2020). Assessment of menthol and nonmenthol cigarette consumption in the US, 2000 to 2018. *JAMA Network Open, 3*(8), e2013601. https://doi.org/10.1001/jamanetworkopen.2020.13601

DeSantis, C. E., Miller, K. D., Dale, W., Mohile, S. G., Cohen, H. J., Leach, C. R., Goding Sauer, A., Jemal, A., & Siegel, R. L. (2019a). Cancer statistics for adults aged 85 years and older, 2019. *CA: A Cancer Journal for Clinicians, 69*(6), 452–467. https://doi.org/10.3322/caac.21577

DeSantis, C. E., Miller, K. D., Goding Sauer, A., Jemal, A., & Siegel, R. L. (2019b). Cancer statistics for African Americans, 2019. *CA: A Cancer Journal for Clinicians, 69*(3), 211–233. https://doi.org/10.3322/caac.21555

Doane, L. D., & Adam, E. K. (2010). Loneliness and cortisol: Momentary, day-to-day, and trait associations. *Psychoneuroendocrinology, 35*(3), 430–441. https://doi.org/10.1016/j.psyneuen.2009.08.005

Drake, E. C., Sladek, M. R., & Doane, L. D. (2015). Daily cortisol activity, loneliness, and coping efficacy in late adolescence: A longitudinal study of the transition to college. *International Journal of Behavioral Development, 40*(4), 334–345. https://doi.org/10.1177/0165025415581914

Erhunmwunsee, L., Seewaldt, V. L., Rebbeck, T. R., & Winn, R. A. (2021). From COVID-19 to cancer, watching social determinants decide life: When will we stop spectating? *Journal of the National Medical Association, 113*(4), 436–439. https://doi.org/10.1016/j.jnma.2021.02.003

Fillmore, N. R., La, J., Szalat, R. E., Tuck, D. P., Nguyen, V., Yildirim, C., Do, N. V., Brophy, M. T., & Munshi, N. C. (2021). Prevalence and outcome of COVID-19 infection in cancer patients: A national veterans affairs study. *Journal of the National Cancer Institute, 113*(6), 691–698. https://doi.org/10.1093/jnci/djaa159

Gardiner, P. S. (2004). The African Americanization of menthol cigarette use in the United States. *Nicotine and Tobacco Research, 6*(suppl 1), S55–65.

Gove, W. R., Hughes, M., & Galle, O. R. (1979). Overcrowding in the home: An empirical investigation of its possible pathological consequences. *American Sociological Review, 44*(1), 59–80. https://doi.org/10.2307/2094818

Henley, S. J., Anderson, R. N., Thomas, C. C., Massetti, G. M., Peaker, B., & Richardson, L. C. (2017). Invasive cancer incidence, 2004–2013, and deaths, 2006–2015, in nonmetropolitan and metropolitan counties—United States. *Morbidity and Mortality Weekly Report Surveillance Summaries, 66*(14), 1–13. https://doi.org/10.15585/mmwr.ss6614a1

Henley, S. J., & Jemal, A. (2018). Rural cancer control: Bridging the chasm in geographic health inequity. *Cancer Epidemiology, Biomarkers, and Prevention, 27*(11), 1248–1251. https://doi.org/10.1158/1055-9965.EPI-18-0807

James, C. V., Moonesinghe, R., Wilson-Frederick, S. M., Hall, J. E., Penman-Aguilar, A., Bouye, K., & National Center for Emerging and Zoonotic Infectious Diseases (U.S.). Division of Vector-Borne

Diseases. (2017, November 17). Racial/ethnic health disparities among rural adults—United States, 2012–2015. *Morbidity and Mortality Weekly Report Surveillance Summaries, 66*(23). https://doi.org/10.15585/mmwr.ss6623a1

Kensler, K. H., Pernar, C. H., Mahal, B. A., Nguyen, P. L., Trinh, Q.-D., Kibel, A. S., & Rebbeck, T. R. (2021). Racial and ethnic variation in PSA testing and prostate cancer incidence following the 2012 USPSTF recommendation, *Journal of National Cancer Institute, 113*(6), 719–726. https://doi.org/10.1093/jnci/djaa171

Kirkwood, M. K., Bruinooge, S. S., Goldstein, M. A., Bajorin, D. F., & Kosty, M. P. (2014). Enhancing the American Society of clinical oncology workforce information system with geographic distribution of oncologists and comparison of data sources for the number of practicing oncologists. *Journal of Oncology Practice, 10*(1), 32–38. https://doi.org/10.1200/JOP.2013.001311

Kish, J. K., Yu, M., Percy-Laurry, A., & Altekruse, S. F. (2014). Racial and ethnic disparities in cancer survival by neighborhood socioeconomic status in surveillance, *Epidemiology, and End Results (SEER) Registries. Journal of National Cancer Institute Monographs, 2014*(49), 236–243. https://doi.org/10.1093/jncimonographs/lgu020

Marmot, M., & Wilkinson, R. G. (2005). Social patterning of individual health behaviours: The case of cigarette smoking. In M. Marmot & R. Wilkinson (Eds.), *Social Determinants of Health* (pp. 224–37). https://doi.org/10.1093/acprof:oso/9780198565895.003.11

Mills, S. D., Henriksen, L., Golden, S. D., Kurtzman, R., Kong, A. Y., Queen, T. L., & Ribisl, K. M. (2018). Disparities in retail marketing for menthol cigarettes in the United States, 2015. *Health Place, 53*, 62–70. https://doi.org/10.1016/j.healthplace.2018.06.011

Moyer, V. A., & U.S. Preventive Services Task Force. (2012, July 17). Screening for prostate cancer: US preventive services task force recommendation statement. *Annals of Internal Medicine, 157*(2), 120–134. https://doi.org/10.7326/0003-4819-157-2-201207170-00459

National Cancer Institute. (2022a). Cancer stat facts: Cancer disparities. https://seer.cancer.gov/statfacts/html/disparities.html

National Cancer Institute. (2022b). Cancer disparities. https://www.cancer.gov/about-cancer/understanding/disparities

Newman, L. A., Winn, R. A., & Carethers, J. M. (2021). Similarities in risk for COVID-19 and cancer disparities. *Clinical Cancer Research, 27*(1), 24–27. https://doi.org/10.1158/1078-0432.CCR-20-3421

Office of Disease Prevention and Health Promotion. (2022a). Healthy people 2030: Cancer. https://health.gov/healthypeople/objectives-and-data/browse-objectives/cancer

Office of Disease Prevention and Health Promotion. (2022b). Increase the proportion of cancer survivors who are living 5 years of longer after diagnosis—C-11: Data methodology and measurement. https://health.gov/healthypeople/objectives-and-data/browse-objectives/cancer/increase-proportion-cancer-survivors-who-are-living-5-years-or-longer-after-diagnosis-c-11/data-methodology

Potter, D., Riffon, M., Kakamada, S., Miller, R. S., & Komatsoulis, G. A. (2020). Disproportionate impact of COVID-19 disease among racial and ethnic minorities in the U.S. Cancer population as seen in CancerLinQ Discovery Data. *Journal of Clinical Oncology, 38*(suppl 29), 84–84. https://doi.org/10.1200/JCO.2020.38.29_suppl.84

Riviere, P., Luterstein, E., Kumar, A., Vitzthum, L. K., Deka, R., Sarkar, R. R., Bryant, A. K., Bruggeman, A., Einck, J. P., Murphy, J. D., Martinez, M. E., & Rose, B. S. (2020). Survival of African American and non-hispanic white men with prostate cancer in an equal-access health care system. *Cancer, 126*(8), 1683–1690. https://doi.org/10.1002/cncr.32666

Schmidt, A. L., Bakouny, Z., Bhalla, S., Steinharter, J. A., Tremblay, D. A., Awad, M. M., Kessler, A. J., Haddad, R. I., Evans, M., Busser, F., Wotman, M., Curran, C. R., Zimmerman, B. S., Bouchard, G., Jun, T., Nuzzo, P. V., Qin, Q., Hirsch, L., Feld, J., …, Doroshow, D. B. (2020). Cancer care disparities during the COVID-19 pandemic: COVID-19 and cancer outcomes study. *Cancer Cell, 38*(6), 769–770. https://doi.org/10.1016/j.ccell.2020.10.023

Selden, T. M., & Berdahl, T. A. (2020). COVID-19 and racial/ethnic disparities in health risk, employment, and household composition. *Health Affairs, 39*(9), 1624–1632. https://doi.org/10.1377/hlthaff.2020.00897

Suran, M. (2022). How cancer will affect the US in 2022. *JAMA, 327*(10), 907–908. https://doi.org/10.1001/jama.2022.2415

Townsend, P., Davidson, N., & Whitehead, M. (Eds.) (1992). *Inequalities in health: The black report and the health divide.* Penguin.

U.S. Department of Health and Human Services, Office of the Surgeon General. (2014). The consequences of smoking—50 years of progress: A report of the surgeon general. https://www.ncbi.nlm.nih.gov/books/NBK179276/pdf/Bookshelf_NBK179276.pdf

U.S. Preventive Services Task Force. (2018, May 8). Final recommendation statement: Prostate cancer screening. https://www.uspreventiveservicestaskforce.org/uspstf/recommendation/prostate-cancer-screening

Wang, Q., Berger, N. A., & Xu, R. (2021). Analyses of risk, racial disparity, and outcomes among US patients with cancer and COVID-19 infection. *JAMA Oncology, 7*(2), 220–227. https://doi.org/10.1001/jamaoncol.2020.6178

World Health Organization. (2013). Global action plan for prevention and control on noncommunicable diseases 2013–2020. https://www.who.int/publications-detail-redirect/9789241506236

World Health Organization. (2021, April 28). Final evaluation of the WHO global coordination mechanism for the prevention and control of noncommunicable diseases (GCM/NCD). https://www.who.int/news/

World Health Organization. (2022). Preventing cancer. https://www.who.int/activities/preventing-cancer

World Health Organization. (n.d.). Social determinants of health. https://www.who.int/health-topics/social-determinants-of-health#tab=tab_1

Yang, L., Chai, P., Yu, J., & Fan, X. (2021). Effects of cancer on patients with COVID-19: A systematic review and meta-analysis of 63,019 participants. *Cancer Biology & Medicine, 18*(1), 298–307. https://doi.org/10.20892/j.issn.2095-3941.2020.0559

Zahnd, W. E., Davis, M. M., Rotter, J. S., Vanderpool, R. C., Perry, C. K., Shannon, J., Ko, L. K., Wheeler, S. B., Odahowski, C. L., Farris, P. E., & Eberth, J. M. (2019). Rural-urban differences in financial burden among cancer survivors: An analysis of a nationally representative survey. *Support Care Cancer, 27*(12), 4779–4786. https://doi.org/10.1007/s00520-019-04742-z

Zahnd, W. E., James, A. S., Jenkins, W. D., Izadi, S. R., Fogleman, A. J., Steward, D. E., Colditz, G. A., & Brard, A. (2018). Rural–urban differences in cancer incidence and trends in the United States. *Cancer Epidemiology, Biomarkers & Prevention, 27*(11), 1265–1274. https://doi.org/10.1158/1055-9965.EPI-17-0430

Zhang, A. Y., Ganocy, S. J., Owusu, C., & Gao, K. (2021). Associations among irritability, high-sensitivity C-reactive protein/interleukin-6, and depression in early-stage breast cancer patients undergoing chemotherapy: A prospective study. *Journal of the Academy of Consultation-Liaison Psychiatry.* https://doi.org/10.1016/j.jaclp.2021.08.012

Zhang, A. Y., Koroukian, S., Owusu, C., Moore, S. E., & Gairola, R. (2022). Socioeconomic correlates of health outcomes and mental health disparity in a sample of cancer patients during the COVID-19 pandemic. *Journal of Clinical Nursing.* https://doi.org/10.1111/jocn.16266

CHAPTER 24

Women and HIV/AIDS in the Kingdom of Eswatini

Tengetile R. Mathunjwa-Dlamini, Nomsa Magagula, and Faye A. Gary

LEARNING OBJECTIVES

- Describe the scope of the HIV and AIDS challenge in Eswatini.

- Describe how gender inequality manifests in Eswatini's culture, economy, politics, and healthcare infrastructure, and how the inequality impacts HIV and AIDS prevalence.

- Discuss the interaction between cultural practices and the healthcare system in relation to HIV and AIDS in Eswatini.

- Explain the role traditional healers play in HIV prevention and care in Eswatini.

- Discuss evidence-based programs that have helped to reduce HIV and AIDS-related mortality and morbidity in Eswatini.

INTRODUCTION

This chapter focuses on the human immunodeficiency virus (HIV) and acquired immunodeficiency syndrome (AIDS) in the Kingdom of Eswatini, which for more than 60 years was known as the Kingdom of Swaziland. Specifically, the chapter highlights the intersection of—and conflicts between—cultural beliefs and practices, traditional healing, and public health interventions. Eswatini continues to have one of the highest HIV prevalence rates in the world. The practice of safer sex is crucial to reducing the incidence and prevalence of the virus; yet, in 2014, UNAIDS reported that women still had challenges negotiating for safer sex (UNAIDS, 2014). This chapter demonstrates how institutionalized gender inequality and cultural practices in the Kingdom of Eswatini impact HIV prevention and treatment. The chapter also highlights several novel, culturally specific programs designed to reduce and eliminate HIV and AIDS in Eswatini.

See Box 24.1 and Figure 24.1 for a description and map of Eswatini.

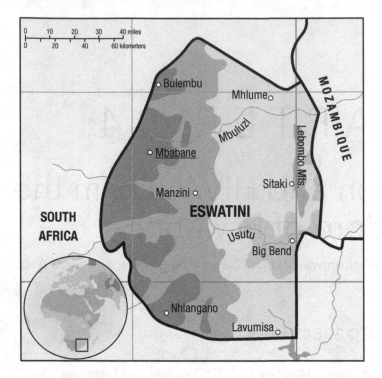

Figure 24.1 Map of Eswatini.

BOX 24.1: A Brief Description of Eswatini

Eswatini (see Figure 24.1) is located in the sub-Saharan region of Africa. It is surrounded by the Republic of South Africa (RSA) to the north, south, and west, and Mozambique to the east. Mbabane is the capital city (World Health Organization [WHO], 2021a). The Kingdom of Eswatini measures 17,400 square kilometers (about 6,718 square miles) and has a population of 1.1 million people (The Commonwealth Secretariat, 2021). It is the last absolute monarchy in Africa. The indigenous language is *Siswati*, but English is the official language. Eswatini is known for its beautiful terrain, wildlife sanctuaries, and game reserves; its dynamic and respectful people; and its colorful traditional celebrations. Poverty is a challenge in Eswatini, with 58.9% of the populace living below the poverty line—defined by The World Bank (2021) as earning less than $1.90 in a day.

GOVERNMENT ARCHITECTURE

His Majesty King Mswati III has led the Kingdom of Eswatini since his inauguration on April 25, 1986. The country adopted a Constitution on July 26, 2005, which acts as the supreme law. Three independent branches compose Eswatini's government, over which the monarch exercises supreme authority: the executive, the legislative, and the judiciary (Eswatini Government, n.d; Shongwe, 2019). Rural Eswatini is governed through 59 *Tinkhundla*, which are further divided into chiefdoms. Chiefdom is patrilineal, with women only eligible to serve in the role when a (male) heir is too young to govern. Urban Eswatini operates under the authority of municipalities, of which there are 14 (Shongwe, 2019).

HEALTH INFRASTRUCTURE

Proximity to health services is relatively high, in part because about 80% of the populace lives within an 8-km radius of a health facility (Ministry of Health, 2015). Hence, the distribution of services skews toward the urban population, suggesting that people in rural areas are less likely to access health services. To address this reality, the Ministry of Health provides care to rural populations through its support of lay and professional health providers: community health workers, epidemiologists, public health nurses, physicians, and others. One fundamental concern, however, is associated with access to clean water (see the Narrative, that follows). For example, 91% of the urban population has access to sanitary water, compared with only 37% of rural residents (WHO, 2018). Consequently, people in rural areas are still negatively impacted by numerous preventable health conditions. For example, dysentery, pneumonia, and other diseases are related to the lack of accessible clean water and the proper disposal of solid waste.

Most health facilities are government owned and subsidize healthcare services. All primary healthcare services (antenatal care, child welfare, family planning, HIV testing, etc.) are free to patients in government-funded health facilities unless they are sick and need additional care. Sick individuals pay approximately $1 for consultation and medication. This is a substantial amount of money for residents living on $1.90/day. Swazi residents also pay for additional services such as laboratory tests, x-rays, and computed tomography. Mandatory retirement for government employees occurs at age 60—thereafter, their healthcare is free and government supported. For others, there is a fee. There are four levels of healthcare services in Eswatini: community-based care, primary care, secondary care, and tertiary care (Magagula, 2017):

1. Community-based care involves rural health motivators, faith-based healthcare providers, volunteers, and traditional birth attendants.
2. Health centers, public health units, rural clinics, and outreach sites compose primary care.
3. Secondary care takes place in Eswatini's five regional hospitals.
4. The Kingdom's three national (referral) hospitals provide tertiary care.

As referenced in item two in this list, Type A clinics offer all public health clinic (PHC) services apart from maternity services. Type B clinics offer all services including maternity. Public health units also provide PHC services, such as antenatal care and family planning; they also support outreach services. Health centers are the base for curative services such as sexually transmitted infections (STIs), malaria, and so forth, and inpatient care that provides acute care and referral to regional hospitals for secondary care. Health centers also offer PHC services (Magagula, 2017).

Because Eswatini is a resource-constrained, low-middle–income country, it receives substantial support through United Nations agencies and bilateral agreements. Agencies including WHO, the United Nations Population Fund (UNFPA), the Joint United Nations Programme on HIV and AIDS (UNAIDS), and the United States Agency for International Development (USAID) provide technical and financial support for health initiatives aimed at preventing diseases and improving the overall health of the Eswatini populace.

NARRATIVE 24.1: WATER IS CRITICAL FOR LIFE

More than 2.2 billion people do not have safe water services throughout the world community, and another 4.2 billion people lack properly managed sanitation services. Approximately 3 billion individuals are without basic handwashing capabilities. As world populations grow, climate variability and pollution continue.

In many world communities, unavailability of water has become a risk to economic progress, the reduction and elimination of poverty, and the sustainability of development. In Africa, for example, water is not available to many communities, and its accessibility is sometimes associated with the "elite." In Eswatini, around 40% of the inhabitants cannot

(continued)

NARRATIVE 24.1: WATER IS CRITICAL FOR LIFE (*CONTINUED*)

gain access to clean water. In some communities, especially rural areas, close to 90% of people experience malfunctioning water pumps and other resources. Maintenance and repairs are delayed for long periods, depriving people and communities of clean water. Hence, people must travel long distances for clean water, which can be expensive, time-consuming, and, at times, dangerous and unattainable. Lack of clean water in Eswatini, much like other world communities, can compromise the health and well-being of a nation. The federal government has begun educating its citizens about using water pumps more effectively; efforts to maintain and repair the water sources are also a high priority across the government and private sectors.

Women and children are often responsible for securing water for their families and frequently walk miles each day to get clean water from streams and ponds. Unfortunately, numerous illnesses are associated with unclean water, including dysentery, pneumonia, trachoma, dengue, and stunted growth (Freeman et al., 2013; Shongwe & Dlamini 2021).

The time lost getting water interferes with the children's education and overall growth and development. Women's daily routines can be consumed with "fetching water" for their households. Thus, securing water demands time, energy, and expenditures, which are major barriers to better health and well-being in Eswatini. Substantial efforts are also being made to improve access to clean water and address the problems associated with open defecation by children and adults (Shongwe & Dlamini, 2021).

Since Africa's population is becoming urbanized at a more rapid rate than any continent on Earth at the rate of 3.5% per year, attention must be given to clean water and solid waste disposal for its population (Nhlengethwa et al., 2020). Policymakers in the Kingdom of Eswatini have begun to systematically examine how the nation can provide safe water and efficient methods of defecation control. The overall efforts to improve water access are essential and intertwined in Eswatini's Sanitation and Hygiene Plan of 2019 to 2023. The objectives of the national program are multifaceted and centered on sanitation and hygiene, which is an essential component for social and economic development at multiple levels: individual, familial, community, and societal levels. Increased access to improved sanitation and hygiene facilities contributes to the population's health and well-being, which, in turn, drives the nation's economy.

The national Sanitation and Hygiene Plan also focuses on educating all communities about the overlap among clean water, sanitation, hygiene, and health outcomes. Training programs and capacity building are evident across the Kingdom. The curricula changes in schools that feature content about sanitation, personal hygiene, hand washing, and waste management are essential and stressed across all sectors. Recycling and the proper disposal of waste are also emphasized and reinforced among private and government segments. WHO (2015) has proclaimed that sanitation is a fundamental human right, and open defecation, especially in rural areas, threatens human health and sustainability. Consequently, the Sanitation and Hygiene Plan emphasizes reducing and eliminating open defecation among people, especially in rural communities (Simelane et al., 2020). For more information, see the National Sanitation and Hygiene Strategy 2019–2023, 2015. www.unicef.org/eswatini/media/886/file/National%20sanitation%20and%20hygiene%20strategy-report-2019.pdf.pdf

HIV IN ESWATINI

Eswatini has been hit hard by the HIV pandemic, with a prevalence rate of 27% (Ministry of Health, 2019). In 1986, Eswatini recorded the first case of HIV (Ministry of Health, 2010) in an anonymous individual. The virus spread like wildfire, particularly among pregnant women (Table 24.1). At the time, epidemiologists used sentinel surveillance data from pregnant women to estimate prevalence for the whole population—the rationale being that this

TABLE 24.1 Kingdom of Eswatini: Key Facts

Indicators	Facts	Source
Crude birth rate	28.5%	2017 Census Preliminary Results
Total fertility rate	3.03 children per woman	World Data Atlas, 2019
Crude death rate	9.38%	
Unemployment rate	22.5%	UNDP Human Development Reports, 2018
Life expectancy at birth (years)	61 Females	
	54 Males	
Literacy rate	76.7%	UN, 2019
Women experiencing GBV	1:3	UNICEF, 2007
Child marriage rate	5.0%	MICS, 2014
Maternal mortality (100,000 live births)	389	WHO, 2018

GBV, gender-based violence; MICS, multiple indicator cluster surveys; UNDP, United Nations Development Programme; UNICEF, United Nations Children's Fund; WHO, World Health Organization.

Source: Data from UNFPA. (2019). *Government of the Kingdom of Eswatini/UNFPA 6th country programme evaluation 2016-2020.* www.unfpa.org/sites/default/files/board-documents/Eswatini_-_CPE_-_Country_programme_evaluation_1.pdf.

TABLE 24.2 HIV Prevalence Among Pregnant Women in Swaziland (Now Eswatini)

Year	1992	1994	1996	1998	2000	2002	2004	2006	2008	2010
Prevalence (%)	3.9	16.1	26.0	31.6	34.2	38.6	42.6	39.2	42.0	41.1

Source: Data from Ministry on Health. (2010). *12th HIV sentinel surveillance.* Mbabane: Webster Print.

population was easy to access. Standard care in Eswatini requires that pregnant women routinely have their blood samples collected during antenatal care visits to assess them for STIs and HIV antibodies (Mathunjwa & Gary, 2006).

Table 24.2 presents data on HIV prevalence among pregnant women from 1992 to 2010. The HIV prevalence began at 3.9% in 1992; however, in 2010 it escalated to 41.1% with a peak of 42.6% in 2004. The prevalence calculated from these data (1992–2010) was significantly higher than that from the population survey in subsequent years (2012 and 2019; Ministry of Health, 2019).

After 2010, the Ministry of Health assessed the data as part of the Swaziland HIV Measurement Surveys I (2010/2011) and II (2016/2017), which evaluated both incidence and prevalence (Ministry of Health, 2012, 2019). Table 24.3 depicts summary data on the incidence and prevalence of HIV in Eswatini based on the Swaziland HIV Measurement Survey's two phases (SHIMS 1 and SHIMS 2). The populace HIV prevalence was stable (27%) in both the 2010 to 2011 and the 2016 to 2017 surveys. However, there was a decline in HIV incidence, from 3.1% in 2010–2011 to 1.36% between 2016 and 2017 (Ministry of Health, 2012, 2019).

Swazi women are disproportionately affected by HIV. The prevalence of HIV among women was 32% compared with 20.4% in men among people age 14 to 49 years (Ministry of Health, 2019). Avert (2020) reported that more women (88.6%) living with HIV are aware of their status, compared with 77.5% of men. One explanation for these differences is that women sometimes test for HIV without disclosing their decision to be tested—or their serostatus—to their partners. Men are reluctant to seek healthcare, and are, accordingly, less likely to undergo

TABLE 24.3 SHIMS 1 and SHIMS 2

Variable	SHIMS 1	SHIMS 2
Year	2012	2019
Prevalence (%)	27	27
Incidence (%)	3.1	1.36

Source: Data from Ministry of Health. (2012). *Swaziland HIV Incidence Measurement Survey (SHIMS): First findings report.* Mbabane. http://ghdx.healthdata.org/record/swaziland-hiv-incidence-measurement-survey-shims-first-findings-report-november-2012; Ministry of Health. (2019). Swaziland HIV Incidence Measurement Survey (SHIMS 2) 2016–2017: Final report. Mbabane. https://phia.icap.columbia.edu/wp-content/uploads/2019/05/SHIMS2_Final-Report_05.03.2019_forWEB.pdf.SHIMS, Swaziland HIV Measurement Survey.

HIV testing. Women also have more opportunities for HIV testing because they are provided child welfare and maternal healthcare services, while men do not attend these services.

HIV affects all population groups in the Kingdom, with widows, sex workers, and adolescents experiencing the highest prevalence. In 2019, HIV incidence and prevalence were estimated from the general population data rather than the sentinel surveillance of pregnant women. The Ministry of Health (2019) reported that of 32% of women who were HIV positive, 74.6% were widows age 15 to 49 years. The prevailing thought is that many of the women might have been infected through their partners. Sex workers have a similarly high prevalence (70%) because they are, at times, forced to engage in unprotected vaginal and anal sex (Parmley et al., 2020). Adolescents frequently have sex with older men—who could also have HIV from previous or concurrent relationships—for money and other favors (Ministry of Health, 2019).

In 1999, His Majesty King Mswati III declared HIV and AIDS a "national disaster" (Disaster Risk Management Information Management System, n.d.). Antiretroviral therapy (ART) was unavailable in Eswatini until 2003, at which time it was dispersed only to those who already had AIDS; an individual is diagnosed with AIDS if they have a CD4 count ≤200 cells/mm³ (Avert, 2020).

Following implementation, in 2016, of a test and treat/test and start initiative, HIV in Eswatini increasingly seems to be a chronic, manageable condition. All individuals who test positive for HIV are now immediately started on ART regardless of their CD4 count (Pell et al., 2018). Remarkably, HIV incidence was reduced from 3.1% in 2012 to 1.36% in 2019 following the implementation of the test and treat/test and start initiative.

Although the Kingdom of Eswatini has made significant progress in the fight against HIV and AIDS, it remains among the leading countries in the world with respect to incidence (Ministry of Health, 2019). The HIV incidence rate in 2019 among individuals age 15 to 49 years was 1.36%; that translates to 7,300 new cases per year (Ministry of Health, 2019). The Government of the Kingdom of Eswatini (2018) reported that 120,000 women and 90,000 men are living with HIV. In addition, it is estimated that 13,000 children are infected. They further estimated that 60% currently suffer TB/HIV co-infection, the mortality rate for which is 14%. Minnery et al. (2020) assert that AIDS is the most common cause of death and disability in Eswatini, with heterosexual sex at 97%,representing the most common cause of transmission (Avert, 2020).

Eswatini's patriarchal social order exacerbates the spread of HIV, as well as the virus's morbidity and mortality. As discussed in the following, the interaction between cultural practices and the healthcare system, while representing a challenge to HIV prevention and treatment, also may offer the most effective solutions to the crisis in the Kingdom.

HIV, Marriage, and Family

Patriarchy is inscribed in Eswatini law, which accords women minority legal status. Getting married reduces the legal status of a woman still further as they are regarded as equivalent to children, according to custom (Swaziland Rural Women Assembly, 2018). Despite this change in status, young girls prefer to get married. In rural settings, neither married nor unmarried women have the right to own land; in urban settings, only unmarried women have property rights. In traditional property transactions, women who want to acquire land require a male relative to act as a surety. Men have and exercise similar decision-making power over women within the bounds of marriage.

At the time of marriage, a bridal price—usually in the form of cattle, but occasionally monetary in nature—is paid to establish a relationship between the two families. Cattle are preferred because, according to Swazi culture, cattle are equated with wealth. Payment of bridal price influences the kind of control husbands have over their wives (Mbaye & Wagner, 2017). Some men believe that, after paying the bridal price, their wife becomes their possession much like any other purchased item and is obligated to work hard for the marital family and bear as many children as possible (Hague & Thiara, 2009).

Two forms of marriage are practiced in the Kingdom of Eswatini: Civil Rights and Swazi Law and Custom. In Civil Rights marriages, husbands are not allowed to have more than one wife. Women in Civil Rights marriages cannot secure bank loans without their husband's approval (Owen, n. d.). In Swazi Law and Custom marriage, the husband is at liberty to marry as many women as he desires—a practice commonly known as polygamy. Men in Swazi Law and Custom marriages cannot be charged with adultery. Women, meanwhile, do not have the option to marry multiple husbands (polyandry); they likewise cannot engage in adultery without the potential for severe reprisals such as dismissal from the marital unit and often return to the parental home.

Because Eswatini's patriarchal social order normalizes polygamous marriages, men in Civil Rights marriages often engage in bigamy; they accomplish this by marrying their first wife under Civil Rights and any subsequent wives under Swazi Law and Custom. Eswatini culture looks upon polygamous marriages as a sign of success and masculinity, in part because, in the past, men who opted for polygamy had to be affluent enough to provide for multiple wives and children. The practice of polygamy is one of the causes of high rates of HIV in the Kingdom of Eswatini. Each additional marriage introduces the possibility of adding an HIV-positive woman to an HIV-negative polygamous cycle (Bechtel, 2016). Moreover, regular screening for STIs of all those involved in polygamous relationships is uncommon.

Another reason for high HIV infection rates is arranged marriages (*kwendzisa*), many of which involve children younger than 18 years. The Sexual Offences and Domestic Violence Act of 2018 has facilitated a decline in arranged marriages; however, abduction of girls by men—an offense punishable by law—still takes place (OECD Development Centre, 2019).

In all forms of Swazi marriage, women lack control over their sexual and reproductive health. For example, Swazi women cannot undergo bilateral tubal ligation without husband's or sister-in-law's consent; some women likewise must obtain consent to undergo HIV testing (personal communication Shongwe, 2021). As a result, when self-testing kits are distributed without the approval of the male partner, some women throw them out. Women lack autonomy and access to care within both allopathic and traditional settings. For example, women are also not allowed to consult traditional healers without permission; if they do so, they are perceived as witches.

Swazi women sometimes endure patriarchal oppression even after their husband dies, as a result of a practice called widow inheritance (*kungenwa*). Like polygamy and arranged marriage, widow inheritance sits at the intersection of cultural practices and HIV and AIDS. In widow inheritance, following the death of the husband, his younger brother assumes the late husband's role. The younger brother who "inherits" the widow should—preferably—be married already (Mhaoldomhnaigh, 2018). Upon marrying his brother's widow, he assumes responsibility for (and authority over) her and her family. While the widow-*cum*-wife remains in her own household, she receives regular visits from her brother-in-law-*cum*-husband. Widow inheritance is a potential driver of HIV because any or all of the parties involved could be HIV positive. The Constitution of 2005 asserts that women should not be forced to engage in any custom against their will. This provision, however, is not supported by any legal instrument to ensure adherence (OECD Development Centre, 2019).

Swazi families are typically organized by kinship. The extended family usually shares a homestead, in which men operate as heads of household. All the members of the extended family take an active role in socializing children and serve as a safety net by providing support in the event of sickness or death (Manala, 2015; Nyambedha, 2004). Unlike their rural counterparts, urban communities tend toward a nuclear family structure. However, most of those families remain linked to relatives in rural areas (Manala, 2015).

These kinship structures are increasingly giving way to child-headed households—especially in rural areas of Eswatini (Mkhatshwa, 2017). This phenomenon frequently happens after parents and elders die of AIDS-related conditions, leaving children to fend for themselves. Although there are Neighbourhood Care Points (NCPs) that provide one meal a day for orphaned children, food security in these households remains a significant problem. Consequently, young people from child-headed households face an elevated risk of poverty, unemployment, homelessness, and sexual exploitation. As a result of sexual abuse, these children are also prone to pregnancy and STIs (Maepa & Ntshalintshali, 2020).

As a patriarchal society, Eswatini's sons are valued above daughters; for instance, female children perform most household chores, for which they do not receive recognition of any kind. Male children, meanwhile, receive goats or cattle upon reaching early adulthood—a reward for tending to their family's herd. Eswatini culture views sons as extending the family line to the next generation (Mathunjwa & Gary, 2006).

Swazi women are expected to perform chores and act as primary caregivers (Asuquo & Akpan-Idiok, 2020). Accordingly, if a family member becomes infected with HIV, a woman must assume the caregiving responsibilities. That work often adversely affects their well-being, because it is physically, emotionally, and psychologically exhausting. The burden of family caregiving is worsened by the fact that formal training for individuals thrust into this new role is rare (Asuquo & Akpan-Idiok, 2020).

Barriers to Safer Sex

Both poverty and the patriarchal social order complicate HIV prevention and treatment efforts in Eswatini. Gender inequality and gender-based violence hinder safer-sex practices among Swazi women. Culturally, women have no control over their sexual and reproductive lives (Mathunjwa & Gary, 2006), which reduces the likelihood of a woman negotiating for safer sex (Turmen, 2003).

Rape and sexual assault likewise deter HIV prevention practices (Ministry of Health, 2019). Sexual violence is common in Eswatini, with an estimated 5% of women being forced into sexual intercourse before age 18 years (UNICEF, 2007). UNAIDS (2014) revealed that 9% of girls between the ages of 14 and 18 years in the kingdom experience rape. In 2014, 48% of women in Eswatini (then Swaziland) reported experiencing sexual violence (UNAIDS, 2014). Incest and marital rape are also common; the International Commission of Jurists (2020) reported that most culprits of sexual abuse were boyfriends or husbands, male relatives, and known community members. Although the 2018 Sexual Offences and Domestic Violence (SODV) Act categorically criminalizes marital rape and incest (International Labour Organization, 2018), conservative Swazi men—and even some Parliamentarians—are resisting the legislation.

Poverty also represents a significant barrier to safer-sex practices. Swazi culture institutionalizes women's dependence on men for financial and physical protection; this makes it difficult, and sometimes impossible, to negotiate for safer sex (Asadhi, 2015). Financial instability pushes many women into sex work, the culture around which disincentivizes HIV prevention practices. Clients of sex workers sometimes offer extra money in exchange for unprotected sex (Parmley et al., 2020). Parmley et al. (2020) also reported that condom use remains uncommon when engaging in anal intercourse. Considering the factors inhibiting condom use, it is perhaps unsurprising that approximately 70% of Swazi sex workers are HIV positive (Parmley et al., 2020). In recent years, the government of Eswatini has introduced programs designed to focus on reducing HIV among sex workers.

In addition to deterring safer sex behaviors, poverty also impacts HIV treatment. While the government greatly subsidizes healthcare services, many people forego healthcare because they lack the funds needed for transportation and copayments to the government (Seervai, 2019). Health facilities sometimes run out of supplies, forcing individuals to purchase their medications from local pharmacies, which are more expensive. Most impoverished individuals cannot afford to go to a pharmacy; as a result, many people default on their treatment, which increases the risk of developing drug resistance and other similarly poor health outcomes.

Cultural Events and Socialization

The way of life for the Eswatini populace is deeply rooted in their rich culture (Shongwe et al., 2019). Cultural patterns have been implicated in the transmission of HIV in sub-Saharan Africa (Mathunjwa & Gary, 2006; UNAIDS, 2016).

According to Swazi culture, boys and young men are socialized by male elders (fathers, uncles, and grandfathers). Girls and young women are commonly socialized by female elders—mainly mothers, grandmothers, and aunts (Mathunjwa & Gary, 2006). The aforementioned socialization happens in the home, fitting the definition of micro-level socialization (Du Toit & Staden, 2009). Female socialization practices used to be carried out at *egumeni*: a place in the yard, between the hut and the windbreakers, where discussions regarding sexual and reproductive health issues were conducted. The cattle byre, or *esangweni*, served the same purpose for boys and young men (Mathunjwa-Dlamini & Mngadi, 2011). Among other issues, elders used these occasions to urge delayed sexual debut, as maintaining virginity until marriage is valued in Eswatini.

Modernization—and the attendant disintegration of family structures—has impacted Eswatini moral values (Mavundla et al., 2015). The forums at the cattle byre and the windbreakers no longer exist due to a combination of factors, among them a decrease in extended-family living arrangements and the resulting lack of social cohesion; free education and resulting changes to children's schedules and family responsibilities; and a growing taboo around parents discussing sexual issues with children. Parents increasingly feel that discussing sexual issues with young people will influence them to engage in sex (Magagula, 2019). The degradation of the sex-education culture in Eswatini causes young people to engage in risky sexual behaviors, with predictable results: teenage pregnancy, STIs, and elevated school drop-out rates.

See Box 24.2 for a description of the national ceremonies of *Umhlanga* and *Incwala* and their role in sex education in Eswatini.

BOX 24.2: Umhlanga and Incwala

There are two national ceremonies that function as socialization strategies: *Umhlanga* (the Reed Dance) for girls, and the *Incwala* ritual for boys. *Umhlanga* is a weeklong national event for girls characterized by the collection of reeds—which are used for building windbreakers for the Royal huts—and traditional dancing. The event encourages young girls to delay sexual intercourse; virgins are distinguished from the rest of the girls by wearing blue and yellow woolen tassels. Girls who are in love relationships wear red and black woolen tassels and are taught to engage in a safer sex practice called *kucencuka* (thigh sex), to prevent pregnancy (Maphanga, 2017). The *Incwala* ceremony is a national event for both men and women. Before the ritual begins, men and boys cut *lusekwane* (shrubs) with which to rebuild the Royal Kraal. Young men are beaten if they carry a shrub that shows signs of wilting, which is believed to indicate they've engaged in sexual intercourse with a woman (Maphanga, 2017; Mathunjwa-Dlamini & Mngadi, 2011). Many organizations use *Umhlanga* and *Incwala* as an opportunity to empower young people about HIV and AIDS-related sexual reproductive health issues. *Khulisa Umntfwana* (Safeguard the Child), for example, seeks to protect children by teaching them about sexual and reproductive health issues, including HIV and AIDS. *Umhlanga* and *Incwala* programming also includes the singing of songs associated with the virus to raise awareness about HIV prevention (Masango, 2008).

Data from http://new.observer.org.sz/details.php?id=10006 (Swazi Observer: August 22, 2019).

Religion and Traditional Healing in HIV Prevention and Treatment

Eswatini is considered a Christian country and is sometimes referred to as the "pulpit of Africa." Religion plays a significant role in HIV prevention and treatment, as some individuals consult religious leaders for healing in all areas of their lives (Wiginton et al., 2019). Health professionals empower religious leaders to discuss HIV with their congregants; for example, they may encourage those who are taking ART to adhere to their regimen *even if* they feel that they have been healed. While religious leaders can facilitate HIV prevention and treatment in Eswatini, some religious beliefs deter prevention strategies such as Voluntary Male Medical Circumcision (VMMC) and condom use (The Government of the Kingdom of Eswatini, 2018).

Various faith-based agencies run home-based care services in the Kingdom. They reportedly contribute to the healing of patients because they provide physical, emotional, and psychological support. In addition, respondents in a study conducted by Root et al. (2017) noted that patients prefer Christian caregivers.

Traditional herbs and healers play a similarly significant role in the prevention and management of HIV and AIDS in Africa, including Eswatini. Some individuals first consult traditional healers for HIV-related ailments before accessing Western-trained practitioners. Others still believe that traditional herbs are the best method for managing HIV (WHO, 2019). Traditional healers are active in the sub-Saharan region, as well as in Eswatini, and play an important role in mitigating the HIV crisis. Traditional healers increasingly encourage the use of condoms; indeed, healthcare workers have trained some traditional healers to educate their patients about the virus. These practitioners also offer psychosocial and physical care to people living with HIV. Traditional healers will treat symptoms to a point, but avoid making incisions when working with HIV-positive patients (Zuma et al., 2017). This practice is related to introducing medications into the body through skilfully induced cuts made with razor blades or other sharp instruments. Incisions in certain areas of the body to insert medications/herbs, such as the forearm, could introduce additional risks for HIV infection—especially when the razor has been used on more than one person. For some individuals, traditional healers are their first point of contact, because these practitioners are readily available in the communities (Mokgobi, 2013). While in the Republic of South Africa, it is legal for traditional healers to refer a client for HIV testing (Audet et al., 2017); the same is not true in Eswatini.

Culturally Specific HIV Prevention Programs

Various innovative programs have contributed to the reduction of HIV and AIDS among women and children in Eswatini. Innovative approaches to HIV testing and the Prevention of Mother-to-Child Transmission (PMTCT) of HIV Program demonstrate how understanding cultural determinants of health paves the way for successful interventions.

HIV testing is the foundation to preventing, treating, and providing care for People Living with HIV (PLWH). All other services such as PMTCT, postexposure prophylaxis (PEP), and ART are accessed only once someone has tested positive for the virus (Eswatini National AIDS Programme, n.d.). Access to HIV testing has improved significantly in Eswatini. In 2003, HIV testing was only offered at 13 sites, most of which were standalone, voluntary-testing areas (Client Initiated HIV Testing). Today, testing happens in all health facilities, and health staff offer to test to all patients, regardless of what service they have come for (provider-initiated HIV testing). Patients have the ability to opt out of testing, thereby preserving their autonomy (Ministry of Health, 2015). Provider-initiated HIV testing not only enables more people to know their status but also reduces stigma and discrimination associated with visiting standalone facilities.

Targeted testing is also carried out as part of Eswatini's efforts to expand HIV testing. There are two types of targeted testing: index and social-network–based testing. Index testing involves offering tests to the family and partner(s) of a person who tests positive.

Social-network–based testing involves follow-up and assessment of both sexual partners and the broader networks of peers within high-risk populations (sex workers, men who have sex with men, etc.; Kitchen et al., 2020; World Health Organization, 2021b).

HIV testing has also been expanded through other approaches. Community-based testing, for example, is a door-to-door approach. Pop-up testing takes place in locations where people converge—at workplaces and bus ranks (major stations), for example. Eswatini also has campaigns like the "Love Test," administered by the Ministry of Health, where couples are encouraged to undergo testing (Eswatini National AIDS Programme, n.d).

It has been recently reported that 92% of Swazi people living with HIV knew their status in 2018, which is close to the global commitment of 95% by 2030 (Avert, 2020). Swati men are significantly less likely to know their status due to poor health-seeking behavior, in addition to their requiring fewer interactions with health services than women. Testing is not mandatory in Eswatini; however, there are circumstances where testing is done to safeguard the life of others—in cases of rape or blood donation, for example (Ministry of Health, 2015). Eswatini's testing infrastructure enables other evidence-based interventions, like the PMTCT program.

By its very nature, a pregnancy indicates that a woman has had at least one unsafe sexual encounter. An HIV-positive woman who becomes pregnant and is not enrolled on ART will likely transmit the virus to the fetus, during pregnancy (transplacental) or the birth process or via breastfeeding (Khumalo et al., 2015). This is one of the reasons that all pregnant women have their blood samples collected and screened for STIs and HIV at their first antenatal care visit.

In 2003, Eswatini—then the Kingdom of Swaziland—introduced the PMTCT program. This is a healthcare scheme wherein all pregnant women who test HIV positive at their first antenatal visit, usually before 14 weeks of pregnancy, are put on ART. The goal of ART is to reduce the mother's viral load, thereby reducing the risk of transmitting HIV to the fetus. Most pregnant Swati women agree to an ART regimen because they want to give birth to healthy babies who will have a long life.

PMTCT is a four-faceted program. This program aims to prevent HIV infection among young women of childbearing age; prevent unintended pregnancy; reduce mother-to-child transmission of HIV among pregnant infected women; and provide ART care and support to HIV-positive women and their families (Ministry of Health and Social Welfare, 2006). It is reported that between 2009 and 2015, PMTCT has contributed to reducing the HIV incidence by 80% among children in Eswatini—then known as Swaziland (UNAIDS, 2016).

There are several factors that have facilitated the development of Eswatini's HIV testing and treatment infrastructure. The first is shared political commitment to the goal of ending HIV. In practice, that commitment is linked to creating dedicated budgets; promptly adapting international HIV guidelines; and receiving support from bilateral partners, UN agencies, nongovernmental organizations, and faith-based organizations (Kitchen et al., 2020). Equally important are the people on the ground and how they work. The Ministry of Health has set up several coordination structures and strengthened its human resources capacity through training and task shifting. By allocating some responsibilities once reserved for health workers, like HIV testing, to nonhealth workers, the Ministry of Health is able to operate more efficiently and use its resources more effectively.

CASE STUDY 24.1: A NURSE'S STORY: PHOPHO SURVIVED HIV/AIDS IN THE KINGDOM OF ESWATINI

I was diagnosed with HIV in 1990 when the disease was rampant, and people were frightened and dying. The annual death rate was about 348,600 internationally, and in Eswatini, it was around 7,000 deaths per year. At that time, there was no ART in Eswatini, and people across the world did not know much about this disease. Being diagnosed with HIV was like

(continued)

CASE STUDY 24.1: A NURSE'S STORY: PHOPHO SURVIVED HIV/AIDS IN THE KINGDOM OF ESWATINI (*CONTINUED*)

a life sentence. Things were complicated, especially for women. Unfortunately, my in-laws disowned me because of my HIV status; however, my husband stuck with me and continued his support. In Eswatini, if the woman discovers that she is infected with HIV before the man, the common belief among people is that the woman is the transmitter of the virus. She is the one who brings the devastating killer into the family and contaminates the polygamous circle of wives and her husband. But my husband was the first to be diagnosed with the disease, and he infected me as a result of his sexual activities with other women. We discovered around the same time that we were infected with HIV. Despite these overwhelming circumstances, my goal was to survive, live, and see my two children grow up and become active citizens in Eswatini. We stayed with my husband, their father.

I was in denial about this disease for several years, but I eventually accepted my status and began an active self-care plan. Because my marital family disowned me, I avoided my in-laws but disclosed my health status to my family and close friends. A balanced diet and exercise became a priority. I joined a support network, the Swaziland AIDS Support Organization (SASO), sponsored by the federal government through the Ministry of Health. In addition, I participated in other health-related groups in the community. The groups provided information and support and stressed coping skills and the use of available resources. To avoid reinfection, I used condoms during sexual activities. When I was not feeling well, I sought medical attention and received flu medications, oral rehydration salts for diarrhea, and other remedies.

After 2002, I could not receive ART because my CD4 count was considered to be too high. When the count requirement changed to 350/cell/mm^3 by the government, some 19 years later (2009), I began the therapy—and, fortunately, by this time, the drugs were available to many more people in the Kingdom. The government provided the medications with support from the Global Fund, an international organization supporting treatments for HIV/AIDS, tuberculosis, malaria, and other diseases.

Over time, my progress was remarkable. Finally, however, I became critically ill and was admitted to the hospital in 2011 with a fungal infection in the brain. The disease caused right-sided paralysis. During this admission, I was diagnosed with AIDS as my CD4 cell count was 3 cells/mm^3. I am grateful to be alive today. The cause of this life-threatening condition and hospitalization was "treatment failure." Although I was religiously taking the ART medications (e.g., tenofovir, lamivudine, efavirenz), I got sick. While in the hospital, I began the second line of treatment and began to heal.

After years of treatment, I sometimes experience neuropathy in the lower extremities, but I can live with this condition. I have also been treated for tuberculosis in the neck glands and survived. Tuberculosis remains a common opportunistic disease among people living with HIV in the Kingdom. I am doing well. I am alive!

SUMMARY

Gender roles, religion, culture, and socioeconomic status influence HIV prevention and treatment. In the Kingdom of Eswatini, gender inequality functions as a determinant of health, with women suffering disproportionately from the virus as a direct result of the country's patriarchal social order. While Swazi culture facilitates the spread of HIV, it is also foundational to many of the country's most successful prevention and treatment programs, from traditional healers encouraging condom use, to the HIV-education activities at the annual *Umhlanga* (Reed Dance), to the Test and Treat Initiative.

DISCUSSION QUESTIONS

1. List three issues that have contributed to HIV/AIDS spread in the Kingdom of Eswatini that are related to cultural practices, economic challenges, and geographic locale.
2. Create a plan of care that addresses the reduction of HIV and AIDS among women and detail culture-specific approaches for gender-congruent comprehensive care.
3. Delineate the characteristics of the health system in the Kingdom of Eswatini and discuss recent interventions—implemented by the government, nongovernmental agencies, and others—that have aided in the reduction and elimination of HIV and AIDS.
4. How would you suggest that the knowledge, traditional practices, and historical perspectives of traditional healers and herbal use be further integrated into current and future family-centered health plans that focus on educating men and women about preventing and treating HIV and AIDS, and one other common health problem in the Kingdom of Eswatini?
5. Develop a 5-year strategic plan with specific pathways and metrics for educating nurses, physicians, and other healthcare providers that focus on eliminating HIV and AIDS among all people in the Kingdom of Eswatini.

ADDITIONAL RESOURCES

Centers for Disease Control and Prevention. (2020). Guidelines for the prevention and treatment of opportunistic infections in adults and adolescents with HIV. https://clinicalinfo.hiv.gov/sites/default/files/guidelines/documents/Adult_OI.pdf

Centers for Disease Control and Prevention. (2021). HIV and women: Prevention challenges. https://www.cdc.gov/hiv/group/gender/women/prevention-challenges.htm

Dlamini, S. Z. (2021). Personal communication. Mbabane.

Enegela, J. E., Paul, O. I., Olaiya, O., Ugba, E., Okoh, P., Ogundeko, O., Fagbemi, A., Akinmade, O., Ibanga, I., & Effiong, A. (2019). Rates of condom use among HIV positive patients on ART in Nasarawa Eggon North Central Nigeria. *Biomedical Journal of Scientific & Technical Research*, 18(5), 13842–13847. https://doi.org/10.26717/BJSTR.2019.18.003201

Eswatini. (2019). Country profile 2019 the local government system in Eswatini. http://www.clgf.org.uk/default/assets/File/Country_profiles/Swaziland.pdf

Godoy, L. (2004). Understanding poverty from a gender perspective. Women and Development Unit of the Economic Commission for Latin America and the Caribbean. https://www.cepal.org/sites/default/files/publication/files/5926/S046466_en.pdf

Hipolito, R. L., de Oliveira, D. C., da Costa, T. L., Marques, S. C., Pereira, E. R., & Gomes, A. M. T. (2017). Quality of life of people living with HIV/AIDS: Temporal, socio-demographic and perceived health relationship. *Revista Latino-Americana de Enfermagem*, 25.

Jewkes, R., Sen, P., & Garcia-Moreno, C. (2002). Chapter 6: Sexual violence. In E. G. Krug, L. L. Dahlberg, J. A. Mercy, A. B. Zwi, & R. Lozano (Eds.), *World report on violence and health*. World Health Organization.

Keyes, K. M., & Galea, S. (2014). Epidemiology matters: A new introduction to methodological foundations. in epidemiology matters. Oxford University Press. https://oxfordmedicine.com/view/10.1093/med/9780199331246.001.0001/med-9780199331246

McGrane Minton, H. A., Mittal, M., Elder, H., & Carey, M. P. (2016). Relationship factors and condom use among women with a history of intimate partner violence. *AIDS and Behavior*, 20(1), 225–234. https://doi.org/10.1007/s10461-015-1189-5

Our World in Data. (n.d.). Eswatini. https://ourworldindata.org/country/swaziland

UNAIDS. (2021). Global HIV & AIDS statistics fact sheet: Preliminary UNAIDS 2021 epidemiological estimates. https://www.unaids.org/en/resources/fact-sheet

The World Bank. (2020). Health system strengthening for human capital development in Eswatini. worldbank.org/curated/ar/667311591296915504/pdf/Eswatini-Health-System-Strengthening-for-Human-Capital-Development-in-Eswatini-Project.pdf

World Health Organization. (2021). HIV data and statistics. Global HIV programme. https://www.who.int/teams/immunization-vaccines-and-biologicals/diseases/tick-borne-encephalitis/hiv

World Health Organization, UNICEF. (2015). Joint monitoring programme for water supply and sanitation. Progress on sanitation and drinking water: 2015 update. WHO. https://www.who.int/water_sanitation_health/publications/9789241563956/en/

REFERENCES

Asadhi, E. O. (2015). *Assessing the factors influencing appropriate use of condoms in South Gem Division, Siaya District*. Post Graduate Diploma in project planning and management at the University of Nairobi.

Asuquo, E. F., & Akpan-Idiok, P. A. (2020). The exceptional role of women as primary caregivers for people living with HIV/AIDS in Nigeria, West Africa. *IntechOpen*, https://doi.org/10.5772/intechopen.93670

Audet, C. M., Ngobeni, S., & Wagner, R. G. (2017). Traditional healer treatment of HIV persists in the era of ART: A mixed methods study from rural South Africa. *BMC Complementary and Alternative Medicine, 17*(1), 434. https://doi.org/10.1186/s12906-017-1934-6

Avert. (2020). Global information and education on HIV and AIDS. https://www.avert.org/professionals/hiv-around-world/sub-saharan-africa/swaziland

Bechtel, S. (2016). The impact of cultural norms on HIV transmission in Swaziland. *Voices in Bioethics*, 2. https://doi.org/10.7916/vib.v2i.5971

The Commonwealth Secretariat. (2021). Kingdom of Eswatini. https://thecommonwealth.org/our-member-countries/kingdom-eswatini

Disaster Risk Management Information Management System. (n. d.). Eswatini. https://drmims.sadc.int/en/profiles/eswatini

Du Toit, D. A., & Van Staden, S. J. (2009). *Nursing sociology*. Van Schaik.

Eswatini National AIDS Programme. (n.d). *HIV/AIDS epidemic in Eswatini*. http://swaziaidsprogram.org/htc/

Freeman, M. C., Ogden, S., Jacobson, J., Abbott, D., Addiss, D. G., Amnie, A. G. et al. (2013). Integration of water, sanitation, and hygiene for the prevention and control of neglected tropical diseases: A rationale for inter-sectoral collaboration. *PLOS Neglected Tropical Diseases, 7*(9), e2439. https://doi.org/10.1371/journal.pntd.0002439

The Government of the Kingdom of Eswatini. (n.d.). http://www.gov.sz/index.php?option=com_content&view=category&id=63

The Government of the Kingdom of Eswatini. (2018). The national multisectoral HIV and AIDS strategic framework (NSF) 2018–2023. https://hivpreventioncoalition.unaids.org/wp-content/uploads/2019/06/Eswatini_NSF-2018-2023_final.pdf

Hague, J., & Thiara, R. (2009). Bride-price, poverty and domestic violence in Uganda. https://citeseerx.ist.psu.edu/viewdoc/download?doi=10.1.1.397.1304&rep=rep1&type=pdf

International Commission of Jurists. (2020). Eswatini: ICJ and partner organization launch guide to reporting gender-based violence for journalists. https://www.icj.org/eswatini-icj-launches-guide-to-reporting-gender-based-violence-for-journalists/

International Labour Organization. (2018). *Sexual offences & domestic violence act, 2018*. Mbabane. https://www.ilo.org/dyn/natlex/natlex4.detail?p_isn=108709&p_lang=en

Kitchen, P. J., Bärnighausen, K., Dube, L., Mnisi, Z., Dlamini-Nqeketo, S., Johnson, C. C., Bärnighausen, T., De Neve J., & McMahon, S. A. (2020). Expansion of HIV testing in Eswatini: Stakeholder perspectives on reaching the first 90. *African Journal of AIDS Research, 19*(3), 186–197. https://doi.org/10.2989/16085906.2020.1790399

Khumalo, N. L., Gary, F. A., Yarandi, H. A., & Mathunjwa-Dlamini, T. R. (2015). Factors influencing HIV-positive expectant mothers' adherence to ARV prophylaxis (PMTCT) in a healthcare facility in the hhohho region, Swaziland. *International Journal of Science & Advanced Technology, 5*(6), 15–27. http://www.ijsat.com

Maepa, M. P., & Ntshalintshali, T. (2020). Family structure and history of childhood trauma: Associations with risk-taking behavior among adolescents in Swaziland. *Frontiers in Public Health*, 8. https://doi.org/10.3389/fpubh.2020.563325

Magagula, N. (2019). Parents' initiated interventions to prevent HIV among adolescents in Swaziland. *Doctor of Literature and Philosophy thesis*. Pretoria: Faculty of Health Studies. University of South Africa.

Magagula, S. V. (2017). A case study of the Swaziland essential health care package (Equinet Discussion Paper 112; p. 31). Regional Network for Equity in Health in East and Southern Africa. https://www.equinetafrica.org/sites/default/files/uploads/documents/Swaziland%20EHB%20case%20study%20rep%20final2017pv.pdf

Manala, M. (2015). African traditional widowhood rites and their benefits and/or detrimental effects on widows in a context of African christianity. *HTS Teologiese Studies/Theological Studies, 71*(3). https://doi.org/10.4102/hts.v71i3.2913

Maphanga, P. (2017). Personal communication. Ezulwini.

Masango, L. P. (2008). *Reading the Swazi reed dance (Umhlanga) as a literary traditional performance art*. Doctor of Philosophy thesis. Johannesburg: Faculty of Humanities, University of the Witwatersrand.

Mathunjwa, T. R., & Gary, F. A. (2006) Women and HIV/AIDS in the Kingdom of Swaziland: Culture and risks. *Journal of National Black Nurses Association*, 17(2), 39–46.

Mathunjwa-Dlamini, T. R., & Mngadi, T. P. (2011). HIV prevention, infection & management of AIDS. Institute of Distance Learning, UNISWA.

Mavundla, S., Dlamini, N., Nyoni, N., & Mac-Ikemenjima, D. (2015). Youth and public policy in Swaziland. https://www.researchgate.net/publication/319403043_Youth_and_Public_Policy _in_Swaziland

Mbaye, L. M., & Wagner, N. (2017). Bride price and fertility decisions: Evidence from rural Senegal. *The Journal of Development Studies*, 53(6), 891–910. https://doi.org/10.1080/00220388.2016.1208178

Mhaoldomhnaigh, R. N. (2018). Putting tamar in her place. *Doctor of Philosophy dissertation*. University of Cambridge Selwyn College.

Ministry of Health. (2019). *Swaziland HIV Incidence Measurement Survey (SHIMS 2) 2016–2017*: Final report. Mbabane. https://phia.icap.columbia.edu/wp-content/uploads/2019/05/SHIMS2_Final -Report_05.03.2019_forWEB.pdf

Ministry of Health. (2015). Standard operational guidelines for community based health volunteers in Swaziland. Swaziland: Print Pak.

Ministry of Health. (2012). Swaziland HIV Incidence Measurement Survey (SHIMS): First findings report. Mbabane. http://ghdx.healthdata.org/record/swaziland-hiv-incidence-measurement -survey-shims-first-findings-report-november-2012

Ministry of Health. (2010). 12th HIV sentinel surveillance. Webster Print.

Ministry of Health and Social Welfare. (2006). Prevention of mother to child transmission of HIV guidelines. https://www.unicef.org/swaziland/sz_publications_2006pmtctguidelines.pdf

Minnery, M., Mathabela, N., Shubber, Z., Mabuza, K., Gorgens, M., Cheikh, N., Wilson, D. P., & Kelly, S. L. (2020). Opportunities for improved HIV prevention and treatment through budget optimization in Eswatini. *PLOS ONE*, 15(7), e0235664. https://doi.org/10.1371/journal.pone.0235664

Mkhatshwa, N. (2017). The gendered experiences of children in child-headed households in Swaziland. *African Journal of AIDS Research*, 16(4), 365–372. https://doi.org/10.2989/16085906.2017.1389756

Mokgobi, M. G. (2013). Towards integration of traditional healing and western healing: Is this a remote possibility? *African Journal for Physical Health Education, Recreation, and Dance*, 2013(suppl 1), 47–57.

National Sanitation and Hygiene Strategy 2019–2023. (2015). Zwane and Magagula. https://www. unicef.org/eswatini/reports/national-hygiene-and-sanitation-strategy

Nhlengethwa, B., Singwane, S. S., Mabaso, S. D., van Zuydam, I. B., & Mamba, S. F. (2020). Assessment of socio-economic impacts of the climate smart gardens project in low-income residential areas in Mbabane City, Eswatini.

Nyambedha, O. E. (2004). Change and continuity in kin-based support systems for widows and orphans among the Luo in Western Kenya. *African Sociological Review/Revue Africaine de Sociologie*, 8(1 special issue), 139–153.

OECD Development Center. (2019). Social institutions and gender index. https://www.genderindex. org/wp-content/uploads/files/datasheets/2019/SZ.pdf

Owen, M. (n.d.). Issues of discrimination in widowhood in Swaziland that require addressing in the context of the CEDAW. Widows for peace through democracy. https://tbinternet.ohchr.org/ Treaties/CEDAW/Shared%20Documents/SWZ/INT_CEDAW_NGO_SWZ_17576_E.pdf; https:// clinicalinfo.hiv.gov/sites/default/files/guidelines/documents/Adult_OI.pdf

Parmley, L., Fielding-Miller, R., Mnisi, Z., & Kennedy, C. E. (2020). Obligations of motherhood in shaping sex work, condom use, and HIV care among Swazi female sex workers living with HIV. *African Journal of AIDS Research*, 18(3), 254–257. https://doi.org/10.2989/16085906.2019.1639521

Pell, C., Vernooij, E., Masilela, N., Simelane, N., Shabalala, F., & Reis, R. (2018). False starts in "test and start": A qualitative study of reasons for delayed antiretroviral therapy in Swaziland. *International Health*, 10(2), 78–83. https://doi.org/10.1093/inthealth/ihx065

Root, R., Wyngaard, A. V., & Whiteside, A. (2017). "We smoke the same pipe": Religion and community home-based care for PLWH in rural Swaziland. *Medical Anthropology*, 36(3), 231–245. https://doi.org/10.1080/01459740.2016.1256885

Seervai, S. (2019, April 19). It's harder for people living in poverty to get health care. Commonwealth Fund. https://doi.org/10.26099/bpv6-7261

Shongwe, M. I., & Dlamini, S. (2021). A systems approach to investigating non-functionality in rural water schemes: A case study. *Sustainable Water Resources Management*, 7(3), 1–10. https://www. worldbank.org/en/topic/water/overview; https://www.worldbank.org/en/topic/water/ overview; https://thewaterproject.org/water-crisis/water-in-crisis-swaziland

Shongwe, M. N. (2019). Traditional institutions and decentralisation, 20 the tinkhundla decentralisation system: Is this a blend of traditional and modern state governance that works? In C. M. Fombad, & N. Steytler (Eds.), *Decentralisation and constitutionalism in Africa*. https://oxcon. ouplaw.com/view/10.1093/law/9780198846154.001.0001/law-9780198846154-chapter-21

Shongwe, S. T., Bhebhe, S., & Nxumalo, Z. G. (2019). The relationship between first language and culture in learning and teaching Siswati as a first language. *European Journal of Education Studies*, 6(6). https://doi.org/10.5281/zenodo.3423110

Shongwe, S. S. (2021). Personal communication.

Simelane, M. S., Chemhaka, G. B., Maphosa, T., & Zwane, E. (2020). Unsafe disposal of faeces and its correlates among children under three years in Eswatini. *South African Journal of Child Health*, 14(4), 217–223.

Swaziland Rural Women Assembly. (2018). Situation of women in Swaziland. https://www.woek.de/fileadmin/user_upload/downloads/publikationen/kasa/emw_2018_swasiland_sibandze_situation_of_women_in_swaziand.pdf

Turmen, T. (2003). Gender and HIV/AIDS. *International Journal of Gynaecology & Obstetrics*, 82(3), 411–418.

UNAIDS. (2016). Swaziland. https://www.unaids.org/sites/default/files/media/documents/UNAIDS_GlobalplanCountryfactsheet_swaziland_en.pdf

UNAIDS. (2014). Swaziland global AIDS response progress reporting 2014. Mbabane. https://www.unaids.org/sites/default/files/country/documents/SWZ_narrative_report_2014.pdf

UNDP-UNCDF. (2020). Making access possible–Eswatini energy and poor. https://www.undp.org/sites/g/files/zskgke326/files/publications/UNDP-UNCDF-eSwatini-Energy-and-the-Poor.pdf

UNFPA. (2019). Government of the Kingdom of Eswatini/UNFPA 6th country programme evaluation 2016–2020. https://www.unfpa.org/sites/default/files/board-documents/Eswatini_-_CPE_-_Country_programme_evaluation_1.pdf

UNICEF. (2007). A national study on violence against children and young women in Swaziland. https://www.unicef.org/swaziland/Violence_study_report.pdf

Wiginton, J. M., King, E. J., & Fuller, A. O. (2019). "We can act different from what we used to": Findings from experiences of religious leader participants in an HIV-prevention intervention in Zambia. *Global Public Health*, 14(5), 636–648. https://doi.org/10.1080/17441692.2018.1524921

The World Bank. (2021). Poverty & equity brief Eswatini. www.worldbank.org/en/country/Eswatini/overview

World Health Organization. (2021a). Eswatini. https://www.afro.who.int/countries/eswatini

World Health Organization. (2021b). How the world's highest HIV-prevalence country turned around, and in record time. https://www.afro.who.int/news/how-worlds-highest-hiv-prevalence-country-turned-around-and-record-time

World Health Organization. (2019). WHO global report on traditional medicine and complementary medicine. https://www.who.int/traditional-complementary-integrative-medicine/WhoGlobalReportOnTraditionalAndComplementaryMedicine2019.pdf

World Health Organization. (2018). Country cooperation strategy at a glance. World Health Organization. http://apps.who.int/iris/bitstream/handle/10665/136886/ccsbrief_swz_en.pdf;jsessionid=CFBC552CE3AC4F2E2F34E7AEE1C2142A?sequence

World Health Organization. (2015). Guideline on when to start antiretroviral therapy and on pre-exposure prophylaxis for HIV. World Health Organization. http://www.ncbi.nlm.nih.gov/books/NBK327115/

Zuma, T., Wight, D., Rochat, T., & Moshabela, M. (2017). Traditional health practitioners' management of HIV/AIDS in rural South Africa in the Era of widespread antiretroviral therapy. *Global Health Action*, 10(1), 1352210. https://doi.org/10.1080/16549716.2017.1352210

CHAPTER 25

Global and Local Poverty and Its Long-Term Impact on Health

Rashmi Sharma, Ricki Sheldon, and Vicken Totten

LEARNING OBJECTIVES

- Analyze the social determinants of health in terms of poverty, gender, and ethnicity.
- Describe the causes of and continuation of global poverty.
- Differentiate the effects of poverty on women and Indigenous people.
- Introduce the concept of historical trauma and its mitigation.
- Provide examples of how social support can mitigate the ill effects of poverty.
- Discuss ongoing efforts to mitigate the social determinants of health and the continuation of poverty.

INTRODUCTION

> *Money can't buy happiness, but it can make you awfully comfortable while you're being miserable.*
>
> *—Clare Boothe Luce*

The social determinants of health (SDOH; Box 25.1) became big news in 2020 when the health disparities suffered by disenfranchised populations were tragically exposed by the COVID-19 pandemic. The causes and results of these injustices are legion and multiply intertwined; however, the common denominator is poverty (Braveman & Gottlieb, 2014). The effects of inequities can last for generations and can be difficult to overcome.

In broad terms, there are three categories of SDOH: physical, social, and economic. The physical environment determines where and how one lives (e.g., food, water, housing, transportation). Social environments include community, customs, religion, and marital and family structures. Economic factors are composed of such factors as income, wealth, and education levels. Of these, the most important determinant of health is wealth—or its converse: poverty. Economic poverty determines, in part, where you live, your local

BOX 25.1: Social Determinants of Health

- Adequate sanitation
- Absence of disease
- Food security
- Nutrition
- Safe drinking water
- Access to healthcare
- Child health
- Maternal health
- Reproductive health
- Gender-related health
- Freedom from trauma
- Freedom from effects of superstition and religious constraints

Source: Adapted from World Health Organization (2008). *Social determinants of health. Report of a regional consultation: Colombo, Sri Lanka, 2-4 October* 2007. https://apps.who.int/iris/handle/10665/206363

environment, what resources are readily available to you, and the safety of your locale (Robitaille & Paquette, 2020; Zahran et al., 2017; see also Chapter 5). For example, do you have access to water? Is your water contaminated with bacteria or heavy metals? Do you have access to nutritious food? Access to good schools?

Note that the specifics vary by location, economic resources, and education. If the only available foods are high calorie and low nutrition, you may stay alive, you may even be obese, but with malnutrition. In larger U.S. cities, like Cleveland or New York City, a poor diet may be a diet rich in processed, carbohydrate-rich foods like potato chips; in Nepal, a poor diet may predominantly consist of boiled rice—also providing calories but with little to sustain good health (Anik et al., 2019; Braveman & Gottlieb, 2014).

Health is defined by the World Health Organization (WHO) as "a state of complete physical, mental, and social well-being, and not merely the absence of disease or infirmity" (WHO, 2022a, para 1). Access to healthcare is often equated with health (Cloninger et al., 2014). Yet, health is not healthcare, nor is healthcare the most important determinant of health. Healthcare rendered *after* health has been impaired does not address the *causes* of ill health (Sinclair & LaPlante, 2019).

For the proper promotion of well-being, healthcare ideally should begin with health promotion and preventive care, which would greatly reduce the need for reactive (after the fact) care. Sinclair and LaPlante (2019) have dubbed reactive care the "whack-a-mole" model of healthcare: treating each new disease as it arises rather than addressing the root causes of these diseases. In the United States, the emphasis is on acute care, which, in the long term, is more expensive than a system of comprehensive health promotion and preventive healthcare would be. Furthermore, acute care is not always readily available. Health promotion addresses such matters as lifestyle issues and nutrition, as these contribute to the achievement of higher levels of health. Increasingly, the SDOH have a profound effect on longevity, even more than healthcare (see Chapter 7 for a more in-depth discussion of the SDOH).

On January 1, 2016, the 17 Sustainable Development Goals (SDGs) of the United Nations 2030 Agenda for Sustainable Development took effect. These goals had been adopted by world leaders at a historic summit the previous year, the first of which was to "end poverty in all its forms" (United Nations, 2015; also see details about the 17 SDGs of the

United Nations in the Resources for More In-Depth Information section at the end of this chapter). Worldwide, policymakers have long been aware that poverty, health, and lifespan are intertwined. The political will to implement change, however, has been less universal. Article 12 of the International Covenant on Economic, Social and Cultural Rights recognizes the "right of everyone to the enjoyment of the highest attainable standard of physical and mental health" including "safe and healthy working conditions," along with other basic rights like safe drinking water, sanitation, adequate nutrition, education, and safe working and living conditions (Pūras, 2017; United Nations General Assembly, 1966a). It was endorsed by most European countries, and signed by President Carter in 1977, but it was never approved by the U.S. Congress (United Nations Treaty Collection, 1966). Instead, the United States ratified the International Covenant on Civil and Political Rights (United Nations General Assembly, 1966b), which allows for democratic rights such as free speech, the right to vote, and free-market rights, but does not recognize the personal rights listed in Article 12 of the International Covenant on Economic, Social and Cultural Rights (Mukherjee, 2018).

Sweden, the United Kingdom, Australia, and even the former United Socialist Soviet Republic have espoused the ideals of the International Covenant on Economic, Social and Cultural Rights by creating a public healthcare system that ensures at least basic services to all citizens (Sinclair & LaPlante, 2019). Several countries instituted reciprocal healthcare agreements, so citizens can receive care abroad as they do at home (Smartraveller, 2022). In countries that have not ratified the International Covenant on Economic, Social and Cultural Rights (like the United States), these personal rights—absent in the International Covenant on Civil and Political Rights—are regarded as "secondary rights" or "privileges" (Mukherjee, 2018; Box 25.2).

In the United States, the difference among insurance plans leads to marked inequities and creates the need for an army of administrators. The result is that the U.S. (non)system is one of the most expensive per capita in the world. Globally, the United States recently ranked 37th—after Costa Rica and Dominica—placing it solidly among those nations with the poorest outcomes (World Population Review, 2022; also see a discussion of the healthcare ranking of nations worldwide in the Resources for More In-Depth Information section at the end of this chapter).

The COVID-19 pandemic has demonstrated to the world what happens when a healthcare system is chronically underfunded and when people do not have resources for both healthcare and basic survival. COVID-19 has also changed the healthcare landscape; while reducing access to in-person primary and specialty care, the pandemic has fostered the rise (in technologically advanced nations) of telehealth. How these changes will progress is unclear at the time of this writing. It is clear that much primary care and health management has been neglected during the pandemic, leading to unnecessary suffering and death (Czeisler et al., 2020).

BOX 25.2: The U.S. Workplace-Based Insurance System

The U.S. workplace-based insurance system depends on:
- The size of the business
  - Optional for businesses with under 50 employees
- The type of insurance
  - Individual plan or family plan
- The status of the employee
  - Full-time or part-time

WHAT IS POVERTY?

Extreme poverty anywhere is a threat to human security everywhere.
      —Kofi Annan, Seventh Secretary-General of the United Nations

Poverty is multidimensional. The phenomena are linked to the absence of material resources to provide the essentials of living for self, family, and/or community (Tackie, 2021). Poverty is rooted in a circumstance where the responsible person or community does not provide for the basic needs that are critical for meeting negligible requirements for survival and well-being (Chen, 2022). Poverty is associated with individuals having inadequate education and the lack of opportunity for attaining it, unemployment and underemployment, and the absence of a worthwhile income for self and family. Access to adequate healthcare is also a major barrier, as are lack of adequate housing, nutrition, and other essentials for survival (Chen et al., 2022; Marmot, 2017; Tackie, 2021).

The scarcity of opportunity is often maintained by unequal laws or disparate enforcement of those laws, and other societal conditions such as prejudice and discrimination against specific persons and groups. Those living in poverty lack social inclusion and are often absent from participating in decision-making (Carney, 1992; Pérez-Muñoz et al., 2015). They do not have access to networks that help to create opportunity and privilege, which are associated with unlocking resources such as credit, education, training, and meaningful employment (Theroux, 2018).

In extreme cases, those living in poverty may not even officially exist. For example, the births of one in four children worldwide younger than 5 years were never registered; therefore, these children do not officially exist (UNICEF, 2021, August). Homeless persons and refugees may have invalid, lost, or expired identification. They may even be considered "non-citizens" in the countries where they have lived for generations. One such example is the seven hill tribes of Thailand. Such people may not have government-issued identification cards or health insurance (Borgen Project, 2015; Chandran, 2020; International Justice Mission, 2022; Ritchie, 2000; United Nations, 2017).

Poverty begets poverty. If a short-term loan to buy food before the next paycheck costs 120% of the amount borrowed, the net effect reduces that next paycheck. Eating cheaply takes time. Buying basic ingredients and cooking takes more time than eating prepared food. Working two jobs to earn food and rent money means less time to prepare quality food and limited time with children and family. If you have a police offense, prison record, bankruptcy claims, or no ID card, then finding a job or a loan may be next to impossible. Getting a place to live might be difficult or next to impossible, too. Homelessness can become very hard to escape (Fowler et al., 2019).

Worldwide, more than 736 million people live in poverty; 10% live in extreme poverty. Extreme poverty means a dearth of access to clean water, food, and sanitation (United Nations, 2020a). Anyone can fall victim to poverty. Unfortunate life circumstances—disasters, accidents, illness, mental health disorders, or posttraumatic stress disorder—can befall anyone (Kraay & McKenzie, 2014).

However, some groups bear a disproportionate burden of poverty. The heavier burdens are born by women of all ethnic groups, Indigenous populations, citizens of developing countries, and persons of color. Natural and man-made disasters can accentuate violence and self-harm, including suicide among women in underresourced communities (Gary et al., 2021). The dynamics that create and maintain these systems are complex, often rooted in history but maintained by those in power for their own advantage (Bernstein et al., 2018). These dynamics primarily are the mechanisms that the wealthy and powerful use to maintain a privileged status quo for themselves and their families (UNICEF, 2020, November).

As of February 2021, an estimated 1.2 million children had been put to work worldwide to support their families during the COVID-19 pandemic. A considerable number of these children will never return to school (Deutschland Welle, 2021; for more information, see a video about the fate of children who have been required to become the family breadwinners in the Resources for More In-Depth Information section at the end of this chapter). In the United States, children relegated to distance learning have lost social opportunities. Those without internet resources have lost a year of schooling, and a sizeable portion of them have not yet returned to the classroom as of this writing (UNICEF, 2020, November).

Poverty is not a problem just found in less developed countries. In the United States, a developed nation, the disparity between the richest (whose personal wealth is measured in billions) and the poorest (who may only own what they carry) is extreme. There are significant parts of the United States that have the problems and profiles of less developed countries. According to the U.S. Census Bureau, depending on the region, 12% to 17% of its citizens live under the poverty threshold (Shrider et al., 2021).

In the Navajo Nation, more than 170,000 persons occupy 27,000 square miles straddling portions of Arizona, New Mexico, and Utah, where there is no electricity, water, or plumbing, even today, for roughly one quarter of the residents. Indigenous Americans at least have government-paid healthcare, when they can access it.

Even impoverished people who are working two jobs to stay above that arbitrary poverty line may still not have access to opportunity-unlocking resources. They may earn too much to qualify for Medicaid yet have no work-related health insurance. For healthcare, the only option, if any, is out-of-pocket payments—which might help to create or maintain the poverty status of the individual or family.

The atrocities and hardships of poverty can be almost unimaginable for some. Often, the only job options are illegal. People may be forced to resort to theft or to selling drugs, sex, and even organs. Helpless children may become goods to buy and sell (Rigby, 2020). "Marrying off" a daughter makes sense when you cannot feed her. Boys join armed gangs or armies to survive (Dudenhoefer, 2016); for example, over the last 50 years in the South American country of Colombia, more than 8,700 children have been recruited into armed groups. Participation in armed groups promises food security and may give these children a sense of belonging. The COVID-19 lockdowns have only exacerbated these desperate situations (Taylor, 2020).

When a person has no good options, the temporary relief of drugs or alcohol may be the best for which they can hope. For people living in poverty, life can become so unstable that thinking beyond tomorrow is difficult. Long-term planning and hope become impossible (Theroux, 2018).

In Bolivia, when the struggle to survive becomes too much, one may check into an "elephant graveyard," where one is given a bucket of high-proof alcohol, a potty bucket, a simple cot, and a lock for the door. The client then may drink themself to death. Although clients may choose to ring a bell to leave, most that do will soon die on the nearby streets anyway (Al Rojo Vivo, 2014; Ollard, 2016; Stewart, 2017). Elephant graveyards are technically illegal in Bolivia; however, the same police who swear to uphold that law often turn their backs to the atrocity, seeing it as the most humane option to deal with homeless people who struggle with alcoholism (Al Rojo Vivo, 2014; also see video by Al Rojo Vivo in the Resources for More In-Depth Information section at the end of this chapter).

Opioids reduce physical and emotional pain. Fatal overdoses are more common among those living in poverty than among the rich, although they are hardly absent there either (Altekruse et al., 2020). Substance users may spend their scarce money to procure drugs, but drug use makes holding a job more difficult; even a history of drug use reduces employability. Addressing the opioid crisis requires confronting the SDOH (Case & Deaton, 2020; National Institute on Drug Abuse, 2017).

Overpopulation is both a cause of and a reaction to poverty. Poverty is associated with increased family size and expanded infant mortality (Mohamoud, 2019; Turner et al., 2020). Many cultures value boys above girls; if the first child is a girl, the family has more children and therefore tends to be poorer (Kugler & Kumar, 2017). In Pakistan, for example, a girl will need a marriage dowry, which is an added expense for the family; a son, on the other hand, will stay at home and care for his parents in their old age. Ironically, a high infant death rate drives high fertility (Mukherjee, 2018). When women's worth is measured only by the number of (boy) children she bears, the resulting children are likely to suffer more malnutrition and infectious disease (Barcellos et al., 2014).

When women receive education and opportunities, then birth rates fall, the gross domestic product (GDP) goes up, and child mortality goes down (Harding et al., 2018; Miller et al., 2017). Therefore, poverty eradication is a moral, ethical, social, political, and economic imperative. Men and women of all ethnic groups need equal access to education and opportunities for financial independence and sustained well-being. An integrated poverty alleviation strategy requires global policies binding on signatory countries to distribute wealth, education, income, and opportunities more equitably (United Nations, 2017).

CAUSES AND CONTINUATION OF GLOBAL POVERTY

In a country well governed, poverty is something to be ashamed of. In a country badly governed, wealth is something to be ashamed of.

—Confucius

The Era of European Exploration (and colonization) started in the 15th century and diminished in the 18th century; it included most regions of the world (Brooks, 2020). This era would better be called the Era of Exploitation. Most colonialized areas have been impoverished by resource extraction and by the deliberate suppression of their native cultures if not by outright genocide. Africa, India, Australia, the Americas, New Zealand, and Tasmania have all suffered (Briney, 2020). In many cases, foreign-owned resource extraction continues to this day, leaving numerous countries without the economic power needed to meet the United Nation's sustainable development goals (SDGs)s (Goldin, 2020). Even in the United States, Native Americans and Alaska Natives do not have the right to benefit from all the resources on their reservations, which are "held in trust" by the U.S government—ostensibly for the Natives, but actually it benefits the government and its donors (Evans, 2020). Native Hawaiians and Pacific Islanders are populations that have experienced disruption of their cultural practices and the extraordinary loss of autonomy, their lands, and opportunities for a higher quality of life (Kaholokula et al., 2019).

The 1978 Alma-Ata International Convention defined the importance of developing international strategies to help impoverished countries advance sustainable public healthcare systems (WHO, 1978). However, without significant international help, those countries were left to figure out how to do this within their own limited budgets. The stark reality was that in some places, such as parts of Africa, the basic economy revolved around average daily wages of less than $5 (Mukherjee, 2018).

Financial aid became available to low- and middle-income countries through World Bank loans. However, since the World Bank is managed by the United States, the support of capitalistic economic policies is prioritized, which in turn promotes privatization of healthcare systems and reduced local and national control (Mukherjee, 2018). Hence, the more developed and powerful countries are benefiting the most from their investments. The resulting market-driven public health systems that World Bank loans have financed do not meet the needs of the people because they focus on a top-down approach that fails to address the community's needs. Instead, the aid prioritizes the development of large, centralized institutions with little outreach to smaller communities. As a result, the health of low- and middle-income country citizens does not much improve (Cloninger et al., 2014).

Profit-driven medical care values the highest return for the least investment. The result is often inadequate quality of medical care. Higher quality and more equitable acute healthcare could save millions of dollars and millions of lives each year (Razzak et al., 2019). These deaths are not because of lack of access to, or less use of, healthcare, but because the care is of low quality. Improper triage, missed diagnoses, and inappropriate treatments result in unnecessary pain and suffering, loss of function, and persistent symptoms (Kruk et al., 2018). Such tragedy can permanently alter a person's life course.

NARRATIVE 25.1: SUDDEN MISFORTUNE

A 16-year-old boy who was rendered quadriplegic during the 2010 Haitian earthquake was brought to a makeshift clinic run by the nonprofit, Remote Area Medical. He was awake and oriented with stable vitals, but he could not perform any self-care. He arrived with a girl. No one knew what their relationship was—sister? girlfriend? Although she cared for him at first, after a few days, she disappeared. He was alone.

The volunteer medical staff did what they could to stabilize him and treat the open wound on his neck. There were no neurosurgical capabilities at this makeshift clinic. Personal protective equipment, sanitation, and pain medications were luxuries. A week later, an American naval ship with a neurosurgery suite came to Port-au-Prince. Because the boy was a Haitian who had been brought to an emergency clinic on Dominican Republic soil, bureaucratic regulations barred him from boarding the ship. Governmental officials took photographs of the patients at Remote Area Medical but took no patients to the hospital ship. This boy was now alone, without treatment options, facing a grim future, helpless and forsaken.

Discussion Questions

1. Misfortune can strike anyone. Can you think of, or do you know, someone who was doing well, and then a life event happened and they ended up in poverty? Describe the optimal timing of and types of intervention that could have prevented this tragedy.
2. What institutional programs could be developed to help cushion the blow of misfortune to prevent unrecoverable poverty situations from developing?
3. What could be done in situations where politics and "red tape" restrict needed healthcare access?

It is indisputable that a strong and healthy workforce is more productive than a chronically ill or malnourished workforce. Likewise, there are ill and injured persons who could be returned to the workforce if their disabilities were quickly and correctly treated. By failing to do so, the resultant incapacitation and death, especially of workers, reduce the economic resources of a country (Alkire et al., 2018). Using macroeconomic modeling, Alkire et al. (2018) estimated that the economic losses from avoidable excess mortality alone due to poor access to high-quality healthcare were in the trillions of dollars. The model further showed that the GDP reduction could be as much as 2.6%, a burden that falls most heavily on low- and middle-income countries. Low-quality healthcare also diminishes public trust and is a waste of valuable resources (Alkire et al., 2018). People do not use care they do not trust (Huang et al., 2018).

COVID-19 IN THE NAVAJO NATION: LESSONS LEARNED

> *I believe if the rest of the country looks at the model that the Navajo Nation has shown, that you can turn things around.*
>
> —Anthony Fauci, Director of NIAID

The COVID-19 pandemic rapidly spread worldwide in 2019 and 2020. Hand and face hygiene, physical distancing, masking, and staying isolated at home were essential protective acts. Many of those living in poverty have been unable to comply with these matters, and protecting themselves and others has not been easily done (Centers for Disease Control and Prevention [CDC], 2022).

The poverty rate in the Navajo Nation is between 38% and 43% (Navajo Nation, 2004). The pandemic hit hard (Christenson, 2020). By summer 2020, the Navajo had the highest infection rate in the United States. Many Navajo are poor, live in small, multigenerational homes (often mud and log hogans or mobile homes), are widely scattered in a dry environment, and often are without electricity or running water (Yellow Horse et al., 2021). Families rely on pickup trucks equipped with 500-gallon tanks to haul water from more than a hundred miles away.

Under these conditions, it is hard to practice frequent hand washing. Physical distancing within the household can be impossible when extended families must share a single small space. However, the Navajo culture also mitigated the effects of COVID-19 in significant ways. Once the reservation government decided that masking, shutting businesses, and staying at home would slow the spread, curfews and home isolation were universally observed, even by those who disagreed. Roadside stands closed. Families took care of each other. Isolation houses were set up for those who needed to isolate or who needed care beyond that which could be provided at home, yet who did not need hospitalization. When vaccinations became available, the Navajo lined up (V. Totten, personal communication, March 2021). As of January 2022, 72.5% of the Navajo were vaccinated with two doses of COVID-19 vaccine (Grigg, 2022; also see the video by Christenson in the Resources for More In-Depth Information section at the end of this chapter).

POVERTY DISPROPORTIONATELY AFFECTS WOMEN

Poverty is relatively cheap to address and incredibly expensive to ignore.

—Clint Borgen

Although Mao Zedong, the founding father of the People's Republic of China, claimed that women "hold up half the sky" (Saba, 1972), women do not control half the world, nor do they manage their fair share of its wealth (Box 25.3). Because women gestate and often raise the next generation of citizens, equity would suggest that women should have greater access to healthcare and social support. Unfortunately, this is not so, and, as women are affected, so are their children (Shaw et al., 2017). By 2030, the United Nations estimates that more than 160 million children across the world will be living in extreme poverty (United Nations, 2020a).

BOX 25.3: Women Lack Equal Legal Protection

Of the 194 countries in the world:

39 do not grant equal inheritance rights to daughters as to sons.

- This is a recommended SDG 5 right.

18 allow husbands to prevent their wives from earning income.

49 lack laws protecting women from domestic violence.

- One in five women and girls worldwide have experienced physical and/or sexual violence by an intimate partner within the last 12 months.

SDG, sustainable development goal.

Source: Adapted from United Nations (2017). *Sustainable development goal 5: Achieve gender equality and empower all women and girls.* https://unstats.un.org/sdgs/report/2017/goal-05

In most cultures, females are less valued than males. Female fetuses are differentially aborted (Agrawal, 2012). Looking only at China and India, for example, as of the early 2000s, there has been a 60 to 100 million reduction of daughters over sons (Hesketh & Xing, 2006; Miller, 2001). Son preference is fueled by the customs of the son carrying on the family name, providing old-age security for parents, and bringing a dowry into the family upon marriage, which continues to this day across many countries in the world (Sivak and Smirnov, 2019).

Women are less politically active. In 2020, women held only 36% of local government seats, and only 25% of national parliament seats—far from parity. However, some (small) progress is being made; in 46 countries, women now hold more than 30% of national parliament seats in at least one chamber (UN Women, 2021).

Women are disproportionately poor. Worldwide, for every 100 men in poverty, there are 122 women in poverty. Women still have less access to property ownership, credit, skill development, education, and employment in parts of the world (United Nations, 2009). Globally, only 13% of agricultural landholders are women. In northern Africa, women hold few paid nonagricultural jobs, although the proportion has increased from 35% in 1990 to 41% in 2015. However, more than 100 of the 194 countries worldwide now track budget allocations by gender. Empowered women benefit entire families and their communities. These benefits are passed to future generations (Cebotari et al., 2020; Clermont, 2017).

Women are more likely to be mutilated or killed. Although widely condemned and usually illegal, misogynistic customs like female genital mutilation (FGM) remain for cultural and religious reasons (Adinew & Mekete, 2017). Wrongly called female circumcision, FGM is the amputation of a portion of a girl's genitalia. This can range from the ritualistic severing of the clitoral hood to complete removal of the labia majora, labia minora, and clitoris, followed by suturing the genital area closed except for a small opening for urine and menses. The cutting instruments and procedures are often not sanitary; the wounds may become infected, and the girls may die. Most common in Africa and the Middle East, at least 200 million girls in 30 countries have been subjected to FGM (United Nations Population Fund, 2022; Utz-Billing and Kentenich, 2008; WHO, 2022b).

In some societies FGM is a rite of passage; in others, it is a prerequisite for marriage, making it difficult for families to decide against having their daughters cut. People who reject the practice may face social denunciation or ostracization, and their daughters may be ineligible for marriage, as in Egypt. Even parents who do not support FGM may feel compelled to participate. Fortunately, the practice is declining (Azeze et al., 2020). In the 30 countries where FGM is concentrated, the proportion of adolescent girls subjected to FGM has dropped from one of two girls in 2000 to one of three girls by 2017 (United Nations Population Fund, 2022). The practice may not die until powerful men prefer to marry women who have not undergone FGM.

Generational wealth is not always redistributed equally between sons and daughters. For example, until 2014 in Nepal, only sons could inherit parental property. It was assumed that all women would marry, and, as wives were their husband's property, they were also his sole responsibility. Progress has been made. The 2014 Nepalese Civil Code bill established equal inheritance laws, after which both sons and daughters would share equally in property inheritance, regardless of marital status (Pun, 2014).

NARRATIVE 25.2: SARITA, A YOUNG WOMAN IN NEPAL

Sarita is 17 years old. She is the oldest daughter in her family. Sarita worked hard in school and dreamed of becoming a schoolteacher someday. However, completing her homework was always difficult as Sarita had to do all the housework before school every day. Her brothers never had to do any of it. Despite not being able to study as much as she would

(continued)

NARRATIVE 25.2: SARITA, A YOUNG WOMAN IN NEPAL (*CONTINUED*)

like, Sarita paid attention in school and always did well. She continued to study diligently and graduated at the top of her class. Eventually, even her ultraconservative parents became proud of her accomplishments. They agreed to allow her to pursue her professional dreams, sending her to Kathmandu to stay with her uncle while pursuing her education.

At first, Sarita's uncle was kind and supportive, but gradually things began to change. He started raping her whenever her aunt was not around. After a few months of this, Sarita stopped menstruating and started getting morning sickness.

Three months later, still feeling sick, she went to a clinic. She had always had an irregular menstrual cycle and had never been taught the symptoms of pregnancy. She was shocked to discover that she was, in fact, 6 months pregnant. She felt alone and helpless and felt that there was no one she could turn to.

Afraid everyone would blame her for ruining the family's reputation, Sarita became desperate. Despite the availability of free abortion clinics locally, Sarita was unaware of how to safely terminate a pregnancy. She bought a toxic potion of chemicals used to kill field mice from the local pharmacy. She had heard from her friends that drinking organophosphorus mouse poison would terminate her pregnancy. That it did, but at the cost of her own life, too.

Discussion Questions

1. Who do you think is responsible for this tragedy? Sarita? Her parents? Her uncle? Her culture?
2. Did poverty play a role in Sarita's situation?
3. What SDOH were involved in Sarita's tragic death?
4. At what levels can we intervene to prevent such a tragedy? Please provide a detailed rationale.
5. How secure are you with providing contraceptive counseling and methods to women?
6. How comfortable are you with performing or assisting in the performance of an abortion? Are you at ease with denying women the right to an abortion? Why?
7. How supportive are you of women having access to approved medical abortion drugs from healthcare providers in their communities?

Women do not always have autonomy. Only 52% of married women may make their own decisions about sexual relations, contraceptives, and health care (WHO, 2020). Yet only women die from pregnancy. Maternal mortality (MM) occurs within a context of gender-based, economic, political, and cultural discrimination and neglect by health care services in both low- and high-income countries (Clermont, 2017; Vilda et al., 2019). Reducing the global maternal mortality rate (MMR) is one of the 17 SDGs of the United Nations. Between 2000 and 2017, the global MMR declined by 2.9% per annum, less than half the 6.4% per annum needed to achieve the SDG of 70 maternal deaths per 100,000 live births by 2030, with no country's MMR more than twice the global average (United Nations, 2015; UNICEF, 2019). An *increase* in MMR in the United States was driven by worsening MM among non-Hispanic Black women (Collier & Molina, 2019). Black women's MM is 37%, compared with 14.7% for White women (CDC, 2020). The United States has some of the highest rates of MM among developed countries for non-White women, including Native American women (Singh, 2021).

The United Nations Population Fund reported that in the least-developed countries, 40% of girls were married before age 18, and 12% before age 15 (UNICEF, 2021). In the 2010 to 2015 period, over 45% of women reported having given birth by age 18. The estimated global adolescent birth rate is 44 births per 1,000 girls. In West and Central Africa, it is 115 births per 1,000 girls (UNICEF, 2019), the highest in the world. Highest among adolescents, lowest in the 20 to 25 age group, and climbing as women near the end of their reproductive life, MM follows a U-shaped curve in relation to age (Blanc et al., 2013; Sedgh et al., 2015). Complications of pregnancy and childbirth are the leading causes of death for teen girls (Zureick-Brown et al., 2013). Deaths from abortions are included as a factor in MM. Worldwide, of the 42,000,000 abortions performed annually, nearly half are procured through unsafe means. Among the 20,000,000 women who have unsafe abortions, 70,000 thousand die and 5,000,000 are disabled, many permanently (Shah & Åhman, 2009).

Other calamities happen too, as illustrated in Narrative 25.3.

NARRATIVE 25.3: BETWEEN A ROCK AND A HARD PLACE: WHEN THE VICTIMS ARE CHILDREN IN BOLIVIA

Talking to residents in certain districts, you can often hear heart-wrenching stories of babies being given away or abandoned by parents in crisis—underage, struggling with addiction, unable to care for an infant due to social conflicts, having too many children to care for already, experiencing familial violence. It is all too common in certain neighborhoods where these poverty-induced situations are rampant. You commonly hear the stories on the news about a baby or newborn found in a trash can near a local hospital, in a public bathroom, or under a park bench (J. Romero, personal communication, 2019; also see Romero, 2019). Local people know where babies tend to be left; they tell you to look for a black trash bag that cries or moves on certain street corners. Sometimes the infants survive and are sent to overpopulated orphanages; sometimes they don't. All these children suffer long-lasting adverse effects from the experience.

The story of one baby that didn't survive was witnessed by a colleague of mine. One night she heard a baby crying. The crying never seemed to stop. The next morning, it was discovered that the infant's mother had given birth during the night. Not wanting to or not able to care for the child, the infant's mother had thrown it out the window, where street dogs had found and dismembered the baby (J. Romero, personal communication, 2019).

Perhaps this parent was irresponsible. Perhaps she was trying to save the infant from a more horrible fate. Rape and home violence are, unfortunately, more common than we like to admit. In 2013, a baby girl of 7 months was raped by a friend of the family in Bolivia. The girl survived and was treated for severe internal injuries that had ruptured various organs and extended into her thoracic cage (Excélsior, 2013). Unfortunately, these horror stories are not unique to Bolivia (Rodríguez, 2018).

Discussion Questions

1. When planning interventions at the policy level, what would be your three highest priorities?
2. Construct an action plan that addresses issues related to culture, public health structure, common practices among women, and immediate and long-term interventions that could be implemented by health professionals and politicians in the communities.
3. How would you link poverty to the parents' practices and their sense of potentially being overwhelmed by the plight of having given birth with limited or no resources for care and support?
4. Using the SDOH framework, how would you construct a brief but powerful concept paper that could be used for planning for three structures: the health system, the health-related workforce, and the patient/family/community?
5. What are five essential themes that ought to be included in curricular reengineering for nurses, physicians, social workers, psychologists, policymakers, community-health workers, and other healthcare providers in Bolivia? In your local culture?

The 2030 UN Agenda for Sustainable Development is one blueprint for achieving global prosperity. The 17 SDGs are intersectional and interlinked. Reducing poverty requires gender equality and equity (United Nations, 2020b). Women must have the same opportunities as men for acquiring education, earning money, accumulating wealth, obtaining quality healthcare, and living autonomously. Unfortunately, women's opportunities have been constrained for centuries by social and cultural customs, laws, and policies.

POVERTY AND INDIGENOUS PEOPLE

American healthcare faces a crisis in quality. There is a dangerous divide between the potential for the high level of quality care that our health system promises and the uneven quality that it actually delivers.

—Risa Lavizzo-Mourey

The Indigenous and Tribal Peoples Convention, also known as C169, was hosted by the International Labour Organization (1989) to de-sanction previous assimilationist attitudes toward Indigenous and Tribal people and to officially recognize their rights and sovereignty over ancestral lands.

Indigenous and tribal people [are any group whose] social, cultural, and economic conditions distinguish them from other sections of the national community and whose status is wholly or partially regulated by their own customs or traditions or by special laws or regulation [and as] people in independent countries who are regarded as Indigenous on account of their descent from the populations which inhabited ... [the] geographical region ... retain[ing] some of their social, economic, cultural and political institutions. (International Labour Organization, 1989, Article 1)

The subsequent Declaration on the Rights of Indigenous Peoples included rights to maintain traditions and religion and rights to equal labor, education, and access to quality community-based healthcare that considered Indigenous traditional cultural and spiritual health providers as a valid resource (International Labour Office, 2013). As a binding international convention, C169 is designed to promote antidiscriminatory socioeconomic equality for the mitigation of historic inequalities and discriminations that have often caused historical trauma.

In Bolivia, 65.8% of the population is Indigenous (Rist & Nuñez del Prado, 2012). Evo Morales, an Indigenous man, was the 65th president of Bolivia, presiding from 2006 to 2019. Upon gaining the presidency, he tried to reverse the economic effects of colonialization, poverty, and the SDOH in his country in a variety of ways. Resources were nationalized, and transnational companies were limited, freeing up profits that could be re-invested in national infrastructure projects, including healthcare. While it was far from a perfect system, public services, including a universal healthcare plan, were created to aid populations at risk of extreme poverty. Traditional Indigenous medicine was recognized and integrated into the universal healthcare system, further expanding healthcare access to most of those living in poverty. The effort improved the lot of traditional healers, who were no longer condemned, but rather paid. Extreme poverty in Bolivia decreased from 38.2% in 2005 to 15.2% in 2018, the greatest decrease in extreme poverty in South America (Instituto Nacional de Estadística, 2019). These shifts have supported huge advances in reducing poverty and meeting millennium development goals (Rist & Nuñez del Prado, 2012; TAC Economics, 2022; United Nations News, 2015).

Historical Trauma

I understand the depression that I suffered and the secretness of it, of the years at boarding school. You don't want to talk to anybody about it. You don't wanna [sic] share these secrets because they're so deep and they're so ... they do something to a person.

—Interview of a sexual abuse survivor by Barbara Charbonneau-Dahlen

For more 100 years, the U.S. government tried to eradicate Native American cultures either through direct genocide or by cultural eradication. Native children were forced to go to government-run boarding schools and forbidden to speak their native languages (Reyhner, 2018). Inadequate basic healthcare resulted in the deaths of children, the alarming numbers of whom have only recently begun to emerge. National Public Radio reported that by July 2021 the remains of more than 1000 children were found at a Canadian government's Indigenous boarding school (National Public Radio, 2021). The Canadian boarding schools were modeled after those in the United States. The United States is now examining its own government boarding schools and the policies and practices that created and maintained devastating outcomes, including high and preventable morbidity and mortality rates (Equal Justice Initiative, 2021; see Chapter 20 for a more detailed discussion of Native Americans and Alaska Natives).

Historical trauma describes the well-documented, generational downward socioeconomic spiral arising from the collective experience of people who have been subjected to extremely traumatic situations (Maxwell, 2014). These factors continue to affect the health of people generations later (Charbonneau-Dahlen et al., 2016), a fact that poignantly surfaced during the COVID-19 pandemic (John-Henderson & Ginty, 2020). The trauma experienced by ancestors has been shown to be related to transgenerational shifts in function in their descendants (Yehuda & Lehrner, 2018). Many peoples have suffered historical trauma: survivors of Nazi death camps, enslaved African people, and most colonized Indigenous communities. Psychological wounding is the mechanism postulated to underlie racial disparities in hypertension (Dolezsar et al., 2014). This wounding is transmitted culturally and epigenetically from generation to generation (Charbonneau-Dahlen et al., 2016). Long-term effects of historical trauma due to the Age of Exploration are still evident worldwide (also see Chapter 20).

For Indigenous peoples in Australia, New Zealand, and the Americas—including Native Hawaiians and Pacific Islanders—historical trauma has arisen due to invaders forcing the eradication of their societal structure and traditions. Cultural practices (including rituals and traditional medicines) were banned under the threat of criminal penalty; children were removed to remote government schools, forbidden their native language and dress, and were taught only the conqueror's religion (Charbonneau-Dahlen et al., 2016; Smith, 2009). Descendants of enslaved African people suffer because their ancestors were brought by force to the Americas, stripped of their native languages and cultures, denied an education and healthcare, and sold as slaves. The result is persons who have an injured sense of self-identity, are without a cultural tradition to fall back on, and may find they have no future in the invader's world (Dubois, 1906/2003; Sotero, 2009).

Native Hawaiians and Pacific Islanders have also lost their land and have experienced disruptions in basic systems that help to define their identities (e.g., cultural rituals, folklore, traditional practices, ways of knowing). Their spiritual, social, and ancestral connections have been severed. In their efforts to revitalize their culture and self-determination, it is important to recognize and embrace their relationship to the land (although much of it has been lost) and Indigenous knowledge about health, wellness, and pathways to resilience (Kaholokula et al., 2019, Spencer et al., 2020).

Historical trauma causes "depression, self-destructive behavior, suicidal thoughts and gestures, anxiety, low self-esteem, anger, and difficulty recognizing and expressing emotions. It may include substance abuse, often an attempt to avoid painful feelings through self-medication" (Brave Heart, 2003, p. 7). Among the adverse effects are sexual risk taking, mental ill-health, problematic alcohol or drug use, and interpersonal and self-directed violence (Hughes et al., 2017).

Historical trauma may not be irreversible. Two Canadian Indigenous communities, Alkali Lake and Hollow Water, broke the chain of historical trauma–induced social problems of alcohol and drug use and sexual abuse that permeated their communities by implementing healing of the entire community based on their own traditional culture. The tribal recovery program included rehabilitation of offenders, offering positive rewards for contributory social behavior, and re-initiation into their community's values, traditions, and roots (Four-Worlds Institute, n.d.; Heal Project, 2020; McCoy, 1988; Woodward, 1986; also see a minidocumentary and a reaction video regarding traditional Indigenous approaches used to successfully combat sexual abuse and substance abuse in the Resources for More In-Depth Information section at the end of this chapter).

Rehabilitation rather than criminalization is a notable difference between the Alkali Lake and Hollow Water approach and the usual Western approach to criminality, mental illness, sexual abuse, and substance use. Rehabilitation supported the SDOH in the lives of the offenders. Pastor Gennadiy Mokhnenko used this same approach when he adopted dozens of Ukraine's drug-addicted and incapacitated street children and organized multiple programs to help them. In his words: "We try to give them a dream. We try to give them something interesting for work. We change the people around them" (Varley, 2016, para 33; also see a video about Mokhnenko's work with the street children of Kiev, Ukraine in the Resources for More In-Depth Information section at the end of this chapter). The success rate of these approaches has been encouraging.

SOCIAL SUPPORT AND CULTURE CAN MITIGATE THE ILL EFFECTS OF POVERTY

> *Poverty is not only about income poverty, it is about the deprivation of economic and social rights, insecurity, discrimination, exclusion, and powerlessness.*
> —Irene Khan, former Secretary-General of Amnesty International

High-quality social support in a safe environment, the antithesis of historical trauma, has been shown to have a protective effect on health (Reblin & Uchino, 2008). With good social support, traumatized individuals are more able to rediscover and maintain their traditions and cultures. Those Native American nations that have been able to maintain a separate identity, such as the Navajo, have fared better than those who, having lost their Indigenous language and culture, have not been fully accepted in mainstream culture (Grayshield et al., 2015).

Indigenous people represent 6.7% of the population in North and South America. Due to difficulty in access to healthcare and poor cultural and logistical preparation for health professionals, most live in poverty with high mortality and morbidity (United Nations News, 2004). Although many lack access to resources and have low incomes, Indigenous cultural traditions can mitigate some of the ill effects of poverty. Remember, poverty is more than just a lack of economic resources.

Many Indigenous cultures believe that the same modern civilization that has improved life in many ways has also caused disease. Science has proven that high-stress lifestyles, human invasions of natural spaces, animal and plant extinctions, armed conflict, processed foods, and pollution all have ill effects on health (Cloninger et al., 2014; Tallman et al., 2020). Such a life is out of balance.

The Kallawaya are an Indigenous culture of doctors and herbalists living amongst the Quechua ethnic group in the mountain valleys north of La Paz, Bolivia. After Bolivia became a signatory to the Indigenous and Tribal People's Convention in 1991, the Kallawaya were no longer persecuted for their practice; instead, their work regained legitimacy. Their methods were integrated into the newly formed National Health Care Plan. Today they are recognized as official medical care providers within the Bolivian public healthcare system and reimbursed for their care rather than chided or ignored (Callahan, 2011).

One treatment to cure grief and sorrow is the Llaki Wijch'una ritual. This cultural rite recognizes the long-lasting effects of grief and misfortune. During this ritual, the soul is called back into the body. Both the body and spirit are cleansed through bathing rituals. The home environment is also cleansed of associations of grief, sorrow, and misfortune (Rösing, 1991). In this way, the patient is returned to harmony with the world, and grief abates.

NARRATIVE 25.4: ABOUT SINCHI

My child's name is Sinchi Wayra, which means Strong Wind in the Quechua language. He was 16 months old when the unthinkable happened. He was hit by a truck and died.

What follows a traumatic death event like that is an experience unequaled and unfathomable by most people who have not gone through such tragedy. Grief victims need a lot of support and help. Not only severe depression, but also physical illness follows. For example, I can't remember much of the first weeks after his death. I couldn't work. And when I could, the effort was so intense that I would get sick for 3 or 4 days after just a half-day of work.

I saw psychiatrists. I tried meditation, churches, exercise, positive thinking—everything to get back on my feet again. But nothing had long-lasting effects—not until I was introduced to a Kallawaya doctor. He had me come to a meditative retreat in the mountains for several months where he performed a series of rituals with me.

The Llaki Wijch'una was one of the rituals that were performed. And I can honestly say, it was key to my healing. I still recall how, following the ceremony, I dreamed of smiling—something I hadn't done for years. And recovery was like a snowball effect. I didn't feel a great difference at first, but as the weeks went by after the ceremony, I could sense how I was getting stronger and thinking clearer. It was something I was unable to do on my own or through other treatments and therapies.

Discussion Questions

1. In your practice, research, and policy making, how do you recognize and connect the physical and psychic components of the human body in the context of wellness, healing, and disease expression?
2. Do you advocate for "traditional" healers in your healthcare delivery system? Are they paid practitioners? Are they considered members of your healthcare team?
3. As health delivery policy and systems embrace intradisciplinary education, research, and practice, how do you envision that your contributions to health and wellness, across a variety of settings, will be enhanced and more impactful? Please be specific and identify five potential outcomes that you envision will occur in your work.

For many thousands of years, practitioners of traditional Indigenous medicine and traditional Chinese medicine (TCM) have successfully treated both acute and chronic conditions by balancing physical, spiritual, and social well-being. TCM is particularly interesting because it has been integrated into modern-day Chinese medical practice. In China, there are both TCM hospitals and hospitals where allopathic and TCM practitioners work together. He and Hou (2013) write:

> Biomedicine [i.e., Western medicine] is very effective when the underlying mechanism… has been well documented and an agent to break down the circle of the pathogen is found. However, it is limited when diseases have either a pathogenous [sic] mechanism that is unknown or the agent to break down the circle of the pathogen (an example can be viral infectious diseases) is unfound [sic]. It is also limited when illness is related to functional defects or diseases with multiple organs, tissue, or system defects. All of these can be overcome by the holistic approach of TCM. (p. 95)

The concept of balance is not completely foreign to Western medicine. The osteopathic concepts of body models and the biopsychosocial model deal with the complexity of the mind/body relationship (Penney, 2013). There is some thought that the integration of these principles could also have Native American influences since the founder of osteopathic medicine, Andrew T. Still, worked with the Shawnee Indigenous people and may have carried their mind/body/spirit healing model into his teaching practice (Zegarra-Parodi et al., 2019).

Allopathic healthcare focuses on physiological illness. Chronic or acute emotional conditions like grief, psychological trauma, depression, and posttraumatic stress disorder are known to be associated with increased risk for long-lasting psychological and social complications, and comorbidities like cancer, cardiovascular disease, and sleep disorders (Treml & Kersting, 2018). Disequilibrium in any one area can cause the other areas to shift out of equilibrium. This is the proposed mechanism for how adverse childhood events (ACEs) can be a root cause of a multitude of physical diseases later in life (Waehrer et al., 2020; see Chapter 22 for an in-depth discussion of ACEs). Yet, until recently, emotional and psychological disorders have, like poverty, been considered personal and moral failings. Conditions caused by lifestyle and external agents that become chronic conditions are treated symptomatically, rather than at their root causes. Improving population health, like the eradication of poverty, requires attention to root causes (Braveman & Gottlieb, 2014; Emanuel, 2020; Marmot, 2015;,2017; Satcher, 2020).

Ina Rösing, a German psychiatrist and anthropologist, described Western medicine as "poor, empty, horribly ordered, dissociated, impersonal, and lacking ritual" (Rösing, 1991, p. 215). Rösing sought to rehumanize Western medicine through documentation of the importance of ritual in healing grief among Indigenous cultures (Alderman, 2018). An interest in the connection between grief and misfortune led her to study the Kallawaya and the Llaki Wijch'una ritual in depth:

> In the world of the Llaki Wijch'una … mourning and the heavy emotions that accompany it attract misfortune and, for this reason, the mourner is in danger [of contracting illness and bad luck]. The Llaki Wijch'una [is a ritual of purification and protection that] expulses, precisely, this danger. (Rösing, 1991, pp. 206–207)

The Kallawaya are not the only people who practice this type of healing. Most Indigenous cultures have rituals to help heal affected individuals of processes like grief. The Navajo Blessing Way is another ritual that seeks to restore a troubled person to harmony with self and the universe (Davis, 2011). A similar healing ritual was used by returning Navajo Code Talkers after World War II to free them of the posttraumatic stress disorders induced by what they had experienced during World War II (Davis, 2011; McClain, 2002; also see NavajoCode videos in the Resources for More In-Depth Information section at the end of this chapter to listen to interviews with Navajo Code Talkers).

Another influential writer who sought to incorporate meaning into Western psychotherapy was Viktor Frankl. In *Man's Search for Meaning*, Frankl (1984) described the importance of finding personal meaning as a strategy for successfully surviving the Nazi concentration camp experience. From these examples, we can see that various traditions and cultures have used healing practices that can support and revitalize communities and individuals, thereby mitigating some of the worst effects of dysfunctional SDOH.

ADDRESSING THE SOCIAL DETERMINANTS OF HEALTH AND THE CONTINUATION OF POVERTY

If poverty is a disease that infects the entire community in the form of unemployment and violence, failing schools and broken homes, then we can't just treat those symptoms in isolation. We have to heal that entire community.

—Barack Obama, 44th President of the United States

Historically, poverty has been considered a moral failure: Those living in poverty are seen as "lazy" and uninterested in bettering themselves. Yet, in every country on Earth, there are those who manage to lift themselves out of poverty, while others are stuck in "poverty traps" (Bowles 2016). Society creates the bulk of these traps through carefully designed laws, policies, and discrimination. The United States exhibits examples aplenty (e.g., redistricting of congressional districts; discriminatory voting laws; food deserts; substandard educational and employment opportunities). Only recently recognized are the roles of macro-level injustices, such as historical traumas, differential credit access, and inequitable enforcement of laws. One example is redlining, by which the U.S. Federal Housing Administration, established in 1934, refused to insure mortgages in and near African American neighborhoods. Persons of color were thereby deprived of access to quality schools and to healthcare. Such discrimination has existed for centuries and continues (Rothstein, 2017; see Chapter 22 for a discussion of redlining).

Corruption at all levels hinders efforts to address the SDOH. Globally, reducing corruption in government has been hard to achieve. It is a never-ending process but has its successes (National Academies of Sciences, 2018). The efforts must continue as all health professionals work toward improving health outcomes for all people.

SDOH are the "causes of the causes" of population health inequality: the inequities in power, money, and resources in which people are born, grow, live, work, and age (Marmot et al., 2008). Environmental exposure to pollutants is an example of an SDOH that contributes to the patterns of disability and mortality arising from noncommunicable diseases (Marmot et al., 2008; Marmot & Bell, 2019). Improving population health requires improving the SDOH. Networking, forming partnerships, developing self-reliance, and capacity building (i.e., creating and enhancing essential knowledge and skillsets, logistics, and resources among individuals and within institutions with the intent of improving outcomes) are the primary instruments of change (WHO, 2008).

The SDOH must be addressed at macro, meso, and micro levels. At the macro levels are largely global and international organizations that set goals and make policies binding on the signatory nations. Of necessity, these are long on ideals and short on specifics; their sights are set years and decades ahead. Global organizations can set long-term goals because they do not need to obsess over the next election cycle. Signatory nations ratify those goals, which become the basis for crafting policies specific to their own people.

At the meso level are organizations, communities, and states working to eliminate poverty in their local areas. These groups may focus on only one aspect, such as improving local schools, feeding the hungry, or advocating for equal rights. Others may try to break the cycle of poverty by offering micro-loans, repatriation, or even crop insurance (Barnett et al., 2008). Other groups might highlight unequal law enforcement or gender-based wage differences. Still others may try to renew poor neighborhoods by promoting trash removal, building parks or sidewalks, or enforcing road maintenance. Planting trees is another example of a meso-level project that improves microclimates, cools cities, and improves psychological well-being. When neighborhoods are more livable and attractive, the people living there may feel more pride.

One meso-level organization supporting microeconomy is the Grameen Bank, founded by Dr. Muhammad Yunus, a Bangladeshi economist (Grameen Bank, 2022). The bank lends to people who do not qualify for traditional loans. Grameen Bank offers reasonable credit to underserved populations (e.g., women, people who are unemployed or live in poverty, people who cannot read), often via a group lending system with weekly installment repayments. Recipients pay off their debt by taking on small-scale initiatives in business or agriculture. These might include buying a cow or seeds or a hand-powered well pump. The bank also offers seasonal agricultural loans and lease-to-own agreements for equipment and livestock (Grameen Bank, 2022). These micro-loans have enabled borrowers to build on existing skills and to earn better income in each cycle of loans.

The stated aims of the bank are to make each of its branch locations free of poverty, as defined by access to adequate food, clean water, and latrines. Tellingly, Grameen Bank lends primarily to women. Yunus found that lending to women generates additional secondary successes. Empowerment of a marginalized segment of society also empowers their children, creating an upward spiral in SDOH (Yunus, 2008). Grameen reports that more than half of its borrowers in Bangladesh (close to 50 million) have risen out of acute poverty; all children of school age are in school; all household members eat three meals a day and have a sanitary toilet, a rainproof house, clean drinking water, and the ability to repay a 300-taka-per-week loan (approximately $4; Grameen Bank, 2022). As of 2017, the bank had about 2,600 branches and 9 million borrowers with a repayment rate of 99.6%.

As a result of these accomplishments, Grameen Bank was awarded the 2006 Nobel Peace Prize. The Nobel Committee affirmed, "Lasting peace cannot be achieved unless large population groups find ways in which to break out of poverty," and, refuting the notion that the poor deserve to be poor, the committee declared "across cultures and civilizations, Yunus and Grameen Bank have shown that even the poorest of the poor can work to bring about their own development" (Nobel Prize Outreach, 2006). The success of Grameen Bank has inspired similar projects in more than 64 countries around the world, including the United States. World Bank now encourages Grameen-type programs globally.

Kiva is an organization that specializes in micro-lending to women. They boast a 96% repayment rate of micro-loans ranging from a few thousand dollars to as little as $25. Even such a tiny investment can be enough to help a woman lift herself out of poverty (Kiva, 2022). These and other ventures promote financial independence with a particular emphasis on women since women traditionally have had less access to ordinary credit lines and incomes.

At the micro level are individuals, couples, families, crowd-funding campaigns, and other small groups. These range from teachers uplifting whole classes, to parent/teacher groups raising money for local schools, to activists advocating for toxin-free water in their neighborhood taps. Amid the maelstrom of danger and scarcity due to natural catastrophes of fire, earthquakes, or massive storms, neighbors are the first responders. Neighbors are the primary providers of emotional support together with material and labor in the absence of and in addition to structured bureaucratic assistance (Drury et al., 2016).

Although a supportive, traditional culture can mitigate poor SDOH, a traditional culture is not the only mitigator of the SDOH. Cultural changes and new cultural norms can bring transformation. HeForShe is a global rallying cry for men to support the empowerment of women (www.heforshe.org/en). In small but encouraging ways, the status of women is improving. Each year, fewer women suffer genital mutilation. More counties legislate women's rights. The #MeToo movement has raised consciousness of sexual harassment and abuse. Powerful figures have fallen due to public outcry against their sexual abuse of women. No single strategy will bring equity to the SDOH, but interventions working from different angles can amalgamate to reduce and eventually bring about the elimination of injustice.

CONCLUSION

> Overcoming poverty is not a gesture of charity. It is an act of justice. It is the protection of a fundamental human right, the right to dignity and a decent life.
> *(Nelson Mandela, former President of South Africa)*

Mitigating global poverty will require action at every level. Supranational organizations need to set goals. Nations must agree to them and develop policies to implement those goals. Solutions may be found in access to micro-finance, secure full employment, improved housing, access to clean water, and high-quality sanitation. Preventive and low-cost curative healthcare at convenient locations can empower currently impoverished populations. Organizations of all kinds need to address the root causes of poverty. Strengthening the weaker sections of society will culminate in a healthy and prosperous future for all members of communities, citizens of nations, and populations worldwide.

See Exhibit 25.1 for further resources.

ADDITIONAL RESOURCES

These additional resources are pertinent to gaining an understanding of global and local poverty and its long-term impact on health and well-being.

Details of the 17 SDGs of the United Nations may be reviewed here:

United Nations, Department of Economic and Social Affairs. (2015). *The 17 goals.* https://sdgs
 .un.org/goals

This 28-minute discussion with Dr. Ezekiel Emanuel, Vice Provost of Global Initiatives at the University of Pennsylvania, is an eye-opener for many who believe their healthcare system to be exceptional in the global ranking:

Emanuel, E. J. (2020). *Which country has the world's best health care? A conversation with Zeke Emanuel.*
 YouTube. www.youtube.com/watch?v=5sttFejWXhA

This 12-minute video shows the dismal fate of children who have been required to become family breadwinners. Many will never return to the classroom, their childhood ended by the COVID-19 pandemic:

Deutschland Welle. (2021, February 22). *COVID-19 special: Child labor surges in pandemic.* YouTube.
 www.youtube.com/watch?v=Gv6LVe2DKN

Do not be discouraged from watching this brief video (2:40) if you are unable to understand Spanish. The graphic depiction clearly illustrates the desperate circumstances compelling hopelessly impoverished people to seek relief and release in the alcohol-induced death chambers known as elephant graveyards:

Al Rojo Vivo. (2014, November 6). *Indigentes se emborrachan hasta morir en bar de Bolivia* [Bolivian
 bar provides service enabling homeless to drink themselves to death]. YouTube. www.youtube
 .com/watch?v=Iol4n6TwRKs

The chief medical officer for Indian Health Services for the Navajo discusses how the COVID-19 pandemic has ravaged the people on the reservation who were already experiencing great hardship (4:44):

Christenson, L. (2020, December 30). *COVID-19 ravages the Navajo Nation.* YouTube. Good Morning
 America. www.youtube.com/watch?v=1Robp8XV5Lg

In this 48-minute documentary, Bonnie Dickie has collected a series of interviews that detail how an Ojibway community in Manitoba chose to tackle widespread sexual abuse in their midst by using traditional healing methods to promote recovery as opposed to punitive methods:

Dickie, B. (2000). *Hollow Water.* www.nfb.ca/film/hollow_water

This is a thoughtful reaction video to the preceding documentary (20:24) in which two young adults discuss their takeaways from the preceding documentary by Dickie:

Heal Project. (2020, July 27). *Hollow Water: Responding to sexual violence without state intervention.*
 YouTube. www.youtube.com/watch?v=beY8wkV61js

This mini documentary (28 minutes) provides a look into the lives of homeless children who live in or under the streets of Kiev, the capital city of Ukraine:

Theroux, M. (2018, February 28). *Ukraine's teens living underground to stay alive | Unreported World.*
 You Tube. www.youtube.com/watch?v=Wq308xBaoGk

This site provides fascinating videotaped interviews with four Navajo Code Talkers (approximately 20 minutes each):

NavajoCode. (2014, April 6). *Keith Little: Real Code Talker interview.* https://navajocodetalkers.org/
 keith-little-real-code-talker-interview

REFERENCES

Adinew, Y. M., & Mekete, B. T. (2017). I knew how it feels but couldn't save my daughter; Testimony
 of an Ethiopian mother on female genital mutilation/cutting. *Reproductive Health, 14*(1), 162.
 https://doi.org/10.1186/s12978-017-0434-y

Agrawal, S. (2012). The sociocultural context of family size preference, ideal sex composition, and induced abortion in India: Findings from India's National Family Health surveys. *Health Care for Women International*, *33*(11), 986–1019. https://doi.org/10.1080/07399332.2012.692413

Alderman, J. (2018, November 28). A tribute to Ina Rösing by a Kallawaya. https://latinamericandiaries.blogs.sas.ac.uk/2019/11/28/a-tribute-to-ina-rosing-by-a-kallawaya/

Alkire, B. C., Peters, A. W., Shrime, M. G., & Meara, J. G. (2018). The economic consequences of mortality amenable to high-quality health care in low- and middle-income countries. *Health Affairs*, *37*(6), 988–996. https://doi.org/10.1377/hlthaff.2017.1233

Al Rojo Vivo. (2014, November 6). Indigentes se Emborrachan Hasta Morir en bar de Bolivia [Bolivian bar provides service enabling homeless to drink themselves to death; Video]. YouTube. https://www.youtube.com/watch?v=Iol4n6TwRKs

Altekruse, S. F., Cosgrove, C. M., Altekruse, W. C., Jenkins, R. A., & Blanco, C. (2020). Socioeconomic risk factors for fatal opioid overdoses in the United States: Findings from the Mortality Disparities in American Communities Study (MDAC). *PLoS One*, *15*(1), e0227966. https://doi.org/10.1371/journal.pone.0227966

Anik, A. I., Rahman, M. M., Rahman, M. M., Tareque, M. I., Khan, M. N., & Alam, M. M. (2019). Double burden of malnutrition at household level: A comparative study among Bangladesh, Nepal, Pakistan, and Myanmar. *PLoS One 14*(8), e0221274. https://doi.org/10.1371/journal.pone.0221274

Azeze, G. A., Williams, A., Tweya, H., Obsa, M. S., Mokonnon, T. M., Kanche, Z. Z., Fite, R. O., & Harries, A. D. (2020). Changing prevalence and factors associated with female genital mutilation in Ethiopia: Data from the 2000, 2005 and 2016 national demographic health surveys. *PLoS One*, *15*(9), e0238495. https://doi.org/10.1371/journal.pone.0238495

Barcellos, S. H., Carvalho, L. S., & Lleras-Muney, A. (2014). Child gender and parental investments in India: Are boys and girls treated differently? *American Economic Journal*, *6*(1), 157–189. https://doi.org/10.1257/app.6.1.157

Barnett, B. J., Barrett, C. B., & Skees, J. R. (2008). Poverty traps and index-based risk transfer products. *World Development*, *36*(10), 1766–1785. https://doi.org/10.1016/j.worlddev.2007.10.016

Bernstein, S. F., Rehkopf, D., Tuljapurkar, S., & Horvitz, C. C. (2018). Poverty dynamics, poverty thresholds and mortality: An age-stage Markovian model. *PLoS One*, *13*(5), e0195734. https://doi.org/10.1371/journal.pone.0195734

Blanc, A. K., Winfrey, W., & Ross, J. (2013). New findings for maternal mortality age patterns: Aggregated results for 38 countries. *PLoS One*, *8*(4), e59864. https://doi.org/10.1371/journal.pone.0059864

Borgen Project. (2015, July 2). Street Children of Thailand. https://borgenproject.org/tag/thailand-street-children/

Bowles, S. (2016). *Poverty traps*. Princeton University Press.

Brave Heart, M. Y. H. (2003). The historical trauma response among natives and its relationship with substance abuse: A Lakota illustration. *Journal of Psychoactive Drugs*, *35*(1), 7–13. https://doi.org/10.1080/02791072.2003.10399988

Braveman, P., & Gottlieb, L. (2014) The social determinants of health: It's time to consider the causes of the causes. *Public Health Reports*, *129*(Suppl. 2), 19–31. https://doi.org/10.1177/00333549141291S206

Briney, A. (2020, January 23). *A brief history of the age of exploration*. https://www.thoughtco.com/age-of-exploration-1435006

Brooks, C. (2020). *Western civilization: A concise history: Chapter 5: European exploration and conquest* (pp. 306–316). Pressbooks.

Callahan, M. (2011). *Signs of the time: Kallawaya medical expertise and social reproduction in 21st century Bolivia*, Doctoral dissertation, University of Michigan. University of Michigan Digital Archive. https://deepblue.lib.umich.edu/bitstream/handle/2027.42/84575/molliec_1.pdf?sequence=1

Carney, P. (1992). The concept of poverty. *Public Health Nursing*, *9*(2),74–80. https://doi.org/10.1111/j.1525-1446.1992.tb00079.x

Case, A., & Deaton, A. (2020). *Deaths of despair and the future of capitalism*. Princeton University Press.

Cebotari, V., Ramful, N., Elezaj, E., & de Neubourg, C. (2020). *Women's empowerment and child wellbeing in Ethiopia* [Research brief]. UNICEF. https://doi.org/10.13140/RG.2.2.11014.11845

Centers for Disease Control and Prevention. (2020, January 30). First data released on maternal mortality in over a decade. https://www.cdc.gov/nchs/pressroom/nchs_press_releases/2020/202001_MMR.htm

Centers for Disease Control and Prevention. (2022, January 20). COVID-19: How to protect yourself and others. https://www.cdc.gov/coronavirus/2019-ncov/prevent-getting-sick/prevention

Chandran, R. (2020, November 1). *'I Waited all my Life': Elderly indigenous people struggle for Thai citizenship. reuters.* https://www.reuters.com/article/us-thailand-migrants-lawmaking-trfn/i-waited-all-my-life-elderly-Indigenous-people-struggle-for-thai-citizenship-idUSKBN27I03G

Charbonneau-Dahlen, B. K., Lowe, J., & Morris, S. L. (2016). Giving voice to historical trauma through storytelling: The impact of boarding school experience on American Indians. *Journal of Aggression, Maltreatment & Trauma*, 25(6), 598–617. https://doi.org/10.1080/10926771.2016.1157843

Chen, J., Sonnenshein, M., & Williams, O. (2022). *Understanding income inequality: poverty definition*. https://www.investopedia.com/terms/p/poverty.asp

Christenson, L. (2020, December 30). *COVID-19 Ravages the Navajo Nation*. YouTube. Good Morning America. https://www.youtube.com/watch?v=1Robp8XV5Lg

Clermont, A. (2017). The impact of eliminating within-country inequality in health coverage on maternal and child mortality: A lives saved tool analysis. *BMC Public Health*, 17(Suppl. 4), 734. https://doi.org/10.1186/s12889-017-4737-2

Cloninger, C. R., Salvador-Carulla, L., Kirmayer, L. J., Schwartz, M. A., Appleyard, J., Goodwin, N., Groves, J., Hermans, M. H. M., Mezzich, J. E., van Staden, C. W., & Rawaf, S. (2014). A time for action on health inequities: Foundations of the 2014 Geneva declaration on person- and people-centered integrated health care for all. *International Journal of Person-Centered Medicine*, 4(2), 69–89. https://doi.org/10.5750/ijpcm.v4i2.471

Collier, A. Y., & Molina, R. L. (2019). Maternal mortality in the United States: Updates on trends, causes, and solutions. *NeoReviews*, 20(10), e561–e574. https://doi.org/10.1542/neo.20-10-e561

Czeisler, M. É., Marynak, K., Clarke, K. E. N., Salah, Z., Shakya, I., Thierry, J. M., Ali, N., McMillan, H., Wiley, J. F., Weaver, M. D., Czeisler, C. A., Rajaratnam, S. M. W., & Howard, M. E. (2020). Delay or avoidance of medical care because of COVID-19–Related concerns—United States. *Morbidity and Mortality Weekly Report*, 69(36), 1250–1257. https://doi.org/10.15585/mmwr.mm6936a4

Davis, P. A. (2011, July 03). *Native American concepts: The blessing way*. https://nativeamericanconcepts.wordpress.com/the-blessing-way/

Deutschland Welle. (2021, February 22). *COVID-19 Special: Child labor surges in pandemic*. YouTube. https://www.youtube.com/watch?v=Gv6LVe2DKNA

Dickie, B. (2000). *Hollow water*. https://www.nfb.ca/film/hollow_water/

Dolezsar, C. M., McGrath, J. J., Herzig, A. J., & Miller, S. B. (2014). Perceived racial discrimination and hypertension: A comprehensive systematic review. *Health Psychology*, 33(1), 20–34. https://doi.org/10.1037/a0033718

Drury, J., Brown, R., González, R., & Miranda, D. (2016). Emergent social identity and observing social support predict social support provided by survivors in a disaster: Solidarity in the 2010 Chile earthquake. *European Journal of Social Psychology*, 46(2), 209–223. https://doi.org/10.1002/ejsp.2146

DuBois, W. E. (1906/2003). The health and physique of the negro American. *American Journal of Public Health*, 93(2):272–276. https://doi.org/10.2105/AJPH.93.2.272

Dudenhoefer, A.-L. (2016, August 16). Understanding the recruitment of child soldiers in Africa. *Conflict Trends*, 2, 45–53. https://www.accord.org.za/conflict-trends/understanding-recruitment-child-soldiers-africa/

Emanuel, E. J. (2020). *Which country has the world's best health care? A conversation with Zeke Emanuel*. YouTube. https://www.youtube.com/watch?v=5sttFejWXhA

Equal Justice Initiative. (2021, July 14). Interior Department to Investigate Abuse of Indigenous Children at American Boarding Schools. https://eji.org/

Evans, T. (2020). Battling for native American lands. *Contexts*, 19(3), 78–79. https://doi.org/10.1177/1536504220950418

Excélsior TV. (2013, September 19). *Conmociona a Bolivia la Violación de un Bebé de Siete Meses: Excélsior Informa con Idaly Ferra* [Bolivians shocked over the rape of a seven-month-old baby: An Excélsior TV interview with Idaly Ferra; Video]. YouTube. https://www.youtube.com/watch?v=YFDIZ6eom2I

Four-Worlds Institute. (n.d.). Part IV-Case Studies. A. the Alkali Lake Community Story; B. the Story of Hollow Water, Manitoba. http://4worlds.org/4w/ssr/Partiv.htm

Fowler, P. J., Hovmand, P. S., Marcal, K. E., & Das, S. (2019). Solving homelessness from a complex systems perspective: Insights for prevention responses. *Annual Review of Public Health*, 40(1), 465–486. https://doi.org/10.1146/annurev-publhealth-040617-013553

Frankl, V. E. (1984). Man's search for meaning: An introduction to logotherapy. Simon & Schuster.

Gary, F. A., Yarandi, H., Hopps, J. C., Hassan, M., Sloand, E. D., & Campbell, J. C. (2021). Tragedy in Haiti: Suicidality, PTSD, and depression associated with intimate partner violence among Haitian women after the 2010 earthquake. *Journal of National Black Nurses' Association*, 32(1), 10–17.

Goldin, I. (2020). Why do some countries develop and others not? In P. Dobrescu (Ed.), *Development in turbulent times* (pp. 13–30). Saint Philip Street Press. https://doi.org/10.1007/978-3-030-11361-2_2

Grameen Bank. (2022). Grameen bank history. https://www.grameen-info.org/history/

Grayshield, L., Rutherford, J. J., Salazar, S. B., Mihecoby, A. L., & Luna, L. L. (2015). Understanding and healing historical trauma: The perspectives of Native American elders. *Journal of Mental Health Counseling*, 37(4), 295–307. https://doi.org/10.17744/mehc.37.4.02

Grigg, N. (2022, January 14). *Navajo nation hits record COVID-19 cases, but vaccination rates climb.* https://www.abc15.com/news/vaccine-in-arizona/navajo-nation-hits-record-covid-19-cases-but-vaccination-rates-climb

Harding, K. L., Aguayo, V. M., Masters, W. A., & Webb, P. (2018). Education and micronutrient deficiencies: An ecological study exploring interactions between women's schooling and children's micronutrient status. *BMC Public Health, 18*(1), 470. https://doi.org/10.1186/s12889-018-5312-1

Heal Project. (2020, July 27). Hollow water: Responding to sexual violence without state intervention. YouTube. https://www.youtube.com/watch?v=beY8wkV61js

He, J., & Hou, X. Y. (2013). The potential contributions of traditional Chinese medicine to emergency medicine. *World Journal of Emergency Medicine, 4*(2), 92–97. https://doi.org/10.5847/wjem.j.issn.1920-8642.2013.02.002

Hesketh, T., & Xing, Z. W. (2006). Abnormal sex ratios in human populations: Causes and consequences. *Proceedings of the National Academy of Sciences of the United States of America, 103*(36), 13271–13275. https://doi.org/10.1073/pnas.0602203103

Huang, E. C., Pu, C., Chou, Y. J., & Huang, N. (2018). Public trust in physicians—Health care commodification as a possible deteriorating factor: Cross-sectional analysis of 23 countries. *Inquiry, 55,* 46958018759174. https://doi.org/10.1177/0046958018759174

Hughes, K., Bellis, M. A., Hardcastle, K. A., Sethi, D., Butchart, A., Mikton, C., Jones, L., & Dunne, M. P. (2017). The effect of multiple adverse childhood experiences on health: A systematic review and meta-analysis. *Lancet, 2*(8), e356–e366. https://doi.org/10.1016/S2468-2667(17)30118-4

Instituto Nacional de Estadística. (2019, December 3). Bolivia Entre los Países de la Region que más se Redujo la Pobreza Extrema [Bolivia among the countries in the region that most reduced extreme poverty]. https://www.ine.gob.bo/index.php/bolivia-entre-los-paises-de-la-region-que-mas-redujo-la-pobreza

International Justice Mission. (2022). More than 900 hill tribe people are now Thai citizens—And That's Just the Beginning. https://www.ijm.org/news/more-than-900-hill-tribe-people-are-now-thai-citizens-and-thats-just-the-beginning

International Labour Office. (2013). Handbook: Understanding the indigenous and tribal peoples convention, 1989 [No. 169]. https://www.ilo.org/

International Labour Organization. (1989). C169-indigenous and tribal peoples convention. https://www.ilo.org/

John-Henderson, N. A., & Ginty, A. T. (2020). Historical trauma and social support as predictors of psychological stress responses in American Indian adults during the COVID-19 pandemic. *Journal of Psychosomatic Research, 139*:110263. https://doi.org/10.1016/j.jpsychores.2020.110263

Kaholokula, J. K. A., Okamoto, S. K., & Yee, B. W. (2019). Special issue introduction: Advancing Native Hawaiian and other Pacific Islander health. *Asian American Journal of Psychology, 10*(3), 197. https://doi.org/10.1037/aap0000167

Kiva. (2022). Loans that change lives. https://www.kiva.org/

Kraay, A., & McKenzie, D. (2014). Do poverty traps exist? Assessing the evidence. *Journal of Economic Perspectives, 28*(3), 127–148. https://doi.org/10.1257/jep.28.3.127

Kruk, M. E., Gage, A. D., Joseph, N. T., Danaei, G., García-Saisó, S., & Salomon, J. A. (2018). Mortality due to low-quality health systems in the universal health coverage era: A systematic analysis of amenable deaths in 137 countries. *Lancet, 392*(10160), 2203–2212. https://doi.org/10.1016/S0140-6736(18)31668-4

Kugler, A. D., & Kumar, S. (2017). Preference for boys, family size, and educational attainment in India. *Demography, 54*(3), 835–859. https://doi.org/10.1007/s13524-017-0575-1

Marmot, M. (2015). *The health gap: The challenge of an unequal world.* Bloomsbury Press.

Marmot M. (2017). The health gap: The challenge of an unequal world: The argument. *International Journal of Epidemiology, 46*(4), 1312–1318. https://doi.org/10.1093/ije/dyx163

Marmot, M., & Bell, R. (2019). Social determinants and non-communicable diseases: Time for integrated action. *BMJ, 364,* 251. https://doi.org/10.1136/bmj.l251

Marmot, M., Friel, S., Bell, R., Houweling, T. A. J., & Taylor, S. (2008). Closing the gap in a generation: Health equity through action on the social determinants of health. *Lancet, 372*(9650), 1661–1669. https://doi.org/10.1016/S0140-6736(08)61690-6

Maxwell, K. (2014). Historicizing historical trauma theory: Troubling the trans-generational transmission paradigm. *Transcultural Psychiatry, 51*(3), 407–435. https://doi.org/10.1177/1363461514531317

McClain, S. (2002). *Navajo weapon: The Navajo code talkers.* Rio Nuevo.

McCoy, K. (1988, April 5). A people in peril: Healing the old wounds. Anchorage Daily. https://www.adn.com/alaska-news/2019/04/05/a-people-in-peril-healing-the-old-wounds/

Miller, B. D. (2001) Female-selective abortion in Asia: Patterns, policies, and debates. *American Anthropologist, 103*(4), 1083–1095. https://doi.org/10.1525/aa.2001.103.4.1083

Miller, L. C., Joshi, N., Lohani, M., Rogers, B., Mahato, S., Ghosh, S., & Webb, P. (2017). Women's education level amplifies the effects of a livelihoods-based intervention on household wealth, child diet, and child growth in rural Nepal. *International Journal for Equity in Health*, 16(1), 183. https://doi.org/10.1186/s12939-017-0681-0

Mohamoud, Y. A., Kirby, R. S., & Ehrenthal, D. B. (2019). Poverty, urban-rural classification and term infant mortality: A population-based multilevel analysis. *BMC Pregnancy and Childbirth*, 19(1). https://doi.org/10.1186/s12884-019-2190-1

Mukherjee, J. S. (2018). *An introduction to global health delivery: Practice, equity, human rights*. Oxford University Press.

National Academies of Sciences, Engineering, and Medicine; Health and Medicine Division; Board on Health Care Services; Board on Global Health; Committee on Improving the Quality of Health Care Globally. (2018). Crossing the global quality chasm: Improving health care worldwide. The critical health impacts of corruption. National Academies Press. https://www.ncbi.nlm.nih.gov/books/NBK535646/

National Institute on Drug Abuse. (2017, October 25). Addressing the opioid crisis means confronting socioeconomic disparities. https://www.drugabuse.gov/about-nida/noras-blog/2017/10/addressing-opioid-crisis-means-confronting-socioeconomic-disparities

National Public Radio. (2021, July 13). More than 160 additional indigenous graves have been found in Canada. https://www.npr.org/2021/07/13/1015823457/more-than-160-additional-indigenous-graves-have-been-found-in-canada

NavajoCode. (2014, April 6). Keith little: Real code talker interview. https://navajocodetalkers.org/keith-little-real-code-talker-interview/

Navajo Nation. (2004). Facts at a glance. http://navajobusiness.com/fastFacts/Overview.htm

Nobel Prize Outreach. (2006). The Nobel Peace Prize for 2006. https://www.nobelprize.org/prizes/peace/2006/press-release/

Ollard, H. (2016, March 28). Elephant cemeteries: Finding death in hidden bars across La Paz. *Bolivian Express*. http://www.bolivianexpress.org/blog/posts/elephant-cemeteries

Penney, J. N. (2013). The biopsychosocial model: Redefining osteopathic philosophy? *International Journal of Osteopathic Medicine*, 16(1), 33–37. https://doi.org/10.1016/j.ijosm.2012.12.002

Pérez-Muñoz, A., Chacón, F., & Martínez Arias, R. (2015). An explanatory model of poverty from the perspective of social psychology and human rights. *Spanish Journal of Psychology*, 18, E99. https://doi.org/10.1017/sjp.2015.104

Pun, W. (2014, November 24). Daughters to get equal share of parental property. *Kathmandu Post*. https://kathmandupost.com/miscellaneous/2014/11/24/daughters-to-get-equal-share-of-parental-property

Pūras, D. (2017, April 7). *Special rapporteur on the right of everyone to the enjoyment of the highest attainable standard of physical and mental health*. United Nations. https://www.ohchr.org/

Razzak, J., Usmani, M. F., & Bhutta, Z. A. (2019). Global, regional and national burden of emergency medical diseases using specific emergency disease indicators: Analysis of the 2015 Global Burden of Disease Study. *BMJ Global Health*, 4(2). https://doi.org/10.1136/bmjgh-2018-000733

Reblin, M., & Uchino, B. N. (2008). Social and emotional support and its implication for health. *Current Opinion in Psychiatry*, 21(2), 201–205. https://doi.org/10.1097/YCO.0b013e3282f3ad89

Reyhner, J. (2018). American Indian boarding schools: What went wrong? What is going right? *Journal of American Indian Education*, 57(1), 58–78. https://doi.org/10.5749/jamerindieduc.57.1.0058

Rigby, J. (2020, September 28). Children for sale: How the pandemic is forcing poverty-stricken parents to make desperate choices. *Telegraph*. https://www.telegraph.co.uk/global-health/climate-and-people/children-sale-pandemic-forcing-poverty-stricken-parents-make/

Rist, S., & Nuñez del Prado, J. , (2012). *The MDGs in Bolivia: Poverty reduction in a post-neoliberal era* [NCCR North-South dialogue 43]. https://doi.org/10.7892/boris.17601

Ritchie, M. A. (2000, September). Evicted & excluded: The struggle for citizenship and land rights by tribal people in Northern Thailand. *Cultural Survival*. https://www.culturalsurvival.org/publications/cultural-survival-quarterly/evicted-excluded-struggle-citizenship-and-land-rights

Robitaille, É., & Paquette, M.-C. (2020). Development of a method to locate deserts and food swamps following the experience of a region in Quebec, Canada. *International Journal of Environmental Research and Public Health*, 17(10), 3359. https://doi.org/10.3390/ijerph17103359

Rodríguez, R. C. (2018, February 2). *An 8-month-old baby fights for her life after being brutally raped by her 28-year-old cousin*. https://www.losreplicantes.com/articulos/bebe-ocho-meses-violada-primo-28-anos-india/

Romero, J. (2019, February 18). *Abandoned babies: The social drama and a crossroads of protocols*. https://www.lostiempos.com/especial-multimedia/20190218/bebes-abandonados-drama-social-encrucijada-protocolos

Rösing, I. (1991). *Las Almas Nuevas del Mundo Callawaya: Analysis de la curación ritual Callawaya para gender penas y tristezas: Tomo II: Datos y Analysis [The new souls of the Callawaya world: Analysis of the*

Callawaya ritual healing for grief and sorrow: Volume II: Data analysis]. Los Amigos del Libro, Bolivia [The Friends of the Book, Bolivia].

Rothstein, R. (2017). *The color of law: A forgotten history of how our government segregated America.* Liveright.

Saba, P. (Transcriber, Ed.), & October League. (1972). *Women hold up half the sky.* Encyclopedia of Anti-Revisionism On-Line. https://www.marxists.org/history/erol/ncm-1/ol-women.htm

Satcher, D. (2020). *My quest for health equity: Notes on learning while leading.* (Health equity in America). Johns Hopkins University Press.

Sedgh, S., Finer, L. B., Bankole, A., Eilers, M. A., & Singh, S. (2015). Adolescent pregnancy, birth, and abortion rates across countries: Levels and recent trends. *Journal of Adolescent Health, 56*(2), 223–230. https://doi.org/10.1016/j.jadohealth.2014.09.007

Shah, I., & Åhman, E. (2009). Unsafe abortion: Global and regional incidence, trends, consequences, and challenges. *Journal of Obstetrics and Gynaecology Canada, 31*(12), 1149–1158. https://doi.org/10.1016/S1701-2163(16)34376-6

Shaw, L. J., Pepine, C. J., Xie, J., Mehta, P. K., Morris, A. A., Dickert, N. W., Ferdinand, K. C., Gulati, M., Reynolds, H., Hayes, S. N., Itchhaporia, D., Mieres, J. H., Ofili, E., Wenger, N. K., & Bairey Merz, C. N. (2017). Quality and equitable health care gaps for women: Attributions to sex differences in cardiovascular medicine. *Journal of the American College of Cardiology, 70*(3), 373–388. https://doi.org/10.1016/j.jacc.2017.05.051

Sinclair, D. A., & LaPlante, M. D. (2019). *Lifespan: Why we age – And why we don't have to.* Atria.

Singh, G. K. (2021). Trends and social inequalities in maternal mortality in the United States, 1969–2018. *International Journal of Maternal and Child Health and AIDS, 10*(1), 29–42. https://doi.org/10.21106/ijma.444

Sivak, E., & Smirnov, I. (2019). Parents mention sons more often than daughters on social media. *Proceedings of the National Academy of Sciences, 116*(6), 2039–2041. https://doi.org/10.1073/pnas.1804996116

Smartraveller. (2022). Reciprocal health care agreements. https://www.smartraveller.gov.au/before-you-go/health/reciprocal-health

Smith, A. (2009, January 26). *Indigenous peoples and boarding schools, a comparative study.* https://www.un.org/esa/socdev/unpfii/documents/IPS_Boarding_Schools.pdf

Sotero, M. (2009). A conceptual model of historical trauma: Implications for public health practice and research. *Journal of Health Disparities Research and Practice, 1*(1), 93–108.

Spencer, M. S., Fentress, T., Touch, A., & Hernandez, J. (2020). Environmental justice, Indigenous knowledge systems, and native Hawaiians and other Pacific islanders. *Human Biology, 92*(1), 45–57. https://doi.org/10.13110/humanbiology.92.1.06

Stewart, H. (2017, May 12). *The scandal behind La Paz's unbelievable elephant cemeteries.* https://theculturetrip.com/south-america/bolivia/articles/the-morbid-story-behind-la-pazs-unbelievable-elephant-cemeteries/

TAC Economics. (2022). MDG monitoring progress towards the millennium development goals: Analysis by country: Bolivia. http://www.mdgtrack.org/index.php?tab=c&c=BOL&g=1#goals

Tackie, D. N. (2021). An examination of poverty: Dimensions, causes, and solutions. *Journal of Rural Social Sciences, 36*(2), Article 2. https://egrove.olemiss.edu/jrss/vol36/iss2/2

Tallman, P. S., Riley-Powell, A. R., Schwarz, L., Salmón-Mulanovich, G., Southgate, T., Pace, C., Valdés-Velásquez, A., Hartinger, S. M., Paz-Soldán, V. A., & Lee, G. O. (2020). Ecosyndemics: The potential synergistic health impacts of highways and dams in the Amazon. *Social Science & Medicine,* 113037. https://doi.org/10.1016/j.socscimed.2020.113037

Taylor, L. (2020, September 10). How Colombia's armed groups are exploiting COVID-19 to recruit children. *New Humanitarian.* https://www.thenewhumanitarian.org/news-feature/2020/09/10/Colombia-conflict-armed-groups-child-recruitment

Theroux, M. (2018, February 28). *Ukraine's teens living underground to stay alive | unreported world.* You Tube. https://www.youtube.com/watch?v=Wq308xBaoGk

Treml, J., & Kersting, A. (2018). Anhaltende trauerstörung [Prolonged grief disorder]. *Der Nervenarzt [The Neurologist], 89*(9), 1069–1078. https://doi.org/10.1007/s00115-018-0577-2

Turner, N., Danesh, K., & Moran, K. (2020). The evolution of infant mortality inequality in the United States, 1960–2016. *Science Advances, 6*(29), eaba5908. https://doi.org/10.1126/sciadv.aba5908

UNICEF. (2019, September). Maternal mortality. https://data.unicef.org/topic/maternal-health/maternal-mortality/

UNICEF. (2020, November). Averting a lost COVID-19 generation: a six-point plan to respond, recover and reimagine a post-pandemic world for every child. https://www.unicef.org/reports/averting-lost-generation-COVID-1919-world-childrens-day-2020-brief

UNICEF. (2021). Research strategy for phase II: UNFPA-UNICEF global programme to end child marriage. https://www.unicef.org/media/104126/file/Child-marriage-research-strategy-2021.pdf

UNICEF. (2021, August). Birth registration: 1 in 4 children under the age of 5 do not officially exist. https://data.unicef.org/topic/child-protection/birth-registration/

United Nations. (2009). 2009 World survey on the role of women in development: women's control over economic resources and access to financial resources, including microfinance. Department of Economic and Social Affairs Division for the Advancement of Women. https://www.un.org/womenwatch/daw/public/WorldSurvey2009.pdf

United Nations. (2017). Sustainable development goal 5: Achieve gender equality and empower all women and girls. https://unstats.un.org/sdgs/report/2017/goal-05/

United Nations. (2020a). Global issues: ending poverty. https://www.un.org/en/global-issues/ending-poverty

United Nations. (2020b). The sustainable development goals report 2020. https://unstats.un.org/sdgs/report/2020/

United Nations, Department of Economic and Social Affairs. (2015). The 17 goals. https://sdgs.un.org/goals

United Nations, General Assembly. (1966a, December 16). International covenant on economic, social and cultural rights. *United Nations Treaty Series*, 993(14531), 3. https://www.refworld.org/docid/3ae6b36c0.html

United Nations, General Assembly. (1966b, December 16). International covenant on civil and political rights. *United Nations Treaty Series*, 993(14668), 171. https://treaties.un.org/Pages/ViewDetails.aspx?src=TREATY&mtdsg_no=IV-4&chapter=4&clang=_en

United Nations News. (2004). Un Mayor Enfoque Intercultural Para Abordar la Salud en los Pueblos Indígenas [A more intercultural approach to addressing health in indigenous peoples]. Pan American Health Organization. https://news.un.org/es/story/2004/08/1039401

United Nations News. (2015, September 25). Evo morales: To eradicate poverty you have to cabaret with capitalism. https://news.un.org/es/story/2015/09/1340281

United Nations News. (2019, April 5). Venezuelans brave torrential border river, face exploitation, abuse—UN urges greater protection. https://news.un.org/en/story/2019/04/1036181

United Nations Population Fund. (2022). Female genital mutilation. https://www.unfpa.org/female-genital-mutilation

United Nations, Treaty Collection. (1966, December 16). Chapter IV: Human rights. https://treaties.un.org/Pages/ViewDetails.aspx?src=TREATY&mtdsg_no=IV-3&chapter=4

UN Women. (2021, January 15). Facts and figures: Women's leadership and political participation. https://www.unwomen.org/en/what-we-do/leadership-and-political-participation/facts-and-figures

Utz-Billing, I., & Kentenich, H. (2008). Female genital mutilation: An injury, physical and mental harm. *Journal of Psychosomatic Obstetrics and Gynecology*, 29(4), 225–229. https://doi.org/10.1080/01674820802547087

Varley, C. (2016, December 14). *Meet the man who Adopts Ukraine's drug-addicted street children*. https://www.bbc.co.uk/bbcthree/article/ec1b151d-2185-42e2-8e9d-63101a2165a3

Vilda, D., Wallace, M., Dyer, L., Harville, E., & Theall, K. (2019). Income inequality and racial disparities in pregnancy-related mortality in the US. *SSM–Population Health*, 9, 100477. https://doi.org/10.1016/j.ssmph.2019.100477

Waehrer, G. M., Miller, T. R., Silverio Marques, S. C., Oh, D. L., & Burke Harris, N. (2020). Disease burden of adverse childhood experiences across 14 states. *PLoS One*, 15(1). https://doi.org/10.1371/journal.pone.0226134

Woodward, R. (1986). The Alkali Lake story: Victory. *Windspeaker*, 4(1), 12–13. https://ammsa.com/publications/windspeaker/alkali-lake-story-victory

World Health Organization. (1978, September 6–12). Declaration of Alma-Ata: International conference on primary health care, Alma-Ata, USSR. https://www.who.int/publications/almaata_declaration_en.pdf

World Health Organization. (2020). Proportion of women aged 15–49 years who make their own informed decisions regarding sexual relations, contraceptive use and reproductive health care (%). https://www.who.int/data/gho/indicator-metadata-registry/imr-details/4986

World Health Organization. (2022a). Constitution. https://www.who.int/about/governance/constitution

World Health Organization. (2022b). Female genital mutilation. https://www.who.int/news-room/fact-sheets/detail/female-genital-mutilation

World Health Organization. (2008). Social Determinants of Health. Report of a Regional Consultation: Colombo, Sri Lanka, 2–4 October 2007. https://apps.who.int/iris/handle/10665/206363

World Population Review. (2022). Best health care in the world: 2022. https://worldpopulationreview.com/country-rankings/best-healthcare-in-the-world

Yehuda, R., & Lehrner, A. (2018). Intergenerational transmission of trauma effects: Putative role of epigenetic mechanisms. *World Psychiatry, 17*(3), 243–257. https://doi.org/10.1002/wps.20568

Yellow Horse, A. J., Yang, T.-C., & Huyser, K. R. (2021, January 19). Structural inequalities established the architecture for COVID-19 pandemic among Native Americans in Arizona: A geographically weighted regression perspective. *Journal of Racial and Ethnic Health Disparities. Advance Online Publication.* https://doi.org/10.1007/s40615-020-00940-2

Yunus, M. (2008). *Banker to the poor: Micro-lending and the battle against world poverty.* Penguin.

Zahran, S., McElmurry, S. P., & Sadler, R. C. (2017). Four phases of the Flint Water crisis: Evidence from blood lead levels in children. *Environmental Research, 157*, 160–172. https://doi.org/10.1016/j.envres.2017.05.028

Zegarra-Parodi, R., Draper-Rodi, J., Haxton, J., & Cerritelli, F. (2019). The Native American heritage of the body-mind-spirit paradigm in osteopathic principles and practices. *International Journal of Osteopathic Medicine, 33*, 31–37. https://doi.org/10.1016/j.ijosm.2019.10.007

Zureick-Brown, S., Newby, H., Chou, D., Mizoguchi, N., Say, L., Suzuki, E., & Wilmoth, J. (2013). Understanding global trends in maternal mortality. *International Perspectives on Sexual and Reproductive Health, 39*(1), 32–41. https://doi.org/10.1363/3903213

Index

A1C test, 285
AACN. *See* American Association of Colleges of Nursing
abuse, 63, 171
ACA. *See* Affordable Care Act
access to healthcare coverage, 149–162, 391
  COVID-19 pandemic, 161
  government programs, 150
  importance, 150–152
  strategies to improve, 157
  types of, 151
  and vulnerable populations, 153–156
    people with disabilities, 153–155
    TGNC, 155–156
    undocumented immigrants, 153
  workforce issues and, 160–161
acculturation, 354
ACEs. *See* adverse childhood experiences
acquired immunodeficiency syndrome (AIDS), 467, 472
ACS. *See* American Cancer Society
acute care, 484
ADCES7 Self-Care Behaviors®, 297
adolescent health, 392
advanced payment methods (APM), 49
adverse childhood experiences (ACEs), 65, 171, 199, 391–406
  child maltreatment, mandatory reporting requirements for, 395–399
    case study, 397–399
    precursor, 395–397
  education, 401–405
  poverty, 399–401
  prevention for, 394
  pyramid, 393
adverse health outcomes, 199
advocacy, 383
Affordable Care Act of 2010 (ACA), 45–46, 65, 150, 265, 328
Agency for Healthcare Research and Quality (AHRQ), 6, 29–30
Agency for Toxic Substances and Disease Registry (ATSDR), 6
AHRQ. *See* Agency for Healthcare Research and Quality
AI. *See* American Indians
AIDS. *See* acquired immunodeficiency syndrome
air pollution, 377
Alaskan Natives (AN), 350–351
  boarding school policies for, 352, 355–356
  colonization of, 351

cultural identity loss, 358–359
historical perspective, 351–356
  acculturation, 354
  assimilation, 354–355
  blood quantum, 352–354
  boarding schools, 355–356
  cultural identity, 355
historical trauma in, 356–363
  cultural identity loss, 358–359
  dispossession, 357
  health disparities related to, 359–362
  IHS, 362–363
Indigenist Stress-Coping Model for, 364–366
population, 351
sweat lodge in, 367
talking circles in, 366–367
treaties for, 352
tribes, 351
Alliance of Nurses for Healthy Environments (AHNE), 382
allostasis, 212
allostatic load, 212, 272
Alma-Ata International Convention (1978), 91, 488
American Association of Colleges of Nursing (AACN), 28
American Cancer Society (ACS), 452–456
An American Health Dilemma (Byrd and Clayton), 249
American Indian and Alaskan Native Research in the Health Sciences Critical Considerations for Review of Research Applications, 356
American Indians (AI), 350–351
  boarding school policies for, 352, 355–356
  colonization of, 351
  cultural identity loss, 358–359
  historical perspective, 351–356
    acculturation, 354
    assimilation, 354–355
    blood quantum, 352–354
    boarding schools, 355–356
    cultural identity, 355
  historical trauma in, 356–363
    cultural identity loss, 358–359
    dispossession, 357
    health disparities related to, 359–362
    IHS, 362–363
  Indigenist Stress-Coping Model for, 364–366
  treaties for, 352
  tribes, 351
American Society for the Prevention of Cruelty to Animals (ASPCA), 396
Amish communities, 229–230

Printed in the United States
by Baker & Taylor Publisher Services

Printed in the United States
by Baker & Taylor Publisher Services